Survival Analysis

Survival analysis is crucial in many fields, including biomedical research, actuarial science, reliability analysis, business and customer analytics, econometrics, and social science. It has witnessed significant advancements in recent decades. However, most of this progress remains in scattered theoretical and applied publications, often focusing on exploratory analysis rather than the design and analysis of clinical trials. Non-proportional hazards are less well addressed. Competing risks are frequently overlooked, and the counting process approach often remains a mystery to many practitioners. Consequently, these critical topics are often not well understood or thoroughly analyzed.

Survival Analysis: Principles and Applications in Clinical Trials and Beyond aims to address these gaps. It provides an up-to-date and reader-friendly account of topics, progressing from the log-rank test, stratified analysis, and Cox regression to more advanced analyses. Heuristic arguments are used, leaving rigorous results to the appendices. The book dedicates separate chapters to topics such as clinical trials basics, modeling and analysis for non-proportional hazards, testing and summarizing treatment effects, trial design and interim monitoring, and the analysis of terminal and non-terminal events. A separate chapter is also devoted to detailed martingale heuristics beyond what is typically offered in other texts. Furthermore, a new contribution to recurrent event analysis is the rigorous formulations of marginal models and an exploration of related properties for statistical applications. The often overlooked one- and two-sample cases are also discussed.

This book provides an exposition of both the theory and practical applications of survival analysis, covering traditional topics and more recent advancements. It illustrates the methods with real-world data, discussing the strengths and limitations of various approaches, and emphasizing modeling assumptions and interpretations. The three appendices offer overviews of modern analytic frameworks pivotal for understanding and developing challenging yet vital statistical solutions. R packages are also available for newer methods. It is an up-to-date, critical, and accessible textbook for graduate students and researchers across industry, government, or academia that will enhance their understanding of complex topics, boosting their confidence in exploring different methods and interpreting the findings. It also encourages a critical evaluation of current literature and motivates the readers to develop new research ideas.

Key Features:

- Emphasis on model interpretations and comparison of different methods
- Intuitive explanations and heuristic derivation of the methods
- Real large trial data applications and R packages for newer methodologies
- Inclusion of more recently researched topics
- Modern analytical methods applied to rigorous asymptotics for key problems (in appendices)

Song Yang has been a senior mathematical statistician in the Office of Biostatistics Research, NHLBI, NIH, since 2003, following his tenure as a full professor and Statistics Coordinator in the Department of Mathematics and Statistics at Texas Tech University. He serves as an associate editor for Lifetime Data Analysis and Statistics and Probability Letters, and has given several short courses at JSM and ICSA meetings on survival analysis and clinical trials. His extensive publications in methodology and clinical research journals reflect his long experience in both areas, including his role as program office statistician on over a dozen large-scale clinical trials.

CHAPMAN & HALL/CRC

Texts in Statistical Science Series

Recently Published Titles

Models for Multi-State Survival Data
Rates, Risks, and Pseudo-Values
Per Kragh Andersen and Henrik Ravn

Spatio–Temporal Methods in Environmental Epidemiology with R, Second Edition
Gavin Shaddick, James V. Zidek, and Alex Schmidt

A Course in the Large Sample Theory of Statistical Inference
W. Jackson Hall and David Oakes

Statistical Inference, Second Edition
George Casella and Roger Berger

Nonparametric Statistical Methods Using R, Second Edition
John Kloke and Joesph McKean

Generalized Linear Mixed Models
Modern Concepts, Methods and Applications, Second Edition
Walter W. Stroup, Marina Ptukhina, and Julie Garai

Analysis of Categorical Data with R, Second Edition
Christopher R. Bilder, Thomas M. Loughin

Applied Nonparametric Statistical Methods, Fifth Edition
Nigel C. Smeeton, Neil H. Spencer, and Peter Sprent

Linear Models with R, Third Edition
Julian J. Faraway

Statistics in Survey Sampling
Jae Kwang Kim

Time Series: A Data Analysis Approach Using R
Robert H. Shumway and David S. Stoffer

Bayesian Statistical Methods: With Applications to Machine Learning
By Brian J. Reich, Sujit K. Ghosh

Experimental Design for Data Science and Engineering
By V. Roshan Joseph

Survival Analysis: Principles and Applications in Clinical Trials and Beyond
Song Yang

For more information about this series, please visit: https://www.routledge.com/Chapman--HallCRC-Texts-in-Statistical-Science/book-series/CHTEXSTASCI

Survival Analysis

Principles and Applications in Clinical Trials and Beyond

Song Yang

CRC Press
Taylor & Francis Group
Boca Raton London New York

CRC Press is an imprint of the
Taylor & Francis Group, an **informa** business
A CHAPMAN & HALL BOOK

Front Cover Image: Song Yang

First edition published 2026
by CRC Press
2385 NW Executive Center Drive, Suite 320, Boca Raton, FL 33431

and by CRC Press
4 Park Square, Milton Park, Abingdon, Oxon, OX14 4RN

CRC Press is an imprint of Taylor & Francis Group, LLC

ISBN: 978-0-367-34186-2 (hbk)
ISBN: 978-1-041-28380-5 (pbk)
ISBN: 978-0-429-32443-7 (ebk)

DOI: 10.1201/9780429324437

Typeset in Ulopia Regular font
by KnowledgeWorks Global Ltd.

Publisher's Note: This book has been prepared from camera-ready copy provided by the author.

This book was written by the author in his private capacity. The views expressed are solely those of the author and do not necessarily reflect the views of the NIH or the United States Government.

To Chunxiao,
Melissa, and Emily

Contents

Preface

Survival analysis provides theoretical foundations and methodologies for designing and analyzing clinical trials with time-to-event outcomes. Beyond clinical trials, its applications extend to diverse fields such as epidemiology, actuarial science, reliability analysis, business and customer analytics, econometrics, and social sciences, where it is often called event history analysis or duration analysis. The broad spectrum of its applications has led to many excellent textbooks covering various aspects of survival analysis.

Progress in the last several decades in the statistical literature, coupled with increasing complexity of data structures, have created a gap in the literature. Few textbooks comprehensively explore the application of these rich and advanced theoretical frameworks to improve the design and analysis of clinical trials or to enhance modeling and analysis of event history data arising from other fields. Furthermore, for survival analysis applications (including clinical trials and other fields), challenges such as non-proportional hazards, competing risks, and counting process models are often not well understood or thoroughly analyzed. This is particularly relevant in an era when traditional methods such as the log-rank test and the Cox model for a single endpoint are becoming increasingly insufficient.

With my training in theoretical statistics and twenty years of teaching in statistics, and subsequent twenty-two years of experience contributing to and overseeing survival analysis in major clinical trials, I have sought to write a book that bridges this gap. My aim is to offer a resource that provides a solid and up-to-date theoretical framework for survival analysis, with practical applications and illustrations from clinical trials. It also addresses the aforementioned complex but crucial issues, making it relevant for broader survival analysis applications across various fields. The book equips readers with fundamental and modern statistical methods for survival analysis, enabling them to confidently explore these methods and interpret their results.

The book introduces key concepts with intuitive explanations and progresses from simple problems to more complex challenges while preserving the motivation behind the work and the intuition of the analysis. Furthermore, it explores different approaches, comparing their strengths, limitations, associated conditions, and the interpretations of their results. It also illustrates these methods using large clinical trial datasets. Such illustrations are particularly informative, as the large samples minimize chance fluctuations and produce more stable, robust, and generalizable results.

This book distills decades of my personal learning and professional experience, which have naturally influenced the selection of topics. It is the kind of reference I would have desired when first exploring survival analysis as a master's or Ph.D. student, or when embarking on a career as a clinical trial researcher or practitioner. Such a resource, had it been available to me during my training or at the beginning of my career at the National Institutes of Health, would have saved considerable time and effort in exploring and gathering information from scattered resources—theoretical and applied, statistical and clinical—and helped me avoid many detours and dead ends.

This book assumes a basic knowledge of calculus-based statistics, though additional training in mathematical statistics will both ease comprehension and deepen understanding. This book is intended for readers at various stages of learning and career development. One group consists of the master's and Ph. D. graduate students in statistics or biostatistics. Another group includes researchers and statisticians in biomedical or other fields, particularly those working in clinical trials who want to expand their understanding beyond basic survival analysis methods such as Kaplan-Meier estimator, log-rank test, and Cox regression. Although the examples are mostly from clinical trials, readers in other fields using survival analysis methods can also benefit from the modeling and analysis approaches, as well as the discussions on the strengths, limitations, and underlying conditions for various methods motivated from different perspectives.

Given the ambition to cater to a diverse readership, organizing the topics and chapters, and determining the presentation style, posed a significant challenge. After considerable thought and revisions, I have settled on the current structure. This book aims to serve as an accessible resource that consolidates information and material that would otherwise require considerable time and effort to collect, filter, and learn from a variety of scattered sources.

Chapter One covers the basics of clinical trials—topics not typically found in survival analysis textbooks. It is not only beneficial for a new graduate or a starting health statistics researcher, but also discusses important topics such as prespecification of analysis plans, multiplicity, and the use of post-randomization variables. While these concepts are fundamental and intuitive in clinical studies, they may be unfamiliar to new researchers, even those with rigorous training in mathematical statistics.

Chapters Two through Fifteen cover survival analysis methods, progressing from simpler problems and methods to more challenging issues and in-depth analyses. In presenting the problems and their solutions, heuristic arguments and informal descriptions are often used. References are provided for readers who wish to delve into the finer points, formal statements, and rigorous analyses. Beyond the traditional scope of univariate analysis (Kaplan-Meier and Nelson-Aalen estimators, log-rank and weighted log-rank tests, parametric regression, and Cox regression models), multivariate survival analysis is also discussed for potentially correlated outcomes subject to independent censoring and competing risks.

This book distinguishes itself by dedicating separate chapters to critical, often-overlooked topics, and by rigorously examining the most recent and impactful methodological advancements.

Following the discussion of Cox multiplicative hazards models in Chapters Five and Six, Chapter Seven examines the model of short-term and long-term hazard ratios. This relatively new model is closely related to the Cox model in its focus on the hazard function. However, while the Cox model specifies constant hazard ratios, this model addresses monotone hazard ratios. Notably, this model encompasses both the Cox and proportional odds models as special cases. Beyond its capacity for analyzing time-varying treatment effects, it offers a compelling alternative to stratification when dealing with covariates exhibiting non-proportional effects. This chapter also presents graphical tools to illustrate how the difference between comparison groups evolves over time.

Chapter Nine addresses the more recently developed methods for testing and summarizing differences between comparison groups. These methods are motivated by the desire to maintain high power for detecting group differences when the proportional hazards condition may or may not hold, and to explore group difference measures that are meaningful and provide different perspectives. Both nonparametric and semiparametric methods are discussed.

Chapter Ten discusses the topics of sample size estimation, power analysis, and interim monitoring in clinical trials. These are essential, yet often underrepresented topics in traditional survival analysis books. Their inclusion reflects the importance of proper design and oversight for clinical trials.

Chapter Fourteen investigates the analysis of terminal and non-terminal events, a topic of growing importance. It addresses key conceptual and methodological challenges, particularly when a terminal event dependently censors non-terminal events. This chapter offers a comprehensive examination of appropriate modeling frameworks, inference methods, required assumptions, and the interpretation of model parameters. It includes a critical assessment and comparison of various methodologies, highlighting their optimal utility and the specific conditions dictating their use. The emphasis is on approaches that make fuller use of available data, accommodate competing risks, and yield model parameters directly relevant to causal inference on treatment effects. This in-depth treatment is vital for researchers and practitioners navigating these increasingly relevant and intricate statistical challenges.

Chapter Fifteen examines the analysis of recurrent events. Besides covering the traditional methods such as the Andersen-Gill model, the Prentice-Williams-Peterson models, and the more recent marginal mean/rate models, the topic of recurrent events analysis in the presence of death or dependent censoring—an area that has garnered significant recent attention—is addressed. A new and crucial contribution of this chapter is its rigorous formulation of definitions for marginal models and its exploration of their implications for statistical properties in practical applications. In the literature, marginal models are typically introduced using informal notations parallel to those for intensity models. However, while intensity models are rigorously supported by counting process and martingale theory, marginal models can no longer rely on that theory. Therefore, it's essential to clarify their meaning and examine the consequential statistical properties. The discussion in Chapter Fifteen addresses this critical gap in the literature, aiming to help readers better understand and feel more comfortable with these models. The often overlooked one- and two-sample cases are discussed, focusing on model meaning, interpretation, bias of the Nelson-Aalen estimator of the mean function, and nonparametric inference.

Furthermore, Chapter Eleven provides an in-depth examination of martingale modeling and analysis approaches. A significant new contribution is the inclusion of more detailed heuristic derivations of key formulas than typically found in other texts, aiming to demystify the counting process and martingale approaches for readers not specializing in theoretical survival analysis. Simultaneously, this chapter encourages readers to critically evaluate the use of intensity models for counting processes, emphasizing the importance of understanding their assumptions and implications, particularly when assessing treatment effects in the presence of internal time-dependent covariates, a complex topic which is also discussed in Chapter Fourteen.

Three appendices follow the main chapters, providing more material than typically found in such sections for three key reasons.

First, they demonstrate how martingale and empirical process theories can rigorously establish the asymptotic properties of the Kaplan-Meier estimator, the weighted log-rank tests, and martingale integrals. In the main text, for readability, asymptotic properties are often mentioned heuristically, and used to form confidence intervals and test hypotheses without proof. For completeness, the appendices illustrate applications of modern theories to the three specific and most basic problems with detailed justifications at a level suitable for Ph. D. students. Most other procedures can be analyzed similarly.

Second, the appendices emphasize rigor at an accessible level. While not all convergence results are new, nor are they always the most general or based on the weakest conditions, the provided proofs are elementary, self-contained, and rely on easily verifiable conditions commonly encountered in practice. Some gaps found in the existing literature are also filled. Furthermore, Propositions B.1, B.2, and C.1, along with Theorem C.2, are general enough to serve as an accessible and easy reference for readers to use in tackling other problems in survival analysis. The appendices also prepare interested readers for more advanced and comprehensive treatments of the theory of counting processes and martingales, and empirical process theory, in books such as Andersen et al. [7], Fleming and Harrington [82], and Van der Vaart and Wellner [310].

Finally, the Riemann-Stieltjes and related integrals presented in Section A.5 of Appendix A are crucial for establishing various properties of rigorously formulated marginal models in Chapter Fifteen, on model interpretation and analysis.

Despite its importance, Riemann-Stieltjes integration theory is not well explored in most survival analysis textbooks. Often, Lebesgue-Stieltjes and Riemann-Stieltjes integrals are used without clear definition or reference, while typical real analysis books do not focus on statistical applications. Given these points, the review in Section A.5 is more in-depth than the review on Lebesgue integration theory in Sections A.1 through A.4. This allows readers to benefit from having relevant results from both real analysis and survival analysis in one place, showing how real analysis tools can intuitively justify various survival models and methods.

Together, the appendices support and validate the intuitive arguments throughout the book, helping readers connect theory with practical application.

Instructors can tailor their use of this book to two different audiences. They can focus on either the practical side of survival analysis, moving at a faster pace to cover more recent topics, or they can spend more time on mathematical derivations and theory for an audience with prior exposure and rigorous training.

For a one-semester introductory course, the focus can be on the practical side of survival analysis. Instructors may cover most of Chapters Two through Six, along with select sections from later chapters based on their interests. The sections marked with an asterisk contain more detailed mathematical derivations. These can be trimmed down or skipped in favor of focusing on the motivation and practical application of the derived inference procedures. A second-semester course can then provide a more in-depth look at recent or advanced topics, such as those in Chapters Thirteen through Fifteen. For a more mathematically oriented course, instructors can dedicate more time to the detailed derivations found in various sections, as well as to Chapter Eleven and material from the appendices.

Chapters Thirteen through Fifteen can also serve as the basis for an independent study, a thesis, or a Master's project. Students majoring in mathematics or probability have the opportunity to develop rigorous model formulations and study related properties, particularly for competing risks or recurrent events data. In particular, Chapter Fifteen presents many intriguing problems in analysis, probability, and statistics ripe for further exploration.

The sections on exercises and complements help readers master the material through practice with basic algebraic and analytic maneuvers in survival analysis, some of which are related to discussions in the text. They also supplement the text by introducing techniques commonly used in research papers, with more details filled out to help readers understand the arguments.

For researchers or practitioners in survival analysis within biomedical or other fields, this book offers content on topics of common interest. These include non-proportional hazards, nonparametric and semiparametric effect size testing and estimation, analysis incorporating competing risks, terminal and non-terminal events, and recurrent events. For aspiring researchers, the three included appendices are a highly beneficial resource. They address many analytic and technical questions, guiding those seeking an in-depth understanding of specific subjects. Crucially, material presented in this book may well propel readers to develop their own novel research ideas, especially when questions linger even after thorough consultation of the appendices and the references provided throughout the book.

To help improve future editions, feedback, comments, and corrections from readers are welcome and greatly appreciated. Please send them to SACTcorrections@gmail.com.

This book has been profoundly shaped by my training and personal perspectives. I am deeply grateful for my education in the Department of Statistics and Probability at Michigan State University.

I fondly recall a time and environment where the pursuit of the unknown was its own reward, and the shared evenings and weekends with an international group of young researchers felt more like a vibrant life than mere work. I would especially like to thank Professor Emeritus Hira Koul, who exemplified the exceptional care, dedication, and invaluable guidance provided by the professors in the department. The stimulating colloquia and visits from many renowned scholars, including Rudolf Beran, David Pollard, L. J. Wei, and Richard Gill, were also profoundly illuminating for graduate students.

My understanding of survival analysis was significantly broadened and deepened through the mentorship and collaboration of Ross Prentice, both during and after my sabbatical at the Fred Hutchinson Cancer Research Center from Texas Tech University.

I am grateful to the many dedicated professionals and experts in the fields of survival analysis, asymptotic theory, and clinical trials, including Odd Aalen, P. K. Andersen, David DeMets, Michael Fay, Thomas Fleming, Dean Follmann, Nancy Geller, Richard Gill, John Kalbfleisch, Michael Kosorok, Gordon Lan, Mei-Ling Ting Lee, Susan Murphy, Danyu Lin, David Oakes, David Pollard, Stuart Pocock, Mike Proschan, James Troendle, Anastasios Tsiatis, Aad van der Vaart, L. J. Wei, Jon Wellner, Zhiliang Ying, and David Zucker, for their ongoing contributions to the scientific discourse. The rich intellectual exchanges and profound insights derived from both direct interactions and their published works have significantly shaped my understanding of these complex areas. I would also like to thank James Troendle, Ao Yuan, and Rui Miao for their helpful discussions and critical feedback on a draft of this book. Additionally, my thanks go to David Grubbs and Soumya Jain at Chapman & Hall/CRC, and Kavitha Sathish and Kumar Shashi at KnowledgeWorks Global, for their help, support and patience throughout the book's development.

Finally, I am deeply indebted to my family, especially my wife Chunxiao, for their enduring patience and encouragement throughout this entire endeavor.

Song Yang
2026

Symbols and Abbreviations

Symbol Description

T	Time-to-event variable.
C	Censoring variable.
$a \wedge b$	Minimum between reals a, b.
X	Censored observation: $X = T \wedge C$.
$I(A)$	Indicator for condition A.
δ	$I(T \leq C)$.
Z	Treatment indicator variable: $Z = 0$—control group, $Z = 1$—treatment group.
$\boldsymbol{W}$	Vector of fixed explanatory variables.
$\boldsymbol{W}(t)$	Vectors of time-dependent explanatory variables.
$\xrightarrow{d}$	Convergence in distribution.
$\xrightarrow{P}$	Convergence in probability.
$A_-(t)$	Left limit of A at t: $A_-(t) = A(t-) = \lim_{\varepsilon \downarrow 0} A(t - \varepsilon)$.
$\Delta A(t)$	Jump of A at t: $\Delta A(t) = A(t) - A_-(t)$.
$dA(t)$	Lebesgue-Stieltjes integral differential.
$\mathfrak{D}A(t)$	Riemann-Stieltjes integral differential.
i.i.d.	independent and identically distributed.
CDF	Cumulative distribution function.
PDF	Probability density function.
F	CDF of T.
S	Survival function of T.
f	PDF of T in the continuous case, probability mass function in the discrete case.
λ	Hazard function of T.
Λ	Cumulative hazard function of T.
F_C	CDF of T in the control group.
F_T	CDF of T in the treatment group.
S_C	Survival function of T in the control group.
S_T	Survival function of T in the treatment group.
λ_C	Hazard function of T in the control group.
λ_T	Hazard function of T in the treatment group.
Λ_C	Cumulative hazard function of T in the control group.
Λ_T	Cumulative hazard function of T in the treatment group.

1

Clinical Trial Basics

1.1 Introduction

Survival analysis has witnessed substantial progress since the later half of the 20th century. Important statistical models and analysis approaches have been developed, applications of which in the design and analysis of clinical trials have been vital in assessing medical treatment and interventions to yield reliable, robust and generalizable study findings. Applications in clinical studies, in turn, have propelled improved and more powerful statistical methods to emerge. All indications are that survival analysis will continue to advance and prosper in the future. After all, time to death or a significant event, such as a major illness or other life change, is arguably one of the most important variables affecting people's lives and well-being, both in biomedical research and other applications of survival analysis.

The models and analysis techniques in this book are applicable to any field where statistical inference with time-to-event data is needed. However, since the book emphasizes applications of survival analysis to clinical trials, with many of the examples from large-scale confirmatory trials, it is beneficial for readers to understand basic concepts and principles of clinical trial research. In this chapter, clinical trial basics are introduced, with emphasis on the statistical aspects. Topics discussed include pre-specification of analysis plans, multiplicity, and the use of post-randomization variables. These subjects may be unfamiliar to new researchers.

To bring the concepts discussed in this book to life, several real-world data sets from clinical trials will be described at the end of this chapter. These data sets will be used to illustrate and discuss various statistical methods in later parts of the book. Readers can better understand discussions and views regarding statistical issues in this chapter after exploring relevant topics in subsequent chapters.

More exposition and discussions on various aspects of clinical trials can be found in books such as Friedman et al. [84], Pocock [236], and the book edited by Piantadosi and Meinert [232]. Guidelines and recommendations for pharmaceutical clinical trials have also been issued by the International Council for Harmonisation of Technical Requirements for Pharmaceuticals for Human Use (ICH) [120],

DOI: 10.1201/9780429324437-1

which has European Commission, U.S. Food and Drug Administration (FDA), and Japan's Ministry of Health, Labour and Welfare as its funding regulatory members.

1.2 Clinical Studies

Clinical studies are frequently conducted to improve medical knowledge concerning the treatment, diagnosis, and prevention of diseases or conditions. They involve human volunteers called participants. Two main types of clinical studies are observational studies and clinical trials.

In an *observational study,* investigators assess health outcomes and gather information on participants according to a research plan called a protocol. Participants may receive interventions as part of their routine medical care, but they are not assigned to specific interventions by the investigators. For example, an observational study may be conducted to observe how different lifestyles are associated with varying cardiac health status. Observational studies may yield findings that are interesting and convincing enough for further confirmatory analysis.

In a *clinical trial,* investigators intend to evaluate a medical, surgical, or behavioral intervention. Often participants are randomly assigned to two groups or *arms,* one receiving the treatment being tested and the other an alternative. These kinds of trials are called *randomized controlled trials,* and the two groups are referred to as the *control group* and the *treatment group,* respectively, or control and treatment arms of the trial. The trial's objective is to learn if a new treatment is more effective and/or has less harmful side effects than what is received in the control group. The treatment could be a new drug, a new diet, a new device, a new detection method, etc. The alternative in the control group could be a placebo with no active ingredients or a currently used standard treatment. It is also possible to have more than two arms. For serious illnesses, when there exists an efficacious treatment, a placebo-controlled trial may be considered unethical, and an active treatment should be used as a control.

1.3 Four Phases of Clinical Trials

Clinical trials are usually conducted in phases sequentially.

A *Phase I trial* provides initial safety data to support further testing with larger samples. It focuses on safety, side effects, and drug dosage of an experimental treatment. The number of participants, or sample size n, is typically in the range of 20–100.

A *Phase II trial* seeks preliminary evidence on whether the drug works and also further evaluates the safety data. A larger group of participants is involved ($n \approx 100$–300). A Phase II drug trial often includes further dose finding to optimize efficacy while maintaining acceptable safety.

A *Phase III trial* aims to confirm the effectiveness of the new treatment in comparison with commonly used treatments and establish an acceptable benefit-risk profile. The sample size n can range from several hundred to many thousands. They are well-controlled and randomized trials, typically involving multiple clinical and research institutions. With a large sample size and rigorously developed protocol, Phase III trials provide a more definitive evaluation of the treatment's efficacy and safety than early phase trials (I and II).

The FDA typically requires Phase I, II, and III trials to be conducted to determine if a drug can be approved for use. Phase III trials may also be based on results from prior observational studies that suggest promising new intervention strategies.

A *Phase IV trial* for a drug or device takes place after the FDA approves its use. These studies evaluate the treatment's long-term effectiveness and safety in large, diverse populations under real-world conditions. Sometimes, the side effects of a drug may not become clear until more people have taken it over a longer period of time. In addition, chronic conditions may require chronic treatment, and the treatment effect may change throughout an individual's lifetime.

1.4 Randomization and Blinding

Randomized controlled trials are the gold standard for determining treatment efficacy. To draw valid conclusions about a treatment's effectiveness compared to a control, participants in the two arms should be as similar as possible with the only difference being the treatment received. This is best achieved by randomly dividing a single sample population into two arms.

Randomization avoids systematic differences between arms in known or unknown baseline variables, such as age, prior history, etc., that could affect the outcomes. The inability to eliminate systematic differences between treatment groups is a major problem of studies without a concurrent randomized control. The unreliability of a trial's findings becomes evident if healthier participants are selected for the treatment arm, or if the treatment arm consists of current participants in the U.S., while the control arm is composed of participants in another country decades ago.

Randomization methods include simple randomization, block randomization, stratified randomization, and covariate adaptive randomization. Simple randomization is based on a single sequence of random assignments. To yield equal sample sizes in the comparison groups, block randomization can be used. Stratified randomization addresses the need to control and balance the influence of covariates. In covariate adaptive randomization, a new participant is sequentially assigned to a particular treatment group by taking into account the specific covariates and previous assignments of participants. Covariate adaptive randomization uses the method of minimization by assessing the imbalance of sample size among several covariates. An overview of these different methods of randomization is given in Suresh [292].

In addition to randomization that minimizes baseline differences, the two arms should also be treated and observed similarly during the trial. In a *double-blind* trial, neither participants nor investigators know participants' assigned treatment. This minimizes potential biases that could result from such knowledge. If medically necessary, however, it is always possible to unblind a participant's treatment assignment.

If double-blinding is not feasible, then the *single-blind* option should be considered. In a single-blind trial, either the participants or the investigators are unaware of the treatment assignment. In some cases only an *open-label* option is possible, in which both investigators and patients know which treatment is given.

For single-blind and open-label trials, it is particularly important to maintain a clear separation between the medical staff who administer the treatment and the investigators who assess clinical outcomes. This ensures that the investigators remain blind to the treatment assignment. Every effort should be made to minimize known sources of bias and to ensure that variables are defined and measured as objectively as possible. Detailed operating procedures should be outlined in the study protocol to maintain consistency and minimize any potential bias.

1.5 Exploratory and Confirmatory Trials

Phase III and IV trials are *confirmatory trials* that are adequately controlled, with pre-specified hypotheses and analysis methods to provide firm evidence of efficacy or safety. In a confirmatory trial, it is also important to estimate the size of treatment effects and to relate these effects to their clinical significance.

The rationale and design of confirmatory trials are typically based on findings from earlier *exploratory* trials, which may have objectives that do not always lead to tests of predefined hypotheses. These exploratory trials may require a more flexible design approach, allowing for adjustments in response to accumulating results. Their analysis may involve data exploration, and while hypothesis testing can be conducted, the choice of hypothesis may be data-dependent. Consequently, such trials cannot serve as the basis for the formal proof of efficacy, although they can contribute to the overall body of relevant evidence.

In most confirmatory trials, the data are also subjected to exploratory analyses. These analyses serve as a basis for explaining or supporting the main trial results and for suggesting further hypotheses for future research.

Exploratory analyses aim to uncover patterns and relationships within the data that may not have been predefined. They allow researchers to generate new hypotheses and research questions based on observed outcomes. However, it is important to interpret exploratory results with caution, as they do not provide definitive evidence of causality.

While confirmatory analyses test predetermined hypotheses and provide evidence for treatment efficacy or safety, exploratory analyses can help predict disease progression and outcomes, uncover complex patterns, refine the analysis for specific subgroups or conditions, and guide future research directions. Both types of analyses are necessary for a comprehensive understanding of a treatment's effects and contribute to the overall body of evidence.

1.6 Trial Protocol and the Need for Pre-Specification

Clinical trials adhere to plans in the *protocol*, which describes the background, rationale, objectives, design, methodology, statistical considerations, and organization of the study. To minimize the risk of spurious findings or selection bias, the trial objectives, outcomes, and data analysis plan must be pre-specified. It is essential to clearly distinguish between the aspects of a trial that will be used for confirmatory proof and those that will provide data for exploratory analysis.

Without adequate pre-specification of these elements, it is unclear whether multiple statistical models and analysis methods are being applied to generate selectively favorable findings. This approach can lead to inflated type I error rates, exaggerated treatment effect estimates, and ultimately, misleading and non-generalizable conclusions [36].

1.7 The Intent-to-Treat Principle

Patients in clinical trials do not always adhere to the protocol. Excluding patients from the analysis who did not get their intended treatment can significantly impact the results and interpretation of a study. *Intention-to-treat* (ITT) analysis is a method for analyzing results in a prospective randomized study where all randomized participants are included in the statistical analysis and analyzed according to the group they were originally assigned, regardless of what treatment (if any) they received. This method enables the investigators to draw unbiased conclusions regarding the treatment effect. It preserves the benefits of randomization, which are not guaranteed under alternative analytic approaches.

In contrast, *per-protocol* (PP) analysis compares treatment groups by including only those participants who strictly adhered to the protocol. The PP analysis estimates the efficacy of the intervention among those who completed treatment as planned. However, because the groups are no longer randomized, the results may be biased.

1.8 Primary and Secondary Analysis

The *primary outcomes* of a trial are the clinical events that provide the most clinically relevant and convincing evidence directly related to the primary objective of the trial. They should be clearly defined in the protocol. The *primary endpoints* are the specific measurements or variables used to analyze those outcomes. While these two terms are often used interchangeably in practice, the endpoint represents the quantifiable data point of the outcome. The *primary analysis* is the statistical procedure specified for testing the hypothesis related to the primary objective of the trial. it is the most important analysis in the trial and must be clearly predefined. When multiple primary endpoints are utilized, there is a risk of inflating the overall type I error rate. This issue is addressed in Section 1.10.

A *secondary analysis* relates to a secondary objective of the trial. Typically, a collection of secondary analyses will be performed in addition to the primary analysis. These analyses provide supportive information related to the primary objective or measurements of effects in important subgroups of participants.

The number of secondary analyses should be limited in a trial. It is also important to pre-specify the secondary analyses and explain their relative importance and roles in interpreting trial results. Sometimes, a *post hoc* secondary analysis may be conducted due to emerging methods or unexpected patterns observed during the trial.

The primary analysis should be clearly distinguished from supporting analyses of the primary or secondary variables. Supporting analyses are considered secondary analyses or sensitivity analyses (see Section 1.19), which are useful for assessing the consistency or robustness of trial results.

Outcome variables or endpoints in a trial can be categorized into two types. *Hard endpoints* are definitive with respect to the disease process and require little or no subjective judgment, such as cardiovascular morbidity and mortality data. *Soft endpoints,* on the other hand, do not relate strongly to the disease process or require subjective assessments by investigators and/or patients. For example, quality of life is often considered a soft endpoint. Additionally, a *surrogate endpoint* is intended to substitute for a direct measure of how a patient feels, functions, or survives.

Using a hard endpoint as a primary endpoint is more straightforward and less controversial. A surrogate endpoint or a soft endpoint may sometimes be included as one of the primary outcomes, but caution is needed to ensure that a well-validated surrogate endpoint is used or to minimize subjectivity in defining a soft endpoint. Analyses of soft and surrogate endpoints are often included in the protocol as secondary analyses.

1.9 Sample Size

Sample size calculation or estimation refers to the determination of the number of subjects required for the primary analysis. The sample size should be large enough to provide a reliable answer to the questions being addressed.

Calculation of sample size depends on the specifications of the test statistic, the null hypothesis, the alternative hypothesis, the probability of type I error (erroneously rejecting the null hypothesis), the probability of type II error (erroneously failing to reject the null hypothesis), and the chance of treatment withdrawals and protocol violations. The assumptions and the method for deriving the sample size should be given in the protocol.

It is important to assess the sensitivity of the sample size estimate to various deviations from the assumptions made. This can be achieved by providing a range of sample sizes that are appropriate for a reasonable range of deviations from these assumptions. In confirmatory trials, the assumptions should generally be based on published data or the results of previous trials, as well as a judgment regarding the minimal effect that has clinical relevance for patient management. Conventionally, the probability of type I error is set at 5% or less, or as dictated by any adjustments necessary for multiplicity considerations discussed in the next section. The probability of type II error is typically set between 10% and 20%.

1.10 Multiplicity

If there is only one primary endpoint and a single test is conducted regarding the treatment effect on that endpoint, then the chance of a false positive or type I error can be controlled by setting the significance level, or the probability of type I error. However, when multiple endpoints are of interest that may be affected by the treatment, there is a potential inflation of the overall type I error rate. This issue is referred to as *multiplicity*.

There is no multiplicity issue if the trial's success depends on all endpoints showing an effect. In this case, the primary objective is considered met only if the null hypothesis for each endpoint is rejected at the same significance level α. Here, the overall type I error rate is less than or equal to α.

However, when the trial's success is defined as the rejection of at least one of the null hypotheses, then multiple testing impacts the overall significance level of the trial. In general, multiplicity arises if there is more than one opportunity to declare success in a trial.

Multiplicity may result in a much larger overall type I error rate. For example, if ten tests are performed, each with a type I error rate of 5%, the overall type I error rate—or the probability of at least one false positive finding—can be as high as $1-(1-0.05)^{10} \approx 0.401$ (or 40.1%) if the events are independent, and reach 50% if the events are disjoint. Although such extreme cases may be unlikely in practice, they illustrate that the overall type I error rate is not guaranteed to be less than or equal to 5% and could be considerably larger.

If a single primary endpoint cannot be selected from multiple measurements associated with the primary objective, a useful strategy is to combine the multiple measurements into a single composite endpoint and then apply a univariate test to the composite. This approach addresses the multiplicity problem without requiring adjustment to the type I error rate. Each component of the composite endpoint is typically analyzed separately as a secondary analysis.

Sometimes, subjective scores are used to assess conditions or responses of participants instead of objective measurements. These scores can be combined to form a global assessment variable that measures the overall safety or efficacy of a treatment. The global assessment variable is typically represented as a scale of ordered categorical ratings.

A drawback of the composite endpoint approach is that if the treatment effects for two components included in the composite variable are in opposite directions, the opposing effects may cancel each other out, resulting in a non-significant overall result even when important differences exist between components. Similarly, a global assessment variable may misleadingly suggest equivalence between treatments that actually have distinct profiles of benefits and adverse effects.

Furthermore, even when a composite endpoint shows an overall favorable result, the treatment might still have a harmful effect on a critical component (e.g., cardiovascular death), while benefiting less critical ones (e.g., hospitalization for heart failure). This indicates a complex situation. It is essential to examine each individual component of a composite endpoint to fully understand the treatment's impact. It is also important to acknowledge the discrepancy in the individual component results and consider potential explanations for the divergent effects.

According to FDA guidelines [308], multiplicity adjustment is unnecessary when the analysis aims to understand the demonstrated composite effect.

However, if the goal is to establish additional, independent effects of the treatment, multiplicity adjustment is required.

Instead of combining endpoints or subjective scores, a global testing procedure can be formed by combining test statistics on individual endpoints. The global null hypothesis is that there is no difference between the treatment and control arms in any of the endpoints involved in the global test. It is rejected if there is significant evidence, at the specified overall error rate level, that the two arms differ in at least one endpoint.

Multiple comparison correction methods, such as the Bonferroni method, can be used to control the overall type I error rate. Alternatively, linear combinations, maximum or χ^2 tests of component test statistics can be considered (see Chapter Fourteen). Typically, compared with the composite outcome or global assessment variable approach, methods such as the Bonferroni test and maximum test are better able to prevent the cancellation/mixing/dilution of effects on component endpoints. But they are less efficient than the linear combination tests if the effect is in the same direction for all component endpoints. Such an efficiency versus robustness trade-off is similar to phenomena observed in many other areas of statistical analysis.

Multiplicity can also happen when there are multiple comparisons of treatments, or when tests are conducted several times with interim data (see Section 1.17). No matter how multiplicity arises or what method is used to deal with it, the overall type I error rate must be controlled and details of the approach should be pre-specified in the protocol for a confirmatory trial.

1.11 One-Sided and Two-Sided Hypothesis Tests

Many hypotheses in medical research are in principle one-sided. Typically, in a randomized controlled trial, the intention is to test whether a new treatment has a better effect than a standard one. However, despite some debate in earlier times, nowadays usually two-sided hypothesis tests are used.

The appeal of a one-sided test is that, at the same significance level, say the usual 5% level, a one-sided test has higher power than its two-sided counterpart since it allocates the type I error probability entirely to only one side. However, we can rarely be certain that an effect in the opposite direction is impossible. Were there such certainty, there probably would be no need for the trial to begin with.

There is, however, a type of trial in which an effect in the opposite direction is of no interest, namely a non-inferiority trial (see Section 1.18). The new treatment will be adopted if it is at least as effective as the standard treatment.

It is important to clarify whether one- or two-sided tests will be used. For one-sided tests, the approach of setting the type I error rate at half the conventional type I error rate used in two-sided tests is the norm in regulatory settings. It ensures consistency with the two-sided confidence intervals that are generally appropriate for estimating the magnitude of the treatment effect.

When the test statistic is asymptotically normal, by symmetry of the normal distribution, a two-sided test at significance level α is equivalent to two one-sided tests, one for benefit/efficacy and one for safety/harm, each at significance level $\alpha/2$. Since the goal of a trial is typically to show benefit rather than harm, and the consequences of type I and type II errors are quite different, it is better to think in terms of the two separate cases. More discussions on efficacy and safety testing can be found in Chapter Ten.

1.12 Covariate Adjustment

For treatment effect assessment with time-to-event outcomes, the treatment group indicator is the most important explanatory variable. Often, there are other variables, referred to as *covariates*, that may influence the time to an event. *Baseline covariates* are variables collected from participants before randomization, such as demographic factors and disease characteristics. These variables are sometimes also called fixed covariates or time-independent covariates.

In many trials, the primary analysis for treatment effect assessment does not adjust for baseline covariates. Such analysis is called an *unadjusted analysis*. While an unadjusted primary analysis has the appeals of simplicity, robustness, and a focus on the overall effect assessment, covariate-adjusted analyses can be valuable, especially as secondary analyses, to understand how treatment and baseline covariates influence outcomes. An unadjusted analysis targets the unconditional treatment effect, whereas a covariate-adjusted analysis typically focuses on the conditional treatment effect specific to covariates.

In non-randomized studies, baseline covariates are often incorporated to reduce bias from chance covariate imbalance between comparison groups. However, this is typically not a concern in large confirmatory randomized trials, where important covariates are often used in the randomization scheme. In these trials, covariate adjustment is mainly considered for potential efficiency gains if covariates are strongly associated with the primary outcome, and for demonstrating treatment effects for individuals with specific baseline characteristics. Covariate-adjusted analyses also support precision medicine by helping to identify subgroups that may benefit more or less from a treatment.

The multivariate model and covariate adjustment details should be prespecified in the protocol, based on solid evidence from prior studies and scientific literature. For a covariate-adjusted primary analysis, only a few well-justified covariates should be used to minimize the risks of multicollinearity and overfitting. When a covariate has many levels (e.g., clinical sites in a large Phase III trial), grouping of sites or covariate levels can be considered. The method of grouping should be pre-specified.

In linear models with continuous outcomes, covariate adjustment often results in smaller variance estimates when covariates are strongly associated with the outcome and the model is correctly specified. For nonlinear models with binary or time-to-event outcomes, covariate adjustment usually yields a point estimate further away from the null hypothesis value, with little change in variance estimate. Therefore, it often results in higher power or smaller P-values.

However, if the association between covariates and outcome is weak, covariate adjustment may have minimal impact or even reduce power, while increase model complexity and the chance of model violation and missing data. In most confirmatory trials, unadjusted and covariate-adjusted analyses yield similar results due to well-designed randomization and large sample sizes.

For linear regression models with completely observed continuous outcomes, inference for the average treatment effect remains valid even under model misspecification [187]. However, the situation is more complex for nonlinear models with time-to-event outcomes. While in some cases the test may still maintain the correct size under the null hypothesis of no treatment effect despite model misspecification [176], its power can be reduced. Moreover, in general, an invalid model makes it difficult, if not impossible, to meaningfully interpret the estimated treatment effect.

Therefore, it's crucial to employ well-justified, validated, and robust models and analytical procedures, and to assess model validity. In its guidelines on statistical principles for clinical trials, the ICH recommends that, when the potential value of an adjustment is uncertain, the unadjusted analysis should be designated as the primary analysis, with the adjusted analysis being supportive [120].

For non-linear models with time-to-event outcomes, recent guidelines from FDA [307] suggest that a covariate-adjusted analysis (without treatment by covariate interactions) can provide more individualized information than the unconditional treatment effect if the model assumption holds, and not otherwise. If a sponsor proposes using nonlinear regression to estimate conditional treatment effects for the primary analysis, they should discuss it with the relevant FDA review divisions. This proactive communication helps ensure proper alignment with regulatory expectations and methodological rigor.

Often, more meaningful power improvements can be achieved through better statistical methods or more efficient data use, rather than covariate-adjusted analysis. Examples are provided in Chapters Six, Seven, and Fourteen.

For primary analysis, given its goal of assessing the overall treatment effect and considering the increased complexity and risks of covariate-adjusted analysis, it's prudent to use either an unadjusted analysis or a covariate-adjusted analysis with a proven, robust model to minimize the risk of model violation.

While a covariate-adjusted model can help predict individual outcomes, a better predictive model often requires more covariates than those pre-specified for the primary analysis. Such predictive models are necessarily considered secondary analyses. Modern machine learning techniques for covariate selection and adjustment can often handle larger numbers of covariates more effectively than traditional statistical approaches. For prediction purposes, statistical significance alone is insufficient for determining covariate inclusion. Efron's work [69] provides insight into prediction versus estimation and attribution/testing.

The potential pitfalls of covariate-adjusted analysis primarily relate to its designation as the primary analysis. As a secondary analysis, it can be valuable in assessing result robustness and can be more exploratory, incorporating statistical advances and emerging data features.

Typically, the primary analysis model does not include treatment by covariate interactions. The European Medicines Agency (EMA) recommends against including such interactions in the primary model, suggesting that if substantial interactions are expected a priori, the trial should be designed to allow separate estimates of treatment effects in specific subgroups [73]. However, interaction effects may be important to assess in supportive analyses.

1.13 Post-Randomization Covariates

The use of post-randomization covariates is potentially dangerous. As these variables may be influenced by the treatment, their inclusion can lead to biased estimates of the treatment effect. If a post-randomization covariate acts as an intermediary in the causal pathway between treatment and outcome, including it in the model can obscure the treatment's overall impact by controlling for an intermediate step. This can lead to an underestimation or even a loss of statistical significance. Moreover, inclusion of a post-randomization covariate makes it difficult to interpret the results, because the analysis is conditional on a variable potentially altered by the treatment.

In its "Guideline on adjustment for baseline covariates in clinical trials" [73], EMA states that covariates measured post-randomization and potentially influenced by the treatment (e.g., treatment duration, compliance, intermediate outcomes, rescue medication) should not be included in the primary analysis in confirmatory trials. In the FDA's guideline on covariate adjustment in clinical trials, the phrase "covariate adjustment" specifically refers to adjustment for baseline covariates.

The issues with using post-randomization covariates are mainly for the scenario when they are included in the primary analysis of a clinical trial. Their use in exploratory analyses can be useful for understanding the mechanism of how the treatment affect the outcome. The EMA acknowledges that post-randomization covariates could be included in exploratory or secondary analyses and might offer useful insights to sponsors during the drug development process. Alternatively, subgroup analyses may offer similar insights.

1.14 Heterogeneity and Subgroup Analyses

Clinical trials often involve heterogeneous populations. Even with strict inclusion criteria, patient prognosis can vary according to baseline characteristics, such as age, sex, or disease severity. A *subgroup analysis* is an evaluation of the treatment effect for a specific subset of patients defined by their baseline characteristics.

Subgroup analyses are typically exploratory. As they often examine one factor at a time, they are subject to the multiplicity problem. To avoid "data dredging," the number of analyses should be controlled, and they should be pre-specified in the protocol. Analyses of subgroups defined by post-baseline characteristics are not recommended in clinical trials, as they can be subject to several types of biases.

Results of subgroup analyses are often over-interpreted. This is primarily due to the fact that the sample size of a clinical trial is typically designed to ensure adequate power for the primary test of the overall treatment effect, but not for detecting effects within particular subgroups.

1.15 Individual Benefit and Risk Assessment

Clinical trials usually aim to assess the overall treatment effect for a targeted patient population, with the effect measure typically being a relative measure such as the hazard ratio (see Chapter Two). Even when there is consistency among subgroup analysis results for a relative measure, there may well be important differences between individuals in absolute treatment benefits [240]. The decision for each person in the targeted population on whether the absolute benefit of an intervention outweighs the risk should be based on a multivariate analysis taking into account the individual's characteristics. Indeed, there are examples in which patients of different age or health status may consider a trial's findings differently [241].

1.16 Data Safety Monitoring Board

A Data Safety Monitoring Board (DSMB) is an independent group of experts that objectively evaluates trial data periodically to ensure the safety of clinical trial participants while preserving the scientific integrity of the trial. The primary responsibilities of a DSMB are to periodically review and evaluate accumulated trial data for participant safety, trial conduct, progress, and efficacy. Based on these reviews, the DSMB makes recommendations to the trial investigators and sponsors concerning the continuation, modification, or termination of the trial.

The panel of scientists in a DSMB is independent of trial investigators, drug or device manufacturers, sponsors, and government officials who will approve the treatment. Its members are clinical trial experts with relevant disciplinary knowledge, including statistics. The National Institutes of Health (NIH) requires the establishment of data safety monitoring boards for multi-site clinical trials involving interventions that may pose risks to participants.

1.17 Interim Analysis and Early Stopping

After the trial start, diligent monitoring of progress is a crucial part of trial management. If outcome data on all participants in a trial can be collected at the same time, then statistical analysis can be performed using all data. However, time-to-event outcomes occur during the course of a trial. Moreover, participants are typically accrued over a few years. Therefore, partial data are available before completion of the trial, or even before completion of the recruitment period.

An *interim analysis* is any analysis with interim data, before a trial ends. Blinded interim analysis maintains study blind and primarily focuses on protocol compliance, safety data and whether the accumulated data at the time of interim analysis are in line with projections on loss to follow-up, event rate or total number of events, etc. based on the pooled data. Unblinded interim analysis compares the treatment groups to assess whether there is overwhelming evidence to support early stopping of the trial. The phrase interim analysis often refers to the latter, unblinded, analysis.

While trial monitoring and management necessitate the conduct of blinded interim analysis, ethical, scientific and economic reasons are behind the practice of unblinded interim analysis. Patients should not be exposed to unsafe, inferior or ineffective treatment, and the trials should not be conducted longer than necessary to establish treatment benefits over a defined time.

Interim analysis can lead to the decision to continue the trial or to stop the trial early if superiority of the treatment is clearly established, if demonstration of a relevant treatment difference has become unlikely, or if unacceptable adverse effects are apparent. These three scenarios are often referred to as stopping for efficacy/benefit/superiority, futility, and safety, respectively.

If an interim analysis can recommend stopping for efficacy, then a multiple testing scenario arises. The multiplicity issue needs to be dealt with to ensure that the overall type I error rate is at the specified level. The major technical challenge is determination of critical values for the interim and final analyses, which depend on the joint distributions of test statistics involved, so that the pre-specified level of the overall type I error rate is met.

If the interim analysis can only recommend stopping the trial for safety or futility, then there is no need for multiplicity adjustment. Statistical methods for interim analysis have been mostly developed and used for Phase III trials, but Phase I and II trials can also employ the methods to add rigor to the analysis plan and to protect trial integrity.

Interim analysis usually makes use of a group sequential design. In general, boundaries for monitoring efficacy require more evidence to terminate a trial early compared with monitoring of safety. When the trial design and monitoring objective involves multiple endpoints, then this aspect of multiplicity should also be taken into account.

Because the number, methods, and consequences of these comparisons affect the interpretation of the trial, all interim analyses should be carefully planned and described in the protocol.

Although interim analysis for benefit has many advantages, there are also associated risks and limitations. Early stopping of a trial means there are less data available for important secondary, subgroup or safety analysis. There is also increased variability in estimates of treatment effects. Therefore early stopping of a trial should not be taken lightly. Often, factors in addition to the stopping boundaries are also considered in the decision making process. These factors include but are not limited to treatment compliance, outcome ascertainment, and benefit versus risk consideration, etc.

1.18 Superiority, Non-Inferiority, and Equivalence Trials

Usually, a trial is aimed at establishing efficacy by demonstrating superiority to a placebo or an active control treatment. This type of trial is referred to as a *superiority trial*.

In some cases, a treatment is compared to an established reference treatment without the objective of showing superiority. Such trials fall into two main categories according to their objectives: equivalence trials and non-inferiority trials.

When a trial is designed to show that the efficacy of a new treatment is no worse than that of the active control, it is called a *non-inferiority trial.* The new treatment may be safer, less invasive, or more cost-effective than the active control.

An *equivalence trial* has the primary objective of showing that the response to two or more treatments differs by an amount that is clinically unimportant. This is usually demonstrated by showing that the true treatment difference is likely to lie between a lower and an upper equivalence margin of clinically acceptable differences.

1.19 Sensitivity Analysis

Sensitivity analysis is an analysis to determine the robustness of a trial's findings by examining how much the results are affected by changes in methods, models, values of unmeasured variables, or assumptions. In a large trial with thousands of participants from dozens of clinical centers, small procedure deviations are likely to occur. Moreover, statistically, the design and analysis of clinical trials often rely on assumptions that may impact the conclusions if they are not met. It is important to assess how these factors can affect the results. The protocol should include pre-specified sensitivity analyses for assessing robustness of the primary and important secondary analyses of the study. In particular, between the options of adjusted and unadjusted analysis, when one is chosen as the primary analysis, the other is often used as a sensitivity analysis. Ideally, a trial's finding should be robust in the sense that small changes in data, minor deviations from assumptions, and change from one reasonable model to another, should not alter the conclusions of the trial. Consistency between results of the primary analysis and the associated sensitivity analysis may strengthen results of the trial [294] and enhance their generalizability. If there are discrepancies between the primary analysis and sensitivity analysis, they should be discussed and explained. A tutorial on sensitivity analyses is given by Thabane et al. [294].

1.20 Clinical Trial Examples

Real clinical trial data will be used to demonstrate most of the statistical concepts, models, and inference methods in this book. This section provides background information for some of the trials. Given that a trial's full name is often lengthy and technical, most trials are commonly referred to by acronyms for ease of reference. The descriptions and results of these trials will involve the definition of specific quantities and statistical models, which will be thoroughly explained in subsequent chapters. For trials funded by National Heart, Lung, and Blood Institute (NHLBI), such as the first four mentioned below, data are available upon request to Biologic Specimen and Data Repository Information Coordinating Center, NHLBI.

1.20.1 SPRINT

The Systolic Blood Pressure Intervention Trial, or SPRINT, was a multi-center, randomized controlled open-label clinical trial [295]. It was conducted at 102 sites in the United States, including Puerto Rico. The primary hypothesis was that, for individuals with a systolic blood pressure of 130 mm Hg or higher and an increased cardiovascular risk, but without diabetes, treatment to reach a systolic blood pressure target of less than 120 mm Hg, as compared with a target of less than 140 mm Hg, would result in a lower rate of cardiovascular morbidity and mortality. There were 9,361 trial participants who were randomly assigned to a systolic blood-pressure target of less than 120 mm Hg (treatment) or a target of less than 140 mm Hg (control). Randomization was stratified according to clinical site. The primary outcome was the composite of myocardial infarction, other acute coronary syndromes, stroke, heart failure, and death from cardiovascular causes.

The trial was designed to have a 2 year recruitment period, with a maximum follow-up of 6 years, and anticipated a loss to follow-up of 2% per year. With an enrollment target of 9,250 participants, the trial was estimated to have 88.7% power to detect a 20% effect for the primary outcome, assuming an event rate of 2.2% per year in the standard treatment group. The primary analysis compared the two study groups using a time-to-event analysis of the primary endpoint, which was defined as the time to the first occurrence of any component event. The stratified Cox proportional hazards regression model (see Chapter Five) was used, with clinic site being the stratifying factor, and treatment group indicator as the only covariate in the model. The primary analysis uses the two-sided likelihood ratio test of zero coefficient for the treatment group indicator at 5% level of significance.

Interim analyses were performed for each meeting of the data and safety monitoring board, with group sequential stopping boundaries defined with the use of the Lan-DeMets method with an O'Brien- Fleming type spending function (see Chapter Ten). The Fine-Gray model [76] for the competing risk of death was used as a sensitivity analysis (see Chapter Thirteen).

The trial was stopped early for benefit on August 20, 2015, at which time the median follow-up was 3.26 years of the planned average of 5 years. Conclusion of the trial was that, among patients at high risk for cardiovascular events but without diabetes, targeting a systolic blood pressure of less than 120 mm Hg, as compared with less than 140 mm Hg, resulted in lower rates of fatal and nonfatal major cardiovascular events and death from any cause, although significantly higher rates of some adverse events were observed in the intensive treatment group. The primary endpoint occurred in 243 of 4678 participants in the intensive treatment group (1.65% per year) and 319 of 4683 patients in the standard treatment group (2.19% per year).

1.20.2 TOPCAT

The Treatment of Preserved Cardiac Function Heart Failure with an Aldosterone Antagonist trial, or TOPCAT, was a multi-center, international, randomized, double-blind, placebo-controlled trial [234]. The primary hypothesis was that, for patients with symptomatic heart failure and a relatively preserved ejection fraction, treatment with spironolactone would improve clinical outcomes. The primary outcome was the composite of death from cardiovascular causes, aborted cardiac arrest, and hospitalization for the management of heart failure. Participants were 3445 patients from 233 clinic sites in the United States, Canada, Brazil, Argentina, Russia, and Georgia. They were randomly assigned to receive either spironolactone or placebo with the use of permuted blocks.

The primary analysis was a time-to-event analysis with the log-rank test (see Chapter Two) on the primary endpoint, defined as the time to the first occurrence of any component event. Cox proportional hazards models were used to obtain unadjusted and covariate-adjusted hazard ratios (see Chapter Five). The trial was designed to have 80% power to detect a 20% relative reduction from a 3-year primary outcome rate of 17.4%, with a type I error of 0.05 (two-sided test).

A total of 22 pre-specified subgroup analyses were conducted for the primary outcome. To assess the homogeneity of study-drug effects across subgroups, a Cox proportional hazards model was used, with the treatment indicator, the subgroup variable, and their interaction as covariates.

At the trial completion with a mean follow-up of 3.3 years, the trial concluded that, treatment with spironolactone did not significantly reduce the incidence of the primary composite outcome in patients with heart failure and a preserved ejection fraction. The primary endpoint occurred in 320 of 1,722 patients in the spironolactone group (18.6%) and 351 of 1,723 patients in the placebo group (20.4%).

1.20.3 WHI E+P

The Women's Health Initiative (WHI) focused on defining the risks and benefits of strategies that could potentially reduce the incidence of heart disease, breast and colorectal cancer, and fractures in postmenopausal women [296]. Between 1993 and 1998, the WHI enrolled 161,809 post-menopausal women, aged 50–79 years, into a set of clinical trials (including trials of a low-fat dietary pattern, calcium and vitamin D supplementation, and two trials of postmenopausal hormone use) and an observational study at 40 clinical centers in the United States.

One of the WHI trials was the trial of combined estrogen and progestin (WHI E+P) in women with a uterus. The trial was designed to assess the major health benefits and risks of the most commonly used combined hormone preparation in the United States. It was a randomized controlled trial with a planned duration of 8.5 years. Participants were randomly assigned to receive either estrogen plus progestin or placebo, using a randomized permuted block algorithm, stratified by clinical center site and age group.

The primary outcome was designated as coronary heart disease (CHD) (nonfatal myocardial infarction and CHD death), with invasive breast cancer as the primary adverse outcome. A global index summarizing the balance of risks and benefits included the two primary outcomes plus stroke, pulmonary embolism (PE), endometrial cancer, colorectal cancer, hip fracture, and death due to other causes. The primary analysis was a time-to-event analysis, on the primary endpoint of the time to the first occurrence of any component event in the primary outcome, based on the hazard ratios from a Cox proportional hazards model stratified by clinical center, age, prior disease, and randomization status in the low-fat diet trial.

On May 31, 2002, after a mean of 5.2 years of follow-up, the Data and Safety Monitoring Board recommended stopping the estrogen plus progestin trial because the test statistic for invasive breast cancer exceeded the stopping boundary for this adverse effect and the global index statistic also provided supporting evidence of risks exceeding benefits [324].

As of April 30, 2002, the primary endpoint occurred in 164 of 8,506 participants in the estrogen plus progestin group (0.37% per year) and 122 of 8,102 participants in the placebo group (0.30% per year). 166 and 124 participants developed invasive breast cancer in the treatment and placebo arms, respectively. For the global index statistic, there were 751 and 637 events in the treatment and placebo arms, respectively.

For the trial, it was postulated in the design that a full-compliance hazards ratio of 70% would be achieved linearly over the first three years after randomization [296]. However, after nine years, the actual data showed a vastly different pattern.

1.20.4 TCD

Graft-versus-host disease (GVHD) reduces the efficacy of unrelated donor bone marrow transplantation in patients with lymphohaemopoietic malignancy. The T-cell Depletion trial (TCD) was a Phase II-III trial to determine the effects of ex-vivo T-cell depletion versus methotrexate and cyclosporine immunosuppression [313].

Patients were randomized to undergo transplantation with either T-cell depleted marrow and cyclosporine A (TCD arm), or methotrexate and cyclosporine A after transplantation of T-replete marrow (M/C arm). The primary outcome was disease-free survival, defined as the minimum time to relapse or death. The primary endpoint was disease-free survival rate at 3 years, which was 27% and 34% for the TCD and M/C arms, respectively.

A modified log-rank statistic was used to assess equality of disease- free survival by treatment due to concerns on non-proportional hazards within the first 6 months [287]. The test had the P-value 0.16. In the final data set, the sample size was 410, with 203 in the TCD arm. The primary outcome was observed in 143 patients in the M/C arm and 153 patients in the TCD arm.

1.20.5 A Gastric Cancer Trial

For patients with locally advanced stage of gastric cancer, a trial was designated in 1974 to compare the therapeutic effectiveness of combined radiation therapy and chemotherapy versus chemotherapy alone on patient survival [106]. Patients were randomized to the two groups taking into account known prognostic factors. After cancellations and exclusion based on eligibility, there were 90 patients, 45 in each group, who were followed until there was evidence of tumor recurrence or progression, or until death. After 8.2 years, there was evidence of an advantage for those patients receiving chemotherapy during the first twelve months of therapy; however, after surviving twelve months of therapy, patients receiving the combined therapy were subsequently subject to a lower risk of death.

This trial was not a large scale confirmatory trial. It is included in the book because the data are publicly available [288] and the data are similar to many observed from cancer or surgical trials in that the phenomenon of crossing survival curves is present, violating the Cox proportional hazards model assumption.

2

Estimation and Comparison of Survival Curves

When analyzing a sample of data, the first task is to estimate the distribution of the variable of interest. In survival analysis, this task is complicated by the fact that the variable is often only partially observed. In clinical trials, the most important question is if there is a significant treatment effect when comparing the treatment and control groups. This chapter focuses on nonparametric methods designed to address these questions.

In this book, the material is presented at a level accessible to readers with basic differentiation and integration knowledge from calculus. However, some notation from the Lebesgue-Stieltjes integral theory will be introduced for a more unified presentation. For readers with calculus training who are mainly interested in the basic problems and analytic approaches, the more general notation and formulas can be interpreted in the context of continuous and discrete cases without hindering their understanding of the material.

For readers who have previous exposure to measure and integration theory, Appendix A provides a convenient overview. It also serves as a valuable resource for those with a calculus background who are interested in understanding how more technical or general results are derived.

2.1 Survival Data and Censoring

Survival analysis is the branch of statistics devoted to analyzing the time from a defined origin to the occurrence of an event. Due to its major applications in biomedical studies and industrial life testing, time-to-event data are often referred to as survival data or failure time data. The term “survival data” is used literally if the event of interest is death, while “failure time data” is particularly relevant in reliability studies where the event is the failure or breakdown of a product.

The time-to-event variable is often only partially observed, with right-censoring being the most common scenario. For consistency and easy reference, throughout this book, the time-to-event variable will be denoted by T, and the

DOI: 10.1201/9780429324437-2

censoring time variable will be denoted by C. There may be subscripts or superscripts associated with T or C to indicate group membership or individual-specific variables.

In the scenario of right-censoring, instead of T, we observe $X = (T \wedge C, \delta)$, where $a \wedge b$ denotes $\min(a,b)$ and δ is an indicator variable which is 1 if $T \le C$ and 0 otherwise. Thus, when $\delta = 1$, T is observed; but when $\delta = 0$, we only have the partial information that $T > C$, not the exact value of T. For easy reference throughout this book, the indicator variable or function will be denoted by $I(A)$, which takes the value 1 if condition A is true, and 0 otherwise. Thus $\delta = I(T \le C)$.

Right censoring is almost inevitable in clinical trial with time-to-event data for several reasons. First, a trial's duration is finite, and some individuals may not experience the event during that time. This type of right censoring is called administrative censoring. Second, individuals may be lost to follow-up due to reasons unrelated to the study, such as relocation. Third, individuals may no longer be under observation due to a terminating event such as death, when an event other than death is of interest. In all these scenarios, and many more, there is a variable C that censors T.

There are several categories of often encountered right-censoring phenomena: type I censoring, type II censoring, and random censoring. Type I censoring occurs when all subjects are followed until a pre-determined, fixed time. That is, the censoring times are constants which may or may not be equal. Type II censoring happens when subjects are followed until a pre-determined number of events have occurred. Random censoring refers to situations where censoring times are independent of the survival times. Therefore, type I censoring is a special case of random censoring.

For discussions on most traditional survival analysis topics, the condition of random censoring is usually assumed in the literature. Chapters Two through Twelve in this book will mostly conform to this convention. When the censoring may be dependent on the survival time, as in the case of censoring by death when the outcome of interest is time to heart failure hospitalization, the situation is more complicated and calls for a more careful analysis and interpretation of the results. Specific forms of dependent censoring frequently encountered in practice will be discussed in detail in Chapters Thirteen through Fifteen, focusing on competing risks data, terminal and non-terminal events, and recurrent events, respectively.

In type II censoring, the censoring variable is an order statistic and therefore dependent on the survival time. However, it's an example of censoring that does not hinder unbiased estimation of the underlying time-to-event distribution. This will be discussed in Sections 2.7, 11.2, and Section B.11 in Appendix B.

In clinical trials, the time origin for T is usually the time of randomization. individuals are followed up until the end of trial unless either the event or censoring occurs before that. Since it may be logistically impossible to recruit participants all at once, a large prospective trial typically starts at a calendar time s_0, and it

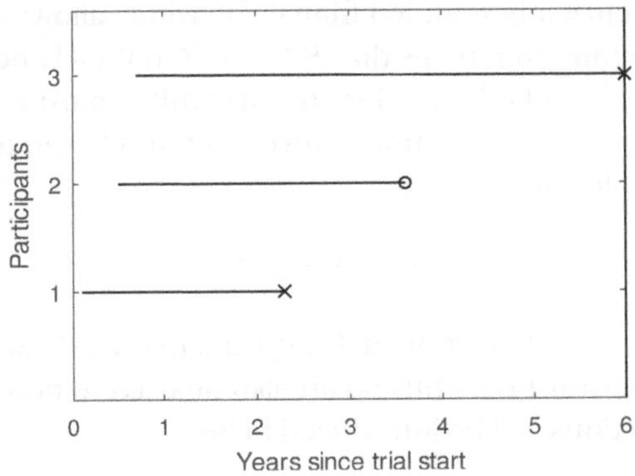

FIGURE 2.1
Follow-up of three participants in a hypothetical trial with two years of recruitment and four year follow-up afterwards ("o" indicates observed event and "x" indicates censoring).

recruits participants during the time interval $[s_0, t_0]$. This phenomenon is called *staggered entry*. After the recruitment period, the trial will end at a time $\tau > t_0$. Thus the minimum follow-up time is $\tau - t_0$ and the maximum is $\tau - s_0$.

Figure 2.1 depicts the scenarios for three individuals in a hypothetical trial that spends two years on recruitment and additional four years of follow-up afterwards. For the scenarios in Figure 2.1, each of the three horizontal lines represents the follow-up duration, from the time of randomization to the time of event or censoring. The trial started at calendar time $t = 0$ (years). Individual #1 was randomized at time $t = .1$, and at time $t = 2.3$ censoring occurred. Therefore, the survival time T_1 is only known to be greater than $2.3 - .1 = 2.2$. Individual #2 was randomized at $t = .5$ and the event occurred at $t = 3.7$. The survival time T_2 was exactly 3.2. Finally, individual #3 was randomized at $t = 0.7$, and neither event nor censoring occurred before trial termination at $t = 6$. Thus, the survival time T_3 is only known to be greater than $6 - 0.7 = 5.3$.

2.2 Fundamental Functions in Survival Data Analysis

The *cumulative distribution function* (CDF) of T is

$$F(t) = P(T \leq t), \quad 0 \leq t < \infty. \tag{2.1}$$

Usually, for convenience it is assumed that $T > 0$, which allows a logarithm transformation. This assumption implies that $F(0) = 0$. F uniquely determines the distribution of T and is the default function to work with in most statistics textbooks.

In survival analysis, it is often more convenient or relevant to work with other functions. For example, the function

$$S(t) = 1 - F(t), \tag{2.2}$$

called the *survivor/survival function* of T, appears frequently and it has a one-to-one correspondence with $F(t)$. Thus it can also be used to describe the distribution of T. Other functions will be introduced below.

2.2.1 Continuous Distributions

Suppose the distribution of T is continuous and it has the *probability density function* (PDF)

$$f(t) = \frac{dF(t)}{dt}. \tag{2.3}$$

Thus f is nonnegative and satisfies

$$\int_0^\infty f(s)ds = 1, \quad F(t+h) - F(t) = \int_t^{t+h} f(s)ds, \ h > 0.$$

When h is small, we have

$$P(t \le T < t+h) = P(t < T \le t+h) \approx f(t)h,$$

where the equality holds since the probability of T taking any one single value is zero by the continuity of F. This kind of approximation is useful in heuristic arguments and in understanding or motivating concepts.

The *hazard function* is

$$\lambda(t) = \lim_{h \downarrow 0} P\big(t \le T < t+h \big| T \ge t\big)/h. \tag{2.4}$$

That is, $\lambda(t)$ gives the instantaneous rate of the event occurring in the immediate future, given it has not happened yet. This function is most easily understood in life insurance analysis, where the premium is partially determined by the rate of death for an individual who has survived to a specific age. Therefore, despite its technical definition, the hazard function is a straightforward and intuitive concept that represents the rate of imminent risk.

The *cumulative hazard function* is

$$\Lambda(t) = \int_0^t \lambda(s)ds. \tag{2.5}$$

To obtain λ and Λ from f, we have, from (2.4) and (2.5), respectively,

$$\lambda(t) = f(t)/[1-F(t)] = f(t)/S(t), \tag{2.6}$$

$$\Lambda(t) = \int_0^t \frac{f(s)ds}{1-F(s)} = -\log[S(t)], \tag{2.7}$$

where "log" denotes the natural logarithm and t satisfies $S(t) > 0$. Verification of (2.6) and (2.7) is left to Exercise 2.1.

Conversely, we have

$$S(t) = \exp[-\Lambda(t)] = \exp\left[-\int_0^t \lambda(s)ds\right], \tag{2.8}$$

$$f(t) = \lambda(t)\exp[-\Lambda(t)], \tag{2.9}$$

for t with $S(t) > 0$. It follows that the hazard function uniquely determines the distribution of T.

Working with the hazard function λ rather than the PDF f often proves more convenient and intuitive in survival analysis for a few key reasons.

First, the criteria for a nonnegative function to be a valid hazard function are less restrictive. Any nonnegative function can serve as a hazard function if its integral on $[0,\tau]$ is finite for some $\tau \le \infty$. In contrast, for a nonnegative function to be a PDF, its integral over $[0,\infty)$ must be 1. This flexibility often makes it easier to model survival distributions through the hazard function.

Another important reason for working with λ is that it arises naturally in various heuristic arguments that will be shown later. Additionally, when there are competing risks—for instance, in a study of cardiovascular death when an individual dies from a non-cardiovascular cause—the concept of the hazard function can be extended in a natural way. However, as will be discussed in Chapter Thirteen, extending the CDF in such scenarios presents a delicate and complex challenge.

2.2.2 Discrete Distributions

When F is discrete, assume that T takes values $s_1 < s_2 < \cdots$ with probability mass function

$$f(s_i) = P(T = s_i), \quad i \ge 1, \tag{2.10}$$

then the CDF and survival functions are

$$F(t) = \sum_{s_i \le t} f(s_i), \quad S(t) = \sum_{s_i > t} f(s_i),$$

respectively. Conversely,

$$f(s_i) = F(s_i) - F_-(s_i) = F(s_i) - F(s_i-), \quad i \ge 1,$$

where $A_-(t)$ or $A(t-)$ denotes the left limit version of a function $A(t)$:

$$A_-(t) = A(t-) = \lim_{h \downarrow 0} A(t-h). \tag{2.11}$$

These notations will also be used throughout the remainder of this book.

The hazard at s_i is defined as the conditional probability of event at s_i given there is no event prior to s_i,

$$\lambda_i = P(T = s_i | T \geq s_i) = \frac{f(s_i)}{S_-(s_i)}, \quad i \geq 1. \tag{2.12}$$

The cumulative hazard function is

$$\Lambda(t) = \sum_{s_i \leq t} \lambda_i. \tag{2.13}$$

Analogous to (2.8) and (2.9), it can be shown that

$$S(t) = \prod_{s_i \leq t} (1 - \lambda_i), \tag{2.14}$$

$$f(s_i) = \lambda_i \prod_{j=1}^{i-1} (1 - \lambda_j), \quad i \geq 1, \tag{2.15}$$

where product over an empty index set is defined to be 1.

Although the equations can be verified algebraically, it is helpful to think intuitively in terms of progression over time. From

$$A_i = A_1 \cap A_2 \cap \cdots \cap A_i, \tag{2.16}$$

where $A_k = \{\text{Event free at time } s_k\}$, $1 \leq k \leq i$, it can be shown that (2.14) follows from (2.16) and the chain rule of probability (Exercise 2.2).

2.2.3 General Distributions*

In the previous two sections, the continuous and discrete cases were discussed separately, similar to the approach taken in most introductory statistics books. This section introduces the general case where the CDF F of T may have both continuous and discrete components. Consideration of the general case is often necessary and advantageous for a more unified notation and for concisely expressing key properties and formulas.

Because this topic involves more advanced mathematical details and notation, it's marked with an asterisk (*). This same notation will be used for a few other sections in this book. Master's students can choose to bypass these sections on a first reading, or focus on the basic concepts and notation without exploring the full details.

In both the continuous or discrete cases, the CDF F of T is increasing and right-continuous with left limit. These properties also hold in the general case. In addition,

$$F(0) = 0, \quad \lim F(t) = 1 \text{ as } t \to \infty.$$

Verification of some of these properties is left as Exercise 2.5.

To define the cumulative hazard function $\Lambda(t)$ of T in the general case, we use the Lebesgue-Stieltjes integral, a concept that extends the Riemann integral of calculus. An overview of Lebesgue-Stieltjes integral is provided in Section A.4 of Appendix A. $\Lambda(t)$ is defined as

$$\Lambda(t) = \int_0^t \frac{dF(s)}{1 - F_-(s)}, \quad \text{for } t \text{ with } F_-(t) < 1, \tag{2.17}$$

where $\int_0^t$ denotes the Lebesgue-Stieltjes integral over the range $(0, t]$.

In the integral, $1/(1 - F_-)$ is called the integrand and F the integrator. The Lebesgue-Stieltjes integral is defined for a right-continuous integrator that can be written as the difference of two increasing functions.

For a general CDF $F(t)$ that may not have derivatives at all t, the concept of absolute continuity from real analysis is fundamental. The definition and some key properties can be found in Section A.4 of Appendix A. This concept is less restrictive than requiring a function to have a derivative at every point; it essentially requires the function to be differentiable "almost everywhere." In particular, a function that has derivatives at all points in a closed interval except for a finite number of points is absolutely continuous.

While more abstract definitions and theories are often needed for a wider range of applications and for theoretical justification, readers can improve their understanding by thinking of any functions involved in data analysis as well-behaved and having necessary smoothness properties to simplify the analysis. In particular, it is usually sufficient to think of an everywhere differentiable function as an example of an absolutely continuous function.

To see how the formulas in Section 2.2.1 for the continuous case can be recovered from the general case, assume that the CDF F is absolutely continuous. This ensures that F has derivative f almost everywhere. Thus, By (A.7) in Appendix A,

$$\int_0^t \frac{dF(s)}{1 - F_-(s)} = \int_0^t \frac{f(s)ds}{1 - F(s)}.$$

By the change of variable formula (A.11) in Appendix A,

$$\int_0^t \frac{f(s)ds}{1 - F(s)} = -\log[S(t)].$$

Therefore, in the absolutely continuous case, (2.17) reduces to (2.7).

For the discrete case, let

$$\Delta A(x) = A(x) - A(x-) = A(x) - A_-(x)$$

for a right-continuous function A at x. Assume that F is discrete with probability mass function $f_i = \Delta F(s_i)$ at s_i, $i \geq 1$. Then by (A.8) in Appendix A,

$$\int_0^t \frac{dF(s)}{1 - F_-(s)} = \sum_{s \leq t} \frac{\Delta F(s)}{S_-(s)} = \sum_{s_i \leq t} \frac{f_i}{S_-(s_i)}.$$

Thus (2.17) reduces to (2.13) in the discrete case.

From the above results, the Lebesgue-Stieltjes integral offers a unified notation for the continuous and discrete cases. This significantly reduces repetition and redundancy. It also makes the formulas for estimators and tests much clearer and more streamlined, as will be seen in later sections.

From (2.17) and (A.9) in Appendix A, for a function g,

$$\int_0^t g(s) d\Lambda(s) = \int_0^t \frac{g(s) dF(s)}{1 - F_-(s)},$$

if the integral exists. The differential notation

$$d\Lambda(s) = \frac{dF(s)}{1 - F_-(s)}$$

offers a succinct way to state this property. Throughout this book, dA will be used to denote the Lebesgue-Stieltjes differential. It follows that $d\Lambda(t) = \lambda(t)dt$ in the continuous case and $d\Lambda(t) = \Delta\Lambda(t)$ in the discrete case.

In the general case, there is still a one-to-one correspondence between F and Λ. That is, there is an inverse for the operation of obtaining Λ from F in (2.17). The inverse operation is called product integration. Given a function Λ, there is a unique F, or equivalently $S = 1 - F$, that satisfies (2.17). It is

$$S(t) = \mathcal{P}_{(0,t]}(1 - d\Lambda), \tag{2.18}$$

where the function on right-hand side is defined as

$$\lim \prod_{k=1}^{L} [1 - \Lambda(u_k) + \Lambda(u_{k-1})], \tag{2.19}$$

with $0 < u_0 < u_1 < \cdots < u_L = t$ being a partition of $(0, t]$ and the limit taken as $\max_i(u_i - u_{i-1}) \to 0$. The term "product integration" arises because it parallels Riemann integration in calculus, except that it works with products instead of sums. Reviews and more detailed discussions are given in Gill and Johansen [99] and Gill [98].

An alternative approach to obtain F or S from Λ is to use Volterra integral equations [312]. By Theorem 5 of Gill and Johansen, S as given in (2.18) is the unique solution of the integral equation

$$\int_0^t S_-(s)d\Lambda(s) = 1 - S(t) \tag{2.20}$$

(see Exercise 2.6 on this). Yang [329] used the integral approach to obtain a few inequalities and integral equation solutions that are useful in various applications [330, 343, 344].

The Lebesgue-Stieltjes integral not only offers a unified notation for the continuous and discrete cases, but it also makes it possible to study $F(t)$ or $\Lambda(t)$ that is a mixture of a continuous part (with derivative λ_c) and a discrete part (that takes values λ_i at s_i, $i \geq 1$). Suppose

$$\Lambda(t) = \int_0^t \lambda_c(s)ds + \sum_{s_i \leq t} \lambda_i, \tag{2.21}$$

for t such that the right side of (2.21) is finite. Then it can be shown (Exercise 2.6) that

$$S(t) = \exp\left[-\int_0^t \lambda_c(s)ds\right] \prod_{s_i \leq t} (1 - \lambda_i). \tag{2.22}$$

Note that (2.22) reduces to (2.8) and (2.14) for the continuous and discrete cases, respectively.

The one-to-one correspondence between F and Λ makes it possible to specify the distribution of T by either F or Λ. In survival analysis, it is often helpful to think in terms of the hazard function. For example, if T represents the age at death for a human population, $\lambda(t)$ typically exhibits a U-shape due to high infant mortality near $t = 0$ and an increasing risk of death at advanced ages. For a clinical trial, depending on the specific time frame and the study population, the hazard can be of any shape.

2.3 Preservation of Stochastic Ordering

An important property of the cumulative hazard function is that it preserves the stochastic ordering. In probability and statistics, *stochastic ordering* is a concept for comparing random variables. It formalizes the idea that one random variable is "larger" than another in a probabilistic sense.

Let X and Y be two random variables, with CDF F_X and F_Y, respectively. X is said to be stochastically greater than Y if

$$F_X(x) \leq F_Y(x)$$

for all $x \in (-\infty, \infty)$. In this case, Y is said to be stochastically less than X. Visually, this condition means that the graph of $F_X(x)$ never rises above the graph of $F_Y(x)$. If, additionally, $F_X(x) < F_Y(x)$ for at least one x, then X is stochastically strictly greater than Y (and Y is stochastically strictly less than X).

Note that the condition of X being stochastically greater than Y is implied by the condition that $X \geq Y$, when X and Y are defined on the same probability space. Also, stochastic ordering is a partial ordering, meaning that it is possible for a pair of random variables to be incomparable. That is, X is stochastically neither greater than nor less than Y. This occurs when F_X and F_Y cross each other.

For applications to survival analysis, to accommodate censoring, X is said to be stochastically greater than Y on $[0, \tau]$, where $0 < \tau \leq \infty$, if

$$F_X(x) \leq F_Y(x)$$

for all $x \in [0, \tau]$.

Let T_1 and T_2 be the time-to-event variables in the control and treatment groups, respectively, or more generally, in two comparison groups. Let the CDF of T_j be F_j, $j = 1, 2$. Then, T_2 is stochastically greater than T_1 on $[0, \tau]$ if

$$F_2(t) \leq F_1(t)$$

for all $t \in [0, \tau]$. This describes an ideal situation where the treatment prolongs life or delays time to the occurrence of a disease.

Let Λ_j be the cumulative hazard function of T_j, $j = 1, 2$. Assume that the distributions are continuous. Suppose $F_j(\tau) < 1$, $j = 1, 2$. Then, since $F_j(t) = 1 - \exp\left(-\Lambda_j(t)\right)$, $j = 1, 2$, T_2 is stochastically greater than T_1 on $[0, \tau]$ if and only if

$$\Lambda_2(t) \leq \Lambda_1(t), \qquad t \in [0, \tau].$$

Therefore, the condition that T_2 is stochastically greater than T_1 on $[0, \tau]$ can be stated in terms of either the CDF or the cumulative hazard function. This means that on $[0, \tau]$, the graph of $F_2(t)$ never rises above that of $F_1(t)$, which is equivalent to the condition that the graph of $\Lambda_2(t)$ never rises above that of $\Lambda_1(t)$.

Note that the cumulative hazard function has the stronger property of equivalence. Not only it preserves the stochastic ordering (i.e., when T_1 and T_2 are stochastically ordered, their cumulative hazards are also ordered), but conversely, if the cumulative hazards are ordered, then stochastic ordering between T_1 and T_2 is implied.

In survival analysis, it is possible to use functions other than the cumulative hazard function that have a one-to-one relationship with the CDF. However, these functions may not necessarily preserve the stochastic ordering. The expected residual life function is one such example (see Exercise 7.12 in Chapter Seven for the definition of expected residual life and related properties).

2.4 Kaplan-Meier Estimator and Nelson-Aalen Estimator as Nonparametric MLEs*

This section presents a heuristic argument to derive an important estimator of F, the Kaplan-Meier estimator. The argument also yields the Nelson-Aalen estimator for the cumulative hazard function Λ.

The derivation is based on an intuitive argument for maximizing a likelihood function along with some algebraic details. Readers with calculus training can focus on the core principles of the derivation and the resulting expressions for the estimators and the variance estimators, without delving into the detailed derivation.

If the time-to-event variable T is observable, then statistical modeling and analysis can proceed as in many conventional statistics textbooks. For example, if a parametric family $\{f_\theta(t) : \theta \in \Theta\}$ is believed to be reasonable for the distribution of T, then the *maximum likelihood estimator* (MLE) can be used to estimate θ. The MLE is a value that maximizes the likelihood function

$$\prod_{i=1}^{n} f_\theta(T_i) \tag{2.23}$$

where $T_1, \ldots, T_n$ is a random sample from a homogeneous population with the distribution of T. On the other hand, if no parametric assumptions are imposed, typically the CDF F of T is estimated by the empirical CDF

$$\tilde{F}_n(t) = \frac{1}{n} \sum_{i=1}^{n} I(T_i \le t), \tag{2.24}$$

where, as mentioned before, $I(A)$ is the indicator function taking the value 1 if A is true and 0 otherwise.

With censored data, a more delicate derivation is needed to obtain a nonparametric estimator of F. For this purpose, available data will be assumed to arise from the following model: there are n positive time-to-event variables $T_1, \ldots, T_n$, that are *independent and identically distributed* (i.i.d.) with CDF F, and nonnegative censoring variables $C_1, \ldots, C_n$ which are independent and also independent of $T_1, \ldots, T_n$. The observed data are $(X_i, \delta_i), 1 \le i \le n$, where

$$X_i = T_i \wedge C_i, \qquad \delta_i = I(X_i = T_i).$$

This model is referred to as the *random censorship model.* The sample is called a randomly censored sample. This model will be used throughout much of this book.

First, assume that F has PDF f, and that the distribution of C_i has PDF g_i and survival function G_i, $1 \le i \le n$. For a pair (X_i, δ_i) with $\delta_i = 1$, we know $T_i = X_i$ and $C_i \ge X_i$. Thus the pair's contribution to the likelihood is, by independence, $f(X_i)G_{i-}(X_i)$, where G_{i-} is the left limit of G_i. Similarly, when $\delta_i = 0$, contribution to the likelihood from the pair (X_i, δ_i) is $g_i(X_i)S(X_i)$. Thus the likelihood function is

$$\prod_{i=1}^{n} [f(X_i)G_{i-}(X_i)]^{\delta_i} [g_i(X_i)S(X_i)]^{1-\delta_i}$$

$$= \Big(\prod_{i=1}^{n} [f(X_i)]^{\delta_i} [S(X_i)]^{1-\delta_i}\Big)\Big(\prod_{i=1}^{n} [G_{i-}(X_i)]^{\delta_i} [g_i(X_i)]^{1-\delta_i}\Big).$$

If the censoring distributions are of no interest and unrelated to F, which is typically the case in survival analysis, then the likelihood function is

$$L_0(F) = \prod_{i=1}^{n} [f(X_i)]^{\delta_i} [S(X_i)]^{1-\delta_i}. \tag{2.25}$$

If F is restricted to have PDF f belonging to a parametric family $\{f_\theta(t) : \theta \in \Theta\}$, then maximization of the likelihood function (2.25) can proceed similarly to the maximization of (2.23). This will be discussed in Chapter Four.

When there is no parametric restriction on F in (2.25), it can be seen that no maximizer of L_0 exists among absolutely continuous F, because for any such F, some maneuver by re-distributing the probability mass can lead to a CDF F^* with $L_0(F^*) > L_0(F)$. Therefore, it is necessary to modify the likelihood function to be, for a discrete CDF F,

$$L(F) = \prod_{i=1}^{n} [\Delta F(X_i)]^{\delta_i} [S(X_i)]^{1-\delta_i}, \tag{2.26}$$

where $\Delta F(X_i) = F(X_i) - F_-(X_i)$. Similarly to the idea of finding a parameter estimator by maximizing the likelihood in (2.23), it seems reasonable to obtain an estimator of F by maximizing $L(F)$. This is the notion of *nonparametric maximum likelihood estimation.*

Let $t_1 < \cdots < t_k$ be the ordered distinct event times (i.e., uncensored times), and

$$\begin{aligned} d_j &= \#\{m : X_m = t_j, \delta_m = 1\}, \\ c_j &= \#\{m : X_m \in [t_j, t_{j+1}), \delta_m = 0\}, \end{aligned}$$

where $t_0 = 0$ and $t_{k+1} = \infty$. d_j and c_j represent the number of tied event times at t_j and the number of censored times in $[t_j, t_{j+1})$, respectively. Furthermore, let

$$n_j = \sum_{m \geq j} (d_m + c_m), \quad 1 \leq j \leq k.$$

n_j denotes the number of individuals at risk at t_j. That is, the number of individuals who have experienced neither event nor censoring before t_j.

If a maximizer of $L(F)$ exists, it must have positive probability at all uncensored times, because $L(F)$ would be zero otherwise. Additionally, the maximizer must not have positive probability at any censored time, as $L(F)$ can be increased by reallocating probabilities at those c_j censored times in $[t_j, t_{j+1})$ to t_j for $j \geq 1$ and to t_1 for $j = 0$ (Exercise 2.7).

It follows that a maximizer should be a discrete distribution with support $\{t_j : 1 \leq j \leq k\}$. Let f_j, S_j and λ_j be the probability, survival and hazard functions at t_j. For the d_j uncensored observations in $[t_j, t_{j+1})$, the contribution to the likelihood is $f_j^{d_j}$. For the c_j censored observations in $[t_j, t_{j+1})$, the contribution to the likelihood is $S_j^{c_j}$. Thus the likelihood function is

$$L(F) = \prod_{j=1}^{k} f_j^{d_j} S_j^{c_j}.$$

By (2.14) and (2.15), we have

$$\begin{aligned} L(F) &= \lambda_1^{d_1}(1-\lambda_1)^{c_1} \cdot \left\{\left[\lambda_2(1-\lambda_1)\right]^{d_2}\left[(1-\lambda_1)(1-\lambda_2)\right]^{c_2}\right\} \cdot \ldots \\ &= \left[\lambda_1^{d_1}(1-\lambda_1)^{\sum_{j\geq 1} c_j + \sum_{j \geq 2} d_j}\right] \cdot \ldots \\ &= \prod_{j=1}^{k} \lambda_j^{d_j}(1-\lambda_j)^{n_j - d_j}. \end{aligned} \tag{2.27}$$

Taking derivative of $\log L$ with respect to λ_j, it can be shown that the likelihood is maximized at

$$\hat{\lambda}_j = d_j / n_j. \tag{2.28}$$

Correspondingly, the estimator for $S = 1 - F$ is

$$\hat{S}(t) = \prod_{t_j \leq t} (1 - \hat{\lambda}_j) = \prod_{t_j \leq t} (1 - \frac{d_j}{n_j}) \tag{2.29}$$

(Exercise 2.8). This estimator was originally proposed by Kaplan and Meier [132] who called it the product limit estimator.

Note that the expression in (2.29) defines $\widehat{S}(t)$ for all $t < \infty$, with $\widehat{S}(t) = \widehat{S}(\max X_i)$ for any $t > \max X_i$. Also, by definition, $d_j \le n_j$. Thus the factors in the product in (2.29) are all positive except possibly for $j = k$. If $d_k = n_k$, then $\widehat{S}(t_k) = 0$, otherwise $\widehat{S}(t_k) > 0$. Therefore, if there is a censored observation larger than all uncensored ones, $\widehat{S}(t)$ will stay positive.

Let $\Lambda(t)$ be the cumulative hazard function corresponding to $F(t)$. From $\hat{\lambda}_j = d_j/n_j$, the estimator for $\Lambda(t)$ is

$$\widehat{\Lambda}(t) = \sum_{t_j \le t} \frac{d_j}{n_j}, \tag{2.30}$$

which is called the Nelson-Aalen estimator [212, 2]. It is important to note that from the derivation of the Kaplan-Meier estimator, the likelihood is re-expressed in terms of the hazard function and is maximized at the Nelson-Aalen estimator. In many applications, it is often more convenient or straightforward to work with the Nelson-Aalen estimator directly. More discussions will be provided in Chapters Nine and Fourteen.

In the above derivation, the hazard $\lambda_j = P(T = t_j | T \ge t_j)$ at t_j is estimated by $\widehat{\lambda}_j = d_j/n_j$, the proportion of events at t_j among the n_j individuals who are at risk of having the event at t_j. Intuitively, this estimator is natural if we believe that individuals who are at risk are representative of the population from which the random sample is drawn. That is, individuals who are censored prior to t_j do not have better or worse survival experience than individuals still at risk. This belief is reasonable in the random censorship model.

2.5 Variance Estimators for Kaplan-Meier Estimator and Nelson-Aalen Estimator

For a heuristic derivation of the asymptotic variance of $\widehat{S}(t)$, assume that T is discrete taking values at $t_j, 1 \le j \le k$. Then $L(F)$ in (2.27) is an ordinary parametric likelihood function in λ_j's. The theory of parametric MLE, to be discussed in Chapter Four, gives $d_i(n_j - d_j)/n_j^3$ as an estimate for the asymptotic variance of $\widehat{\lambda}_j$, and 0 as an estimate for the asymptotic covariance between $\widehat{\lambda}_j, \widehat{\lambda}_m, 1 \le j, m \le k, j \ne m$ (see Exercise 2.9). From the delta method as stated in Exercise 2.10, it follows that the asymptotic variance of $\hat{\Lambda}(t)$ can be estimated by

$$\widehat{V}_\Lambda = \sum_{t_j \le t} \frac{d_i(n_j - d_j)}{n_j^3}. \tag{2.31}$$

Equation (2.14) and one more application of the delta method shows that the asymptotic variance of $\widehat{S}(t)$ can be estimated by

$$\widehat{\sigma}^2(t) = \widehat{S}^2(t) \sum_{t_j \le t} \frac{d_j}{n_j(n_j - d_j)}. \tag{2.32}$$

Details of the argument are left to Exercise 2.10.

Although formulas (2.31) and (2.32) are derived under the assumption of a discrete F in the heuristic argument above, they are valid more generally, without restricting to a discrete F. Proofs for this and the asymptotic normality of $\widehat{\Lambda}(t)$ and $\widehat{S}(t)$ are given in Section B.11 of Appendix B and Section C.7 of Appendix C. Formula (2.32) is called Greenwood's formula [105]. Since $\widehat{F} = 1 - \widehat{S}$, formula (2.32) is also the variance formula for $\widehat{F}(t)$.

Note that if $d_k = n_k$, then at t_k, the denominator $n_k - d_k = 0$. Since $\widehat{S}(t_k) = 0$ in that case, with the convention $0/0 = 0$, $\widehat{\sigma}^2(t_k) = 0$. In applications, for making inference about $F(t)$ or $\Lambda(t)$ themselves directly, the interest is usually on t values not close to the end of data range. However, inference procedures sometimes involve the behavior of $\widehat{S}(t)$ for t in the maximal possible range. The works of Gill [97] and Yang [331] are useful in those situations, as demonstrated in Hellinger distance estimation [328].

Alternative variance formulas for continuous F are also given by (B.40) and (B.41) in Appendix B. In the notations here, they can be written as

$$\widetilde{V}_\Lambda = \sum_{t_j \le t} \frac{d_i}{n_j^2}, \qquad \widetilde{\sigma}^2(t) = \widehat{S}^2(t) \sum_{t_j \le t} \frac{d_j}{n_j^2}, \tag{2.33}$$

respectively.

An asymptotic 95% confidence interval for $S(t)$ is

$$\widehat{S}(t) \mp 1.96\widehat{\sigma}(t).$$

To avoid negative values, it's common to transform $S(t)$ to a function that does not have any range restrictions. By the delta method, the asymptotic variance of $\log \widehat{S}(t)$ can be estimated by

$$\widehat{Var}[\log \widehat{S}(t)] = \sum_{t_j \le t} \frac{d_j}{n_j(n_j - d_j)}.$$

However, $\log S(t)$ still has the range restriction of $(-\infty, 0]$. Thus it is necessary to use the logarithm transformation one more time and consider $\log[-\log S(t)]$, which takes values in $(-\infty, \infty)$. By the delta method again, the asymptotic variance of $\log[-\log \widehat{S}(t)]$ can be estimated by

$$\widehat{v}^2(t) = \widehat{Var}[\log \widehat{S}(t)] / [\log \widehat{S}(t)]^2.$$

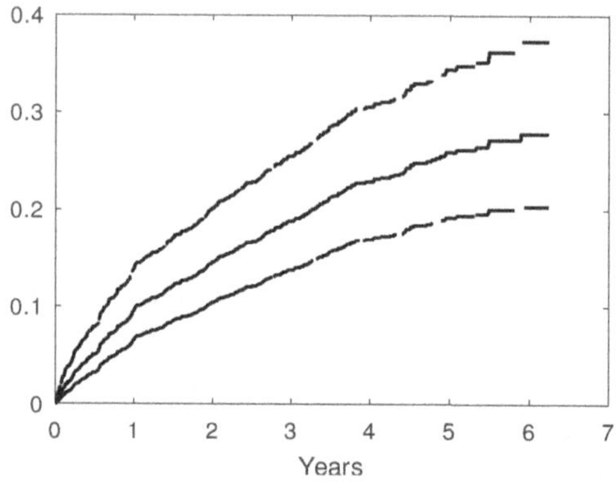

FIGURE 2.2
Kaplan-Meier estimates of the event probabilities and the associated 95% confidence intervals for the primary endpoint in the control group of the TOPCAT trial.

Thus an asymptotically correct 95% confidence interval for $\log[-\log S(t)]$ is

$$\log\left[-\log \widehat{S}(t)\right] \mp 1.96\widehat{v}(t).$$

For $-\log[S(t)]$, the corresponding confidence interval is

$$\left[-\log \widehat{S}(t)\right] \exp[\mp a(t)] = -\log[\widehat{S}(t)]^{\exp[\mp a(t)]},$$

where

$$a(t) = 1.96\widehat{v}(t).$$

This yields the 95% confidence interval

$$\left[\widehat{S}(t)\right]^{\exp[\pm a(t)]}$$

for $S(t)$. From this, a 95% confidence interval for $F(t)$ is

$$1 - \left[\widehat{S}(t)\right]^{\exp[\mp a(t)]}.$$

Example 2.1. Unless mentioned otherwise, throughout this book, all numerical computations are performed using GNU Octave [67]. The TOPCAT trial was described in Section 1.20.2. For the primary endpoint of the control group in TOPCAT, the Kaplan-Meier estimate of the event probability $F(t)$ and the 95% confidence interval, for t in the data range, are plotted in Figure 2.2. In particular, at the three specific time points $t = 1, 3, 5$, in years, the event probabilities and confidence intervals are given in Table 2.1.

With the alternative variance formula in (2.33), the confidence intervals are indistinguishable from those in Figure 2.2. Typically, for moderate sample sizes

TABLE 2.1
Estimated event probabilities at year 1, 3 and 5, with associated 95% confidence intervals, for the primary endpoint of the control group in TOPCAT.

t	$\widehat{F}(t)$	95% CI
1	0.10	0.07–0.14
3	0.19	0.14–0.25
5	0.26	0.19–0.35

and t not near the end of the data range, the difference between the two variance formulas are negligible for practical purposes. For small samples and t near the end of the data range, Greenwood's formula often leads to a smaller bias [7, p.260]. However, in those situations, the results are only descriptive with either formula, as the finite sample behavior may not be approximated well by the asymptotic normality.

Also, note that the band formed by the confidence intervals at all t values may give the wrong impression that the band contains the true function with high probability. From k confidence intervals, we have

$$P(\theta_j \in [L_j, U_j]) = 1 - \alpha, \qquad j = 1, \ldots, k.$$

These results can only ensure that

$$P(\theta_j \in [L_j, U_j], \ \ j = 1, \ldots, k) \geq 1 - k\alpha.$$

With increasing k, the simultaneous coverage probability can go down rapidly. This is related to the multiplicity issue in multiple testing. More discussions on relevant problems will be given in Chapters Six and Seven.

In general, a Kaplan-Meier curve is descriptive only and is often plotted without the confidence intervals. To test the hypothesis that two survival functions are the same, procedures such as the log-rank test, to be discussed in the next section, are typically used. Use of test statistics based on survival curves or Nelson-Aalen curves will be discussed in Chapter Nine.

2.6 Comparison of Survival Curves

2.6.1 Log-Rank Test

Comparison of survival experiences for participants is often the most important task in a clinical trial. Statistically this translates to comparing the survival distributions or hazard functions. The *log-rank* test, a nonparametric test first proposed by Mantel [195], is a widely used method for this purpose. A heuristic derivation of this test will be given below.

Suppose there are two independent randomly censored samples from two survival functions $S_m, m = 1,2$, respectively. Based on the samples, one would like to test the hypothesis that $S_1 = S_2$. Let $t_1 < \cdots < t_k$ be the distinct event times from the pooled sample. Let n_j, d_j be the number of participants at risk and the number of events, respectively, at t_j, $1 \le j \le k$. For the mth sample define n_{jm}, d_{jm} analogously to n_j, d_j, $m = 1,2$.

To facilitate understanding of the test statistic and its asymptotic distribution, assume furthermore that S_m is discrete with hazard λ_{jm} at t_j, $1 \le j \le k$, $m = 1,2$. From the derivation of the Kaplan-Meier estimator, the second sample gives an estimate d_{j2}/n_{j2} for the hazard at t_j. On the other hand, under the hypothesis that $S_1 = S_2$, the pooled sample yields an estimate d_j/n_j. The two estimates should be close to each other when $S_1 = S_2$. Thus the weighted sum

$$\sum_j w_j \left(\frac{d_{j2}}{n_{j2}} - \frac{d_j}{n_j} \right) \tag{2.34}$$

should be close to 0, where the weights w_j's are positive. If S_1, S_2 are not equal, and S_2 is the survival function of the treatment group for a treatment that lowers the hazard at t_j, then, using $n_j = n_{j1} + n_{j2}$, $d_j = d_{j1} + d_{j2}$, $1 \le j \le k$, one obtains

$$\frac{d_{j2}}{n_{j2}} - \frac{d_j}{n_j} = \frac{n_{j1}}{n_j} \left(\frac{d_{j2}}{n_{j2}} - \frac{d_{j1}}{n_{j1}} \right).$$

This difference will tend to be negative since d_{jm}/n_{jm} estimates λ_{jm}, $m = 1,2$, and $\lambda_{j2} < \lambda_{j1}$. Thus the weighted sum in (2.34) is a reasonable test statistic for testing $S_1 = S_2$.

In particular, if $w_j = n_{j2}$, then

$$w_j \left(\frac{d_{j2}}{n_{j2}} - \frac{d_j}{n_j} \right) = d_{j2} - \frac{n_{j2}}{n_j} d_j.$$

The above expression has a connection with the hypergeometric distribution via a conditioning argument. A review on conditional probability is provided in Appendix B. Let $\mathscr{F}_j$ be the collection of information on each participant's history prior to time t_j. Then given $\mathscr{F}_j$ and d_j, the variable d_{j2} is the number of events from the second sample among the total d_j events.

Under the hypothesis $S_1 = S_2$, the d_j events can be viewed as being randomly drawn from the set of n_j participants among whom n_{j2} are from the second sample, it follows that d_{j2} has a hypergeometric distribution with mean

$$e_j = \frac{n_{j2}}{n_j} d_j$$

and variance

$$v_j = e_j \frac{(n_j - d_j)(n_j - n_{j2})}{n_j(n_j - 1)}.$$

A detail worth pointing out is that since $d_j \geq 1$, when $n_j = 1$, we have $d_j = 1$, thus $v_j = 0$ with the convention that $0/0 = 0$.

Rewrite d_{j2} as $o_j, 1 \leq j \leq k$. The log-rank test statistic is

$$\sum_j \left(d_{j2} - \frac{n_{j2}}{n_j} d_j\right) = \sum_j (o_j - e_j), \tag{2.35}$$

the sum of differences between observed and expected numbers of events from the second sample at t_j, $1 \leq j \leq k$.

To obtain the variance of $\sum_j (o_j - e_j)$ under the hypothesis $S_1 = S_2$, the covariance between $o_j - e_j$ and $o_\ell - e_\ell$ is needed, $1 \leq j < \ell \leq k$. Given $\mathscr{F}_\ell$, $o_j - e_j$ is completely determined since $j < \ell$. By the law of iterated expectations and the product rule of conditional expectation, or (B.5) and (B.3) in Appendix B, respectively,

$$\begin{aligned} E\left[(o_j - e_j)(o_\ell - e_\ell)\right] &= EE\left[(o_j - e_j)(o_\ell - e_\ell)\middle|\mathscr{F}_\ell\right] \\ &= E\left\{(o_j - e_j)E\left[(o_\ell - e_\ell)\middle|\mathscr{F}_\ell\right]\right\}. \end{aligned}$$

Now by (B.4),

$$\begin{aligned} E\left[(o_\ell - e_\ell)\middle|\mathscr{F}_\ell\right] &= E\left\{E\left[(o_\ell - e_\ell)\middle|\mathscr{F}_\ell, d_\ell\right]\middle|\mathscr{F}_\ell\right\} \\ &= 0. \end{aligned}$$

Thus $E\left[(o_j - e_j)(o_\ell - e_\ell)\right] = 0$ and the variance of $\sum_j (o_j - e_j)$ is

$$\sum_j v_j = \sum_j \frac{n_{j2}}{n_j} \frac{d_j(n_j - d_j)(n_j - n_{j2})}{n_j(n_j - 1)}. \tag{2.36}$$

By the central limit theorem, for large samples,

$$\frac{\sum_j (o_j - e_j)}{\sqrt{\sum_j v_j}} \xrightarrow{d} N(0,1), \tag{2.37}$$

where $\xrightarrow{d}$ denotes convergence in distribution and $N(0,1)$ denotes the standard normal distribution. At a significance level α, the log-rank test rejects the hypothesis $S_1 = S_2$ if

$$\frac{|\sum_j (o_j - e_j)|}{\sqrt{\sum_j v_j}} > z(\alpha/2),$$

where $z(\gamma)$ denotes the upper γth percentile of $N(0,1)$.

It turns out that for the log-rank test, the asymptotic result in (2.37) is valid for general survival functions $S_m, m = 1,2$, without the restriction that S_1, S_2 are discrete. Rigorous statements and proofs are given in Section B.11 of Appendix B.

2.6.2 Stratified Log-Rank Test

There is almost always heterogeneity in populations from which the survival data are drawn, with individuals varying in characteristics such as age, sex, race, and medical history. If these factors impact survival experiences and there is an imbalance of the factors between the two samples, the log-rank test may incorrectly reject the hypothesis of equal survival distributions. This can occur simply because one sample happens to include more participants with favorable characteristics (e.g., younger or healthier individuals) than the other.

To reduce the influence of such confounding variables, the samples can be stratified such that participants have similar characteristics within each stratum. The log-rank test can be modified to account for these stratified samples.

Suppose there are b strata. Define $o_{j\xi}, e_{j\xi}, v_{j\xi}$ analogously to o_j, e_j, v_j for each stratum, $1 \le \xi \le b$. Then the stratified log-rank test statistic is $\sum_\xi \sum_j (o_{j\xi} - e_{j\xi})$, with variance $\sum_\xi \sum_j v_{j\xi}$. Similarly to (2.37), for large samples,

$$\frac{\sum_\xi \sum_j (o_{j\xi} - e_{j\xi})}{\sqrt{\sum_\xi \sum_j v_{j\xi}}} \xrightarrow{d} N(0,1). \tag{2.38}$$

The stratified log-rank test rejects the hypothesis $S_1 = S_2$ if the standardized test statistic exceeds $z(\alpha/2)$.

The stratified log-rank test is most effective when there are a small number of strata, each stratum having a reasonable sample size and homogeneity within. If the number of strata is large, then the stratified log-rank test has little advantage or may even have lower statistical power than the unstratified version. In large clinical trials, randomization typically helps balance heterogeneity factors between the treatment groups. Thus the unstratified and stratified versions of the log-rank test often yield very similar results.

When the heterogeneity factor considered for stratification is a continuous variable, stratification requires discretizing it into several groups. While this simple method is often used in practice, it is prone to various problems, including loss of information about individual differences, loss of effect size and power, or spurious statistical significance and overestimation of effect size. These issues are discussed in MacCallum et al. [193]. It is preferable to use the original data with alternative methods, as illustrated in Chapters Six and Seven.

2.6.3 Weighted Log-Rank Test

For two survival functions $S_1(t)$ and $S_2(t)$, let the corresponding hazard functions be $\lambda_1(t)$ and $\lambda_2(t)$. From the heuristic derivation, the log-rank test should work well if λ_2 is consistently lower or higher than λ_1 at all time points, i.e., if S_1 and S_2 are stochastically ordered.

It turns out that the log-rank test is asymptotically the most powerful test if the hazard functions are proportional, i.e., the hazard ratio $h(t) = \lambda_2(t)/\lambda_1(t)$ is constant in t [95, 82]. More discussion on this will be given in Chapter Ten.

Often, survival data from two treatment groups have a hazard ratio that varies mildly over time t, in which case the log-rank test works well. However, there are situations where the hazard ratio exhibits more pronounced deviations from constancy. For example, the treatment effect may be large initially but diminish over time, in which case $h(t)$ converges to one and the two survival cures close in as t increases.

Conversely, the treatment may take effect gradually over time, in which case $h(t)$ deviates slowly from one and the two survival cures gradually separate as t increases. In these situations, a weighted log-rank test may have higher power to detect the group difference.

For possibly data-dependent nonnegative weights $w_1, \ldots, w_k$, the weighted log-rank test statistic is $\sum_j w_j(o_j - e_j)$. From the heuristic derivation, if the weight function $w(t)$ depends only on censoring and survival information before t at each time point t, then similarly to the derivation of (2.36), the variance of $\sum_j w_j(o_j - e_j)$ is

$$\sum_j w_j^2 v_j.$$

Under certain regularity conditions, this can be rigorously justified using the counting process and martingale theory, an overview of which is provided in Appendix B.

Various weights can be used for situations where the hazards are non-proportional. These weights include the Gehan weight $w_j = n_j$ [87] and the Peto-Prentice weight $w_j = S_{j-}$ where S_{j-} is the left limit of the Kaplan-Meier estimator from the pooled sample at t_j [228, 245]. Harrington and Fleming [82] also proposed the $G^{\rho,\gamma}$ family of weights $w_j = S_{j-}^{\rho}(1 - S_{j-})^{\gamma}$, $\rho \geq 0$, $\gamma \geq 0$.

Note that the left limit version S_{j-} is used in the weights mentioned above. This allows applications of the counting process and martingale theory in asymptotic analysis. It often leads to better small sample behavior than the right limit version S_j which is also asymptotically valid.

TABLE 2.2
P-vales of the log-rank test and several weighted log-rank tests for the TOPCAT primary endpoint. LR–log-rank; G–Gehan; PP–Peto-Prentice; CPP–complement Peto-Prentice.

Test	LR	G	PP	CPP
P-value	0.14	0.08	0.12	0.58

Weighted log-rank tests offer simple and intuitive ways to compare two survival distributions. Various aspects of the tests will be discussed throughout the book.

Example 2.2. In the TOPCAT trial, the log-rank test was used to test the primary hypothesis that, for patients with symptomatic heart failure and a relatively preserved ejection fraction, treatment with spironolactone would improve clinical outcomes. The test had a P-value of 0.14. This result indicates that there was no statistically significant difference between the spironolactone and placebo groups in the primary outcome.

Table 2.2 gives the P-values for various tests: the log-rank test and weighted log-rank tests with Gehan weight, Peto-Prentice weight, and the complement Peto-Prentice weight $w_j = 1 - S_{j-}$. These tests correspond to the abbreviations LR, G, PP, and CPP, respectively. The log-rank test has a connection with the Cox model that will be discussed in Chapter Five [51]. The Gehan weighted log-rank test has a connection with the win ratio [79, 238] that will be discussed in Chapter Fourteen, and the PP and CPP weighted log-rank tests have a connection with the model of short-term and long-term hazard ratios developed by Yang and Prentice that will be discussed in Chapter Seven [344].

All the P-values are non-significant at the significant level 0.05. Further analysis of the data, as discussed in Chapter Seven, indicates that the treatment effect is more pronounced early and gradually diminishes over time. Given this phenomenon, a weighted log-rank test that assigns more weight to early events should be better able to detect the group difference.

Figure 2.3 presents plots of the weights for those weighted log-rank tests used in Table 2.2. Among the three weights, the Gehan weight assigns the most weight to early time points, while the complement Peto-Prentice weight assigns the least weight to these early events. This pattern explains the behavior of the corresponding P-values.

In clinical trials, the analysis plan must be pre-specified before data unblinding. Therefore, it is beneficial to have a general understanding of how the treatment effect may vary over time. If no clear pattern is anticipated, or if robustness across several possible treatment effect scenarios is desired, combinations of

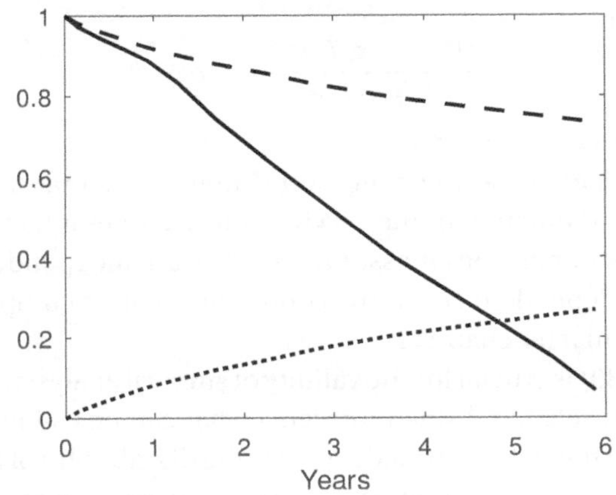

FIGURE 2.3
Weight functions for various weighted log-rank tests of the primary outcome in TOPCAT. Solid—Gehan; dashed—Peto-Prentice; dotted—complement Peto-Prentice.

weighted log-tests or adaptively weighted log-rank tests can be considered. These topics are discussed in Chapter Nine.

2.7 Random Censoring and Independent Censoring

The random censorship model assumes that the pairs $(T_i, C_i), 1 \le i \le n$, are independent, and T_i, C_i are independent within each pair, $1 \le i \le n$. Often, for simpler notation and analysis, additionally the censoring distributions will be assumed to be identical. Sometimes an analysis may also be conditional on the censoring variables, effectively reducing the case of random C_i's to type I censoring. This conditioning argument may offer some flexibility in certain situations [203, 243]. In the literature, depending on the context, either approach may be adopted. The random censorship model will be used for most of the book for easier heuristic argument and simpler presentation. However, the independence assumptions may not be satisfied in cases such as type II censoring, which violates both independence assumptions.

Intuitively, since the hazard function determines the distribution, inference procedures remain valid as long as the censoring does not alter the hazard function. The *independent censoring condition* assumes that $T_1, \ldots, T_n$ are i.i.d. with cumulative hazard function $\Lambda(t)$, and that the censoring variables $C_1, \ldots, C_n$ satisfy the condition

$$\frac{dP(T_i \le x, T_i \le C_i)}{P(T_i \wedge C_i \ge x)} = d\Lambda(x), \tag{2.39}$$

when $P(T_i \wedge C_i \ge x) > 0,\ 1 \le i \le n$.

The independent censoring condition simply states that the censoring does not alter the hazard function of the survival times. It does not assume that T_i and C_i are independent, nor does it assume that C_i's are independent among themselves. Various independent censoring conditions in more complicated situations will be discussed in later chapters.

Condition (2.39) is crucial for the validity of survival analysis on censored time-to-event data. The left-hand side represents what can be estimated from the observed data, while the right-hand side reflects the distribution of the time-to-event variable, which is of primary interest. Further discussions related to this topic will be given in Chapter Eleven.

Under the independent censoring condition, with the martingale techniques outlined in Appendix B, it can be shown that the Kaplan-Meier estimator, the Nelson-Aalen estimator and the log-rank test continue to have properties such as consistency and asymptotic normality.

When both T_i and C_i have absolutely continuous distributions, (2.39) is equivalent to the condition

$$\lim_{h \downarrow 0} P\big(t \le T_i < t+h \big| T_i \ge t, C_i \ge t\big)/h = \lambda(t). \tag{2.40}$$

Verification of this is left to Exercise 2.16. With the definition of hazard function in (2.4), this condition in turn can be rewritten as

$$\begin{aligned} & \lim_{h \downarrow 0} P\big(t \le T_i < t+h \big| T_i \ge t, C_i \ge t\big)/h \\ = \ & \lim_{h \downarrow 0} P\big(t \le T_i < t+h \big| T_i \ge t\big)/h, \end{aligned} \tag{2.41}$$

for t such that $P(T_i \wedge C_i \ge t) > 0,\ 1 \le i \le n$. Thus, given that there is neither event or censoring before time t, the instantaneous rate of event at time t is $\lambda(t)$, identical to the rate in the absence of censoring.

Independent censoring requires that, given there is neither event nor censoring in $[0, t)$, the instantaneous rate of event is $\lambda(t)$, the same rate as if there were no censoring. That is, individuals who are censored should have the same survival experience as those who are still at risk.

Therefore, it would violate the independent censoring condition if individuals are censored because their risk of event is either higher or lower than the average level of the population.

The condition of independent censoring is weaker than the independence assumptions in the random censorship model, since it can be verified that the random censorship model satisfies the condition (Exercise 2.17). It can also be checked that type II censoring is an independent censoring model and the likelihood function is of the form (2.25) in the absolutely continuous case (Exercise 2.18).

2.8 Counting Process and Lebesgue-Stieltjes Integral Notations

At a pre-calculus level, sums of random variables based on observed data are often encountered, with the sample mean and the sample variance as two familiar examples. At the calculus level, integrals are frequently used, such as for calculating population mean and population variance.

Using counting process and Lebesgue-Stieltjes integral notations, formulas can be written in a convenient and unified manner, which also facilitate the use of more sophisticated mathematical tools. This is especially important for survival analysis, as censoring and the use of hazard function could lead to quite messy formulas if we adhere to elementary pre-calculus notations. Thus, even though informal and heuristic arguments are often used in this book to motivate various estimators and tests, it is beneficial to become familiar with counting process and Lebesgue-Stieltjes integral notations.

We have already seen in Section 2.2.3 that the Lebesgue-Stieltjes integral notation gives a unified definition of the cumulative hazard function. Below, we further demonstrate how estimators and test statistics discussed in Sections 2.4 through 2.6 can be written in more compact expressions. These expressions also lend themselves to analysis with more powerful tools.

For $i = 1, \ldots, n$ and $t > 0$, let T_i, $N_i(t)$, and $Y_i(t)$ be, respectively, the time to event, the number of events observed in $[0, t]$, and the at-risk process for the ith individual, where the at-risk process $Y_i(t)$ is the indicator that the ith individual is under observation before t (neither event nor censoring has occurred before t). Under the random censorship model described in Section 2.4, we have

$$N_i(t) = \delta_i I(X_i \le t), \qquad Y_i(t) = I(X_i \ge t), \tag{2.42}$$

where $T_i$is the time to event for the ith individual.

The function $N_i(t)$ is an example of a counting process, the precise definition of which is given in Section B.3 of Appendix B. $N_i(t)$ is right-continuous at any $t \ge 0$ with left limit at each $t > 0$. This property of right-continuity with left limit will be given the acronym *cadlag*, from abbreviation of the phrase in French. In contrast, $Y_i(t)$ is left continuous at any $t > 0$ with right limit at each $t \ge 0$. This property of left continuity with right limit will be called *caglad*, parallel to the cadlag property of $N_i(t)$.

Define

$$H(t) = \sum_{i=1}^{n} N_i(t), \quad K(t) = \sum_{i=1}^{n} Y_i(t), \quad t > 0. \tag{2.43}$$

Then $H(t)$ is a cadlag step function and $H(t) = \sum_{t_j \le t} d_j$, where t_j's are the ordered distinct event times and d_j is the number of tied event times at t_j, as described in Section 2.4. Also, $K(t)$ is a caglad step function which is the number of individuals who are at risk at t, i.e., who have neither had the event nor been censored before t. For any $t > 0$, H, K are monotone and bounded on $[0, t]$.

2.8.1 Nelson-Aalen and Kaplan-Meier Estimators

The counting process N_i is discrete with the only possible jump δ_i at X_i. It will remain identically 0 if $\delta_i = 0$. From (A.8) in Appendix A, for a bounded function g, we have

$$\int_{(0,t]} g(s)dN_i(s) = \sum_{s \le t} g(s)\Delta N(s) = \delta_i g(T_i) I(T_i \le t).$$

Thus

$$\int_{(0,t]} g(s)dH(s) = \sum_{i=1}^{n} \int_{(0,t]} g(s)dN_i(s) = \sum_{i=1}^{n} \delta_i g(T_i) I(T_i \le t).$$

In particular, the Nelson-Aalen estimator of the cumulative hazard function in (2.30) can be written

$$\widehat{\Lambda}(t) = \int_0^t \frac{dH(s)}{K(s)}, \tag{2.44}$$

where and throughout this book the notation $\int_l^u = \int_{(l,u]}$ is adopted. Since $dH(s)$ has no mass when $K(s) = 0$, with the convention $0/0 = 0$, the integral is well defined and $\widehat{\Lambda}(t) = \widehat{\Lambda}(\max X_i)$ for any $t > \max X_i$.

Now for the Kaplan-Meier estimator $\widehat{F}(t)$ of $F(t)$, from (2.29) and corresponding to (2.18), $\widehat{F}(t)$ can be written

$$\widehat{F}(t) = 1 - \mathcal{P}_{(0,t]}(1 - d\widehat{\Lambda}). \tag{2.45}$$

The estimator for the variance of $\widehat{\Lambda}(t)$, given in (2.31), can now be written

$$\widehat{V}_\Lambda(t) = \int_0^t \frac{1}{K(s)^2}\left[1 - \frac{\Delta H(u)}{K(s)}\right] dH(s). \tag{2.46}$$

The Greenwood formula in (2.32) for the variance of $\widehat{S}(t) = 1 - \widehat{F}(t)$ can be written

$$\widehat{\sigma}^2(t) = [1 - \widehat{F}(t)]^2 \int_0^t \frac{1}{K(s)[K(s) - \Delta H(s)]} dH(s). \tag{2.47}$$

For $\widehat{F}$ and $\widehat{\Lambda}$, there is a very important identity:

$$\frac{\widehat{F}(t)-F(t)}{1-F(t)}=\int_0^t \frac{1-\widehat{F}_-(x)}{1-F(x)}d\big[\widehat{\Lambda}(x)-\Lambda(x)\big].$$

The precise statement is (A.14) in Appendix A. This identity is useful in rigorously establishing the asymptotic distribution of $\widehat{F}$ and obtaining a consistent variance estimator via the counting process and martingale approach.

2.8.2 Log-Rank Test and Weighted Log-Rank Tests

Weighted log-rank tests are widely used in time-to-event analysis. In addition to clinical trials, they have been applied in situations where the two groups are not formed via random assignment of group membership.

For a more clear and unified presentation, in this section we formulate the two sample comparison problem and weighted log-rank tests with notations which will be used repeatedly later. For clinical trial, this is the setup conditional on the treatment group membership variables. This approach may be more convenient in two sample comparison problems.

Label the two groups control and treatment, with cumulative hazard functions Λ_C and Λ_T, respectively. Then the null hypothesis of $S_1 = S_2$ in Section 2.6.1 is now expressed as

$$H_0 : \Lambda_T = \Lambda_C.$$

Let the pooled time-to-event variables be $T_1,\ldots,T_n$, with the first n_1, $n_1 < n$, variables from the control group and the remaining variables from the treatment group.

The available data are independent pairs $(X_i,\ \delta_i), i = 1,\ldots,n$, with $X_i = T_i \wedge C_i$, $\delta_i = I(X_i = T_i)$, and C_i the time-to-censoring variable, $1 \le i \le n$. It is also assumed that T_i, C_i are independent, $1 \le i \le n$.

For more flexibility, the pairs $(X_i,\ \delta_i), i = 1,\ldots,n$, are in general not assumed to be identically distributed. However, for simplified analysis, in the literature it is often assumed that the censoring variables are identically distributed within each treatment group. That simplifying assumption may also be used for certain situations in this book.

Let

$$z_i = I(i > n_1), \qquad 1 \le i \le n.$$

That is, $z_i = 1$ if the ith individual is in the treatment group, and $z_i = 0$ otherwise. For the control and treatment groups, the at-risk processes are defined by

$$K_C(t)=\sum_{i=1}^n (1-z_i)Y_i(t), \qquad K_T(t)=\sum_{i=1}^n z_i Y_i(t), \tag{2.48}$$

respectively. It follows that $K_C + K_T = K$, for K in (2.43). In the context here, K represents the at-risk process of the pooled sample. The log-rank test statistic in (2.35) can now be written as

$$\sum_{i=1}^{n}\int_0^{\infty}\left[z_i - \frac{K_T(t)}{K(t)}\right]dN_i(t)$$

$$= \sum_{i=1}^{n}\delta_i\left[z_i - \frac{\sum_{m=1}^{n} z_m I(X_m \geq X_i)}{\sum_{m=1}^{n} I(X_m \geq X_i)}\right]. \quad (2.49)$$

From (2.49), it can be seen that the log-rank statistic is a *rank statistic* which is determined by the ranks and not the exact values of $X_1,\ldots,X_n$. Most nonparametric tests and estimators in introductory statistics books are rank-based. Such property makes rank statistics less sensitive to outliers in data than statistics that depend on the exact values of $X_1,\ldots,X_n$.

In the extreme case when the largest X_i is uncensored, then a large increase in that observation does not have any impact on the log-rank test, while other quantities, such as the mean of X_i's, can be dramatically changed. This scenario may not be as unlikely or irrelevant as it seems, as long time survivors are often present in clinical trials or observational studies.

The variance formula (2.36) under H_0 can be expressed as

$$\int_0^{\infty}\frac{K_C(t)K_T(t)}{K(t)}\left[1 - \frac{\Delta H(t) - 1}{K(t) - 1}\right]d\widehat{\Lambda}(t), \quad (2.50)$$

where $\widehat{\Lambda}(t)$ is as in (2.44). In the context here, $\widehat{\Lambda}(t)$ is the estimator from the pooled sample of the common cumulative hazard function under the null hypothesis $S_T = S_C$, where S_T and S_C are the survival functions of the treatment and control groups, respectively.

Similar to (2.49), the weighted log-rank statistics can be written as

$$U_{\Phi} = \sum_{i=1}^{n}\int_0^{\infty}\Phi(t)\left[z_i - \frac{K_T(t)}{K(t)}\right]dN_i(t), \quad (2.51)$$

where the weight function Φ is nonnegative, possibly data-dependent, and satisfies certain regularity conditions. It is typically required to be predictable, as defined in Section B.3 of Appendix B.

Loosely speaking, $\Phi(t)$ being predictable means that at each time $t > 0$, $\Phi(t)$ is determined given information on event and censoring up to but not including t. This requirement is satisfied for the Gehan weight $K(t)$ and weights $\widehat{S}_-^{\rho}(t)(1 - \widehat{S}_-(t))^{\gamma}$, ρ, $\gamma \geq 0$, from the $G^{\rho,\gamma}$ family of Harrington and Fleming [82], where $\widehat{S}_-$ is the left continuous version of the Kaplan-Meier estimator from the pooled sample.

Similarly to (2.50), the variance estimator of U_Φ under H_0 is

$$\int_0^\infty \Phi^2(t)\frac{K_C(t)K_T(t)}{K(t)}\left[1-\frac{\Delta H(t)-1}{K(t)-1}\right]d\widehat{\Lambda}(t). \tag{2.52}$$

In this book, we primarily deal with the case of continuous survival distributions, in which there are no ties in observed event times and the variance estimator reduces to

$$\begin{aligned} V_\Phi &= \int_0^\infty \Phi^2(t)\frac{K_C(t)K_T(t)}{K(t)}d\widehat{\Lambda}(t) \\ &= \sum_{i=1}^n \int_0^\infty \Phi^2(t)\frac{K_C(t)K_T(t)}{K^2(t)}dN_i(t) \end{aligned} \tag{2.53}$$

In practice, for large samples, formulas (2.52) and (2.53) typically give numerical values that differ by a negligible amount.

For an alternative expression of the weighted log-rank test statistics, let

$$H_C(t) = \sum_{i=1}^n (1-z_i)N_i(t), \qquad H_T(t) = \sum_{i=1}^n z_i N_i(t), \tag{2.54}$$

the counting processes for the two groups, respectively. Then $H_C + H_T = H$ for H in (2.43) which, in the context here, is the counting process of the pooled sample. With some algebraic simplification, the weighted log-rank test statistics can be expressed as

$$\begin{aligned} U_\Phi &= \int_0^\infty \frac{\Phi(t)K_C(t)}{K(t)}dH_T(t) - \int_0^\infty \frac{\Phi(t)K_T(t)}{K(t)}dH_C(t) \\ &= \int_0^\infty \frac{\Phi(t)K_C(t)K_T(t)}{K_C(t)+K_T(t)}d\left[\widehat{\Lambda}_T(t)-\widehat{\Lambda}_C(t)\right], \end{aligned} \tag{2.55}$$

where

$$\widehat{\Lambda}_C(t) = \int_0^t \frac{dH_C(t)}{K_C(t)}, \qquad \widehat{\Lambda}_T(t) = \int_0^t \frac{dH_T(t)}{K_T(t)}. \tag{2.56}$$

$\widehat{\Lambda}_C(t)$ and $\widehat{\Lambda}_T(t)$ are the Nelson-Aalen estimators of the cumulative hazard functions $\Lambda_C(t)$ and $\Lambda_T(t)$ of the two groups, respectively. Verification of this alternative expression is left to Exercise 2.22.

2.9 Exercises and Complements

2.1 Assume that the CDF F is differentiable and the PDF f is continuous, show that

$$\lambda(t) = \frac{f(s)}{1-F(s)}, \quad \int_0^t \frac{f(s)ds}{1-F(s)} = -\log[S(t)],$$

for t satisfying $S(t) > 0$.

2.2 (a) Verify (2.14). (*Hint*: Write down $\lambda_1, \lambda_2, \ldots$ in terms of $f(s_i)$ and then simplify the product in (2.14)).

(b) Use (2.14) to verify (2.15).

(c) Verify (2.14) using (2.16) and the chain rule of probability

2.3 (a) Suppose T is a discrete random variable taking integer values $1, 2, \cdots$, and its hazard is constant:

$$\lambda_j = c, j \geq 1,$$

for some $c > 0$. Obtain the cumulative hazard function and the CDF.

(b) Suppose T is a discrete random variable taking integer values $1, 2, \cdots, k$, for some integer $k > 1$, and the hazard is

$$\lambda_j = j/k, \ 1 \leq j \leq k,$$

Obtain the cumulative hazard function and the CDF.

2.4 (a) Suppose T is discrete, taking values $s_1 < s_2 < s_3$ with the probability mass function

$$P(T = s_j) = f_j, \quad j = 1, 2, 3,$$

where $f_j > 0, \ \ j = 1, 2, 3$ and $f_1 + f_2 + f_3 = 1$. Obtain the CDF $F(t)$ of T, plot it and verify that it is increasing and right-continuous with left limit.

(b) Obtain the cumulative hazard function $\Lambda(t)$ and plot it.

2.5 (a) If two events A and B in a probability space are disjoint ($A \cap B = \emptyset$), then $P(A \cup B) = P(A) + P(B)$. Use this to show that for any random variable X, its CDF $F_X(x) = P(X \leq x)$ is increasing. That is,

$$F_X(x) \leq F_X(y) \ \text{ if } \ x < y.$$

(b) By the monotone convergence theorem, if a sequence is either increasing and bounded from above, or decreasing and bounded from below, it converges. Use this to show that for the CDF F_X in (b), both its right and left limits exist at any point x. That is, $\lim_{x_n \uparrow x} F_X(x_n)$ and $\lim_{x_n \downarrow x} F_X(x_n)$ exist.

(c) Let

$$f_n(x) = I(X \le x - \epsilon_n), n \ge 1,$$

where $\epsilon_n \downarrow 0$. Note that $\lim_n f_n(x) = I(X < x)$. Additionally, $f_n(x) \le 1$, $P(X \le x - \epsilon_n) = Ef_n(x)$, and expectation is an integral with respect to the probability measure. Applying the dominated convergence theorem (property #7 in Section A.3 of Appendix A), we have

$$\lim_n P(X \le x - \epsilon_n) = \lim_n Ef_n(x) = E\lim_n f_n(x) = EI(X < x) = P(X < x).$$

This proves that the left limit exists, and it also gives the value of the limit. Use an analogous argument to show that F is right-continuous.

2.6 The assertion that S in (2.18) is the unique function satisfying (2.20) for Λ in (2.17) can be proved using integration by parts formula. Decompose Λ as in (2.21). Let

$$\Lambda_c(t) = \int_0^t \lambda_c(s)ds, \quad \Lambda_d(t) = \sum_{s_i \le t} \lambda_i.$$

and $S(t) = S_c(t)S_d(t)$, $F(t) = 1 - S(t)$, where

$$S_c(t) = \exp\left[-\int_0^t \lambda_c(s)ds\right]. \quad S_d(t) = \prod_{s_i \le t} (1 - \lambda_i).$$

Then $\Lambda = \Lambda_c + \Lambda_d$. By the discussions on the continuous and discrete cases in Sections 2.2.1 and 2.2.2,

$$\Lambda_c(t) = \int_0^t \frac{d[1 - S_c(s)]}{S_{c-}(s)}, \quad \Lambda_d(t) = \int_0^t \frac{d[1 - S_d(s)]}{S_{d-}(s)}.$$

The integration by parts formula gives

$$dF = -dS = -(S_c dS_d + S_{d-} dS_c).$$

Thus

$$\begin{aligned} \frac{dF}{S_-} &= -\frac{S_c dS_d + S_{d-} dS_c}{S_{c-} S_{d-}} \\ &= d\Lambda_d - \frac{dS_c}{S_{c-}} = d(\Lambda_d + \Lambda_c) = d\Lambda, \end{aligned}$$

where, in obtaining the second-last and the third-last equalities, the definition of $\Lambda_d(t)$ and the fact $S_{c-} = S_c$ have been used. It follows that $-dS/S_- = dF/S_- = d\Lambda$. By (A.9) in Appendix A, $-dS = S_- d\Lambda$. It follows that S satisfies (2.20).

To prove uniqueness of S, suppose A also satisfies (2.20), or $-dA = A_- d\Lambda$. Let $D = S - A$. Then

$$D_- d\Lambda = -dD$$

which, from $d\Lambda = -dS/S_-$, can be rewritten as

$$\frac{D_-}{S_-} dS = dD. \tag{2.57}$$

(a) Use the integration by parts formula with $D = (D/S)S$ to show that (2.57) becomes

$$\frac{D_-}{S_-} dS = \frac{D_-}{S_-} dS + Sd\left(\frac{D}{S}\right).$$

Thus $Sd(D/S) = 0$ or, $D(t)/S(t)$ is a constant.

(b) Use the fact that $D(t)/S(t)$ is a constant to prove that $S(t) = A(t)$. (*Hint:* $S(0) = 1$).

(c) For $S(t)$ in (2.18), note that

$$S(t) = S_-(t)\left[1 - \Delta\Lambda(t)\right] = S_-(t) - S_-(t)\Delta\Lambda(t).$$

It can be verified that

$$dS(t) = -S_-(t)d\Lambda(t).$$

Show that $S(t)$ satisfies (2.20). Conclude that $S(t)$ is the product $S_c(t)S_d(t)$.

(d) Let

$$\Psi_c(t) = \exp\left[\int_0^t \lambda_c(s)ds\right]. \quad \Psi_d(t) = \prod_{s_i \le t}(1 + \lambda_i),$$

and

$$\Psi(t) = \Psi_c(t)\Psi_d(t).$$

We have

$$d\Psi_c(t) = \Psi_c(t)\lambda_c(t)dt = \Psi_{c-}(t)d\Lambda_c(t),$$

where the last equality is due to the continuity of $\Psi_c(t)$. For $\Psi_d(t)$, we have

$$\Psi_d(t) = \Psi_{d-}(t)\left[1 + \Delta\Lambda_d(t)\right] = \Psi_{d-}(t) + \Psi_{d-}(t)\Delta\Lambda_d(t).$$

Thus

$$d\Psi_d(t) = \Psi_{d-}(t)d\Lambda_d(t),$$

Use these results and an argument analogous to those for parts (a) and (b) to show that

$$d\Psi(t) = \Psi_-(t)d\Lambda(t)$$

and that $\Psi(t)$ is the unique solution to

$$\int_0^t \Psi_-(s)d\Lambda(s) = \Psi(t).$$

2.7 Prove the assertion in Section 2.3 that a maximizer of $L(F)$ in (2.26) should not have positive probability at any censored time.

2.8 Show that the likelihood function (2.27) is maximized by $\widehat{S}(t)$ in (2.29).

2.9 Assume that F is discrete with hazard λ_j at t_j, $1 \le j \le k$. Obtain the second order partial derivative matrix

$$\Omega = \left(\frac{\partial^2 A}{\partial\lambda_\ell \partial\lambda_m}\right)_{k\times k},$$

where A is the logarithm of $L(F)$ in (2.27). From the theory of parametric MLE in Chapter Four, for $\widehat{\theta} = (\hat{\lambda}_1, \ldots, \hat{\lambda}_k)^{\mathrm{T}}$ and $\theta = (\lambda_1, \ldots, \lambda_k)^{\mathrm{T}}$ where V^{T} denotes the transpose for a vector V,

$$\sqrt{n}(\widehat{\theta} - \theta) \xrightarrow{d} N(0, \Sigma),$$

where $N(0, \Sigma)$ denotes the normal distribution with mean 0 and covariance matrix Σ. The covariance matrix Σ can be estimated by $(-n\Omega)^{-1}$. Show that the latter is a diagonal matrix with (j, j) element $d_j(n_j - d_j)/n_j^2$.

2.10 (*Delta method*[135, 64]) Suppose

$$\sqrt{n}(\widehat{\boldsymbol{\theta}} - \boldsymbol{\theta}) \xrightarrow{d} N(0, \boldsymbol{\Sigma}),$$

where $\widehat{\boldsymbol{\theta}}$, $\boldsymbol{\theta}$ are k dimensional and $\boldsymbol{\Sigma}$ a $k \times k$ covariance matrix. If g is differentiable with continuous gradient

$$\nabla g(\boldsymbol{\theta}) = \left(\frac{\partial g}{\partial \theta_1}, \ldots, \frac{\partial g}{\partial \theta_k}\right)^{\mathrm{T}},$$

Then

$$n^{1/2}[g(\widehat{\boldsymbol{\theta}}) - g(\boldsymbol{\theta})] \xrightarrow{d} N\Big(0, \nabla g(\boldsymbol{\theta})^{\mathrm{T}} \boldsymbol{\Sigma} \nabla g(\boldsymbol{\theta})\Big). \tag{2.58}$$

This method establishes the asymptotic normality of a smooth function of $\widehat{\boldsymbol{\theta}}$ from that of $\widehat{\boldsymbol{\theta}}$. More general versions are given in (4.14) in Chapter Four and in Section C.6 of Appendix C.

(a) Use (2.58) and the results of Exercise 2.9 to show that for $\widehat{\Lambda}(t)$ in (2.30), in the discrete case,

$$n^{1/2}[\widehat{\Lambda}(t) - \Lambda(t)] \xrightarrow{d} N(0, s^2)$$

where $s^2 = \lim_n n\widehat{V}_\Lambda$ for $\widehat{V}_\Lambda$ in (2.31).

(b) Show that for $\widehat{S}(t)$ in (2.29), in the discrete case,

$$n^{1/2}[\widehat{S}(t) - S(t)] \xrightarrow{d} N(0, \tilde{s}^2)$$

where $\tilde{s}^2 = \lim_n n\widehat{\sigma}^2(t)$ for $\widehat{\sigma}^2(t)$ in (2.32).

2.11 Suppose a censored sample from a homogeneous population has the following data:

$$x_1, x_2^*, x_3, x_4$$

where $x_1 < x_2 < x_3 < x_4$ and * denotes a censored observation.

(a) Show that the estimated hazard function is

$$\widehat{\lambda}(x_1) = 1/4, \quad \widehat{\lambda}(x_3) = 1/2, \quad \widehat{\lambda}(x_4) = 1$$

and that the Kaplan-Meier estimator $\widehat{S}$ is

$$\widehat{S}(x_1) = 3/4, \quad \widehat{S}(x_3) = 3/8, \quad \widehat{S}(x_4) = 0.$$

(b) (*Redistribution to the right algorithm*) if there were no censoring, the empirical CDF would assign probability 1/4 to each of the four time points x_1 through x_4. But x_2 is right censored, randomly. It makes sense to re-assign the initial mass 1/4 at x_2 to observed event times larger than x_2, equally. Thus the probability at x_3, x_4 would each be updated to $1/4 + 1/4 \cdot 1/2 = 3/8$. The final probability mass function is

$$P(T = x_1) = 1/4, \quad P(T = x_k) - 3/8, k = 3, 4.$$

This is the redistribution to the right algorithm of Efron [68]. Show that this probability mass function is identical to the one associated with $\widehat{S}$ in (a).

(c) Suppose the mean of time-to-event variable is of interest. Explain if it makes sense to estimate it by

$$(x_1 + x_2^* + x_3 + x_4)/4 \tag{2.59}$$

or by

$$(x_1 + x_3 + x_4)/3. \tag{2.60}$$

If not, what are the expectations of quantities in (2.59) and (2.60)?

2.12 (a) Suppose T is discrete, taking positive values $a_1 < a_2 < a_3$, and with the probability mass function

$$P(T = a_j) = f_j, \quad j = 1,2,3,$$

where $f_j > 0$, $j = 1,2,3$, and $\sum_j f_j = 1$. Verify that

$$\int_0^\infty S(t)dt = ET.$$

Then also verify that

$$\int_0^\infty S_-(t)dt = ET.$$

(b) Show that, for a nonnegative random variable T with finite expectation,

$$\int_0^\infty S(t)dt = ET. \tag{2.61}$$

Hint: $S(t) = P(T > t) = EI(T > t)$. Also assume that the order of integration and expectation can be interchanged.

(c) Apply (b) to Exercise 2.11 to obtain an estimate of ET. Compare it to the two proposals in Exercise 2.11.

2.13 Instead of $\ln[-\ln x]$ used in Section 2.5, use the transformation $\ln[x/(1-x)]$ and the delta method to derive a confidence interval for $S(t)$. Are there other transformations you can think of?

2.14 Imitate derivation of the Kaplan-Meier estimator to show that the empirical CDF in (2.17) is the nonparametric MLE for F when i.i.d. $T_1, \ldots, T_n$ are observable, i.e., when there is no censoring.

2.15 Consider the random censorship model with $C_i \equiv \tau, 1 \le i \le n$, for some constant $\tau > 0$. Suppose that the observed distinct event times are $t_1 < \cdots < t_k$ and that d_j is the number of events at t_j, $j \le k$. Note that $t_k < \tau$.

(a) Let $c_0 = 0$ and

$$c_m = d_1 + \cdots + d_m, \quad 1 \le m \le k.$$

Show that

$$\widehat{\Lambda}(t_j) = \sum_{m=1}^{j} \frac{d_m}{n - c_{m-1}}, \quad j \le k.$$

(b) Show that

$$\widehat{S}(t_j) = 1 - \frac{c_j}{n}, \quad j \le k.$$

That is, the Kaplan-Meier estimator reduces to the empirical cumulative distribution function.

(c) Assume that there are no ties. That is, $d_j = 1$ for all $j \le k$. Simplify $\widehat{S}(t)$ and the variance estimator in (2.32). Note that in this case, by the harmonic number approximation

$$\frac{1}{1} + \cdots + \frac{1}{n} \approx \log(n) + \gamma$$

where γ is the Euler-Mascheroni constant ≈ 0.577, we have

$$\widehat{\Lambda}(t_j) = \frac{1}{n} + \cdots + \frac{1}{n-j+1} \approx \log\left(\frac{n}{n-j}\right)$$

for $j/n \to a \in (0,1)$.

2.16 Assume that both T_i and C_i have absolutely continuous distribution. Show that (2.39) and (2.40) are equivalent.

2.17 Assume that T_i and C_i are independent and both have absolutely continuous distribution. Show that

$$\begin{aligned} & \lim_{h\downarrow 0} P\big(t \le T < t+h \big| T \ge t, C \ge t\big)/h \\ = \quad & \lim_{h\downarrow 0} P\big(t \le T < t+h \big| T \ge t\big)/h, \end{aligned}$$

for t such that $P\big(\min(T,C) > t\big) > 0$. That is, the condition of independent censoring is implied by independence between T and C.

2.18 Assume that $T_i, i = 1, \ldots, n$ are i.i.d. copies of absolutely continuous T and that they are censored by $T_{(k)}$, the kth order statistic of the sample, for $k > 1$, where $T_{(1)} < \cdots < T_{(n)}$. Then

$$\{T_{(k)} \ge t\} = \bigcup_{m=n-k+1}^{n} A_m,$$

where

$$A_m = \{m \text{ of } T_i\text{'s} > t, \text{ the other observations} < t\}.$$

Now consider the event $\{T_1 \ge t, T_{(k)} \ge t\}$. In this event, T_1 is one of those observations $\ge t$.

(a) Show that

$$\begin{aligned} & P(T_1 \ge t, T_{(k)} \ge t) \\ = \quad & \sum_{m=n-k}^{n-1} C_m^{n-1} S^{m+1}(t) F^{n-m-1}(t), \end{aligned}$$

where C_j^{ℓ} is the number of ways to choose j items from a set of ℓ.

(b) Show that

$$\begin{aligned} & P\big(T_1 \in [t, t+\varepsilon), T_{(k)} \ge t\big) \\ = \quad & \sum_{m=n-k}^{n-1} C_m^{n-1} S^m(t) F^{n-m-1}(t) \big[F(t+\varepsilon) - F(t)\big], \end{aligned}$$

where $\varepsilon > 0$.

(c) Show that

$$\lim_{\varepsilon \downarrow 0} P\big(T_1 \in [t, t+\varepsilon) \big| T_1 \geq t, T_{(k)} \geq t\big)/\varepsilon = \lambda(t).$$

Since the T_i's are i.i.d., this result shows that type II censoring satisfies the independent censoring condition (2.40).

(d) Show that the joint p.d.f of $T_{(1)} < \cdots < T_{(k)}$ is

$$\frac{n!}{(n-k)!} f(y_1) \cdot \cdots \cdot f(y_k) [1 - F(y_k)]^{n-k}.$$

2.19 Show that (2.36) and (2.50) are the same.

2.20 Rewrite the test statistic and variance for the stratified log-rank test using the counting process and integral notations.

2.21 (a) Let X, Y be independent variables with PDF f and g, respectively, and $\phi(y) = Eh(X, y)$. Show that

$$Eh(X, Y) = E\phi(Y). \tag{2.62}$$

This result is valid more generally, in the form of (B.7) in Appendix B.

(b) Let T and C be independent random variables, and $a(X)$ a bounded function of $X = T \wedge C$. Also, let $\delta = I(T \leq C)$. Then

$$E\big(\delta a(X)\big) = E\big((1 - G_-(T))a(T)\big). \tag{2.63}$$

Verify this result in the continuous case, assuming that T and C have PDFs f and g, respectively. Note that from (2.63),

$$P(X \leq t, \delta = 1) = EI(X \leq t, \delta = 1) = E\big(\delta I(X \leq t)\big) = \int_0^t \big[1 - G_-(x)\big] dF(x).$$

(c) Verify the equivalence of (2.40) and (2.41) when the joint distribution of each pair (T_i, C_i) is continuous with a joint density function. Although unnecessary, smoothness and boundedness of relevant densities can be assumed to simplify the proof.

2.22 Verify that the weighted log-rank test statistics can be rewritten as the expression in (2.55) (*Hint:* Split the integration range

$$(0, \infty) = (0, a] \cup (a, b] \cup (b, \infty),$$

where a, b are the maximum X_i's in the control and treatment groups, with a

being the smaller one. Remember that $0/0 = 0$, K_C, $K_T > 0$ on $(0, a]$, and z_i is either 0 or 1).

2.23 Suppose a censored sample is as below:

1 2* 2* 4 5 6 7 8*

where * denotes a censored observation.

(a) Manually obtain and plot the Kaplan-Meier and Nelson-Aalen curves.

(b) Obtain and plot confidence intervals for the Kaplan-Meier estimator.

2.24 Consider the continuous distribution case and the setup for stochastic ordering in Section 2.3. Then $F_i(t) = 1 - \exp\left(-\Lambda_j(t)\right), j = 1.2$. Show that

$$\Lambda_2(t) \le \Lambda_1(t), \quad t \in [0, \tau]$$

if and only if

$$F_2(t) \le F_1(t), \quad t \in [0, \tau].$$

2.25 Suppose T is discrete, taking positive values $a_1 < a_2 < a_3$, and with the probability mass function

$$P(T = a_j) = f_j, \quad j = 1,2,3,$$

where $f_j > 0$, $j = 1,2,3$, and $\sum_j f_j = 1$. Express $\Lambda(a_j)$ in terms of $S(a_1)$, $S(a_2)$, and $S(a_3)$, $j = 1,2,3$.

2.26 Consider the special case of random censorship model in which the censoring variables are i.i.d. with common CDF G satisfying $G(\tau) = 1$ for some $\tau > 0$. Yang [331] established convergence of the Kaplan-Meier estimator $\widehat{F}(t)$ on the interval $[0, \tau]$, which is the maximum possible interval by the assumption $G(\tau) = 1$. One of the conditions required is

$$\int_0^\tau \frac{dF(t)}{1 - G_-(t)} < \infty, \tag{2.64}$$

which is weaker than conditions needed for alternative methods, and is often necessary. For the staggered entry problem, suppose the time to randomization is a random variable ξ in $[0, A]$ and the trial concludes at time $\tau = A + B$. Then the censoring variable is $C = \tau - \xi$.

(a) Suppose $P(\xi = 0) > 0$. That is, there is a portion of individuals who are randomized at time 0. Show that (2.64) is satisfied.

(b) Suppose $P(\xi = 0) = 0$. Show that $G_-(\tau) = 1$. Thus (2.64) fails to hold when F has an exponential distribution. This result shows that for clinical trials with staggered entry, convergence of $\widehat{F}(t)$ on the maximum interval $[0, \tau]$ is generally impossible unless $P(\xi = 0) > 0$.

(c) Suppose ξ is uniform$[0,2]$ and $\tau = 6$. Obtain the CDF of C.

(d) Suppose that ξ has CDF $(t/2)^2$ for $t \in [0,2]$. and $\tau = 6$. Obtain the CDF of C.

(e) Suppose that ξ has CDF $\sqrt{t/2}$ for $t \in [0,2]$. and $\tau = 6$. Obtain the CDF of C.

3

Parametric Distributions

The Kaplan-Meier estimator and the weighted log-rank tests introduced in Chapter Two are nonparametric. They are applicable under quite general settings for survival data, without imposing assumptions on the shape or functional form of the survival distributions. Sometimes, parametric models and inferences can be used. They often result in closed-form expressions for various functions and also play important roles in generating data for simulations which help evaluate and compare statistical procedures.

In this chapter, some parametric models for survival data are discussed. Since the logarithm transformation is often used in survival analysis, descriptions will be given for either T or $Y = \log T$, depending on the motivation and mathematical convenience in specifying these distributions. Parametric models for homogeneous populations will be discussed first, followed by extensions to include explanatory variables.

3.1 Univariate Distributions

3.1.1 Exponential Distribution

In terms of the hazard function, the exponential distribution is the simplest, with a constant hazard: $\lambda(t) = \eta > 0$. The cumulative hazard function, survival function and PDF of T are, respectively,

$$\Lambda(t) = \eta t, \qquad S(t) = e^{-\eta t}, \qquad f(t) = \eta e^{-\eta t}. \tag{3.1}$$

Under the exponential model, the plot of $\Lambda(t)$ versus t should approximate a straight line in the data range. This gives a simple graphical method to check model validity.

In applications, often the exponential distribution can fit the data well except for the part near the end of the data range. This is similar to the situation of fitting the normal distribution to data with outliers. However, the exponential distribution has larger tail probability than the normal distribution. Consequently, extrapolation near or beyond the upper end of the data range is more problematic with the exponential distribution. Caution should be exercised when interpreting results near the upper end of the data range.

DOI: 10.1201/9780429324437-3

The PDF of $Y = \log T$ is

$$e^y f(e^y) = \exp[y - a - \exp(y - a)], \quad -\infty < y < \infty, \tag{3.2}$$

where $a = -\log\eta$. Verification of this claim is left to Exercise 3.1. The distribution in (3.2) is an extreme value distribution, which derives the name from being the limiting distribution of a standardized minimum of a sample from a continuous distribution [129].

3.1.2 Weibull Distribution

The Weibull distribution extends the exponential distribution with an additional power parameter, resulting in the hazard function

$$\lambda(t) = \eta\nu(\eta t)^{\nu-1}, \quad t > 0, \quad \eta, \nu > 0. \tag{3.3}$$

This distribution allows more diverse hazard patterns than the exponential for the hazard: constant when $\nu = 1$ (exponential), decreasing from ∞ to 0 when $\nu < 1$, and increasing from 0 to ∞ when $\nu > 1$.

The survival and cumulative hazard functions are, respectively,

$$S(t) = \exp[-(\eta t)^\nu], \quad \Lambda(t) = (\eta t)^\nu. \tag{3.4}$$

Since

$$\log\Lambda(t) = \nu(\log t + \log\eta),$$

a graphical way to check model validity is to plot $\log\Lambda(t)$ versus $\log t$ and assess if it approximates a straight line. If so, the slope and intercept of the line provide estimates of ν and $-\log\eta$, respectively.

For the distribution of Y, it can be shown (Exercise 3.2) that Y can be written as $a + bY_0$, where $a = -\log\eta$, $b = \nu^{-1}$, and Y_0 has the extreme value distribution with PDF

$$\exp[y - \exp(y)], \quad -\infty < y < \infty. \tag{3.5}$$

The two parameters η, ν are scale and power parameter, respectively. Careful attention and maneuver is needed for stable and efficient numerical calculation of an estimator of ν [47, 12].

3.1.3 Log-Normal Distribution

T has a log-normal distribution if $Y = \log T$ can be written $Y = \mu + \sigma Y_0$ where μ, σ are real, $\sigma > 0$, and Y_0 has the standard normal distribution with PDF

$$\phi(y) = \frac{1}{\sqrt{2\pi}} \exp(-\frac{1}{2}y^2), \quad -\infty < y < \infty. \tag{3.6}$$

Let Φ be the CDF of the standard normal distribution. Then the CDF of T is

$$\Phi\Big(\frac{\log t-\mu}{\sigma}\Big)$$

and the PDF of T is

$$\frac{d}{dt}\Phi\Big(\frac{\log t-\mu}{\sigma}\Big)=\frac{1}{t\sigma\sqrt{2\pi}}\exp\Big(-\frac{(\log t-\mu)^2}{2\sigma^2}\Big).$$

The hazard function $\lambda(t)$ can be obtained from the CDF and the PDF, although there is no simple closed form. It can be shown that $\lim_{t\downarrow 0}\lambda(t)=0$, and that $\lambda(t)$ initially increases to a maximum value, then decreases to 0 as $t\to\infty$. This hazard pattern is opposite to that of the human aging process. However, it can gives a good fit for fatigue-stress testing in reliability studies and for analysis of insurance claims in an actuarial setting.

3.1.4 Gamma Distribution

T has a gamma distribution with shape parameter α and rate parameter β if it has the PDF

$$f(t)=\frac{\beta^\alpha t^{\alpha-1}\exp(-\beta t)}{\Gamma(\alpha)}\qquad t>0, \tag{3.7}$$

where $\alpha,\beta>0$, and Γ is the gamma function

$$\Gamma(\alpha)=\int_0^\infty t^{\alpha-1}e^{-t}dt.$$

The survival function is

$$S(t)=1-\frac{\gamma_\alpha(\beta t)}{\Gamma(\alpha)}$$

with the incomplete gamma function

$$\gamma_\alpha(x)=\int_0^x t^{\alpha-1}\exp(-t)dt.$$

The hazard function is

$$\lambda(t)=\frac{\beta^\alpha t^{\alpha-1}\exp(-\beta t)}{\Gamma(\alpha)-\gamma_\alpha(\beta t)}.$$

If $\alpha=m$, a positive integer, then $\Gamma(\alpha)=(m-1)!$ and the expressions for $f(t)$, $\lambda(t)$ can be simplified a little. In particular, $m=1$ gives rise to the exponential distribution, and the sum of m independent exponential variables with hazard λ has a gamma distribution with shape m and rate λ.

The hazard function is increasing from 0 if $\alpha>1$, decreasing from ∞ if $\alpha<1$, and in both cases approaches β as $t\to\infty$.

The rth moment is

$$ET^r = \frac{\Gamma(\alpha + r)}{\beta^r \Gamma(\alpha)}, \qquad r > 0. \tag{3.8}$$

For a nonnegative random variable X, or equivalently the associated distribution, its Laplace transformation is the function

$$\mathfrak{L}_X(s) = E\exp(-sX),$$

for real values of s where the function is well defined. It is left to Exercise 3.4 to verify that the Laplace transformation of a gamma variable T is

$$E\exp(-sT) = \left(\frac{\beta}{\beta + s}\right)^{\alpha}, \qquad s > -\beta. \tag{3.9}$$

These properties make the gamma distribution a convenient choice for studying association between random variables via the notion of *frailty*. This will be discussed in Chapter Ten.

3.1.5 Log-Logistic Distribution

The log-logistic and log-normal variables share the property that their natural logarithm has a distribution belonging to a location-scale parametric family. For T to have a log-logistic distribution, its natural logarithm $Y = \log T$ must have the form $Y = \mu + \sigma Y_0$, where μ, σ are real, $\sigma > 0$, and Y_0 has the standard logistic distribution with symmetric PDF

$$\frac{\exp(y)}{[1 + \exp(y)]^2}, \qquad -\infty < y < \infty. \tag{3.10}$$

Y_0 has mean 0 and variance $\pi^2/3$. The PDF of T is

$$f(t) = \frac{\alpha\beta(\alpha t)^{\beta - 1}}{[1 + (\alpha t)^\beta]^2}, \tag{3.11}$$

where $\alpha = \exp(-\mu)$ and $\beta = 1/\sigma$. The survival, hazard and cumulative hazard functions are, respectively,

$$S(t) = \frac{1}{1 + (\alpha t)^\beta}, \qquad \lambda(t) = \frac{\alpha\beta(\alpha t)^{\beta - 1}}{1 + (\alpha t)^\beta}, \qquad \Lambda(t) = \log[1 + (\alpha t)^\beta]. \tag{3.12}$$

The hazard function is decreasing from ∞ to 0 if $\beta < 1$, decreasing from α to 0 if $\beta = 1$. If $\beta > 1$, the hazard function increases from 0 to a maximum at $t = (\beta - 1)^{1/\beta}/\alpha$ and then decreases toward 0 as $t \to \infty$. Compared to the log-normal distribution, the log-logistic distribution has simpler expressions for the survival and hazard functions, but heavier tail probabilities.

3.1.6 Gompertz-Makeham Distributions

In addition to the ones discussed so far, other continuous parametric distributions can be used. For example, the Gompertz distribution [102] with hazard

$$\lambda(t) = \eta \exp(\nu t), \qquad t > 0,\ \eta,\ \nu > 0$$

has been found to provide a good fit for certain human mortality studies. The hazard function increases from η to ∞. As $t \to \infty$, it increases more rapidly than the hazard function for the Weibull distribution with $\nu > 1$.

The Makeham generalization [194], with hazard function

$$\lambda(t) = \alpha + \eta \exp(\nu t),$$

incorporates one additional parameter for an improved fit.

For all the distributions except the exponential, the hazard function $\lambda(t)$ has 0 or ∞ as the limiting value for t near one or both ends of the range $(0,\infty)$. Also, the parameters are often described as shape or tuning parameters in the distribution for T or the log-transformed Y.

A new distribution will be introduced next that has certain desirable parameter interpretations.

3.1.7 A New Class of Hazard Focused Distributions

The exponential distribution is the simplest for time-to-event data, with one parameter that is the constant hazard. However, survival data in general have non-constant hazard. Many of the other distributions can be viewed as extensions of the exponential distribution for non-constant hazard situations. Most of these distributions have two parameters that control the shape of the distribution, but the parameters themselves do not necessarily have simple interpretations.

In the case of the Weibull distribution, perhaps the most widely used extension of the exponential distribution, a power parameter, or equivalently a scale parameter for the logarithm transformed data, is added. As noted before, care is needed for stable numerical estimate of the additional parameter. In addition, the hazard either monotonically decreases from ∞ to 0 or monotonically increases from 0 to ∞.

Define a new parametric distribution by the hazard function

$$\lambda(t) = \alpha\left[1 - F_0(t)\right] + \beta F_0(t), \qquad t > 0,\ \alpha,\ \beta > 0, \tag{3.13}$$

where F_0 is a known CDF. This distribution also has two parameters. Its hazard function varies monotonically between α and β for $t \in (0,\infty)$, and

$$\lim_{t \downarrow 0} \lambda(t) = \alpha, \qquad \lim_{t \to \infty} \lambda(t) = \beta. \tag{3.14}$$

Therefore α, β can be interpreted as the short-term and long- term hazards, respectively. This distribution will be referred to as the short- and long-term hazards distribution. The exponential distribution is a special case of the new distribution with $\alpha = \beta$.

The parameters in this new model are more intuitive than generic shape parameters. Together they specify the range of $\lambda(t)$, which is bounded, unlike the Weibull distribution where $\lambda(t)$ spans $(0, \infty)$. In model (3.13), $\lambda(t)$ monotonically varies between $\min(\alpha, \beta)$ and $\max(\alpha, \beta)$.

Let $\Phi_0(t) = \int_0^t F_0(x)dx$. The cumulative hazard function is

$$\Lambda(t) = \alpha\left[t - \Phi_0(t))\right] + \beta\Phi_0(t), \quad t > 0, \ \alpha, \ \beta > 0, \tag{3.15}$$

Various simulation studies and applications to trial data have shown that the function

$$F_0(t) = \frac{t}{1+t} \tag{3.16}$$

is often a good choice.

As an alternative to (3.13), the model

$$\lambda(t) = \exp\left\{\alpha\left[1 - F_0(t)\right] + \beta F_0(t)\right\}, \quad t > 0, \ \alpha, \ \beta \text{ real}, \tag{3.17}$$

can also be considered. A drawback of this model is that the expression of $\Lambda(t)$ is more complicated.

The distributions discussed thus far exhibit diverse shapes for their hazard functions. For easy reference, Table 3.1 summarizes various hazard patterns and identifies suitable distributions for each pattern.

3.1.8 Threshold Parameter

For any of the previously mentioned parametric distributions, an additional parameter ξ can be introduced with the assumption that the event cannot happen before ξ. The parameter is called the threshold parameter. If it is known, the parametric distributions can be modified simply by replacing T with $T - \xi$. If it is unknown, the analysis is much more difficult. Therefore, usually it is not included as a free parameter in the distribution.

3.1.9 Discrete Distributions

Parametric distributions in Sections 3.1.1 through 3.1.7 are for a continuous time-to-event variable. Sometimes, discrete survival data can arise, either because the event time is naturally discrete or due to the grouping of a continuous time variable. Discrete distributions also play an important role in motivating the log-rank test and the variance formula for the Kaplan-Meier estimator as discussed in Chapter Two.

TABLE 3.1
Hazard patterns and suitable distributions (a and b are positive constants).

Hazard Patterns	Cases	Distributions
Constant		Exponential
Increasing	0 to ∞	Weibull
	a to ∞	Gompertz, Makeham
	0 to a	Gamma
	a to b	Short- & Long-Term Hazards
Decreasing	∞ to 0	Weibull, Log-Logistic
	∞ to a	Gamma
	a to 0	Log-Logistic ($\beta = 1$)
	a to b	Short- & Long-Term Hazards
Increase from 0 to $a(> 0)$, then decrease to 0		Log-Logistic, Log-Normal

A discrete time-to-event model or distribution can be derived from any continuous parametric distribution by partitioning the time axis. Such discrete distributions from grouping are often preferred for discrete survival data analysis over common discrete distributions in introductory statistics, such as the binomial or Poisson. These common discrete distributions typically have less flexible hazard shapes than those of discrete distributions obtained through grouping, and their survival and hazard functions usually do not have simple expressions.

Suppose T is a continuous time-to-event variable that follows a parametric distribution with survival function $S(t;\boldsymbol{\theta})$. Let $0 = a_0 < a_1 \cdots < a_k = \infty$, and define

$$T^{\#} = a_m \quad \text{if } T \in [a_m, a_{m+1}), \quad m = 0, \ldots, k-1.$$

Then $T^{\#}$ is a discrete survival time variable with parametric survival function

$$S^{\#}(a_m) = P(T^{\#} > a_m) = P(T \geq a_{m+1}) = S(a_{m+1};\boldsymbol{\theta})$$

and probability mass function

$$f^{\#}(a_m) = P(T^{\#} = a_m) = P(T \in [a_m, a_{m+1})) = S(a_m;\boldsymbol{\theta}) - S(a_{m+1};\boldsymbol{\theta}).$$

The hazard at a_m is

$$\lambda^{\#}(a_m) = \frac{f^{\#}(a_m)}{S^{\#}_{-}(a_m)} = 1 - \frac{S(a_{m+1};\boldsymbol{\theta})}{S(a_m;\boldsymbol{\theta})}.$$

3.2 Regression Models

The two primary goals of a clinical trial are to test if there is a treatment effect and, if so, to quantify the size of that effect. In an unadjusted analysis for a two-arm trial, the log-rank test or its variants are commonly used methods for testing treatment effect. For the second task of quantifying the size of treatment effect, a summary measure is needed to represent the overall effect. In standard statistics books, for a continuous outcome, the mean difference between groups is the most used measure.

In a covariate-adjusted analysis, a regression analysis on the conditional mean of the outcome given explanatory variables is often employed. However, in survival analysis, estimating the mean can be biased or unstable due to censoring, and alternative regression models are often used.

Typically, a regression model postulates a specific form for the conditional distribution of T given certain explanatory variables. Since we focus on survival analysis in clinical trials, the treatment indicator is the most important explanatory variable. Throughout the book, the treatment indicator will be denoted by Z. In a two-arm trial, $Z = 1$ for the treatment group and $Z = 0$ for the control group.

Here we focus on regression models with explanatory variables consisting of Z and a vector $\boldsymbol{B}$ of baseline covariates. For brevity, such a model will be referred to as *regression with fixed covariates*. Both Z and $\boldsymbol{B}$ remain constant once the trial starts, in contrast to post-treatment variables such as intermediate outcomes or time-dependent covariates. Further discussions on post-treatment covariates are provided in Chapters Six and Fourteen.

In this section, we discuss parametric regression models. Semiparametric regression models will be covered on Chapters Five through Eight. In an adjusted analysis with age, the conditional distribution of T given (Z, age) is of interest. This conditional distribution may be a function of a parametric linear combination $\theta_1 Z + \theta_2 age$. Sometimes higher order terms may be included. For example, a model may assume that the conditional distribution given Z and age is $\theta_1 Z + \theta_2 age + \theta_3 age^2$.

Let a^{T} be the transpose of a vector a. For a regression model with fixed covariates, the vector of explanatory variables will be denoted by $\boldsymbol{W}$, also referred to as a covariate vector for brevity. $\boldsymbol{W}$ may be Z, or $(Z, \boldsymbol{B})^{\mathrm{T}}$ with $\boldsymbol{B}$ being the collection of baseline covariates. $\boldsymbol{W}$ may also include higher order terms built from $(Z, \boldsymbol{B})^{\mathrm{T}}$. In the example where the conditional distribution involves age and age^2, note that the conditional distribution of T given $\boldsymbol{W} = (Z, age, age^2)^{\mathrm{T}}$ is the same as the conditional distribution of T given (Z, age) since age completely determines age^2.

To extend parametric models in the previous section to the regression setting, let $f(t; \boldsymbol{w})$, $S(t; \boldsymbol{w})$ be the conditional PDF and survival function of T given $\boldsymbol{W} = \boldsymbol{w}$, respectively. The conditional hazard function is

$$\lambda(t; \boldsymbol{w}) = \lim_{h \downarrow 0} P(t \le T < t + h \big| T \ge t, \boldsymbol{W} = \boldsymbol{w}) / h. \tag{3.18}$$

Similarly to (2.6) and (2.8),

$$\lambda(t; \boldsymbol{w}) = \frac{f(t; \boldsymbol{w})}{S(t; \boldsymbol{w})}, \quad S(t; \boldsymbol{w}) = \exp\big[-\int_0^t \lambda(s; \boldsymbol{w}) ds \big]. \tag{3.19}$$

The regression models can be described by either the PDF or the hazard function.

Suppose that $\boldsymbol{W}$ is a p- dimensional vector with components $W_1, \ldots, W_p$, $p \ge 1$. To simplify the presentation, notation such as $\lambda(t; \boldsymbol{W}) = \boldsymbol{\beta}^{\mathrm{T}} \boldsymbol{W}$, with a p- dimensional parameter $\boldsymbol{\beta} = (\beta_1, \ldots, \beta_p)^{\mathrm{T}}$, will be used which means that the conditional hazard function of T given $\boldsymbol{W} = \boldsymbol{w}$ is $\boldsymbol{\beta}^{\mathrm{T}} \boldsymbol{w}$.

3.2.1 Exponential Regression

The exponential regression model specifies that

$$\lambda(t; \boldsymbol{W}) = C_{\boldsymbol{W}}.$$

That is, the hazard function is constant in t but the constant depends on $\boldsymbol{W}$. For example, with $\boldsymbol{W}$ having two components $W_1 = Z$ and $W_2 = age - 50$, one could specify that

$$\lambda(t; \boldsymbol{W}) = \eta(1 + \beta_1 W_1 + \beta_2 W_2) \tag{3.20}$$

or

$$\lambda(t; \boldsymbol{W}) = \eta \exp(\beta_1 W_1 + \beta_2 W_2), \tag{3.21}$$

where η $(> 0), \beta_1, \beta_2$ are unknown parameters. Model (3.21) is more natural, as the expression on the right-hand side is always positive. However, depending on particular circumstances, other forms may be used.

Under model (3.21),

$$\frac{\lambda(t; \boldsymbol{W})\big|_{\boldsymbol{W}=(1, W_2)^{\mathrm{T}}}}{\lambda(t; \boldsymbol{W})\big|_{\boldsymbol{W}=(0, W_2)^{\mathrm{T}}}} = \exp(\beta_1).$$

That is, for two participants with the same age, one in the treatment arm and one in the control arm, their hazards differ by a multiple of $\exp(\beta_1)$. Therefore, β_1 is the log hazard ratio for the treatment versus control comparison, holding age fixed.

Since

$$\frac{\lambda(t;\boldsymbol{W})\big|_{\boldsymbol{W}=(W_1,\widetilde{W}_2)^{\mathrm{T}}}}{\lambda(t;\boldsymbol{W})\big|_{\boldsymbol{W}=(W_1,W_2)^{\mathrm{T}}}} = \exp\left[\beta_2(\widetilde{W}_2 - W_2)\right],$$

it follows that β_2 is the log hazard ratio for two participants who are in the same arm and whose ages differ by 1. Finally the parameter η is the hazard of a participant in the control group whose age is 50.

Reparametrizing with $\beta_3 = \log\eta$, model (3.21) can be written

$$\lambda(t;\boldsymbol{W}) = \exp(\boldsymbol{\beta}^{\mathrm{T}}\boldsymbol{W}), \tag{3.22}$$

with a new covariate $\boldsymbol{W} = (Z, age - 50, 1)^{\mathrm{T}}$ and new parameter $\boldsymbol{\beta} = (\beta_1, \beta_2, \beta_3)^{\mathrm{T}}$, both being 3-dimensional vectors.

In terms of the log survival time $Y = \ln T$, model (3.22) can be written

$$Y = -\boldsymbol{\beta}^{\mathrm{T}}\widetilde{\boldsymbol{W}} + Y_0, \tag{3.23}$$

where Y_0 has the extreme value distribution with PDF in (3.5). Thus model (3.22) is a log-linear model, *i.e.*, Y obeys a linear model with a specific error distribution.

3.2.2 Weibull Regression

Similarly to (3.21), the Weibull distribution can be generalized to the regression setting. In the example with $\boldsymbol{W} = (W_1, W_2)^{\mathrm{T}}$ where $W_1 = Z$ and $W_2 = age - 50$, the Weibull regression model specifies the conditional hazard function to be

$$\lambda(t;\boldsymbol{W}) = \nu\eta^{\nu} t^{\nu-1}\exp(\beta_1 W_1 + \beta_2 W_2) \tag{3.24}$$

The corresponding cumulative hazard function is

$$\Lambda(t;\boldsymbol{W}) = \left[\eta\exp(\boldsymbol{\beta}^{\mathrm{T}}\boldsymbol{W}/\nu)t\right]^{\nu}. \tag{3.25}$$

where $\boldsymbol{\beta} = (\beta_1, \beta_2)^{\mathrm{T}}$.

Similarly to the reparametrization in (3.22), model (3.25) can be written

$$\Lambda(t;\widetilde{\boldsymbol{W}}) = \left[\exp(\widetilde{\boldsymbol{\beta}}^{\mathrm{T}}\widetilde{\boldsymbol{W}})t\right]^{\nu} \tag{3.26}$$

where $\widetilde{\boldsymbol{W}} = (\boldsymbol{W}^{\mathrm{T}}, 1)^{\mathrm{T}}$ and $\widetilde{\boldsymbol{\beta}} = \left(\boldsymbol{\beta}^{\mathrm{T}}/\nu, \log\eta\right)^{\mathrm{T}}$. From this, it follows that model (3.26) is a log-linear model, with

$$Y = -\widetilde{\boldsymbol{\beta}}^{\mathrm{T}}\widetilde{W} + \frac{1}{\nu}Y_0 \tag{3.27}$$

where Y_0 has PDF in (3.5).

3.2.3 Parametric Regression

The exponential and Weibull regression models suggest two ways to generalize parametric distributions to regression setting. The first is to specify that effect of $\boldsymbol{W}$ is a multiplicative factor on the hazard function:

$$\lambda(t;\boldsymbol{W}) = \lambda_0(t)\exp(\boldsymbol{\beta}^{\mathrm{T}}\boldsymbol{W}) \tag{3.28}$$

where $\lambda_0(t)$ is a parametric baseline hazard function. For exponential regression, $\lambda_0(t) = \eta$ as illustrated by (3.21). For Weibull regression, $\lambda_0(t) = \nu\eta^{\nu}t^{\nu-1}$, as illustrated by (3.24). Models of the form (3.28) with $\lambda_0(t)$ a known parametric hazard function will be referred to as parametric multiplicative hazards models.

The second way to obtain a regression model is to specify that the effect of $\boldsymbol{W}$ is an additive term in the expression for Y:

$$Y = \boldsymbol{\beta}^{\mathrm{T}}\boldsymbol{W} + Y_0 \tag{3.29}$$

where Y_0 is independent of $\boldsymbol{W}$ and has a parametric distribution. This is illustrated by (3.23) and (3.27), for exponential regression and Weibull regression, respectively. Models of the form (3.29) are called parametric log-linear or accelerate failure time models.

Exponential and Weibull regression models are both multiplicative hazards models and log-linear models. It can be shown that they are the only models having this property.

To accommodate heterogeneity in data, stratified versions can be considered. Suppose data are partitioned into J strata or mutually exclusive subsets according to participants' characteristics. Examples include partitioning by sex, age, or a combination of both. Then the stratified multiplicative hazards model specifies that within stratum j, $1 \le j \le J$, the conditional hazard function is

$$\lambda_j(t;\boldsymbol{W}) = \lambda_{0j}(t)\exp(\boldsymbol{\beta}^{\mathrm{T}}\boldsymbol{W}), \tag{3.30}$$

where $\lambda_{0j}(t)$ is the baseline hazard for the jth stratum. It follows that for two participants in the jth stratum with covariates $\widetilde{\boldsymbol{W}}$ and $\boldsymbol{W}$, respectively, ratio of the conditional hazard functions is

$$\frac{\lambda_j(t;\widetilde{\boldsymbol{W}})}{\lambda_j(t;\boldsymbol{W})} = \exp\left[\boldsymbol{\beta}^{\mathrm{T}}(\widetilde{\boldsymbol{W}} - \boldsymbol{W})\right],$$

which depends on $\widetilde{\boldsymbol{W}} - \boldsymbol{W}$, but neither on time t nor the stratum j. However, if two participants are in different strata, then the baseline hazard functions do not cancel and ratio of the conditional hazard functions is much more complicated and depends on t, $\widetilde{\boldsymbol{W}}$ and $\boldsymbol{W}$.

Similarly, stratified log-linear models can also be considered. For the jth stratum,

$$Y = \boldsymbol{\beta}^{\mathrm{T}} \boldsymbol{W} + Y_{0j} \tag{3.31}$$

where Y_{0j} has a parametric distribution depending on j.

In addition to the multiplicative hazards and log-linear models, other parametric regression models are possible. Some related semi-parametric versions are discussed in Chapters Seven and Eight.

3.3 Exercises and Complements

3.1 (a) Obtain the CDF of $Y = \log T$, where T has an exponential distribution.

(b) Verify that the PDF of Y is given by (3.2).

3.2 (a) Suppose that T has the survival function

$$P(T > t) = S_0\big((\eta t)^{\nu})\big),$$

where S_0 is a survival function. Show that $Y = \log T$ has the survival function

$$P(Y > x) = \widetilde{S}_0\big((x-a)/b\big),$$

where $\widetilde{S}_0(x) = S_0(e^x)$ and

$$a = -\log\eta, \; b = 1/\nu.$$

(b) Obtain the survival function and PDF of $Y = \log T$ where T has the Weibull distribution.

3.3 For the hazard function $\lambda(t)$ of the log-normal distribution, show that

$$\lim_{t\downarrow 0} \lambda(t) = 0, \qquad \lim_{t\to\infty} \lambda(t) = 0.$$

3.4 Suppose T has the gamma distribution.

(a) Verify (3.8).

(b) Use the formula

$$ET^n = (-1)^n \frac{d^n}{ds^n} Ee^{-sT}\big|_{s=0}$$

to obtain the mean and variance of the Gamma distribution.

(c) Verify that the Laplace transform $E\exp(-sT)$ is given by (3.9).

3.5 (a) Obtain the Laplace transform $E\exp(-sT)$ for an experiential random variable T with survival function $S(t) = \exp(-\beta t)$.

(b) Obtain the Laplace transform $E\exp(-sT)$ for $T = T_1 + \cdots + T_m$, where T_j's are independent random variables with survival function $S(t) = \exp(-\beta t)$.

(c) Show that T in (b) above has the Gamma distribution with shape parameter m and rate parameter β.

3.6 For the log-Logistic distribution, verify that

(a) the PDF in (3.10) is symmetric;

(b) the PDF, survival, hazard, and cumulative hazard functions are given by (3.11) and (3.12).

3.7 For the Makeham distribution, obtain the cumulative hazard and survival functions.

3.8 (a) For $F_0(t) = t/(1+t)$, derive the hazard, cumulative hazard, and survival functions for $\lambda(t)$ in (3.13). Then obtain the PDF. In particular, show that the survival function is $S(t) = e^{-\beta t}(1+t)^{\beta-\alpha}$.

(b) For $F_0(t) = 1 - \exp(-t)$, derive the hazard, cumulative hazard, and survival functions for $\lambda(t)$ in (3.13). Then obtain the PDF.

3.9 Suppose that T_1 and T_2 are independent random variables following exponential distributions with parameters η_1 and η_2, respectively.

(a) Obtain the PDF, survival, and hazard functions of $\min(T_1, T_2)$.

(b) Obtain the PDF, survival, and hazard functions of $\max(T_1, T_2)$.

3.10 Suppose that T_1 and T_2 are independent random variables following Weibull distributions with parameters (η_1, ν_1) and (η_2, ν_2), respectively.

(a) Obtain the PDF, survival, and hazard functions of $\min(T_1, T_2)$.

(b) Obtain the PDF, survival, and hazard functions of $\max(T_1, T_2)$.

3.11 Suppose that T is a discrete random variable following the geometric distribution, with probability mass function

$$f(k) = p(1-p)^{k-1}, \quad k \geq 1,$$

for some $p \in (0,1)$. Obtain the survival and hazard functions of T.

3.12 Suppose T has the log-logistic distribution with survival function

$$S(t) = \frac{1}{1 + (\alpha t)^\beta}.$$

Derive $f^\#$, $S^\#$ and $\lambda^\#$ for the discrete variable $T^\#$ obtained from T through grouping.

3.13 Suppose T has the parametric hazard function in (3.13), with $F_0(t) = t/(1+t)$. Derive $f^{\#}$, $S^{\#}$ and $\lambda^{\#}$ for the discrete variable $T^{\#}$ obtained from T through grouping.

3.14 Suppose T has the exponential distribution with survival function

$$S(t) = \exp(-\beta t),$$

and the partition of the time axis is

$$[0,\infty) = [0,1) \cup [1,2) \cup \cdots.$$

Derive $f^{\#}$, $S^{\#}$ and $\lambda^{\#}$ for the discrete variable $T^{\#}$ obtained from T through grouping. Show that the distribution of $T^{\#}$ is the geometric distribution.

3.15 Suppose T has the survival function

$$S(t) = \exp[-\beta(t-A)], \quad t \geq A$$

where A, $\beta > 0$. Obtain the PDF, the hazard and the cumulative hazard functions.

3.16 Suppose T has the hazard function

$$\lambda(t) = \begin{cases} \theta_1, & \text{if } t < a \\ \theta_2, & \text{if } t \geq a \end{cases}$$

where a, θ_1, $\theta_2 > 0$. Obtain the PDF, the survival and the cumulative hazard functions.

3.17 Suppose T has the hazard function

$$\lambda(t) = \begin{cases} \theta t/a, & \text{if } t < a \\ \theta, & \text{if } t \geq a \end{cases}$$

where a, $\theta > 0$. Obtain the PDF, the survival and the cumulative hazard functions.

4

Large-Sample Theory for Inference in Parametric Models

As mentioned previously, censoring is often encountered in dealing with survival data. Even when the censoring mechanism is simple, closed-form expressions for parameter estimators and exact distributions of the estimators are usually difficult to obtain. Thus asymptotic theory for estimation and testing plays a vital role. This chapter is devoted to applications of the asymptotic theory to statistical inference under parametric models with survival data.

While semiparametric inference based on partial likelihood under the Cox model, to be discussed in Chapter Five, is more commonly used, maximum likelihood estimation theory remains a foundational pillar in statistics. Familiarity with it also provides a clearer theoretical basis for understanding partial likelihood inference theory. Some of the procedures will be illustrated with data from a recent large clinical trial. Robust estimation is also briefly covered.

4.1 Large-Sample Theory for Likelihood Inference

4.1.1 Maximum Likelihood Estimation and Large-Sample Theory

Consider the *random censorship model with fixed covariates,* in which observed data from n individuals are $(X_i, \delta_i, \boldsymbol{W}_i)$, where $X_i = T_i \wedge C_i$ and $\delta_i = I(X_i = T_i)$, with T_i, C_i, $\boldsymbol{W}_i$ being, respectively, the time to event, time to censoring, and a $p \times 1$ vector built from baseline explanatory variables for the ith participant, $p \geq 1$, $i = 1, \cdots, n$. The pairs $(T_i, \boldsymbol{W}_i)$, $i = 1, \cdots, n$ are i.i.d. and the triplets $(T_i, \boldsymbol{W}_i, C_i)$, $i = 1, \cdots, n$ are independent, and, given $\boldsymbol{W}_i$, T_i and C_i are independent, $i = 1, \cdots, n$.

In the development below, we will focus on the absolutely continuous case. The theory for the discrete case is similar with proper modifications. Furthermore, since large-sample theory for the random censorship model without explanatory variables (as considered in Section 3.1) is similar, it will be omitted as well. A convenient way is to think of the case without explanatory variables as the special case when the covariate is identically 0 and the coefficient is 0, thus formulas for

DOI: 10.1201/9780429324437-4

the case without explanatory variables are obtained by simply dropping all the terms involving covariates in the corresponding formulas given in this section.

To use parametric models for inference, first the parameter needs to be estimated. Let $f(t;\boldsymbol{\theta},\boldsymbol{w}_i)$, $S(t;\boldsymbol{\theta},\boldsymbol{w}_i)$ and $\lambda(t;\boldsymbol{\theta},\boldsymbol{w}_i)$ be the conditional PDF, survival and hazard functions of T_i given $\boldsymbol{W}_i=\boldsymbol{w}_i$, respectively. Similar to (2.25) in Chapter Two, by the conditional independence of T_i and C_i given $\boldsymbol{W}_i$, the likelihood of data conditional on $\boldsymbol{W}_1,\cdots,\boldsymbol{W}_n$, is

$$L(\boldsymbol{\theta})=\prod_{i=1}^{n}L_i(\boldsymbol{\theta})$$

where

$$L_i(\boldsymbol{\theta})=f(X_i;\boldsymbol{\theta},\boldsymbol{W}_i)^{\delta_i}S(X_i;\boldsymbol{\theta},\boldsymbol{W}_i)^{1-\delta_i}.$$

For the random censorship model considered here, with

$$\begin{aligned}
\lambda(t;\boldsymbol{\theta},\boldsymbol{W}_i) &= f(t;\boldsymbol{\theta},\boldsymbol{W}_i)/S(t;\boldsymbol{\theta},\boldsymbol{W}_i),\\
\Lambda(t;\boldsymbol{\theta},\boldsymbol{W}_i) &= \int_0^t \lambda(u;\boldsymbol{\theta},\boldsymbol{W}_i)du,\\
S(t;\boldsymbol{\theta},\boldsymbol{W}_i) &= \exp\big[-\Lambda(t;\boldsymbol{\theta},\boldsymbol{W}_i)\big],
\end{aligned}$$

it can be shown that

$$\begin{aligned}
L(\boldsymbol{\theta}) &= \prod_{i=1}^{n}\Big\{\lambda(X_i;\boldsymbol{\theta},\boldsymbol{W}_i)^{\delta_i}\exp\big[-\Lambda(X_i;\boldsymbol{\theta},\boldsymbol{W}_i)\big]\Big\}\\
&= \Big[\prod_{i=1}^{n}\lambda(X_i;\boldsymbol{\theta},\boldsymbol{W}_i)^{\delta_i}\Big]\exp\Big[-\int_0^\infty\sum_{i=1}^{n}I(X_i\ge u)\lambda(u;\boldsymbol{\theta},\boldsymbol{W}_i)du\Big]\\
&= \Big[\prod_{i=1}^{n}\lambda(X_i;\boldsymbol{\theta},\boldsymbol{W}_i)^{\delta_i}\Big]\exp\Big[-\int_0^\infty\sum_{i\in R(u)}\lambda(u;\boldsymbol{\theta},\boldsymbol{W}_i)du\Big] \qquad (4.1)
\end{aligned}$$

where $R(u)=\{i: X_i\ge u\}$ is called the *risk set* at u. It is the set of individuals at risk at time u, i.e., neither event nor censoring has occurred before u. A *maximum likelihood estimate* (MLE) $\widehat{\boldsymbol{\theta}}$ is a maximizer of $L(\boldsymbol{\theta})$ over the parameter space.

When there is no censoring, under certain regularity conditions, typically $\widehat{\boldsymbol{\theta}}$ exists asymptotically and has good properties such as consistency, asymptotic normality and efficiency for having asymptotic variance achieving the Cramér-Rao lower bound [55, 257]. A summary of asymptotic likelihood theory can be found in many books, including Cox and Hinkley [53] and Hogg, McKean and Craig [114]. A review on the history of maximum likelihood theory is given by Stigler [289]. Although the i.i.d. setup is typically used in the asymptotic likelihood theory, extensions to independent but not identically distributions observations are also available [231, 167].

In the setting here with right censored data, analogous results can also be obtained. Let $\boldsymbol{U}_i(\boldsymbol{\theta})$ be the score vector for the ith individual:

$$\boldsymbol{U}_i(\boldsymbol{\theta}) = \frac{\partial}{\partial \boldsymbol{\theta}} \log L_i(\boldsymbol{\theta}).$$

Under the regularity conditions that the true parameter value $\boldsymbol{\theta}_0$ is in the interior of the parameter space and that $L(\boldsymbol{\theta})$ is sufficiently smooth with proper boundedness conditions, the order of expectation and differentiation can be interchanged. Therefore, $\boldsymbol{U}_i(\boldsymbol{\theta}_0)$ has expectation 0 and $p \times p$ covariance matrix

$$E[\boldsymbol{U}_i(\boldsymbol{\theta}_0)\boldsymbol{U}_i^{\mathrm{T}}(\boldsymbol{\theta}_0)] = \mathscr{I}_i(\boldsymbol{\theta}_0), \tag{4.2}$$

where

$$\mathscr{I}_i(\boldsymbol{\theta}) = -\left(E\frac{\partial^2 \log L_i}{\partial \theta_j \partial \theta_\ell}\right)_{p\times p},$$

the negative of expectation of the Jacobian matrix of $\boldsymbol{U}_i(\boldsymbol{\theta})$. Verification of (4.2) when there is no censoring is left to Exercise 4.1.

Although regularity conditions for (4.2) are flexible enough to have a wide range of applications, they fail to hold for parameters defining the support set of a distribution, such as threshold and range parameters. Exercise 4.2 describes a case where the asymptotic theory is different from what is presented here.

Define the score function $\boldsymbol{U}(\boldsymbol{\theta})$ and the Fisher information matrix $\mathscr{I}(\boldsymbol{\theta})$ by

$$\boldsymbol{U}(\boldsymbol{\theta}) = \sum_{i=1}^{n} \boldsymbol{U}_i(\boldsymbol{\theta}), \quad \mathscr{I}(\boldsymbol{\theta}) = \sum_{i=1}^{n} \mathscr{I}_i(\boldsymbol{\theta}). \tag{4.3}$$

Since $\boldsymbol{U}(\boldsymbol{\theta})$ is a sum of independent random vectors, by the central limit theorem, under certain regularity conditions, at the true parameter value $\boldsymbol{\theta}_0$, $\mathscr{I}(\boldsymbol{\theta}_0)/n$ converges in probability to a positive definite matrix $\mathbf{V}(\boldsymbol{\theta}_0)$, and

$$n^{-1/2}\boldsymbol{U}(\boldsymbol{\theta}_0) \xrightarrow{d} N\big(0, \mathbf{V}(\boldsymbol{\theta}_0)\big), \tag{4.4}$$

where $N(\mu, \boldsymbol{B})$ denotes the normal distribution with mean μ and covariance matrix $\boldsymbol{B}$.

To simplify the presentation, some notations will be introduced. For a sequence of $p \times 1$ random vectors X_n, suppose

$$a_n^{-1}(X_n - \mu) \xrightarrow{d} N\big(0_p, \Sigma\big),$$

where μ is a $p \times 1$ vector, a_n is a scaling constant, 0_p is the $p \times 1$ zero vector and Σ is a $p \times p$ covariance matrix. For brevity, X_n is said to be asymptotically normal with mean μ and covariance matrix $a_n^2\Sigma$. Such property will also be denoted by

$$X_n \sim N(\mu,\ a_n^2\Sigma).$$

Furthermore, if $\widehat{\Sigma}$ is a consistent estimator of Σ, the convergence result will also be denoted by

$$X_n \sim N(\mu,\ a_n^2\widehat{\Sigma}).$$

Using these notations, we have

$$\boldsymbol{U}(\boldsymbol{\theta}_0) \sim N\big(0,\ \mathscr{I}(\boldsymbol{\theta}_0)\big). \tag{4.5}$$

To use the asymptotic normality of $\boldsymbol{U}(\boldsymbol{\theta}_0)$ for inference, often further approximations are needed. This is because $\mathscr{I}(\boldsymbol{\theta})$ is an expectation which involves the censoring distributions. Denote the observed information matrix by

$$\mathbb{I}(\boldsymbol{\theta}) = -\sum_{i=1}^{n}\left(\frac{\partial^2 \log L_i}{\partial\theta_j\partial\theta_\ell}\right)_{p\times p}.$$

Then

$$\boldsymbol{U}(\boldsymbol{\theta}_0) \sim N\big(0,\ \mathbb{I}(\boldsymbol{\theta}_0)\big).$$

The asymptotic normality remains valid if $\mathbb{I}(\boldsymbol{\theta}_0)$ is replaced by $\mathbb{I}(\widehat{\boldsymbol{\theta}})$. Note that $\mathbb{I}(\boldsymbol{\theta})$ depends only on $\boldsymbol{\theta}$ and the observed data.

For the asymptotic distribution of $\widehat{\boldsymbol{\theta}}$, by the mean value theorem and smoothness of $\mathscr{I}(\boldsymbol{\theta})$,

$$-\boldsymbol{U}(\boldsymbol{\theta}_0) = \boldsymbol{U}(\widehat{\boldsymbol{\theta}}) - \boldsymbol{U}(\boldsymbol{\theta}_0) \approx \mathscr{I}(\boldsymbol{\theta}_0)(\widehat{\boldsymbol{\theta}} - \boldsymbol{\theta}_0).$$

Thus if $\mathscr{I}(\boldsymbol{\theta})$ has inverse $\mathscr{I}^{-1}(\boldsymbol{\theta})$, then

$$\widehat{\boldsymbol{\theta}} - \boldsymbol{\theta}_0 \approx -\mathscr{I}^{-1}(\boldsymbol{\theta}_0)\boldsymbol{U}(\boldsymbol{\theta}_0).$$

It follows that

$$\widehat{\boldsymbol{\theta}} \sim N\big(\boldsymbol{\theta}_0,\ \mathscr{I}^{-1}(\boldsymbol{\theta}_0)\big). \tag{4.6}$$

That is, $n^{1/2}(\widehat{\boldsymbol{\theta}} - \boldsymbol{\theta}_0)$ converges in distribution to the normal distribution with mean 0 and covariance $\lim_n\big(n\mathscr{I}^{-1}(\boldsymbol{\theta}_0)\big)$. Similar to the case for $\boldsymbol{U}(\boldsymbol{\theta})$, $\mathscr{I}^{-1}(\boldsymbol{\theta}_0)$ in (4.6) can be replaced by $\mathbb{I}^{-1}(\boldsymbol{\theta}_0)$ or $\mathbb{I}^{-1}(\widehat{\boldsymbol{\theta}})$.

The above asymptotic results can be rigorously justified using modern statistical theory. Andersen et al. provides a rigorous statement of sufficient conditions and proofs of the asymptotic results in a counting process formulation [7, Section VI.1], as well as applications of the results to parametric regression models [7, Section VII.6]. Rigorous asymptotic analysis can also be obtained using empirical process theory [310, 139]. An overview of the counting process and martingale theory is given in Appendix B, while an overview of the empirical process theory is presented in Appendix C.

In addition to $\boldsymbol{U}(\boldsymbol{\theta})$ and $\widehat{\boldsymbol{\theta}}$, the likelihood ratio, defined by

$$R(\boldsymbol{\theta}) = \frac{L(\widehat{\boldsymbol{\theta}})}{L(\boldsymbol{\theta})}, \tag{4.7}$$

can also be used for parameter inference. Under the regularity conditions for the maximum likelihood theory, the asymptotic distribution of $2\log R(\boldsymbol{\theta}_0)$ is χ^2_p, the χ^2 distribution with p degrees of freedom.

4.1.2 Hypothesis Testing

To test the hypothesis that the parameter is a specific known vector $\boldsymbol{\theta}_0$, consider $H_0 : \boldsymbol{\theta} = \boldsymbol{\theta}_0$. Traditionally, three approaches can be taken. Under H_0,

$$\boldsymbol{U}^{\mathrm{T}}(\boldsymbol{\theta}_0)\mathscr{I}^{-1}(\boldsymbol{\theta}_0)\boldsymbol{U}(\boldsymbol{\theta}_0)$$

has an asymptotic χ^2_p distribution. This yields a version of the score test that rejects H_0 if

$$\boldsymbol{U}^{\mathrm{T}}(\boldsymbol{\theta}_0)\mathscr{I}^{-1}(\boldsymbol{\theta}_0)\boldsymbol{U}(\boldsymbol{\theta}_0) > \chi^2_p(\alpha),$$

where$\chi^2_p(\alpha)$ is the upper αth percentile of χ^2_p. This test is asymptotically correct at significance level α. In applications, $\mathscr{I}(\boldsymbol{\theta}_0)$ is usually approximated by $\mathbb{I}(\boldsymbol{\theta}_0)$. This results in the version of the score test that rejects H_0 if

$$\boldsymbol{U}^{\mathrm{T}}(\boldsymbol{\theta}_0)\mathbb{I}^{-1}(\boldsymbol{\theta}_0)\boldsymbol{U}(\boldsymbol{\theta}_0) > \chi^2_p(\alpha), \tag{4.8}$$

Since $\mathscr{I}(\boldsymbol{\theta}_0)$ depends on the assumed censoring distributions while $\mathbb{I}(\boldsymbol{\theta}_0)$ does not, the simpler score test using $\mathbb{I}(\boldsymbol{\theta}_0)$ may also be more robust. Note that $\widehat{\boldsymbol{\theta}}$ is not needed for the test in (4.8).

Alternatively, the Wald test is based on the asymptotic normality of $\widehat{\boldsymbol{\theta}}$. The hypothesis H_0 is rejected if

$$(\widehat{\boldsymbol{\theta}} - \boldsymbol{\theta}_0)^{\mathrm{T}}\mathbb{I}(\widehat{\boldsymbol{\theta}})(\widehat{\boldsymbol{\theta}} - \boldsymbol{\theta}_0) > \chi^2_p. \tag{4.9}$$

The third option is the likelihood ratio test which rejects H_0 if

$$2\log R(\boldsymbol{\theta}_0) > \chi^2_p(\alpha).$$

This test is often considered as the gold standard. For small samples, It is typically more accurate than other options.

Asymptotically, the MLE-based score test, Wald test, and likelihood ratio test are equivalent. However, The likelihood ratio test has the advantage that it is invariant under a one-to-one reparametrization. This property ensures consistency across different parameter scales. The likelihood ratio test is generally preferred for its invariance properties and robustness across sample sizes.

In simple models and with large clinical trials, the likelihood ratio, score and Wald tests typically yield very similar results for both hypothesis testing and confidence regions. However, differences emerge in more complex scenarios or with smaller sample sizes. For inference procedures based on the score test or Wald test, if necessary and feasible, it is useful to consider a parameter transformation that stabilizes the variance of the transformed parameter estimator.

Between the score test and the Wald test, the former often demonstrates greater stability and robustness when there is limited information on part of the parameter vector. This is because changes in that part of the parameter vector only result in small changes in the score function, but may lead to relatively larger changes in the Wald statistic.

Sometimes only part of the parameter is of interest. Suppose $\boldsymbol{\theta}$ consists of $\boldsymbol{\theta}_1$ and $\boldsymbol{\theta}_2$, which are q and $p-q$ dimensional vectors, respectively ($1 \le q < p$). Correspondingly, decompose $\widehat{\boldsymbol{\theta}}$ as $\widehat{\boldsymbol{\theta}} = (\widehat{\boldsymbol{\theta}}_1, \widehat{\boldsymbol{\theta}}_2)$, and $\mathbb{I}^{-1}(\boldsymbol{\theta})$ as

$$\mathbb{I}^{-1}(\boldsymbol{\theta}) = \begin{pmatrix} \mathbb{I}^{11}(\boldsymbol{\theta}) & \mathbb{I}^{12}(\boldsymbol{\theta}) \\ \mathbb{I}^{21}(\boldsymbol{\theta}) & \mathbb{I}^{22}(\boldsymbol{\theta}) \end{pmatrix},$$

where $\mathbb{I}^{11}(\boldsymbol{\theta})$ has dimension $q \times q$. Then $(\widehat{\boldsymbol{\theta}}_1 - \boldsymbol{\theta}_{01})^{\mathrm{T}}\big(\mathbb{I}^{11}(\boldsymbol{\theta}_0)\big)^{-1}(\widehat{\boldsymbol{\theta}}_1 - \boldsymbol{\theta}_{01})$ has an asymptotic χ^2_q distribution under the hypothesis $H_{01} : \boldsymbol{\theta}_1 = \boldsymbol{\theta}_{01}$. Thus an asymptotically level α test rejects H_{01} if

$$(\widehat{\boldsymbol{\theta}}_1 - \boldsymbol{\theta}_{01})^{\mathrm{T}}[\mathbb{I}^{11}(\widehat{\boldsymbol{\theta}})]^{-1}(\widehat{\boldsymbol{\theta}}_1 - \boldsymbol{\theta}_{01}) > \chi^2_q(\alpha). \tag{4.10}$$

The likelihood ratio statistic can also be used to test H_{01}. Split $\boldsymbol{U}(\boldsymbol{\theta})$ into two parts $\boldsymbol{U}^{(1)}(\boldsymbol{\theta})$ and $\boldsymbol{U}^{(2)}(\boldsymbol{\theta})$, corresponding to $\boldsymbol{\theta}_1$, $\boldsymbol{\theta}_2$, respectively. Let $\widetilde{\boldsymbol{\theta}}_2(\boldsymbol{\theta}_{01})$ be the MLE of $\boldsymbol{\theta}_2$ with $\boldsymbol{\theta}_1$ fixed at $\boldsymbol{\theta}_{01}$. That is, $\widetilde{\boldsymbol{\theta}}_2(\boldsymbol{\theta}_{01})$ is the solution in $\boldsymbol{\theta}_2$ of the equation

$$\boldsymbol{U}^{(2)}(\boldsymbol{\theta}_{01}, \boldsymbol{\theta}_2) = 0.$$

Under H_{01}, $2\log R\Big(\big(\boldsymbol{\theta}_{01}, \widetilde{\boldsymbol{\theta}}_2(\boldsymbol{\theta}_{01})\big)\Big)$ has a limiting χ^2_q distribution. Thus H_{01} is rejected if

$$2\log R\Big(\big(\boldsymbol{\theta}_{01}, \widetilde{\boldsymbol{\theta}}_2(\boldsymbol{\theta}_{01})\big)\Big) > \chi^2_q(\alpha). \tag{4.11}$$

The likelihood ratio test statistic for H_{01} requires numerical root finding twice, once for the MLE $\widehat{\boldsymbol{\theta}}$ without any constraint, and once for the MLE $\widetilde{\boldsymbol{\theta}}_2(\boldsymbol{\theta}_{01})$ under the constraint $\boldsymbol{\theta}_1 = \boldsymbol{\theta}_{01}$.

To use the score function $\boldsymbol{U}(\boldsymbol{\theta})$ for testing H_{01}, Let $\widetilde{\boldsymbol{U}}^{(1)}(\boldsymbol{\theta}_{01}) = \boldsymbol{U}^{(1)}\Big(\big(\boldsymbol{\theta}_{01}, \widetilde{\boldsymbol{\theta}}_2(\boldsymbol{\theta}_{01})\big)\Big)$ and $\widetilde{\mathbb{I}}^{11}(\boldsymbol{\theta}_{01}) = \mathbb{I}^{11}\Big(\big(\boldsymbol{\theta}_{10}, \widetilde{\boldsymbol{\theta}}_2(\boldsymbol{\theta}_{01})\big)\Big)$. Then the test statistic is

$$\widetilde{\boldsymbol{U}}^{(1)}(\boldsymbol{\theta}_{01})^{\mathrm{T}}\widetilde{\mathbb{I}}^{11}(\boldsymbol{\theta}_{01})\widetilde{\boldsymbol{U}}^{(1)}(\boldsymbol{\theta}_{01}), \tag{4.12}$$

which has a limiting χ^2_q distribution under H_{01}.

Sometimes certain functions of $\boldsymbol{\theta}$, such as linear combinations $l_1,\ldots,l_q$ of components of $\boldsymbol{\theta}$, are of interest. It is possible to reparametrize such that the new parameter is θ^* which has $l_1,\ldots,l_q$ as its first q components. Then the procedures in (4.10) through (4.12) can be applied.

More generally, the delta method can be used. Let

$$\boldsymbol{\xi} = (\xi_1,\ldots,\xi_q)^{\mathrm{T}} \tag{4.13}$$

be a vector function from the p dimensional parameter space to a q dimensional space, $1 \le q \le p$, with continuous first order $q \times p$ partial derivative matrix

$$\boldsymbol{A}(\boldsymbol{\theta}) = \left(\frac{\partial \xi_j}{\partial \theta_\ell}\right)_{q\times p}.$$

Then, at the true parameter $\boldsymbol{\theta}_0$,

$$n^{1/2}[\boldsymbol{\xi}(\widehat{\boldsymbol{\theta}}) - \boldsymbol{\xi}(\boldsymbol{\theta}_0)] \xrightarrow{d} N\big(0, \lim_n n\mathbf{V}(\boldsymbol{\theta}_0)\big) \tag{4.14}$$

where $\mathbf{V}(\boldsymbol{\theta}) = \boldsymbol{A}(\boldsymbol{\theta})\mathscr{I}^{-1}(\boldsymbol{\theta})\boldsymbol{A}(\boldsymbol{\theta})^{\mathrm{T}}$. Now a test of $H_{\xi_0} : \boldsymbol{\xi} = \boldsymbol{\xi}_0$ is to reject H_{ξ_0} if

$$\big[\boldsymbol{\xi}(\widehat{\boldsymbol{\theta}}) - \boldsymbol{\xi}_0\big]^{\mathrm{T}} \widehat{\mathbf{V}}^{-1} \big[\boldsymbol{\xi}(\widehat{\boldsymbol{\theta}}) - \boldsymbol{\xi}_0\big] > \chi^2_k, \tag{4.15}$$

where $\widehat{\mathbf{V}} = \boldsymbol{A}(\widehat{\boldsymbol{\theta}})\mathbb{I}^{-1}(\widehat{\boldsymbol{\theta}})\boldsymbol{A}(\widehat{\boldsymbol{\theta}})^{\mathrm{T}}$.

4.1.3 Confidence Regions and Intervals

Confidence regions of $\boldsymbol{\theta}$ can be obtained by inverting the score test or likelihood test. This is known as the test inversion method. Using the score function, an asymptotic $100(1-\alpha)\%$ confidence region for the true parameter $\boldsymbol{\theta}_0$ is

$$\left\{\boldsymbol{\theta} : \boldsymbol{U}^{\mathrm{T}}(\boldsymbol{\theta})\mathscr{I}^{-1}(\boldsymbol{\theta})\boldsymbol{U}(\boldsymbol{\theta}) \le \chi^2_p(\alpha)\right\}, \tag{4.16}$$

With $\mathscr{I}$ and $\boldsymbol{\theta}$ replaced by their estimators, we also have the confidence region

$$\left\{\boldsymbol{\theta} : \boldsymbol{U}^{\mathrm{T}}(\boldsymbol{\theta})\mathbb{I}^{-1}(\boldsymbol{\theta})\boldsymbol{U}(\boldsymbol{\theta}) \le \chi^2_p(\alpha)\right\} \tag{4.17}$$

or

$$\left\{\boldsymbol{\theta} : \boldsymbol{U}^{\mathrm{T}}(\boldsymbol{\theta})\mathbb{I}^{-1}(\widehat{\boldsymbol{\theta}})\boldsymbol{U}(\boldsymbol{\theta}) \le \chi^2_p(\alpha)\right\}. \tag{4.18}$$

Corresponding to the likelihood ratio statistic, we have the confidence region

$$\left\{\boldsymbol{\theta} : 2\log R(\boldsymbol{\theta}) \le \chi^2_p(\alpha)\right\}, \tag{4.19}$$

The MLE $\widehat{\boldsymbol{\theta}}$ yields the confidence region

$$\left\{\boldsymbol{\theta} : (\widehat{\boldsymbol{\theta}} - \boldsymbol{\theta})^{\mathrm{T}}\mathbb{I}(\widehat{\boldsymbol{\theta}})(\widehat{\boldsymbol{\theta}} - \boldsymbol{\theta}) \le \chi^2_p\right\}. \tag{4.20}$$

This is the simplest and most often used form of the confidence region, a p dimensional ellipsoid. Other confidence regions are not guaranteed to be convex or even connected.

For $\boldsymbol{\xi}$ in (4.13), the confidence region is

$$\left\{\boldsymbol{\zeta}:\ [\boldsymbol{\zeta}-\boldsymbol{\xi}(\widehat{\boldsymbol{\theta}})]^{\mathrm{T}}\widehat{\mathbf{V}}^{-1}[\boldsymbol{\zeta}-\boldsymbol{\xi}(\widehat{\boldsymbol{\theta}})] \le \chi_q^2\right\}. \tag{4.21}$$

When $p \ge 3$, it is not easy to visualize or display the ellipsoidal confidence regions. Let θ_{0j}, $\widehat{\theta}_j$ be the jth component of $\boldsymbol{\theta}_0$, $\widehat{\boldsymbol{\theta}}$, respectively, and v_j be the jth diagonal element of $\mathbb{I}^{-1}(\widehat{\boldsymbol{\theta}})$, $1 \le j \le p$. Then from (4.14) with $\xi = \theta_j$,

$$\frac{\widehat{\theta}_j - \theta_{0j}}{\sqrt{v_j}} \xrightarrow{d} N(0,1).$$

Thus an asymptotic $100(1-\alpha)\%$ confidence interval for θ_{0j} is

$$\widehat{\theta}_j \mp z(\alpha/2)\sqrt{v_j}. \tag{4.22}$$

Each of the intervals in (4.22) has an asymptotic confidence level $1-\alpha$, but the probability that they simultaneously cover $\theta_1, \cdots, \theta_p$ could be much less that $1-\alpha$. To achieve simultaneous coverage probability $1-\alpha$, let $\boldsymbol{X} = (X_1, \ldots, X_p)^{\mathrm{T}}$ be a p-variate normal random vector with mean 0 and covariance matrix Υ which is the correlation matrix of $\lim_n \left(n\mathscr{I}^{-1}(\boldsymbol{\theta})\right)$ at the true parameter, and $c_\alpha(\Upsilon)$ the critical value such that

$$P\Big(\max_{1\le 1j\le p} |X_j| \le c_\alpha(\Upsilon)\Big) = 1-\alpha. \tag{4.23}$$

Define the intervals

$$[a_j,\ b_j] = \left[\widehat{\theta}_j - c_\alpha(\hat{\Upsilon})\sqrt{v_j},\ \widehat{\theta}_j + c_\alpha(\hat{\Upsilon})\sqrt{v_j}\right], \quad 1 \le j \le p,$$

where $\hat{\Upsilon}$ is the correlation matrix of $n\mathbb{I}^{-1}(\widehat{\boldsymbol{\theta}})$. Then as $n \to \infty$,

$$P\Big(\theta_j \in [a_j, b_j],\ 1 \le j \le p\Big) \to 1-\alpha$$

Therefore $[a_j,\ b_j]$, $1 \le j \le p$, are simultaneous confidence intervals for $\theta_{01}, \ldots, \theta_{0p}$.

To obtain $c_\alpha(\hat{\Upsilon})$, numerical integration is needed. Alternatively, $c_\alpha(\hat{\Upsilon})$ can be approximated by the sample upper αth percentile of $\max_{1\le j\le p}|X_{ij}^*|$ from a sample of $\boldsymbol{X}_i^* = (X_{i1}^*, \ldots, X_{ip}^*)^{\mathrm{T}}$, $i = 1, \ldots, B$, with large B, where $\boldsymbol{X}_i^*$ is defined similarly to $\boldsymbol{X}$, but with $\lim_n \left(n\mathscr{I}^{-1}(\boldsymbol{\theta})\right)$ replaced by $n\mathbb{I}^{-1}(\widehat{\boldsymbol{\theta}})$.

Use of the simultaneous confidence intervals in estimation and testing has been shown to have certain robustness property in different contexts such as combining several tests [342] or analyzing multiple correlated time-to-event outcomes [348, 349].

4.2 Illustrations with the TOPCAT Data

In this section, we illustrate some of the inference procedures with the TOPCAT primary outcome data, starting with fitting the exponential model to the primary endpoint in the control group. The MLE for the exponential distribution is one rare case where the estimator has a closed form and various inference procedures have simple expressions. The hazard and cumulative hazard functions are

$$\lambda(t) = \theta, \qquad \Lambda(t) = \theta t,$$

and the log likelihood function is

$$L(\theta) = \sum_{i=1}^{n} \left[\delta_i \log \lambda(X_i) - \Lambda(X_i)\right] = \sum_{i=1}^{n} \delta_i \log\theta - \theta \sum_{i=1}^{n} X_i.$$

Let

$$S_d = \sum_{i=1}^{n} \delta_i, \; S_x = \sum_{i=1}^{n} X_i.$$

The score function is

$$U(\theta) = \sum_{i=1}^{n} \delta_i/\theta - \sum_{i=1}^{n} X_i = S_d/\theta - S_x,$$

and the observed information is

$$\mathbb{I}(\theta) = \sum_{i=1}^{n} \delta_i/\theta^2 = S_d/\theta^2.$$

Thus the MLE is

$$\hat{\theta} = S_d S_x^{-1} = 0.066,$$

and

$$\hat{\theta} \sim N(\theta_0, \theta^2 S_d^{-1}),$$

where θ_0 is the true parameter value. That is,

$$\sqrt{n}(\hat{\theta} - \theta_0) \xrightarrow{d} N(\theta_0, \lim_n \theta^2 n S_d^{-1}).$$

The limiting variance $\lim_n \theta^2 n S_d^{-1}$ has a factor of θ^2. By the delta method, for $\xi = \ln\theta$, we have

$$\sqrt{n}(\hat{\xi} - \xi_0) \xrightarrow{d} N(\theta_0, \lim_n n S_d^{-1}),$$

where $\xi_0 = \ln\theta_0$ and the limiting variance $\lim_n n S_d^{-1}$ does not involve the parameter anymore.

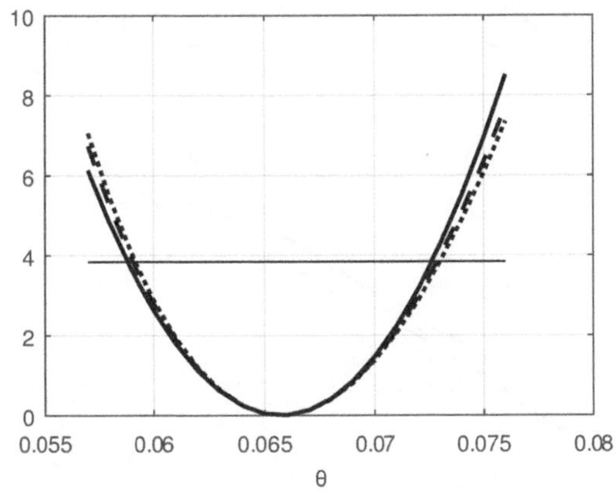

FIGURE 4.1
The interval-producing functions in (4.24) through (4.26). Solid— Wald; dotted—Wald with the log transformation; dashed—likelihood ratio.

With the original parameter θ, the Wald test gives the 95% confidence interval

$$\left\{\theta: \ S_d(\widehat{\theta}-\theta)^2/\widehat{\theta}^2 \leq 3.84\right\}. \tag{4.24}$$

For the new parameter ξ, the Wald test gives the 95% confidence interval

$$\left\{\xi: S_d(\xi-\widehat{\xi})^2 \leq 3.84\right\}$$

That is,

$$\left\{\theta: S_d(\log\theta-\log\widehat{\theta})^2 \leq 3.84\right\} \tag{4.25}$$

The likelihood ratio test gives the 95% confidence interval

$$\left\{\theta: 2\log\frac{L(\widehat{\theta})}{L(\theta)} \leq 3.84\right\} \tag{4.26}$$

Figure 4.1 exhibits the interval-producing functions in (4.24) through (4.26). The horizontal line is at the level 3.84. The log transformation yields a curve hardly distinguishable from that of the likelihood ratio method. The curve of the untransformed Wald method is also very close. When rounding to three decimal places, the three confidence intervals in (4.24) through (4.26) yield the same interval: $(0.059, 0.073)$. Other methods also yield virtually the same results.

Next, for TOPCAT data from the two arms, consider regression models with Z being the only baseline variable. For exponential regression, the hazard and cu-

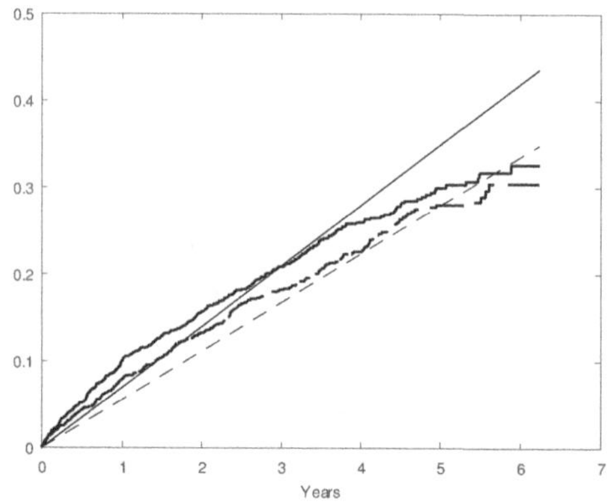

FIGURE 4.2
Estimated CDF for the TOPCAT primary endpoint. Thick solid: control group, Kaplan-Meier; thick dashed: treatment group, Kaplan-Meier; thin solid: control group, exponential; thin dashed: treatment group, exponential.

mulative hazard functions are

$$\lambda(t; Z_i) = \exp(\alpha + \beta Z_i), \qquad \Lambda(t; Z_i) = t\exp(\alpha + \beta Z_i). \tag{4.27}$$

It is left to Exercise 4.5 to obtain the score vector, information matrix, and the MLEs. Figure 4.2 displays the Kaplan-Meier CDF estimates and those based on model (4.27). Compared to the Kaplan-Meier curves, the curves from the exponential regression under-estimate at early event times, and over-estimate at late event times.

To fit the Weibull regression model, for simpler algebra and a more stable numerical algorithm, it is often advantageous to separate the parameters. Thus instead of (3.26), we use the following Weibull parametrization

$$\Lambda(t; Z_i) = \exp\left[\nu Z_i + \alpha + e^{\beta}\log t\right]. \tag{4.28}$$

It is left to Exercise 4.6 to find the score vector. The MLE no longer has a closed form. Commonly used numerical techniques such as Newton's or quasi-Newton methods can be employed to obtain the MLE.

Let $\widehat{\boldsymbol{\theta}} = (\widehat{\alpha}, \widehat{\beta}, \widehat{\nu})$ be the MLE of (α, β, ν). Since the score function is smooth, the observed information matrix $\mathbb{I}(\boldsymbol{\theta})$ can be obtained numerically which saves the potentially tedious and error-prone manual calculation. The step size $\Delta = 10^{-8}$ typically yields reliable approximation of $f(x)$ by $\left[f(x+\Delta) - f(x)\right]\Delta^{-1}$.

To find $\widehat{\boldsymbol{\theta}}$, a good initial value can often lead to a more stable algorithm and faster convergence. Note that

$$\log \Lambda_C(X_i) = \alpha + e^{\beta}\log X_i, \tag{4.29}$$

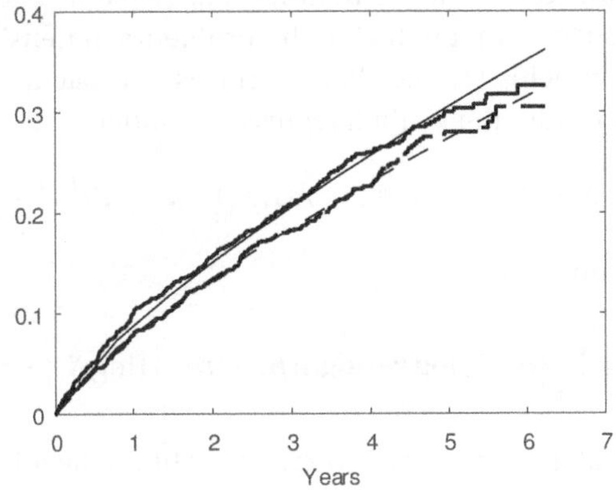

FIGURE 4.3
Estimated CDF for the TOPCAT primary endpoint. Thick solid: control group, Kaplan-Meier; thick dashed: treatment group, Kaplan-Meier; thin solid: control group, Weibull; thin dashed: treatment group, Weibull.

where Λ_C is the cumulative hazard function of the control group which can be estimated by the Nelson-Aalen estimator. Thus a good initial value for α, β can be obtained using the least squares method based on (4.29) which is linear in α and e^{β}. Given that a clinical trial is typically powered to detect 20% or so reduction in event rate, a good initial value of v is ln(0.8). The resulting algorithm typically works well.

In the case here, we obtain

$$\widehat{\boldsymbol{\theta}} = (-2.43, -.26, -.11)$$

and

$$\mathbb{I}(\widehat{\boldsymbol{\theta}}) = \begin{bmatrix} 425.9 & 100.1 & 251.7 \\ 100.1 & 45.7 & 70.0 \\ 251.7 & 70.0 & 321.7 \end{bmatrix}.$$

From these results, the estimated hazard ratio for the treatment effect is $e^{\widehat{v}} = 0.90$, with a 95% confidence interval 0.77–1.04. For the null hypothesis of no treatment effect $H_0 : v = 0$, the Wald test yields a P-value of 0.16.

Figure 4.3 displays the Kaplan-Meier CDF estimates and the Weibull model-based estimates. The fit is much improved compared with the exponential regression model. For t close to the upper end of data range, there is still some noticeable discrepancy between the Kaplan-Meier and model-based estimates. However, since data are sparse there and the Kaplan-Meier estimates are known to be less stable in that region, this is not a big concern.

The power parameter β may sometimes still cause issues in the algorithm. Research findings suggest that reducing the problem's dimension by eliminating some variables often helps [47, 12]. Based on this approach, we will develop an algorithm below. Consider the Weibull regression model

$$\Lambda(t;Z_i)=\nu^{Z_i}\alpha t^{\beta}, \quad \lambda(t;Z_i)=\nu^{Z_i}\alpha\beta t^{\beta-1}. \tag{4.30}$$

The log likelihood function is

$$\ell(\alpha,\beta,\nu)=\sum_{i=1}^{n}\left\{\delta_i\left[Z_i\log\nu+\log(\alpha\beta)+(\beta-1)\log X_i\right]-\nu^{Z_i}\alpha X_i^{\beta}\right\}.$$

Setting the partial derivatives of ℓ to zero, we obtain the following three equations

$$\sum_{i=1}^{n}\delta_i = \alpha\Big[\sum_C X_i^{\beta}+\nu\sum_T X_i^{\beta}\Big], \tag{4.31}$$

$$\frac{\sum_{i=1}^{n}\delta_i}{\beta}+\sum_{i=1}^{n}\delta_i\log X_i = \alpha\Big[\sum_C X_i^{\beta}\log X_i+\nu\sum_T X_i^{\beta}\log X_i\Big], \tag{4.32}$$

$$\sum_T\delta_i = \alpha\nu\sum_T X_i^{\beta}, \tag{4.33}$$

where $\sum_C$, $\sum_T$ are summations over i for which $Z_i=0$ and $Z_i=1$, respectively.

From (4.31) and (4.33), we obtain

$$\alpha=\frac{\sum_C\delta_i}{\sum_C X_i^{\beta}} \tag{4.34}$$

and

$$\nu=\frac{\sum_T\delta_i}{\alpha\sum_T X_i^{\beta}}=\frac{\sum_T\delta_i}{\sum_C\delta_i}\cdot\frac{\sum_C X_i^{\beta}}{\sum_T X_i^{\beta}}. \tag{4.35}$$

From (4.32), (4.34) and (4.35), we obtain the following equation involving only the parameter β:

$$\beta=\frac{\sum_{i=1}^{n}\delta_i}{R_C\sum_C X_i^{\beta}\log X_i+R_T\sum_T X_i^{\beta}\log X_i-\sum_{i=1}^{n}\delta_i\log X_i}, \tag{4.36}$$

where

$$R_C=\frac{\sum_C\delta_i}{\sum_C X_i^{\beta}}, \quad R_T=\frac{\sum_T\delta_i}{\sum_T X_i^{\beta}}.$$

Denote the right-hand side of (4.36) by $A(\beta)$. Based on (4.34) through (4.36), the following algorithm can be obtained:

1. Start with an initial guess for β, say $\beta_{(1)} = 1$.

2. After $\beta_{(k)}$, obtain $\beta_{(k+1)} = A(\beta_{(k)})$, for $k \geq 1$, until the convergence criterion is met. The final value of β is $\widehat{\beta}$.

3. Obtain $\widehat{\alpha}$ and $\widehat{\nu}$ from $\widehat{\beta}$ via (4.34) and (4.35), respectively.

For the TOPCAT data, this iterative procedure converges to a vector that is virtually the same as $\widehat{\boldsymbol{\theta}}$ after reparametrization.

To fit the short- and long-term hazards regression model, let

$$\lambda(t; Z_i) = e^{\nu Z_i}\left[e^{\alpha} S_0(t) + e^{\beta} F_0(t)\right], \tag{4.37}$$

for $F_0(t) = t/(1+t)$, $S_0(t) = 1 - F_0(t)$. In this parametrization, there is no range restriction for (α, β, ν). The cumulative hazard function is

$$\Lambda(t) = e^{\nu Z_i}\left\{e^{\alpha}\Psi_0(t) + e^{\beta}\left[t - \Psi_0(t)\right]\right\},$$

where $\Psi_0(t) = \ln(1+t)$.

For this model,

$$\Lambda_C(X_i) = e^{\alpha}\Psi_0(X_i) + e^{\beta}\left[X_i - \Psi_0(X_i)\right]. \tag{4.38}$$

Thus, similar to the case for the Weibull regression model, a good initial value for α, β can be obtained using the least squares method based on (4.38).

It is left to Exercise 4.8 to find the score vector under model (4.37). The estimated hazard ratio for the treatment effect is $e^{\widehat{\nu}} = 0.90$, with a 95% confidence interval 0.77–1.04. For $H_0 : \nu = 0$, the Wald test yields a P-value of 0.16. These results, rounded to two decimal places, are identical to those for Weibull regression.

Figure 4.4 displays Kaplan-Meier CDF estimates and those based on model (4.37). The plots look very similar to those in Figure 4.3. The model-based estimates show slightly better agreement with the Kaplan-Meier estimates at the upper end of the data range.

The short- and long-term hazards regression model contains intuitive parameters, and numerical algorithms typically are stable and fast. Thus it provides a useful and simple alternative to the Weibull regression model.

4.3 Robust Estimation

Maximum likelihood estimation is a standard approach to parameter inference in statistics. Its asymptotic theory is well established and is familiar to many statisticians. When the model is correctly specified, there is little incentive to look beyond MLE due to its asymptotic efficiency.

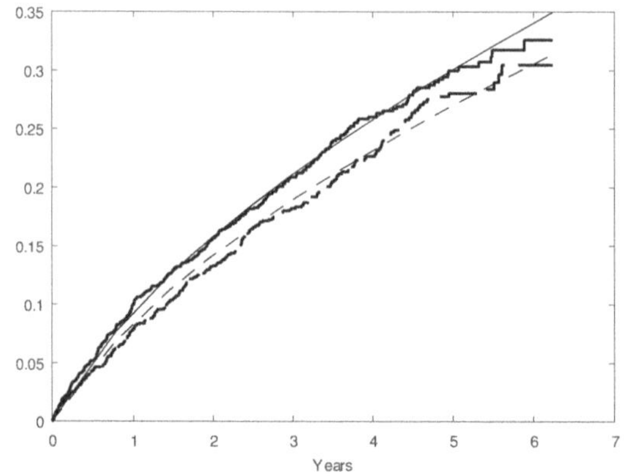

FIGURE 4.4
Estimated CDF for the TOPCAT primary endpoint. Thick solid: control group, Kaplan-Meier; thick dashed: treatment group, Kaplan-Meier; thin solid: control group, short-term and long-term hazards model; thin dashed: treatment group, short-term and long-term hazards model.

However, although we hope that a parametric model is reasonably adequate, various factors, such as lack of information, mathematical approximations, data contamination, makes it almost certain that the model is not strictly correct. Instead, it may be close to the truth in some sense.

In light of this recognition, the minimum distance estimation method emerged as a heuristically effective tool for parameter estimation in the 1980s [20, 221, 142]. In particular, the minimum Hellinger distance estimation procedure proposed by Beran [20] is asymptotically efficient within the specified parametric family of densities. Additionally, it is also robust in a minimax sense in a small Hellinger metric neighborhood of the given family.

While most results of minimum distance estimation were derived for completely observed data, there were some extensions of the method to inference with censored data. Yang [328] extended Beran's procedure and showed that the asymptotic efficiency at the model and the minimax robustness property continue to hold. Ying [354] proposed an alternative extension using the Hellinger distance between hazard functions instead of density functions, and established asymptotic efficiency at the model. Both works used kernel estimation, for density and hazard functions, respectively.

In survival analysis, semiparametric models, which will be discussed in Chapters Five through Eight, have been the mainstream approach to address issues of model flexibility. Related inference procedures, such as partial likelihood inference and pseudo-likelihood inference, to be discussed in Chapter Five, have been quite successful and widely adopted. More discussions can be found in the relevant chapters.

4.4 Exercises and Complements

4.1 When there is no censoring,

$$\boldsymbol{U}_i(\boldsymbol{\theta}) = \frac{1}{f_{\boldsymbol{\theta}}(T_i)} \frac{\partial f_{\boldsymbol{\theta}}(T_i)}{\partial \boldsymbol{\theta}}.$$

In this case, verify that at the true parameter $\boldsymbol{\theta}_0$,

$$E\boldsymbol{U}_i(\boldsymbol{\theta}_0)\boldsymbol{U}_i(\boldsymbol{\theta}_0)^{\mathrm{T}} = -E\Big(\frac{\partial^2 \log L_i}{\partial \theta_j \partial \theta_\ell}\Big)_{p\times p}\Big|_{\boldsymbol{\theta}=\boldsymbol{\theta}_0}.$$

Hint: Take partial derivatives in $\boldsymbol{\theta}$ on both sides of the identity

$$\int_0^\infty f_{\boldsymbol{\theta}}(t)dt = 1$$

to establish

$$\int_0^\infty \frac{\partial^2 f_{\boldsymbol{\theta}}(t)}{\partial \theta_j \partial \theta_\ell} dt = 0$$

(assume that the order of integration and expectation can be interchanged).

4.2 Suppose $T_1, \ldots, T_n$ are i.i.d. uniform random variables on $[0, \theta]$.

(a) Show that $\hat{\theta} = \max_i T_i$ is the MLE and $n(\theta - \hat{\theta})$ converges in distribution to the exponential distribution with survival function $\exp(-t/\theta)$. Contrary to the central limit theorem, the limiting distribution here is not normal and the rate of convergence is n^{-1} rather than $n^{-1/2}$.

Hint: Show that

$$\lim_n P(n(\theta - \hat{\theta}) \le t) = 1 - e^{-t/\theta},$$

by using $P(\hat{\theta} \le c) = (c/\theta)^n$, $c > 0$, and

$$\lim_n \left(1 - \frac{a}{n}\right)^n \to e^{-a}, \quad a > 0.$$

(b) Let $Y_n = \min_i T_i$. Show that nY_n converges in distribution to the exponential distribution with survival function $\exp(-t/\theta)$.

4.3 Suppose $T_1, \ldots, T_n$ are i.i.d. exponential with survival function $S(t) = \exp(-\beta t)$.

(a) Let $X_n = \max_i T_i$. Show that $\beta X_n - \log n$ converges in distribution to the standard Gumbel distribution. That is,

$$\lim_n P\big(\beta X_n - \log n \le t\big) = e^{-e^{-t}}.$$

(b) Obtain the limiting distribution of $\exp(\beta X_n)/n$.

(c) Let $Y_n = \min_i T_i$. Show that nY_n has the exponential distribution with survival function $S(t) = \exp(-\beta t)$.

4.4 Suppose $T_1, \ldots, T_n$ are i.i.d. log-logistic with survival function

$$S(t) = \frac{1}{1 + (\alpha t)^\beta}.$$

(a) Let $X_n = \max_i T_i$. Show that $[(\alpha X_n)^\beta + 1]/n$ converges in distribution to a Fréchet distribution with CDF $F(t) = e^{-1/t}$. That is,

$$\lim_n P\Big(\frac{1 + (\alpha X_n)^\beta}{n} \le t\Big) = e^{-1/t}.$$

(b) Show that $(\alpha X_n)^\beta / n$ converges in distribution to the distribution with CDF $F(t) = e^{-1/t}$.

Hint: Use Slutsky's theorem (property #6 in Section B.9 of Appendix B).

(c) Let $Y_n = \min_i T_i$, $Z_n = (\alpha Y_n)^\beta$ and $W_n = nZ_n/(1 + Z_n)$. Show that W_n converges in distribution to the standard exponential distribution.

(d) Show that

$$nZ_n = \frac{W_n}{1 - W_n/n}.$$

From this and Slutsky's theorem, conclude that nZ_n converges in distribution to the same distribution as W_n.

4.5 (a) For the exponential regression model in (4.27), derive the score vector and the information matrix.

(b) Verify that the MLEs are

$$\hat{\alpha} = \log(S_{1d} S_{1x}^{-1}), \quad \hat{\beta} = \log\{S_{2d} S_{1x} [S_{2x} S_{1d}]^{-1}\},$$

where

$$S_{1d} = \sum_{i=1}^n (1 - Z_i)\delta_i, \quad S_{1x} = \sum_{i=1}^n (1 - Z_i) X_i,$$

$$S_{2d} = \sum_{i=1}^n Z_i \delta_i, \quad S_{2x} = \sum_{i=1}^n Z_i X_i.$$

(c) Obtain the likelihood ratio test of the hypothesis $H_0 : \beta = 0$.

4.6 Derive the score function for the Weibull model in (4.28).

4.7 Verify the results (4.31) through (4.36).

4.8 Derive the score function for the short- and long-term hazards model in (4.37).

4.9 Consider the model

$$\lambda(t; Z_i) = \begin{cases} e^{\beta Z_i + \gamma_1}, & \text{if } t < a \\ e^{\beta Z_i + \gamma_2}, & \text{if } t \geq a \end{cases}$$

where $a > 0$ is a known constant.

(a) Show that the corresponding cumulative hazard function is

$$\Lambda(t; Z_i) = e^{\beta Z_i}\{e^{\gamma_1} t I(t < a) + [e^{\gamma_1} a + e^{\gamma_2}(t - a)] I(t \geq a)\}.$$

(b) Derive the score function and the observed information matrix.

4.10 Consider the model

$$\lambda(t; Z_i) = e^{\beta Z_i}(e^{\gamma_1} + e^{\gamma_2} t).$$

Derive the score vector and the information matrix.

4.11 Consider the model

$$\lambda(t; Z_i) = \begin{cases} \frac{t}{a} e^{\beta Z_i}, & \text{if } t < a \\ e^{\beta Z_i}, & \text{if } t \geq a \end{cases}$$

where $a > 0$ is a known constant. Derive the score vector and the information matrix.

5

Cox Proportional Hazards Model

5.1 Introduction

The previous two chapters described various parametric models and the theory of maximum likelihood for parametric inference. In applications, the unknown parameters can often be divided into two parts. The first part is of primary interest, while the second part, although necessary to completely specify the model, is not. The latter are called "nuisance parameters." For example, in clinical trials or other two-sample comparison problems, the focus is usually on a single parameter that describes the group difference.

In a covariate-adjusted analysis for a two-arm trial, we may use exponential, Weibull or other regression models as illustrated in Chapter Three. Regardless of the model used, the primary interest usually lies in β_1, the coefficient of the treatment indicator Z in the model.

It is desirable to consider models that lump all the nuisance parameters into an unspecified baseline function. A model that contains a parameter vector as well as an unspecified baseline function, or an infinite dimensional parameter, is called a *semiparametric model.* In addition to the convenience of lumping all the nuisance parameters into an unspecified baseline function, a more important consideration of semiparametric modeling and analysis is that, typically, the model is more flexible and the resulting inference procedures are more robust than those derived under parametric models.

The Cox model [51] specifies that, given covariate $\boldsymbol{W}$, the conditional hazard function of T is

$$\lambda(t;\boldsymbol{W}) = \lambda_0(t)\exp[h(\boldsymbol{W},\boldsymbol{\beta})], \tag{5.1}$$

where $\lambda_0(t)$ is an unknown baseline hazard function, $\boldsymbol{\beta}$ is a regression parameter, and $h(\boldsymbol{W},\boldsymbol{\beta})$ is a specific known function. In this chapter we focus on the case when $h(\boldsymbol{W},\boldsymbol{\beta})$ is time independent, i.e., it does not involve t. In Chapter Six, more general forms of $h(\boldsymbol{W},\boldsymbol{\beta})$ will be discussed.

Under model (5.1), for two different levels $\boldsymbol{W}$ and $\widetilde{\boldsymbol{W}}$ of the covariate vector, the ratio of the two corresponding conditional hazard functions is

$$\frac{\lambda(t;\widetilde{\boldsymbol{W}})}{\lambda(t;\boldsymbol{W})} = \exp\left[h(\widetilde{\boldsymbol{W}},\boldsymbol{\beta}) - h(\boldsymbol{W},\boldsymbol{\beta})\right], \tag{5.2}$$

DOI: 10.1201/9780429324437-5

which does not depend on time t. Thus the model is often called the *proportional hazards (PH) model.*

For most applications, $h(\boldsymbol{W},\boldsymbol{\beta})$ is taken to be $\boldsymbol{\beta}^{\mathrm{T}}\boldsymbol{W}$, in which case

$$\frac{\lambda(t;\widetilde{\boldsymbol{W}})}{\lambda(t;\boldsymbol{W})} = \exp\left[\boldsymbol{\beta}^{\mathrm{T}}(\widetilde{\boldsymbol{W}}-\boldsymbol{W})\right]. \tag{5.3}$$

For an unadjusted analysis in a two-arm trial, $\boldsymbol{W}=Z$ and the model is

$$\lambda(t;Z) = \lambda_0(t)\exp(\beta Z). \tag{5.4}$$

Thus

$$\frac{\lambda(t;Z=1)}{\lambda(t;Z=0)} = \exp(\beta). \tag{5.5}$$

That is, β is the log hazard ratio of treatment over control. For an adjusted analysis in a two-arm trial with $\boldsymbol{W}^{\mathrm{T}}=(Z,\boldsymbol{B}^{\mathrm{T}})$ where $\boldsymbol{B}$ is a vector of baseline covariates, let β_1 be the coefficient of Z in $\boldsymbol{\beta}^{\mathrm{T}}\boldsymbol{W}$. Then

$$\frac{\lambda(t;Z=1,\mathbf{V})}{\lambda(t;Z=0,\mathbf{V})} = \exp(\beta_1). \tag{5.6}$$

Thus, β_1 is the log hazard ratio of treatment over control, holding the covariates fixed at the same level. In either case, $\exp(\beta)$ or $\exp(\beta_1)$ is a reasonable summary measure that describes the treatment effect or group difference, with or without covariate adjustment, respectively.

With $h(\boldsymbol{W},\boldsymbol{\beta})=\boldsymbol{\beta}^{\mathrm{T}}\boldsymbol{W}$, model (5.1) reduces to the exponential regression model in (3.21) if $\lambda_0(t)=\eta$, and to the Weibull regression model in (3.24) if $\lambda_0(t)=\nu\eta^{\nu}t^{\nu-1}$. By leaving the baseline function $\lambda_0(t)$ unspecified, model (5.1) is more flexible than specific models such as exponential or Weibull regression.

This flexibility provides important improvements over parametric approaches and is one reason that the Cox proportional hazards model has been the most widely model in survival analysis. More generally, semiparametric models are the main tools for formulating and analyzing covariate effects with survival data, as they provide a good compromise between parametric and nonparametric approaches, yielding a reasonable trade-off between efficiency and robustness.

The form $h(\boldsymbol{W},\boldsymbol{\beta})=\boldsymbol{\beta}^{\mathrm{T}}\boldsymbol{W}$ implies that $h(\boldsymbol{W},\boldsymbol{\beta})$ is linear in the parameter $\boldsymbol{\beta}$. However it is not necessarily linear in the baseline variables, since $\boldsymbol{W}$ may contain higher order terms such as age^2.

Corresponding to (5.1), the cumulative hazard function is

$$\Lambda(t;\boldsymbol{W}) = \int_0^t \exp\left[h(\boldsymbol{W},\boldsymbol{\beta})\right]\lambda_0(x)dx = \exp[h(\boldsymbol{W},\boldsymbol{\beta})]\Lambda_0(t), \tag{5.7}$$

where $\Lambda_0(t)=\int_0^t\lambda_0(s)ds$. The conditional survival function of T given $\boldsymbol{W}$ is

$$S(t;\boldsymbol{W}) = \left[S_0(t)\right]^{\exp\left[h(\boldsymbol{W},\boldsymbol{\beta})\right]}, \tag{5.8}$$

where

$$S_0(t) = \exp\left[-\int_0^t \lambda_0(s)ds\right].$$

The conditional PDF is

$$f(t; \boldsymbol{W}) = \lambda_0(t)\exp\left[h(\boldsymbol{W},\boldsymbol{\beta})\right]\left[S_0(t)\right]^{\exp\left[h(\boldsymbol{W},\boldsymbol{\beta})\right]}. \tag{5.9}$$

The survival function in (5.8) is obtained by raising a baseline function to a power. Such a class of models is known as a *Lehmann class* [164].

In applications, the exponential form $\exp(\boldsymbol{\beta}^{\mathrm{T}}\boldsymbol{W})$ is most widely used for $\exp\left[h(\boldsymbol{W},\boldsymbol{\beta})\right]$, and it will be used in this book unless otherwise indicated. Other forms have also appeared in the literature [251], such as $1+\boldsymbol{\beta}^{\mathrm{T}}\boldsymbol{W}$ or $(1+\boldsymbol{\beta}^{\mathrm{T}}\boldsymbol{W})^{-1}$. In those situations care is needed in both theoretical development and numerical computation to ensure that the quantity is well-defined and positive.

Model (5.1) implies proportional covariate effect in terms of the hazard function. The proportional hazards assumption provides an adequate approximation in many situations, in which the hazard ratio gives a simple and useful summary measure, even if the hazard ratio is moderately time-dependent [250]. Models and analysis for non-proportional hazards situations will be discussed in Chapters Six through Eight.

5.2 Partial Likelihood Inference on $\boldsymbol{\beta}$

For model (5.1), Cox proposed an inference method based on a partial likelihood function. It was speculated that inference based on the partial likelihood could proceed as if the partial likelihood were a true likelihood function, with the resulting estimator of β enjoying properties of a usual MLE. This turned out to be the case. A heuristic argument is given below to derive the partial likelihood.

Consider the random censorship model with fixed covariates as described in Section 4.1.1 in Chapter Four. Assume there are no ties and $t_1 < \cdots < t_k$ are the ordered distinct event times among a randomly censored sample of n individuals. For $\ell = 1, \ldots, k$, and $\varepsilon > 0$, suppose t_ℓ comes from individual $i(\ell)$, and

$$\begin{aligned}
A_\ell &= \text{individual } i(\ell) \text{ experiences event in } [t_\ell, t_\ell+\varepsilon),\\
B_\ell &= \text{one individual experiences event in } [t_\ell, t_\ell+\varepsilon),\\
\mathscr{F}_\ell &= \text{information on participants' history prior to time } t_\ell.
\end{aligned}$$

Also define the *risk set*

$$\mathscr{R}(t) = \{j : \text{the } j\text{th individual is still under observation prior to } t\}.$$

Consider the conditional probability $P(A_\ell|\mathscr{F}_\ell, B_\ell)$. Since $A_\ell \subset B_\ell$, for small ε we have

$$P(A_\ell|\mathscr{F}_\ell, B_\ell) = \frac{P(A_\ell|\mathscr{F}_\ell)}{P(B_\ell|\mathscr{F}_\ell)} \approx \frac{\lambda(t_\ell, \boldsymbol{W}_{i(\ell)})}{\sum_{m\in\mathscr{R}(t_\ell)} \lambda(t_\ell, \boldsymbol{W}_m)},$$

where the approximation follows from the definition of hazard function. Since an index m is in $\mathscr{R}(t_\ell)$ if and only if $T_m \geq t_\ell$, we have

$$\sum_{m\in\mathscr{R}(t_\ell)} \lambda(t_\ell, \boldsymbol{W}_m) = \sum_{m=1}^{n} Y_m(t_\ell)\lambda(t_\ell, \boldsymbol{W}_m),$$

with the at-risk process $Y_i(t) = I(X_i \geq t)$ defined in (2.42).

The *partial likelihood* is

$$\begin{aligned} L(\boldsymbol{\beta}) &= \prod_{\ell=1}^{k} \frac{\lambda(t_\ell, \boldsymbol{W}_{i(\ell)})}{\sum_{m\in\mathscr{R}(t_\ell)} \lambda(t_\ell, \boldsymbol{W}_m)} = \prod_{\ell=1}^{k} \frac{\lambda(t_\ell, \boldsymbol{W}_{i(\ell)})}{\sum_{m=1}^{n} Y_m(t_\ell)\lambda(t_\ell, \boldsymbol{W}_m)} \\ &= \prod_{\ell=1}^{k} \frac{\exp(\boldsymbol{\beta}^{\mathrm{T}}\boldsymbol{W}_{i(\ell)})}{\sum_{m=1}^{n} Y_m(t_\ell)\exp(\boldsymbol{\beta}^{\mathrm{T}}\boldsymbol{W}_m)} \\ &= \prod_{i=1}^{n} \left[\frac{\exp(\boldsymbol{\beta}^{\mathrm{T}}\boldsymbol{W}_i)}{\sum_{m=1}^{n} Y_m(X_i)\exp(\boldsymbol{\beta}^{\mathrm{T}}\boldsymbol{W}_m)}\right]^{\delta_i}, \end{aligned} \tag{5.10}$$

where the second last equality follows from cancelling out the common factor $\lambda_0(t_\ell)$ in both numerator and denominator.

From the derivation, the partial likelihood approximates a product of conditional probabilities. Such an idea of progressive conditioning has been used previously in motivating the survival function formula (2.14) and the log-rank test variance formula (2.36).

Define the score function

$$\boldsymbol{U}(\boldsymbol{\beta}) = \frac{\partial}{\partial \boldsymbol{\beta}} \log L(\boldsymbol{\beta}). \tag{5.11}$$

Then the partial likelihood estimator $\widehat{\boldsymbol{\beta}}$ of the true parameter is the zero of $\boldsymbol{U}(\boldsymbol{\beta})$. From (5.10), $\widehat{\boldsymbol{\beta}}$ is a rank estimator, determined by ranks but not exact values of $X_1, \ldots, X_n$.

Let

$$S^{(m)}(\boldsymbol{\beta}, t) = n^{-1} \sum_{i=1}^{n} Y_i(t)\exp(\boldsymbol{\beta}^{\mathrm{T}}\boldsymbol{W}_i)\boldsymbol{W}_i^{\otimes m} \tag{5.12}$$

for $m = 0, 1, 2$, where for a vector $\mathbf{V}$,

$$\mathbf{V}^{\otimes 0} = 1, \ \ \mathbf{V}^{\otimes 1} = \mathbf{V} \text{ and } V^{\otimes 2} = \mathbf{V}\mathbf{V}^{\mathrm{T}}. \tag{5.13}$$

Then

$$\boldsymbol{U}(\boldsymbol{\beta}) = \sum_{i=1}^{n} \delta_i \left[\boldsymbol{W}_i - E(\boldsymbol{\beta}, X_i)\right] = \sum_{i=1}^{n} \int_0^{\infty} \left[\boldsymbol{W}_i - E(\boldsymbol{\beta}, t)\right] dN_i(t), \tag{5.14}$$

where $E(\boldsymbol{\beta}, t) = S^{(1)}(\boldsymbol{\beta}, t)/S^{(0)}(\boldsymbol{\beta}, t)$ and the counting process and Lebesgue-Stieltjes integral notations in Section 2.8 have been used. The score vector behaves very much like its parametric counterpart in Chapter Four.

If $\boldsymbol{\beta}$ and $\boldsymbol{W}_i$ are $p \times 1$ vectors with jth component β_j and W_{ij}, respectively, then $\boldsymbol{U}(\boldsymbol{\beta})$ is also $p \times 1$, with jth component

$$\boldsymbol{U}_j(\beta) = \sum_{i=1}^{n} \delta_i \left\{ W_{ij} - \frac{\sum_{m=1}^{n} W_{mj} I(X_m \geq X_i) \exp(\boldsymbol{\beta}^{\mathrm{T}} \boldsymbol{W}_m)}{\sum_{m=1}^{n} I(X_m \geq X_i) \exp(\boldsymbol{\beta}^{\mathrm{T}} \boldsymbol{W}_m)} \right\}.$$

Define the information matrix

$$\mathscr{I}(\boldsymbol{\beta}) = -\sum_{i=1}^{n} \left(E \frac{\partial^2 \log L}{\partial \beta_j \partial \beta_\ell} \right)_{p \times p}. \tag{5.15}$$

Under certain regularity conditions, analogously to (4.5) and (4.6), it can be shown that at the true parameter value $\boldsymbol{\beta}_0$,

$$\boldsymbol{U}(\boldsymbol{\beta}_0) \sim N\big(0, \mathscr{I}(\boldsymbol{\beta}_0)\big), \tag{5.16}$$

and that

$$\widehat{\boldsymbol{\beta}} \sim N\big(\boldsymbol{\beta}_0, \mathscr{I}^{-1}(\boldsymbol{\beta}_0)\big). \tag{5.17}$$

Furthermore, $\mathscr{I}(\boldsymbol{\beta}_0)$ in (5.16) and (5.17) can be replaced by either $\mathbb{I}(\boldsymbol{\beta}_0)$ or $\mathbb{I}(\widehat{\boldsymbol{\beta}})$, where $\mathbb{I}(\boldsymbol{\beta})$ is the observed information matrix:

$$\mathbb{I}(\boldsymbol{\beta}) = -\sum_{i=1}^{n} \left(\frac{\partial^2 \log L}{\partial \beta_j \partial \beta_\ell} \right)_{p \times p}.$$

Also, it can be shown (Exercise 5.3) that

$$\mathbb{I}(\boldsymbol{\beta}) = \sum_{i=1}^{n} \delta_i \mathbf{V}(\boldsymbol{\beta}, X_i) = \sum_{i=1}^{n} \int_0^{\infty} \mathbf{V}(\boldsymbol{\beta}, t) dN_i(t), \tag{5.18}$$

where $\mathbf{V}(\boldsymbol{\beta}, t)$ is a $p \times p$ matrix given by

$$\mathbf{V}(\boldsymbol{\beta}, t) = S^{(2)}(\boldsymbol{\beta}, t)/S^{(0)}(\beta, t) - E(\boldsymbol{\beta}, t)^{\otimes 2}.$$

Now inference on $\boldsymbol{\beta}$ can be based on these asymptotic results. Tests and confidence intervals can be constructed similarly to how they are obtained in Chapter Four under a parametric model.

For an unadjusted analysis, where $\boldsymbol{W}_i = Z_i$, the statistic $\boldsymbol{U}(0)$ yields the same numeric result as the log-rank test statistic in (2.49). The setting here is for a regression analysis, while the setting in Section 2.8.2 is for an analysis conditional on the Z_i's with a rearrangement of labels so that the first n_1 observations constitute the control group. Either way, the test statistic and the variance estimator remain unchanged (Exercise 5.2).

5.3 Estimation of Baseline Cumulative Hazard and Survival Functions

Inference on $\boldsymbol{\beta}$ based on the partial likelihood is appealing because it proceeds quite similarly to the parametric likelihood inference. Additionally, its asymptotic properties can be rigorously justified. Relevant discussions are given in Chapter Eleven and Appendices B and C. Compared with exponential regression or any other parametric regression, relative covariate effect represented by $\boldsymbol{\beta}$ can be estimated without having to specify the baseline distribution by a particular parametric form.

In some situations, the absolute covariate effect is of interest. For instance, a trial participant may wish to know what impact a new treatment would have on, say, five-year survival. Furthermore, reductions in hazard from 0.1 to .08 and from 0.001 to .0008, although both resulting in a hazard ratio of .8, may have different implications for collective decision-making in health management and policy issues, as well as for the individual decision-making of a potential treatment recipient. For these reasons, it is important to estimate the baseline cumulative hazard and survival functions.

For data $(X_i, \delta_i, \boldsymbol{W}_i), i = 1, \ldots, n$, from the random censorship model with fixed covariates, denote the conditional survival function of C_i given $\boldsymbol{W}_i = \boldsymbol{w}$ and the marginal survival function of $\boldsymbol{W}_i$ by $\widetilde{S}_i(t; \boldsymbol{w})$ and $A(\boldsymbol{w})$, respectively. Also recall that the conditional PDF, hazard and survival functions of T_i given $\boldsymbol{W}_i = \boldsymbol{w}$ are $f(t; \boldsymbol{w})$, $\lambda(t; \boldsymbol{w})$ and $S(t; \boldsymbol{w})$, respectively. Let $\widetilde{S}_{i-}(t; \boldsymbol{w})$ be the left limit version of the conditional survival function of C_i given the covariate. From the result of Exercise 2.16 (b), under model (5.1) with $h(\boldsymbol{W}, \boldsymbol{\beta}) = \boldsymbol{W}^{\mathrm{T}}\boldsymbol{\beta}$, we have

$$\begin{aligned}
EN_i(t) &= P\big(T_i \le t, T_i \le C_i\big) \\
&= \int P\big(T_i \le t, T_i \le C_i \big| \boldsymbol{W}_i = \boldsymbol{w}\big) dA(\boldsymbol{w}) \\
&= \int \int_0^t \widetilde{S}_{i-}(x; \boldsymbol{w}) dF(x; \boldsymbol{w})\ dA(\boldsymbol{w}) \\
&= \int \int_0^t \widetilde{S}_{i-}(x; \boldsymbol{w}) S(x; \boldsymbol{w}) \lambda(x; \boldsymbol{w}) dx\ dA(\boldsymbol{w}) \\
&= \int \int_0^t \widetilde{S}_{i-}(x; \boldsymbol{w}) S(x; \boldsymbol{w}) \exp(\boldsymbol{w}^{\mathrm{T}}\boldsymbol{\beta}_0) \lambda_0(x) dx\ dA(\boldsymbol{w}), \qquad (5.19)
\end{aligned}$$

for $i = 1, \ldots, n$, where $\boldsymbol{\beta}_0$ is the true parameter value. Also,

$$ES^{(0)}(\boldsymbol{\beta}_0, t) = \frac{1}{n} \sum_{i=1}^{n} \int \widetilde{S}_{i-}(t; \boldsymbol{w}) S(t; \boldsymbol{w}) \exp(\boldsymbol{\beta}_0^{\mathrm{T}} \boldsymbol{w}) dA(\boldsymbol{w}). \qquad (5.20)$$

Verification of (5.19) and (5.20) is left as Exercise 5.4. The Breslow estimator of $\Lambda_0(t)$ is $\widehat{\Lambda}_0(t;\widehat{\boldsymbol{\beta}})$, where

$$\widehat{\Lambda}_0(t;\boldsymbol{\beta}) = \sum_{i=1}^{n} \frac{\delta_i I(X_i \le t)}{\sum_{\ell=1}^{n} Y_\ell(X_i)\exp(\boldsymbol{\beta}^{\mathrm{T}}\boldsymbol{W}_\ell)} = \int_0^t \frac{d\sum_{i=1}^{n} N_i(s)}{nS^{(0)}(\boldsymbol{\beta}, s)}. \tag{5.21}$$

For large n, $\widehat{\Lambda}_0(t;\boldsymbol{\beta}_0)$ should be close to

$$\int_0^t \frac{d\sum_{i=1}^{n} EN_i(s)}{nES^{(0)}(\boldsymbol{\beta}_0, s)} = \Lambda_0(t), \tag{5.22}$$

where the equality follows from (5.18) and (5.19). It follows that the Breslow estimator $\widehat{\Lambda}_0(\theta;\widehat{\boldsymbol{\beta}})$ is a reasonable estimator of $\Lambda_0(t)$ since $\widehat{\Lambda}_0(\theta;\boldsymbol{\beta})$ is a smooth function in $\boldsymbol{\beta}$ and $\widehat{\boldsymbol{\beta}}$ is close to the true parameter $\boldsymbol{\beta}_0$. Breslow obtained the estimator from a nonparametric maximum likelihood argument, treating $\lambda_0(t)$ as piecewise constant between adjacent observed event times. The derivation of Breslow estimator as a nonparametric maximum likelihood estimator in the semiparametric model (5.1) will be discussed in Section 5.5. The application of Breslow-type estimators in various semiparametric models was reviewed and discussed in Lin [173].

Corresponding to the Breslow estimator, the estimator for conditional survival function of T given $\boldsymbol{W} = \boldsymbol{w}$ is

$$\widehat{S}(t;\boldsymbol{w}) = \exp\Big[-\int_0^t \exp(\widehat{\boldsymbol{\beta}}^{\mathrm{T}}\boldsymbol{w})\, d\widehat{\Lambda}_0(t;\widehat{\boldsymbol{\beta}})\Big]. \tag{5.23}$$

To obtain a confidence interval for $S(t;\boldsymbol{w})$ at a specific t, a variance estimator is needed. Andersen and Gill [8] provided a rigorous justification of the asymptotic normality of $\widehat{\Lambda}(t;\widehat{\boldsymbol{\beta}})$ and a consistent variance estimator. Then results on $\widehat{S}(t;\boldsymbol{w})$ follow from the delta method. More discussions will be given in Chapter Six.

Example 5.1. Consider model (5.4) for the TOPCAT trial primary endpoint. The log partial likelihood is

$$\ln L(\beta) = \sum_{i=1}^{n} \delta_i \Big\{\beta Z_i - \ln\Big[\sum_{m=1}^{n} I(X_m \ge X_i)\exp(\beta Z_m)\Big]\Big\},$$

and the score function is

$$U(\beta) = \sum_{i=1}^{n} \delta_i \left\{ Z_i - \frac{\sum_{m=1}^{n} Z_m I(X_m \ge X_i)\exp(\beta Z_m)}{\sum_{m=1}^{n} I(X_m \ge X_i)\exp(\beta Z_m)} \right\}.$$

The estimated hazard ratio is $e^{\widehat{\beta}} = 0.89$, with a 95% confidence interval 0.77–1.04. For the null hypothesis of no treatment effect, $H_0 : \beta = 0$, the Wald test has a P-value of 0.14, which is identical to that from the log-rank test, and slightly smaller

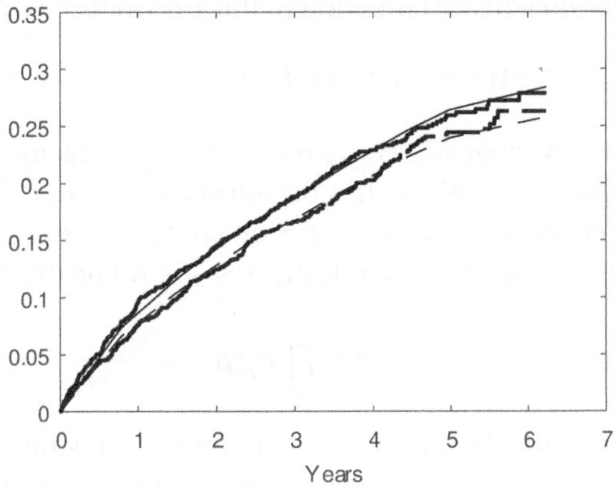

FIGURE 5.1
Estimated CDF for the TOPCAT primary endpoint. Thick solid: control group, Kaplan-Meier; thick dashed: treatment group, Kaplan-Meier; thin solid: control group, model (5.4); thin dashed: treatment group, model (5.4).

than the value of 0.16 obtained from fitting either the Weibull or the short-term and long-term hazards model.

Figure 5.1 displays the Kaplan-Meier CDF estimates and those based on model (5.4). The flexibility of leaving the baseline hazard unspecified, combined with the partial likelihood method, yield estimators of $\lambda_0(t)$ and the corresponding CDFs that better capture the pattern in the data. As a result, overall, the agreement between the Kaplan-Meier and model-based estimates is improved compared to the results from fitting parametric models in Chapter Four.

Covariate-adjusted analysis can also be considered. However, it turns out that the resulting models do not fit the data well, as will be discussed in Example 6.3 of Chapter Six.

5.4 Stratified Analysis

For each covariate included in the covariate vector $\boldsymbol{W}$, from (5.2) the effect is proportional on the hazard function. Sometimes there are covariates which do not have this proportional hazards property. Stratification is a simple option to deal with this situation.

Suppose that there is one or more covariates with non-proportional effect and that they are all discrete. Then the sample can be stratified into r strata for some integer r, corresponding to distinct sets for those covariate values. In the stratified analysis, the conditional hazard function in the jth stratum is modeled to be

$$\lambda_j(t;\breve{\boldsymbol{W}}) = \lambda_{0j}(t)\exp(\boldsymbol{\beta}^{\mathrm{T}}\breve{\boldsymbol{W}}), \quad j = 1,\ldots,r, \tag{5.24}$$

where the covariate $\breve{\boldsymbol{W}}$ does not contain the stratifying factors. In this stratified model, each component of $\breve{\boldsymbol{W}}$ still has proportional effect on the hazard in each stratum, and the effect is the same across all strata. However, each stratum has a different baseline hazard function $\lambda_{0j}(t), 1 \le j \le r$. For this model, the partial likelihood is

$$L(\boldsymbol{\beta}) = \prod_{j=1}^{r} L_j(\boldsymbol{\beta}), \tag{5.25}$$

where $L_j(\boldsymbol{\beta})$ in the partial likelihood function for the jth stratum. Thus the score vector $\boldsymbol{U}^s(\boldsymbol{\theta})$ and the information matrix $\mathcal{I}^s(\boldsymbol{\theta})$ are simply the sum of score vectors and information matrices from each stratum, respectively, After the partial likelihood estimator $\widehat{\boldsymbol{\beta}}^s$ is obtained from solving $\boldsymbol{U}^s(\boldsymbol{\beta}) = 0$, baseline cumulative hazard and survival functions can be estimated by the methods in Section 5.3 for each stratum separately.

To test $\boldsymbol{\beta} = \boldsymbol{0}$ in (5.24), where $\boldsymbol{0}$ is the $p \times 1$ vector with all components 0, Wald test, score test and likelihood ratio test can be used similarly to the results in Section 4.3. Tests on only part of $\boldsymbol{\beta}$ can also be considered. It is left to Exercise 5.5 to show that, in the case $\boldsymbol{W}_i = Z_i$, the stratified score test is the stratified log-rank test.

If it is believed that the effect of $\breve{\boldsymbol{W}}$ varies from one stratum to the next, then different models can be fit to each stratum:

$$\lambda_j(t;\breve{\boldsymbol{W}}) = \lambda_{0j}(t)\exp(\boldsymbol{\beta}_j^{\mathrm{T}}\breve{\boldsymbol{W}}), \quad j = 1,\ldots,r, \tag{5.26}$$

Thus effectively there are r independent samples, one for each stratum, and each sample follows a separate proportional hazards model. Inference for each stratum can be carried out independently of all other strata.

For the stratified model, it is ideal that the number of strata r is not too large. Otherwise the loss of efficiency may be substantial. Even when the number of strata r is small, the stratified analysis may still lose some efficiency, because there are r unspecified baseline hazard functions instead of one for an unstratified analysis.

When applying a stratified analysis to a continuous covariate with non-proportional effect, the covariate needs to be discretized, which leads to further loss of efficiency. Discretization loses information about individual differences, and individuals close to the outpoints can be characterized as being very different rather than very similar. Furthermore, the results are dependent on the arbitrary and subjective way of discretizing the covariate. It also makes it difficult to compare or aggregate findings across studies. MacCallum et al. [193, 266] discussed various issues with dichotomization, the simplest discretization method.

TABLE 5.1
Point estimate ($\widehat{\beta}$), 95% confidence interval (CI), standardized z-score and P-value for β_1 through β_4 in the stratified model (5.27).

	$\widehat{\beta}$	CI	z-score	P-value
Z	0.90	0.77–1.04	-1.42	0.16
W_1	1.54	1.25–1.91	3.99	< 0.0001
W_2	1.25	1.04–1.51	2.33	0.02
W_3	1.03	0.87–1.21	0.33	0.74

In a stratified analysis, since stratum effects are modeled nonparametrically, there are no straightforward methods to evaluate the effect of the stratifying factor on survival or the interaction between the stratifying factor and other variables. Alternative approaches for dealing with non-proportional hazards will be discussed in Chapters Six, Seven, and Eight.

Example 5.2. The TOPCAT trial had a pre-specified covariate-adjusted analysis that used the Cox model with 3 covariates: age (as a continuous variable), diabetes history at baseline (insulin–treated, not insulin–treated, or no history of diabetes), and whether or not the participant had been hospitalized in the twelve months prior to enrollment with management of heart failure as a major component. It will be shown in Example 6.3 that there is evidence of model violation, with age showing non-proportional hazards. To remedy this, we stratify according to whether age is > 69 or otherwise, where 69 is the median age. The stratified model is

$$\lambda_j(t;\breve{\boldsymbol{W}}) = \lambda_{0j}(t)\exp(\beta_1 Z + \beta_2 W_1 + \beta_3 W_2 + \beta_4 W_3), \qquad j = 1.2, \tag{5.27}$$

where the first stratum denoted individuals with age ≤ 69, Z is the treatment group indicator, and W_1, W_2, W_3 are the indicators for, respectively, diabetes history, insulin-treated; diabetes history, not insulin-treated; and hospitalized in the twelve months prior to enrollment with management of heart failure as a major component. Table 5.1 gives the results of parameter estimation for β_1 through β_4.

From Table 5.1, the test for the null hypothesis of no treatment effect, $H_0 : \beta_1 = 0$, yields a P-value of 0.16. Note that this P-value is actually slightly larger than the P-value of 0.14 for the unadjusted analysis in Example 5.1. This example illustrates that there may not always be a gain in power with a covariate-adjusted or stratified analysis over the unadjusted analysis. Furthermore, the chance of model violation and loss of efficiency is increased due to inclusion of additional variables in the model and/or stratification.

In Example 7.5 of Chapter Seven, a different model is employed to address the non-proportionality issue with the covariate age, without using stratification.

5.5 Pseudo-Likelihood Estimator

The Cox proportional hazards model (5.1) is specified by the parametric component β and the nonparametric component $\lambda_0(t)$. With $\lambda_0(t)$ unspecified, the model offers more flexibility than a parametric regression model. At the same time, inference based on the partial likelihood avoids the technical challenges in dealing with the unknown $\lambda_0(t)$, allowing estimation and testing to parallel their counterparts in parametric models. These properties contribute to making the Cox model with partial likelihood inference the most popular approach for analyzing survival data.

However, there are situations that call for other models as will be discussed in Chapters Seven and Eight. An important feature of the Cox model is that the partial likelihood does not contain the unknown baseline function $\lambda_0(t)$. This property typically no longer holds in other models, and the partial likelihood approach does not yield a simple estimating function.

In this section, we show that a different inference procedure, called pseudo-likelihood estimation, leads to the same estimator for $\boldsymbol{\beta}$ under the Cox model. Pseudo-likelihood estimation is useful in analyzing the models in Chapters Seven and Eight.

Suppose that $\lambda_0(t)$ is known and let $L(\boldsymbol{\beta}, \lambda_0)$ be the likelihood of the observed data. Then the score function is $\boldsymbol{S}(\boldsymbol{\beta}, \lambda_0) = \frac{\partial}{\partial \boldsymbol{\beta}} \ln L(\boldsymbol{\beta}, \lambda_0)$. That is,

$$\boldsymbol{S}(\boldsymbol{\beta}, \lambda_0) = \sum_{i=1}^{n} \boldsymbol{W}_i \left[\delta_i - \exp(\boldsymbol{\beta}^{\mathrm{T}} \boldsymbol{W}_i) \Lambda_0(X_i) \right]. \tag{5.28}$$

The zero of $\boldsymbol{S}(\boldsymbol{\beta}, \lambda_0)$ is the MLE of the true parameter.

In reality $\lambda_0(t)$ and therefore $\Lambda_0(t)$ is unknown. From (5.21), $\widehat{\Lambda}_0(t; \boldsymbol{\beta})$ at the true parameter is close to $\Lambda_0(t)$. Thus it is reasonable to replace $\Lambda_0(t)$ in (5.28) by $\widehat{\Lambda}_0(t; \boldsymbol{\beta})$, which results in the estimating function

$$\widetilde{\boldsymbol{U}}(\boldsymbol{\beta}) = \sum_{i=1}^{n} \boldsymbol{W}_i \left[\delta_i - \exp(\boldsymbol{W}_i^{\mathrm{T}} \boldsymbol{\beta}) \widehat{\Lambda}_0(X_i; \boldsymbol{\beta}) \right]. \tag{5.29}$$

The pseudo-likelihood estimator of $\boldsymbol{\beta}$ is the zero of $\widetilde{\boldsymbol{U}}$. With some algebra (Exercise 5.6), it can be shown that $\widetilde{\boldsymbol{U}}$ is the same as the score function in (5.14).

The pseudo-likelihood estimator here is somewhat related to but different from the pseudo-maximum likelihood estimator proposed in Gong and Samaniego [103], where the nuisance parameter is a real number and is replaced by a consistent estimator in the estimating function. In comparison, the approach here deals with the unknown $\Lambda_0(t)$ as an infinite dimensional nuisance parameter which is replaced by $\widehat{\Lambda}_0(t;\boldsymbol{\beta})$. The latter is not an estimator as it involves the argument $\boldsymbol{\beta}$ in the estimating function. Nonetheless, both approaches involve approximation of the nuisance parameter that leads to a reasonable estimator for the parameter of interest.

5.6 Nonparametric Maximum Likelihood Estimation*

Nonparametric maximum likelihood estimation was mentioned in Chapter Two and used to obtain the Kaplan-Meier estimator. It can also be used for model (5.1). The idea is to view an appropriate likelihood as a function of $\boldsymbol{\beta}$ as well as $\Lambda_0(t)$, and maximize the likelihood to simultaneously obtain estimators of $\boldsymbol{\beta}$ and $\Lambda_0(t)$. Applications of the nonparametric maximum likelihood approach to semiparametric models have been discussed by various authors [21, 7, 50, 210, 139, 359, 361, 260, 62]. Because there is a finite-dimensional parameter and an unspecified baseline function involved, this method is also called semiparametric maximum likelihood estimation.

For illustration, let $\exp\left[h(\boldsymbol{W},\boldsymbol{\beta})\right] = \exp(\boldsymbol{\beta}^{\mathrm{T}}\boldsymbol{W})$. From (4.1) and (5.1), the likelihood is

$$\prod_{i=1}^{n}\Big\{\big[\lambda_0(X_i)\exp(\boldsymbol{\beta}^{\mathrm{T}}\boldsymbol{W}_i)\big]^{\delta_i}\exp\big[-\Lambda_0(X_i)\exp(\boldsymbol{\beta}^{\mathrm{T}}\boldsymbol{W}_i)\big]\Big\}. \tag{5.30}$$

As in Chapter Two, there is no maximizer of this likelihood if Λ_0 is restricted to be absolutely continuous. On the other hand, the maximizer exists if Λ_0 is restricted to be discrete and the likelihood is modified accordingly to be

$$\prod_{i=1}^{n}\Big\{\big[\Delta\Lambda_0(X_i)\exp(\boldsymbol{\beta}^{\mathrm{T}}\boldsymbol{W}_i)\big]^{\delta_i}\exp\big[-\Lambda_0(X_i)\exp(\boldsymbol{\beta}^{\mathrm{T}}\boldsymbol{W}_i)\big]\Big\}, \tag{5.31}$$

where $\Delta\Lambda_0(X_i) = \Lambda_0(X_i) - \Lambda_0(X_i-)$. To further simplify the derivation, assume that there are no ties among data and $X_1 < \cdots < X_n$. The latter requirement is equivalent to assuming that data have been re-arranged according to the order statistics. Let $J_i = \Lambda_0(X_i) - \Lambda_0(X_i-)$. Then $\Lambda_0(X_i) = \sum_{m\le i} J_m$ and the likelihood in (5.31), as a function of $\boldsymbol{\beta}$ and $J_1,\ldots,J_n$, can be maximized to obtain estimators of $\boldsymbol{\beta}$ and Λ_0. For the moment assume all factors are positive so that logarithm can be taken.

Then the log-likelihood is

$$\ell(\boldsymbol{\beta}, J_1, \ldots, J_n) = \sum_{i=1}^{n} \delta_i \left(\log(J_i) + \boldsymbol{\beta}^{\mathrm{T}} \boldsymbol{W}_i \right) - \sum_{i=1}^{n} \sum_{m \le i} J_m \exp\left(\boldsymbol{\beta}^{\mathrm{T}} \boldsymbol{W}_i\right). \tag{5.32}$$

Setting the partial derivatives of ℓ with respect to $J_1, \ldots, J_n$ and $\boldsymbol{\beta}$, to zero, we obtain

$$\frac{\delta_k}{J_k} - \sum_{i \ge k} \exp(\boldsymbol{\beta}^{\mathrm{T}} \boldsymbol{W}_i) = 0, \quad k = 1, \ldots, n, \tag{5.33}$$

$$\sum_{i=1}^{n} \delta_i \boldsymbol{W}_i - \sum_{i=1}^{n} \sum_{m \le i} J_m \exp(\boldsymbol{\beta}^{\mathrm{T}} \boldsymbol{W}_i) \boldsymbol{W}_i = 0. \tag{5.34}$$

From (5.33),

$$J_k = \frac{\delta_k}{\sum_{i \ge k} \exp(\boldsymbol{\beta}^{\mathrm{T}} \boldsymbol{W}_i)}, \quad k = 1, \ldots, n. \tag{5.35}$$

Since

$$\frac{\partial^2 \ell}{\partial J_k \partial J_q} = -\frac{\delta_k I(k = q)}{J_k^2}, \quad 1 \le k, q \le n, \tag{5.36}$$

the solution (5.35) is indeed the maximizer of ℓ in $J_1, \ldots, J_n$ for fixed $\boldsymbol{\beta}$. It can be seen that the cumulative hazard function from (5.35) jumps only at the uncensored times and is the Breslow estimator in (5.21) for $\Lambda_0(t)$.

Now, plugging the solution (5.35) into (5.34), it can be seen that the resulting estimating equation for $\boldsymbol{\beta}$ coincides with that in (5.14). Thus for model (5.1) with $\exp\left[h(\boldsymbol{W}, \boldsymbol{\beta})\right] = \exp(\boldsymbol{\beta}^{\mathrm{T}} \boldsymbol{W})$, nonparametric maximum likelihood estimation leads to the partial likelihood estimator for $\boldsymbol{\beta}$ and the Breslow estimator for $\Lambda_0(t)$.

However, the above heuristic argument has a flaw: the logarithm is taken for J_i which is zero when $\delta_i = 0$. Nevertheless, if δ_i's are positive, then the solution is justified. Note that both the log likelihood function (5.32) and the solution (5.35) are continuous functions of $\delta_1, \ldots, \delta_n$. Therefore, by passing to the limit as in Exercise (5.7), the Breslow estimator indeed maximizes the likelihood for fixed $\boldsymbol{\beta}$.

For the Cox model (5.1), pseudo-likelihood, nonparametric likelihood and the partial likelihood all lead to the same estimating function which does not contain the unknown baseline hazard. This appealing feature helps make the model the most widely used one for analyzing survival data. This situation is somewhat analogous to the role of the normal distribution, where various reasonable perspectives lead to the same simple estimator, the sample mean, as an estimator for the population mean.

For a wide variety of semiparametric models, an appropriate likelihood $L(\boldsymbol{\theta}, \eta)$ can be constructed, where $\boldsymbol{\theta}$ is the finite-dimensional parameter and η the unspecified baseline function. Under certain regularity conditions, the nonparametric MLE $(\widehat{\boldsymbol{\theta}}, \widehat{\eta})$ exists and can be shown to be consistent and asymptotically normal, with the asymptotic covariance matrix $\Sigma_{\boldsymbol{\theta}}$ of $\widehat{\boldsymbol{\theta}}$ achieving the efficiency lower bound [21, 7, 210, 139]. However, in more complicated semiparametric models such as those that will be discussed in Chapters Seven and Eight, the nonparametric MLE of η often does not have a closed form such as (5.35).

When the interest is in the finite-dimensional parameter $\boldsymbol{\theta}$, Murphy and van der Vaart [210] investigated the profile likelihood approach. For a likelihood $L(\boldsymbol{\theta},\eta)$, the profile likelihood is

$$pl(\boldsymbol{\theta}) = \sup_{\eta} L(\boldsymbol{\theta},\eta), \tag{5.37}$$

and the profile MLE is the maximizer of $pl(\boldsymbol{\theta})$. The profile MLE is the nonparametric MLE for $\boldsymbol{\theta}$, as it is obtained by "taking the maximum in two steps." Murphy and van der Vaart [210] showed that the profile likelihood behaves much like the ordinary likelihood. In particular, the limiting covariance matrix $\Sigma_{\boldsymbol{\theta}}$ can be consistently estimated by inverting the observed Fisher information matrix, and the likelihood ratio statistic has the familiar asymptotic χ^2 distribution.

As discussed in Andersen et al. [7, pp. 221–226], there are multiple approaches to constructing likelihood functions that can yield slightly different estimators. Ren and Zhou [260] worked with a likelihood that is expressed as a function of $\boldsymbol{\beta}$ and the CDF F_0 corresponding to Λ_0. They obtained a profile likelihood for $\boldsymbol{\beta}$ by maxing out F_0 similarly to (5.37), and the nonparametric/profile MLE for $\boldsymbol{\beta}$ is obtained by maximizing the profile likelihood. Among several considerations that motivated the work of Ren and Zhou, their approach can be extended more easily to other types of censored data such as doubly censored data and interval censored data, for which it is more natural to work with the CDF rather than the hazard function. Their work also demonstrated some advantages for small samples.

5.7 Generalized Rank Estimators

The discussion in this section is restricted to the two-sample problem. Suppose that data are available under the two-sample setup described in Section 2.8.2, with $\lambda_T(t)$, $\lambda_C(t)$ the hazard functions of the two groups, where the subscripts T and C refer to the treatment and control groups, respectively. Consider the two-sample model that for some $\theta > 0$,

$$\lambda_T(t) = \theta\lambda_C(t), \ \ t > 0. \tag{5.38}$$

Let $\Lambda_T(t)$ and $\Lambda_C(t)$ be the cumulative hazard functions of the two groups, with corresponding Nelson-Aalen estimators $\widehat{\Lambda}_T(t)$ and $\widehat{\Lambda}_C(t)$, respectively. Gill's statistics of class $\mathscr{K}$ [95] is a class of statistics

$$\int_0^\infty \Psi(t)d\big[\widehat{\Lambda}_T(t) - \widehat{\Lambda}_C(t)\big], \tag{5.39}$$

where Ψ satisfies certain regularity conditions. In particular, it is nonnegative, predictable and vanishes whenever $\min\big(K_C(t), K_T(t)\big) = 0$.

Under model (5.38), from the statistics of class $\mathscr{K}$, a class of estimators of θ is given by

$$\widehat{\theta}_\Psi = \frac{\int_0^\infty \Psi(t)d\widehat{\Lambda}_T(t)}{\int_0^\infty \Psi(t)d\widehat{\Lambda}_C(t)}. \tag{5.40}$$

Estimators of the form (5.40) are called *generalized rank estimators* (GRE) [18, 6]. For

$$\Psi(t) = \frac{\Phi(t)K_C(t)K_T(t)}{K_C(t) + K_T(t)}, \tag{5.41}$$

where 0/0 is defined to be 0 as in Chapter Two, the GRE with Ψ is related to the weighted log-rank test statistics with weight Φ in that they are the ratio and difference of $\int_0^\infty \Phi(t)d\widehat{\Lambda}_T(t)$ and $\int_0^\infty \Phi(t)d\widehat{\Lambda}_C(t)$, respectively. Examples of Ψ for the GRE include

$$\Psi_{LR} = \frac{K_T K_C}{K_T + K_C}$$

and

$$\Psi_{PP} = \frac{K_T K_C}{K_T + K_C}\widehat{S}_-$$

where $\widehat{S}_-$ is the left limit version of the Kaplan-Meier estimator calculated from the pooled sample. These two choices of the integrand correspond to the log-rank test and the Peto-Prentice test, respectively.

Under (5.38),

$$\theta = \frac{\int_0^\infty \Psi(t)d\Lambda_T(t)}{\int_0^\infty \Psi(t)d\Lambda_C(t)}.$$

Thus

$$\begin{aligned}\widehat{\theta}_\Psi - \theta \quad &= \quad \left\{\int_0^\infty \Psi(t)d\big[\widehat{\Lambda}_T(t) - \Lambda_T(t)\big] - \theta\int_0^\infty \Psi(t)d\big[\widehat{\Lambda}_C(t) - \Lambda_C(t)\big]\right\} \\ &\quad \cdot\left[\int_0^\infty \Psi(t)d\widehat{\Lambda}_C(t)\right]^{-1}. \end{aligned} \tag{5.42}$$

Using the counting process and martingale theory, which will be discussed in Chapter Eleven, it can be shown that $\sqrt{n}(\widehat{\theta}_\Psi - \theta)$ converges in distribution to a mean zero normal distribution whose variance v_Ψ can be estimated by

$$\begin{aligned}\widehat{v}_\Psi &= n\Big[\int_0^\infty \Psi^2(t)\frac{d\widehat{\Lambda}_T(t)}{K_T(t)} + \widehat{\theta}_\Psi^2 \int_0^\infty \Psi^2(t)\frac{d\widehat{\Lambda}_C(t)}{K_C(t)}\Big] \\ &\quad \cdot \Big[\int_0^\infty \Psi(t)d\widehat{\Lambda}_C(t)\Big]^{-2}. \end{aligned} \tag{5.43}$$

Based on the asymptotic normality, an asymptotic $100(1-\alpha)\%$ confidence interval for θ is

$$\Big[\big(\widehat{\theta}_\Psi - z(\alpha/2)\sqrt{\widehat{v}_\Psi/n}\big)_+,\ \widehat{\theta}_\Psi + z(\alpha/2)\sqrt{\widehat{v}_\Psi/n}\Big], \tag{5.44}$$

where $a_+ = \max(a, 0)$. An asymptotic level α test of $H_0 : \theta = 1$ rejects H_0 if the confidence interval excludes 1. To avoid 0 as the lower limit of the confidence interval, a proper transformation can be used. Related discussions can be found in Chapter Fourteen.

At $\theta = 1$, or $\Lambda_T(t) = \Lambda_C(t)$, with an argument similar to those in [95, 100], it can be shown that the GRE with $\Psi = \Psi_{LR}$ has the smallest asymptotic variance among all GREs (see Exercise 5.13). This GRE will be referred to as the log-rank GRE. Compared with the partial likelihood estimator of θ, the log-rank GRE is in closed form and does not require numerical rooting-finding. In large samples, the two estimators typically are very close to each other.

In Section 6.6.1 and Chapter Fourteen, more discussions on the GREs will be found, in applications to model assessment and semi-competing risks analysis, respectively.

5.8 Time-to-Event Analysis Versus Binomial Approximation

Sometimes, binomial approximations are used to simplify the analysis and to obtain quick results. For example, for a comparison between the treatment and control groups, proportion of events in the two groups are obtained as

$$\widehat{p}_j = \frac{\#\text{ of events in group } j}{n_j},$$

where the subscript j refers to the group ($j = 1$ for the control group), and the control and treatment group sizes are n_1 and n_2, respectively. Then, $\widehat{p}_j$ estimates the probability of observing the event for a randomly selected individual from group j. The hypothesis of no treatment effect is the hypothesis of equal proportions,

$p_2 = p_1$, which is rejected at 5% significance level if

$$\frac{|\widehat{p}_2 - \widehat{p}_1|}{\sqrt{\widehat{p}_p(1-\widehat{p}_p)\cdot\left(\frac{1}{n_1}+\frac{1}{n_2}\right)}} > 1.96, \tag{5.45}$$

where $\widehat{p}_p = (n_1\widehat{p}_1 + n_2\widehat{p}_2)/(n_1+n_2)$.

However, note that

$$p_j = P(T_j \le C_j),$$

where T_j and C_j represent the time-to-event variable and the censoring variable in group j, respectively. Therefore, the null hypothesis $p_2 = p_1$ depends on the censoring distributions in the two groups.

Consequently, a significant test result from (5.45) might stem from differences in the censoring distributions rather than the distributions of the time-to-event variable in the two groups. Conversely, a non-significant test from (5.45) could be due to differences in the censoring distributions that obscure distinct characteristics in the time-to-event variable distributions across the two groups. It's worth noting that the partial likelihood inference under model (5.4) is asymptotically valid for the random censorship model with fixed covariates in Section 4.1.1, which does not require equal censoring distributions.

Example 5.3. For the primary endpoint in the TOPCAT trial, Example 5.1 gives the results on point and interval estimates of the hazard ratio, as well as the P-value for testing the hypothesis of no treatment effect, $\beta = 0$. From the binomial approximation mentioned above, the ratio of event proportions, treatment over control, is 0.91. The test in (5.45) for the hypothesis of no treatment effect, $p_2 = p_1$, yields a P-value of 0.185.

Now consider two scenarios of additional artificial censoring of outcomes:

A. The additional artificial censoring is only in the treatment group, by a variable C_a which is 50 times a standard exponential variable independent of the data. This results in about 10 fewer events in the treatment group.

B. The additional artificial censoring is only in the control group, by a variable C_a which is 50 times a standard exponential variable independent of the data. This results in about 10 fewer events in the control group.

Table 5.2 summarizes the results of an analysis under model (5.4) and the binomial test in (5.45), using the original data and with the additional censoring, as described in scenario A, across 10 runs.

Note that for the time-to-event analysis, the point and interval estimates in the 10 runs are close to the results for the original data. The P-values are also mostly close to the p-value of 0.14 for the original data. For the binomial approximation, the ratios $\widehat{p}_2/\widehat{p}_1$ in the 10 runs tend to be smaller than the ratio using the original data. Furthermore, the P-values in the 10 runs are much closer to the threshold

TABLE 5.2
Comparison of time-to-event analysis (model 5.4) and binomial approximation: original TOPCAT data and 10 runs under scenario A. Model (5.4): $e^{\hat{\beta}}$ and CI are the point and 95% interval estimates of the hazard ratio, and P-Cox is the P-value for testing $\beta = 0$; binomial approximation: $\hat{p}_2/\hat{p}_1$ is the ratio of proportions of events, and P-Bin is the P-value for testing $p_2 = p_1$.

	$e^{\hat{\beta}}$	CI	P-Cox	$\hat{p}_2/\hat{p}_1$	P-Bin
Original	0.89	0.77–1.04	0.14	0.91	0.19
Run 1	0.89	0.77–1.04	0.15	0.88	0.07
Run 2	0.88	0.76–1.03	0.11	0.88	0.06
Run 3	0.90	0.78–1.05	0.20	0.90	0.12
Run 4	0.90	0.77–1.05	0.18	0.88	0.08
Run 5	0.88	0.76–1.03	0.11	0.87	0.047
Run 6	0.89	0.76–1.03	0.12	0.88	0.06
Run 7	0.89	0.77–1.04	0.14	0.88	0.06
Run 8	0.89	0.76–1.04	0.13	0.88	0.06
Run 9	0.89	0.77–1.04	0.15	0.89	0.09
Run 10	0.91	0.78–1.06	0.22	0.90	0.11
10-run Average	0.89	0.77–1.04	0.15	0.88	0.08

0.05 than the P-value for the original data, and one run has a significant P-value at 0.047.

Next, consider scenario B. Table 5.3 summarizes the results of an analysis under model (5.4) and the binomial test in (5.45), using the original data and with the additional censoring, as described in scenario B, across 10 runs.

From Table 5.3, for scenario B, in the 10 runs, the time-to-event analysis continues to yield point and interval estimates close to the results for the original data, and the P-values are also mostly close to the P-value of 0.14 for the original data. For the binomial approximation, the ratios $\hat{p}_2/\hat{p}_1$ in the 10 runs are in general larger than the ratio of 0.91 for the original data. Furthermore, the P-values in the 10 runs are substantially larger than those for either scenario A or the original data.

TABLE 5.3
Comparison of time-to-event analysis (model 5.4) and binomial approximation: original TOPCAT data and 10 runs under scenario B. Model (5.4): $e^{\widehat{\beta}}$ and CI are the point and 95% interval estimates of the hazard ratio, and P-Cox is the P-value for testing $\beta = 0$; binomial approximation: $\widehat{p}_2/\widehat{p}_1$ is the ratio of proportions of events, and P-Bin is the P-value for testing $p_2 = p_1$.

	$e^{\widehat{\beta}}$	CI	P-Cox	$\widehat{p}_2/\widehat{p}_1$	P-Bin
Original	0.89	0.77–1.04	0.14	0.91	0.19
Run 1	0.89	0.76–1.04	0.14	0.95	0.44
Run 2	0.89	0.76–1.03	0.12	0.93	0.30
Run 3	0.91	0.78–1.06	0.22	0.96	0.55
Run 4	0.89	0.76–1.03	0.12	0.93	0.30
Run 5	0.90	0.78–1.05	0.20	0.96	0.58
Run 6	0.90	0.77–1.05	0.19	0.95	0.49
Run 7	0.88	0.76–1.03	0.11	0.93	0.32
Run 8	0.88	0.76–1.03	0.11	0.93	0.32
Run 9	0.89	0.76–1.03	0.13	0.94	0.37
Run 10	0.89	0.77–1.04	0.15	0.94	0.39
10-run Average	0.89	0.77–1.04	0.15	0.94	0.41

From these results, the binomial test in (5.45) is very sensitive to differences in the censoring distributions between the two groups. This can distort the test result in either direction. For other variations of the binomial approximation, the situation is similar. In comparison, a time-to-event analysis under model (5.4) is asymptotically valid without requiring the equality of the censoring distributions in the two groups, and is often much more robust against the influence of censoring than the binomial test.

5.9 Exercises and Complements

5.1 For $L(\boldsymbol{\beta})$ in (5.10), take the second order derivatives of its logarithm to verify that the observed information matrix $\mathbb{I}(\boldsymbol{\beta})$ can be written in the form given in (5.18).

5.2 For an un-adjusted analysis with $\boldsymbol{W} = Z$, show that the information in (5.18) is the same as the variance of the log-rank test given in (2.53) with $\Phi(t) \equiv 1$.

5.3 When $\boldsymbol{\beta}$ is $p \times 1$, show that the observed information matrix

$$\mathbb{I}(\boldsymbol{\beta}) = -\sum_{i=1}^{n} \left(\frac{\partial^2 \log L}{\partial \beta_j \partial \beta_\ell} \right)_{p \times p}$$

has (j,k) element $\sum_{i=1}^{n} \delta_i (v_{ijk} - \mu_{ij}\mu_{ik})$, where

$$v_{ijk} = \frac{\sum_{m=1}^{n} W_{mj} W_{mk} I(X_m \geq X_i) \exp(\boldsymbol{\beta}^{\mathrm{T}} \boldsymbol{W}_m)}{\sum_{m=1}^{n} I(X_m \geq X_i) \exp(\boldsymbol{\beta}^{\mathrm{T}} \boldsymbol{W}_m)},$$

$$\mu_{ij} = \frac{\sum_{m=1}^{n} W_{mj} I(X_m \geq X_i) \exp(\boldsymbol{\beta}^{\mathrm{T}} \boldsymbol{W}_m)}{\sum_{m=1}^{n} I(X_m \geq X_i) \exp(\boldsymbol{\beta}^{\mathrm{T}} \boldsymbol{W}_m)}.$$

This verifies (5.18).

5.4 Use the results of Exercise 2.21 to verify (5.19) and (5.20).

5.5 (a) Prove (5.25).

(b) In the case $\boldsymbol{W}_i = Z_i$, show that the stratified score test is the stratified log-rank test.

5.6 Shown that $\widetilde{\boldsymbol{U}}$ in (5.29) is the same as the score function in (5.14).

5.7 (a) Let $A(x,c)$ be a continuous function defined for $x \geq 0$, $c \geq 0$. Suppose for each fixed $c > 0$, $A(x,c)$ is maximized at $x = \widehat{x}(c)$, where $\widehat{x}(c)$ is a continuous function of c for $c \geq 0$. Show that $A(x,0)$ is maximized at $x = \widehat{x}(0)$.

Hint: Write down the relevant inequality involving $\widehat{x}(c)$, then take limit as $c \downarrow 0$.

(b) Use (a) above to justify that (5.35) is the maximizer of the likelihood function for fixed $\boldsymbol{\beta}$. For simplicity assume there are no ties and $X_1 < \cdots < X_n$.

5.8 (a) Verify (5.33) and (5.34) by calculating the partial derivatives of ℓ with respect to $J_1, \ldots, J_n$ and $\boldsymbol{\beta}$.

(b) Verify that the solution in (5.35) is the Breslow estimator in (5.21).

(c) Verify (5.36).

5.9 (a) Write out the details of the partial likelihood $L(\boldsymbol{\beta})$ in (5.25) for the stratified model (5.24).

(b) Obtain the score function and observed information matrix for model (5.24).

5.10 Consider a variation of Cox model by specifying that, given covariate $\boldsymbol{W}$, the conditional hazard function of T is

$$\lambda(t;\boldsymbol{W}) = \lambda_0(t)(1+\boldsymbol{\beta}^{\mathrm{T}}\boldsymbol{W}). \tag{5.46}$$

(a) Parallel to (5.10), derive the partial likelihood.

(b) Obtain the score function and observed information matrix.

(c) Adapt the Breslow estimator in (5.21) to model (5.46).

5.11 Consider the random censorship model described in Section 2.4. Suppose $w_1,\cdots,w_n$ are nonnegative constants and with probability 1,

$$\lim_n \sum_{i=1}^n w_i Y_i(\tau) > 0$$

for some $\tau > 0$, where the at-risk process $Y_i(t)$ is defined in (2.42). Define

$$\begin{aligned} H_w(t) &= \sum_{i=1}^n w_i N_i(t), \\ K_w(t) &= \sum_{i=1}^n w_i Y_i(t), \end{aligned}$$

for $t \in [0,\tau]$, where the counting process $N_i(t)$ is defined in (2.42).

(a) Show that

$$\begin{aligned} EH_w(t) &= \sum_{i=1}^n w_i \int_0^t G_{i-}(s)dF(s), \\ EK_w(t) &= \sum_{i=1}^n w_i G_{i-}(t)S_-(t), \end{aligned}$$

where $G_{i-}(t) = P(C_i \geq t)$ and $S(t)$ is the survival function of T. Conclude that

$$\int_0^t \frac{dEH_w(s)}{EK_w(s)} = \Lambda(t).$$

This shows that

$$\widehat{\Lambda}_w(t) = \int_0^t \frac{dH_w(s)}{K_w(s)} \tag{5.47}$$

is a reasonable estimator of $\Lambda(t)$.

(b) Assume that F is continuous. Let $J(t) = I(K_w(t) > 0)$. By the counting process and martingale theory in Appendix B, we have

$$Var\big(\widehat{\Lambda}_w(t) - \int_0^t J(s)d\Lambda(s)\big) = E\int_0^t \frac{\sum_{i=1}^n w_i^2 Y_i(s)}{\big[\sum_{i=1}^n w_i Y_i(s)\big]^2} J(s)d\Lambda(s).$$

Use the Cauchy-Schwartz inequality to show that

$$\frac{\sum_{i=1}^n w_i^2 Y_i(s)}{\big[\sum_{i=1}^n w_i Y_i(s)\big]^2} \geq \frac{1}{\sum_{i=1}^n Y_i(s)},$$

with equality achieved when $w_i = 1$ for all i.

Therefore, there is nothing to be gained from using $\widehat{\Lambda}_w(t)$ in (5.47) instead of the Nelson-Aalen estimator in the one-sample case. However, in regression models, Yang [332, 334] proposed weighted Nelson-Aalen estimators and weighted Kaplan-Meier estimators using this type of result. These weighted estimators have been applied in various regression models [334, 343, 336].

5.12 (a) Let $A(t)$ be a strictly increasing differentiable function on $[0,\infty)$, with inverse $B(t)$. Suppose that the hazard function of T is $\lambda(t)$. Define the new random variable $\widetilde{T} = A(T)$.

(a) Show that the hazard function of $\widetilde{T}$, denoted by $\widetilde{\lambda}(t)$, is

$$\lambda(B(t))\frac{dB(t)}{dt}.$$

(b) Suppose the conditional hazard function of T given $\boldsymbol{W}$ satisfies model (5.1). Show that the conditional hazard function of $\widetilde{T}$ given $\boldsymbol{W}$ is

$$\widetilde{\lambda}(t;\boldsymbol{W}) = \widetilde{\lambda}_0(t)\exp[h(\boldsymbol{W},\boldsymbol{\beta})],$$

where

$$\widetilde{\lambda}_0(t) = \lambda_0(B(t))\frac{dB(t)}{dt}.$$

That is, $(\widetilde{T},\boldsymbol{W})$ satisfies model (5.1) with the same $\boldsymbol{\beta}$ but different baseline hazard function. In particular, for $h(\boldsymbol{W},\boldsymbol{\beta}) = \beta Z$, β remains the log hazard ratio, treatment over control, for the transformed variable $\widetilde{T}$.

5.13 Consider the null hypothesis $H_0: \theta = 1$ for θ in model (5.38). Denote the common value of Λ_C and Λ_T by Λ_0 under H_0. Then $\widehat{v}_\Psi$ in (5.43) is approximately

$$v(\Psi) = n\Big[\int_0^\infty \Psi^2(t)\frac{d\Lambda_0(t)}{K_T(t)} + \int_0^\infty \Psi^2(t)\frac{d\Lambda_0(t)}{K_C(t)}\Big]\cdot\Big[\int_0^\infty \Psi(t)d\Lambda_0(t)\Big]^{-2}.$$

Use the Cauchy-Schwartz inequality to show that

$$v(\Psi) \geq \left\{ \int_0^\infty \frac{K_C(t)K_T(t)}{K_C(t)+K_T(t)} d\Lambda_0(t) \right\}^{-1},$$

with equality achieved when

$$\Psi(t) = \frac{K_C(t)K_T(t)}{K_C(t)+K_T(t)}.$$

6

Time-Dependent Covariates and Cox Multiplicative Hazards Model

6.1 Introduction

The previous chapter focused on proportional hazards regression analysis, where the effects of baseline variables are assessed similarly to a traditional regression analysis in introductory statistics books. Survival analysis using hazard function provides the opportunity to work with *time-dependent* covariates.

The possibility of using time-dependent multiplicative factor was noted when Cox first introduced the hazard-based model [51]. In the model, the conditional hazard function given covariate $\boldsymbol{W}$ is

$$\lambda(t;\boldsymbol{W}) = \lambda_0(t)\exp\left[h(\boldsymbol{W},\boldsymbol{\beta})\right],$$

where $\lambda_0(t)$ is an unspecified baseline hazard function and $h(\boldsymbol{W},\boldsymbol{\beta})$ is a possibly time-dependent deterministic parametric function of $\boldsymbol{W}$. To distinguish it from the model studied in Chapter Five, here the model will be explicitly written as

$$\lambda(t;\boldsymbol{W}) = \lambda_0(t)\exp\left[h(t;\boldsymbol{W},\boldsymbol{\beta})\right]. \tag{6.1}$$

When $h(t;\boldsymbol{W},\boldsymbol{\beta})$ does not depend on t, model (6.1) reduces to model (5.1).

In Cox [51], a time-dependent $h(t;\boldsymbol{W},\boldsymbol{\beta})$ is used in non-proportional hazards situations. For an unadjusted analysis of a two-arm trial where the assumption of proportional hazards is questionable, one option is to consider the model

$$\lambda(t;Z) = \lambda_0(t)\exp(\beta_1 Z + \beta_2 Zt). \tag{6.2}$$

This model contains an additional artificially defined time-dependent covariate Zt and yields the hazard ratio for treatment

$$\frac{\lambda(t;Z=1)}{\lambda(t;Z=0)} = \exp(\beta_1 + \beta_2 t). \tag{6.3}$$

This hazard ratio is monotone in t, starting from $\exp(\beta_1)$ at $t = 0$ and increases or decreases as t increases.

DOI: 10.1201/9780429324437-6

As another example, if it is believed that the treatment gradually achieves its full effect after t_0 time units, one may consider the model

$$\lambda(t;Z) = \lambda_0(t)\exp\{\beta Z[t/t_0 I(t \le t_0) + I(t > t_0)]\}. \tag{6.4}$$

The hazard ratio is

$$\frac{\lambda(t;Z=1)}{\lambda(t;Z=0)} = \exp\{\beta[t/t_0 I(t \le t_0) + I(t > t_0)]\}, \tag{6.5}$$

which is 1 at $t = 0$, increases or decreases to $\exp(\beta)$ as t increases to t_0, and remains constant afterwards.

Another option is to let $h(t;Z,\boldsymbol{\beta})$ be piecewise constant, yielding the model

$$\lambda(t;Z) = \lambda_0(t)\exp\Big[\sum_{j=1}^{J} \beta_j Z I(t \in I_j)\Big], \tag{6.6}$$

where intervals $I_1, \ldots, I_J$ form a partition of time axis in the data range. Thus

$$\frac{\lambda(t;Z=1)}{\lambda(t;Z=0)} = \exp(\beta_j), \ \ t \in I_j, \ j = 1, \ldots, J. \tag{6.7}$$

That is, β_j is the log hazard ratio over interval I_j, $1 \le j \le J$. Here the model uses J artificially defined time-dependent covariates $ZI(t \in I_j)$, $1 \le j \le J$.

Corresponding to (6.1), the cumulative hazard function is

$$\Lambda(t;\boldsymbol{W}) = \int_0^t \exp[h(x;\boldsymbol{W},\boldsymbol{\beta})]\lambda_0(x)dx, \tag{6.8}$$

the conditional survival function of T given $\boldsymbol{W}$ is

$$S(t;\boldsymbol{W}) = \exp\Big[-\int_0^t \exp[h(x;\boldsymbol{W},\boldsymbol{\beta})]\lambda_0(x)dx\Big], \tag{6.9}$$

and the conditional PDF is

$$f(t;\boldsymbol{W}) = \lambda_0(t)\exp[h(t;\boldsymbol{W},\boldsymbol{\beta})]\exp\{-\int_0^t \exp[h(x;\boldsymbol{W},\boldsymbol{\beta})]\lambda_0(x)dx\}. \tag{6.10}$$

When $h(t;\boldsymbol{W},\boldsymbol{\beta})$ does not depend on t, these functions reduce to (5.6), (5.7), and (5.8), respectively.

As in Chapter Five, the exponential form $\exp[h(t;\boldsymbol{W}.\boldsymbol{\beta})]$ is most widely used for the multiplicative factor. However, other forms, such as $1 + h(t;\boldsymbol{W}.\boldsymbol{\beta})$, are also possible. Again, in those situations, care is needed in both theoretical development and numerical computation to ensure that the quantity is nonnegative.

Although the use of defined time-dependent covariates gives a simple solution in non-proportional hazards situations, it has several limitations, such as being restrictive and data driven, as has been observed in the literature [361]. Chapters Seven and Eight will discuss alternative approaches to addressing non-proportional hazards.

6.2 Time-Dependent Covariates

In the previous section, the covariates were assumed not to change over time, although artificially defined time-dependent covariates were used in the model. However, in certain situations, the covariates themselves may vary over time. Let $\boldsymbol{W}(t)$ be the covariate vector at time t and let $\boldsymbol{W}^h(t)$ be the covariate history from 0 up to, but not including, time t: $\boldsymbol{W}^h(t) = \{\boldsymbol{W}(s), 0 \le s < t\}$. Models can be defined in terms of the conditional hazard function given $\boldsymbol{W}^h(t)$.

With a slight misuse of notation, this conditional hazard function will be denoted by $\lambda[t; \boldsymbol{W}(t)]$ and is given by

$$\lambda[t; \boldsymbol{W}(t)] = \lim_{c \downarrow 0} P\left[t \le T < t + c \middle| T \ge t, \boldsymbol{W}^h(t)\right]/c. \tag{6.11}$$

When models are defined using this conditional hazard function, usually a vector $\mathbf{V}(t)$ that is a function of $\boldsymbol{W}^h(t)$ and t, is used, as in the model $\lambda[t; \boldsymbol{W}(t)] = \alpha + \boldsymbol{\beta}^{\mathrm{T}}\mathbf{V}(t)$. To simplify notation, this model will be written as $\lambda[t; \mathbf{V}(t)] = \alpha + \boldsymbol{\beta}^{\mathrm{T}}\mathbf{V}(t)$, or, to be consistent with previous notations, $\lambda[t; \boldsymbol{W}(t)] = \alpha + \boldsymbol{\beta}^{\mathrm{T}}\boldsymbol{W}(t)$.

At each t, the covariate $\boldsymbol{W}(t)$ is a random vector. Such a collection of random variables or vectors indexed by time t over an interval is called a stochastic process. With this terminology, the time-dependent $\boldsymbol{W}(t)$ will sometimes be called a *covariate process*, and a realization of the process is a *covariate path.* Often there is a technical assumption that $\boldsymbol{W}(t)$ is predictable, which is satisfied when $\boldsymbol{W}(t)$ is left continuous. Precise definitions related to processes are given in Section B.3 of Appendix B.

Two broad categories of time-dependent covariates were introduced by Kalbfleisch and Prentice [131]. A covariate $\boldsymbol{W}(t)$ is *external* if

$$\begin{aligned} & \lim_{c \downarrow 0} P\left[(t \le T < t + c \middle| T \ge t, \boldsymbol{W}^h(t)\right]/c \\ = \quad & \lim_{c \downarrow 0} P\left[t \le T < t + c \middle| T \ge t, \boldsymbol{W}^h(x)\right]/c \end{aligned} \tag{6.12}$$

for any $x \ge t$. This property will be denoted by $\lambda[t; \boldsymbol{W}(t)] = \lambda[t; \boldsymbol{W}(x)],\ x \ge t$.

When $\boldsymbol{W}(t)$ is external, denote the entire covariate path $\{\boldsymbol{W}(s), s \ge 0\}$ by $\boldsymbol{W}^*$ and let $\lambda(t; \boldsymbol{W}^*)$ be the hazard function of T given $\boldsymbol{W}^*$. Then

$$\lambda[t; \boldsymbol{W}(t)] = \lambda(t; \boldsymbol{W}^*).$$

A covariate that is not external is called *internal.*

A fixed covariate $\boldsymbol{W}$, such as those in Chapter Four, is clearly external. Artificially defined covariates, like those in (6.2), (6.4), and (6.6), are also external because the only random component is Z. In these cases, the covariate path is predetermined for each individual. One more such example with predetermined covariate path is age, defined as the time from birth to time t, whether or not the individual is alive. A third type of external covariate is called *ancillary*. This type is determined by a stochastic process external to the individual under study and governed by a probability mechanism that does not share parameters with the model being studied [131]. Examples of this type include the air pollution level in a study of asthma, and a factor under control of researchers that varies externally to the individual under study.

For external covariate $\boldsymbol{W}(t)$, $\lambda[s;\boldsymbol{W}(s)] = \lambda[s;\boldsymbol{W}(t)]$ for $0 \le s \le t$. The latter is a conditional hazard function given the covariate $\boldsymbol{W}^h(t)$ that does not change over $s \in [0,t]$. Thus

$$\begin{aligned} \exp\{-\int_0^t \lambda[s;\boldsymbol{W}(s)]ds\} &= \exp\{-\int_0^t \lambda[s;\boldsymbol{W}(t)]ds\} \\ &= P\big(T > t \big| \boldsymbol{W}^h(t)\big), \end{aligned} \tag{6.13}$$

where the last quantity will be denoted by $S\big[t;\boldsymbol{W}(t)\big]$. The result (6.13) shows that the way the conditional hazard and survival functions determine each other is the same as in the case of fixed covariates. From $\lambda[t;\boldsymbol{W}(t)] = \lambda(t;\boldsymbol{W}^*)$, and (6.13), we also have

$$P\big(T > t \big| \boldsymbol{W}^*\big) = \exp\{-\int_0^t \lambda[s;\boldsymbol{W}^*]ds\} = S\big[t;\boldsymbol{W}(t)\big]. \tag{6.14}$$

So additional information in the covariate path after time t alters neither the hazard function nor the survival function.

An internal covariate is a random process generated by the individual under study, such as blood pressure. Typically, an internal covariate is observed only if the individual has experienced neither event nor censoring. Care is needed for handling internal covariates. Although the conditional hazard function is still defined by (6.11), the relationship (6.13) with the conditional survival function no longer holds. In particular,

$$P\big(T \ge t \big| \boldsymbol{W}^h(t)\big) = 1 \tag{6.15}$$

if $\boldsymbol{W}^h(t)$ indicates that the individual is alive prior to t. More discussions and examples can be found in Kalbfleisch and Prentice[131] and Fisher and Lin [80].

6.3 Cox Multiplicative Hazards Model with Time-Dependent Covariates

Suppose that $\boldsymbol{W}(t)$ is a $p \times 1$ time-dependent covariate vector process. The Cox proportional hazards model $\lambda(t;\boldsymbol{W}) = \lambda_0(t)\exp(\boldsymbol{W}^{\mathrm{T}}\boldsymbol{\beta})$ in (5.3) can be extended to

$$\lambda\left[t;\boldsymbol{W}(t)\right] = \lambda_0(t)\exp\left[\boldsymbol{\beta}^{\mathrm{T}}\boldsymbol{W}(t)\right], \tag{6.16}$$

where components of $\boldsymbol{W}(t)$ may be internal or external. In (6.16), the multiplicative factor has the form $\exp\left[\boldsymbol{\beta}^{\mathrm{T}}\boldsymbol{W}(t)\right]$ as in most applications, although other forms can be considered.

Under certain regularity conditions, the construction of the partial likelihood function, inference for $\boldsymbol{\beta}$ based on the partial likelihood, and the Breslow estimator of the baseline cumulative hazard function $\Lambda_0(t) = \int_0^t \lambda_0(s)ds$, can all be extended to model (6.16), whether $\boldsymbol{W}(t)$ is internal or external [52, 7, 131]. Many other hazard-based procedures can also be extended. Related discussions can be found in Chapters Eleven, Fourteen and Appendix B.

If all covariates are external, the baseline survival function $S_0(t) = \exp\left[-\int_0^t \lambda_0(s)ds\right]$ can be estimated. However, if $\boldsymbol{W}(t)$ contains internal covariates, there is no simple interpretation for $S_0(t)$, therefore the results of statistical analysis should be given in terms of $\Lambda_0(t)$.

An internal covariate is a post-randomization covariate, likely responsive to treatment, which complicates the interpretation of treatment effects. For example, if $\boldsymbol{W}(t) = (Z, V(t))^{\mathrm{T}}$ for the treatment indicator Z and an external covariate $V(t)$ in (6.16), then the coefficient of Z in (6.16), say β_1, is the log hazard ratio of treatment over control, holding $V(t)$ fixed at the same level. However, when $V(t)$ is an internal covariate responsive to treatment, "holding $V(t)$ fixed at the same level" is no longer feasible, and interpretation of β_1 as a measure of treatment effect is no longer valid.

In general, when a possibly treatment-affected internal covariate is included, although model (6.16) provides the conditional instantaneous event rate given the survival experience history, treatment assignment, and covariates, it is not straightforward or even clear how the treatment effect should be measured in the model. Since this book focuses on survival analysis in clinical trials, typically the covariate process $\boldsymbol{W}(t)$ will not include an internal covariate. This approach is consistent with guidelines from the FDA, EMA, and ICH on covariate-adjusted analysis of treatment effects [307, 73, 120].

Nevertheless, time-dependent internal covariates in model (6.16) can offer insights into the mechanism by which the treatment operates. If the internal covariate affects survival but is not affected by treatment—a scenario that is difficult to envision but may still occur—then model (6.16) can be used, and β_1 can be interpreted as the log hazard ratio of treatment over control while holding other covariates fixed at the same levels.

If the internal covariate affects survival and is also influenced by treatment, then model (6.16) describes the conditional instantaneous event rate given $\boldsymbol{W}(t)$, although the treatment effect on this rate can no longer be explained by a simple parameter. In the extreme case where an internal covariate $V(t)$ affects survival and the treatment effect is primarily on lowering or raising values of $V(t)$, it is possible that the treatment has effect on survival, yet β_1, the coefficient of Z, shows little or no treatment effect.

If there is interest in studying the treatment effect both through $V(t)$ and otherwise, it is possible to adopt the approach of joint modeling of longitudinal and time-to-event data [303, 262], although the joint modeling approach was mainly developed to assess within-subject patterns of change in the internal covariate $V(t)$ and the relationship between $V(t)$ and the time-to-event variable T, rather than the treatment effect on the distribution of T [303].

Here we consider the random censorship model with time-dependent external covariate, leaving the discussion on models with internal covariates to Chapter Eleven. The available data from n individuals are $(X_i, \delta_i, \boldsymbol{W}_i)$, where $X_i = T_i \wedge C_i$, $\delta_i = I(T_i \le C_i)$, with T_i, C_i, $\boldsymbol{W}_i(t)$ being, respectively, time to event, time to censoring, and $p \times 1$ time-dependent external covariate process for the ith participant, $p \ge 1$, $i = 1, \cdots, n$. The triplets $\left(T_i,\ C_i,\ \{\boldsymbol{W}_i(t) : t \ge 0\}\right)$, $i = 1, \ldots, n$ are i.i.d. Within each triplet, T_i and C_i are conditionally independent of each other given the entire covariate path $\boldsymbol{W}_i^* = \{\boldsymbol{W}_i(t) : t \ge 0\}$.

Under the above setup, the conditional probability argument in Chapter Five motivating the partial likelihood still applies, except that the participants' history $\mathscr{F}_\ell$ now also contains the covariate path information prior to t_ℓ. The partial likelihood now is

$$\begin{aligned} L(\boldsymbol{\beta}) &= \prod_{i=1}^{n} \left[\frac{\lambda[X_i; \boldsymbol{W}_i(X_i)]}{\sum_{m=1}^{n} Y_m(X_i) \lambda[X_i; \boldsymbol{W}_m(X_i)]} \right]^{\delta_i} \\ &= \prod_{i=1}^{n} \left[\frac{\exp[\boldsymbol{\beta}^{\mathrm{T}} \boldsymbol{W}_i(X_i)]}{\sum_{m=1}^{n} Y_m(X_i) \exp[\boldsymbol{\beta}^{\mathrm{T}} \boldsymbol{W}_m(X_i)]} \right]^{\delta_i}. \qquad (6.17) \end{aligned}$$

Similarly, the score function and information matrix can be extended. The quantities $S^{(m)}(\boldsymbol{\beta}, t)$ in (5.12) are extended to

$$S^{(m)}(\boldsymbol{\beta}, t) = n^{-1} \sum_{i=1}^{n} Y_i(t) \exp[\boldsymbol{\beta}^{\mathrm{T}} \boldsymbol{W}_i(t)] \boldsymbol{W}_i(t)^{\otimes m},$$

for $m = 0, 1, 2$, and the $p \times 1$ score function $\boldsymbol{U}(\boldsymbol{\beta})$ is extended to

$$\boldsymbol{U}(\boldsymbol{\beta}) = \sum_{i=1}^{n} \delta_i [\boldsymbol{W}_i(X_i) - E(\boldsymbol{\beta}, X_i)] = \sum_{i=1}^{n} \int_0^{\infty} [\boldsymbol{W}_i(t) - E(\boldsymbol{\beta}, t)] dN_i(t), \tag{6.18}$$

with

$$E(\boldsymbol{\beta}, t) = S^{(1)}(\boldsymbol{\beta}, t)/S^{(0)}(\boldsymbol{\beta}, t). \tag{6.19}$$

The partial likelihood estimator $\widehat{\boldsymbol{\beta}}$ of $\boldsymbol{\beta}$ is the zero of $\boldsymbol{U}(\boldsymbol{\beta})$. The information matrix is

$$\mathscr{I}(\boldsymbol{\beta}) = -\left(E\frac{\partial^2 \log L}{\partial \beta_j \partial \beta_\ell}\right)_{p\times p}. \tag{6.20}$$

Under certain regularity conditions, at the true parameter value $\boldsymbol{\beta}_0$,

$$\boldsymbol{U}(\boldsymbol{\beta}_0) \sim N\big(0, \mathscr{I}(\boldsymbol{\beta}_0)\big), \tag{6.21}$$

and

$$\widehat{\boldsymbol{\beta}} \sim N\big(\boldsymbol{\beta}_0, \mathscr{I}^{-1}(\boldsymbol{\beta}_0)\big). \tag{6.22}$$

Again, $\mathscr{I}(\boldsymbol{\beta}_0)$ in (6.21) and (6.22) can be replaced with the observed information matrix $\mathbb{I}(\widehat{\boldsymbol{\beta}})$, where

$$\mathbb{I}(\boldsymbol{\beta}) = -\left(\frac{\partial^2 \log L}{\partial \beta_j \partial \beta_\ell}\right)_{p\times p},$$

and $\mathbb{I}(\boldsymbol{\beta})$ can be written as

$$\mathbb{I}(\boldsymbol{\beta}) = \sum_{i=1}^{n} \delta_i \mathbf{V}(\boldsymbol{\beta}, X_i) = \sum_{i=1}^{n} \int_0^{\infty} \mathbf{V}(\boldsymbol{\beta}, t) dN_i(t) \tag{6.23}$$

where

$$\mathbf{V}(\boldsymbol{\beta}, t) = S^{(2)}(\boldsymbol{\beta}, t)/S^{(0)}(\boldsymbol{\beta}, t) - E(\boldsymbol{\beta}, t)^{\otimes 2}. \tag{6.24}$$

Inference on $\boldsymbol{\beta}$ can proceed as in Chapter Five.

Likewise, for the baseline cumulative hazard function $\Lambda_0(t) = \int_0^t \lambda_0(s)ds$, the Breslow estimator is $\widehat{\Lambda}_0(t; \widehat{\boldsymbol{\beta}})$, where

$$\widehat{\Lambda}_0(t; \boldsymbol{\beta}) = \sum_{i=1}^{n} \frac{\delta_i I(X_i \le t)}{\sum_{m=1}^{n} Y_m(X_i) \exp\left[\boldsymbol{\beta}^{\mathrm{T}} \boldsymbol{W}_m(X_i)\right]} = \sum_{i=1}^{n} \int_0^t \frac{dN_i(s)}{nS^{(0)}(\boldsymbol{\beta}, s)}. \tag{6.25}$$

With time-dependent covariate $\boldsymbol{W}(t)$, evaluation of the partial likelihood $L(\boldsymbol{\beta})$ in (6.17) requires availability of $\boldsymbol{W}_m(X_i)$ for (m, i) such that $X_m \ge X_i$ and $\delta_i = 1$. If all participants get randomized at the same calendar time, then each time when $X_{(i)}$ occurs with associated censoring indicator $\delta_{(i)} = 1, i = 1, \ldots, n$, where $X_{(1)} < \cdots < X_{(n)}$ are the order statistics of X_i's, measurements need to be taken for $\boldsymbol{W}$ on the individuals still in the trial (with neither event nor censoring before $X_{(i)}$). This is logistically already very difficult to achieve. In real clinical trials,

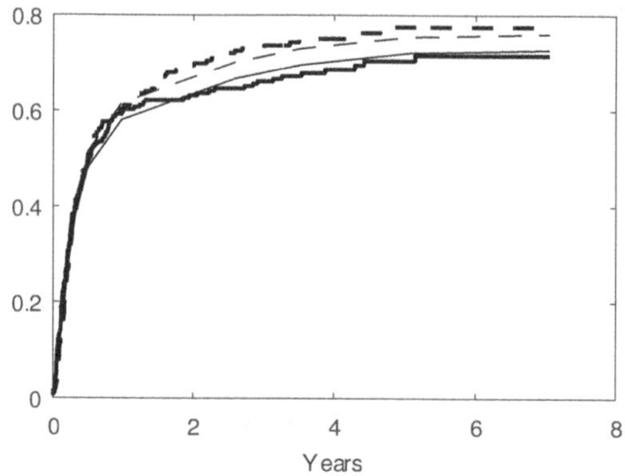

FIGURE 6.1
Estimated CDF for the TCD trial. Thick solid: control group, Kaplan-Meier; thick dashed: treatment group, Kaplan-Meier; thin solid: control group, model (5.4); thin dashed: treatment group, model (5.4).

typically individuals enter the trial in a staggered entry fashion. This makes measurement of $\boldsymbol{W}$ even harder. Practically, measurements of $\boldsymbol{W}$ are only available intermittently, and the "last value carried forward" method is often used in which $\boldsymbol{W}_m(X_i)$ is replaced by the most recent value of $\boldsymbol{W}_m$ before X_i. The concern over bias caused by this method is a major motivating factor behind the approach of joint modeling of longitudinal and time-to-event data [303].

To justify the asymptotic validity of partial likelihood inference, an elegant approach is based on the counting process and martingale theory, an overview of which is given in Appendix B. Andersen and Gill [8] used this approach to establish asymptotic properties for estimators of $\boldsymbol{\beta}$ and $\Lambda_0(t)$ under quite general conditions. More discussions on martingales will be found in Chapters Seven and Eleven. Additionally, modern empirical process theory can also be utilized for asymptotic analysis [310].

Example 6.1. The TCD trial, described in Section 1.20.4, used 3-year disease-free survival as the primary endpoint. This choice does not reflect the survival rate at other time points. The less common approach was adopted due to concerns about non-proportional hazards within the first 6 months [313]. As will be shown in Example 6.2, there is strong evidence of non-proportional hazards. For a visual inspection, consider model (5.4) for data on time to event, defined as the minimum of relapse or death. Figure 6.1 displays the Kaplan-Meier and model-based CDF estimates. The model-based estimates consistently underestimate the group difference for $t > 2$ years.

Now consider model (6.2). Let $\mathbf{0} = (0,0)^{\mathrm{T}}$. For testing $H_0 : \boldsymbol{\beta} = \mathbf{0}$, where $\boldsymbol{\beta} = (\beta_1, \beta_2)^{\mathrm{T}}$, the score test $\boldsymbol{U}(\mathbf{0})^{\mathrm{T}}\mathbb{I}^{-1}(\mathbf{0})\boldsymbol{U}(\mathbf{0})$, where $\boldsymbol{U}$ and $\mathbb{I}$ are the score and observed

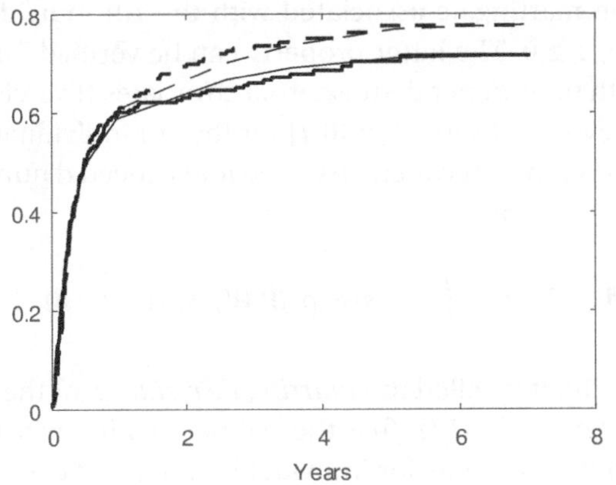

FIGURE 6.2
Estimated CDF for the TCD trial. Thick solid: control group, Kaplan-Meier; thick dashed: treatment group, Kaplan-Meier; thin solid: control group, model (6.2); thin dashed: treatment group, model (6.2).

information in (6.18) and (6.23), respectively, yields a P-value 0.31. The Wald test $\widehat{\boldsymbol{\beta}}^{\mathrm{T}}\mathbb{I}(\mathbf{0})\widehat{\boldsymbol{\beta}}$ has a P-value of 0.33, and the likelihood ratio test has a P-value of 0.50.

Unlike the case for parametric models in Chapter Four, these P-values show some noticeable differences among them. In non-proportional hazards situations, results from the score test, Wald test and likelihood ratio test often show large differences, reflecting the challenges associated with non-proportional hazards analysis. The likelihood ratio test also tends to be more conservative.

The Kaplan-Meier CDF estimates and model-based estimates are displayed in Figure 6.2. The agreement with the Kaplan-Meier estimates is improved for $t > 4$ year. However, between year 2 and year 4, the model-based estimates still consistently underestimate the group difference. An approach with improved fit will be discussed in Chapter Seven.

6.4 Estimating Functions Based on Martingale Residuals

For asymptotic analysis under models to be discussed in Chapters Seven and Eight, it helps to relate the score vector in (6.18) to martingales. Consider the multiplicative hazards model (6.16) with time-dependent covariates. For the ith individual, let

$$M_i(t) = N_i(t) - \int_0^t Y_i(s)\exp(\boldsymbol{\beta}_0^{\mathrm{T}}\boldsymbol{W}_i(s))\,d\Lambda_0(s). \tag{6.26}$$

$M_i(t)$ is called the martingale associated with the ith individual. Under model (6.16), $EM_i(t) \equiv 0,\ t \geq 0$. The latter property can be verified for the random censorship model with time-dependent external covariates (Exercise 6.7). Since $N_i(t)$ is the number of events observed in $[0, t]$ for the ith individual, $M_i(t)$ can be interpreted as the difference between observed and expected numbers of events for individual i in $[0, t]$. Define

$$\widehat{M}_i(t;\boldsymbol{\beta}) = N_i(t) - \int_0^t Y_i(s)\exp(\boldsymbol{\beta}^{\mathrm{T}}\boldsymbol{W}_i(s))d\widehat{\Lambda}_0(s;\boldsymbol{\beta}),\ 1 \leq i \leq n,$$

with $\widehat{\Lambda}_0(s;\boldsymbol{\beta})$ in (6.25). It is called the *martingale residual* for the ith individual under model (6.16), Note that $\widehat{M}_i(t;\widehat{\boldsymbol{\beta}})$ is the estimated difference between observed and expected number of events for individual i in $[0, t]$. It can be verified that the score function in (6.18) can be rewritten as

$$\sum_{i=1}^{n}\int_0^{\infty} \boldsymbol{W}_i(t)\widehat{M}_i(ds;\boldsymbol{\beta}). \tag{6.27}$$

That is, the partial likelihood estimator $\widehat{\boldsymbol{\beta}}$ is zero of the function in (6.27). More generally, a class of estimators can be obtained as zeros of the estimating functions

$$\sum_{i=1}^{n}\int_0^{\infty} \boldsymbol{\Phi}_i(t;\boldsymbol{\beta})\widehat{M}_i(ds;\boldsymbol{\beta}) \tag{6.28}$$

for appropriate data-dependent $p \times 1$ vector functions $\boldsymbol{\Phi}_i, i = 1, \ldots, n$.

The martingale residuals have been extensively used for model checking purposes [15, 297, 178]. They have also been used to generate estimating functions in various models as will be seen in Chapters Seven and Eight.

6.5 Confidence Bands and Monte Carlo Methods

Consider model (6.16) with time-dependent external covariates. From (6.13), for a specific $\boldsymbol{W} = \boldsymbol{w}$ and at the true parameter value $\boldsymbol{\beta}_0$, the survival function is $S(t;\boldsymbol{w}) = \exp\left[-\Lambda(t;\boldsymbol{w})\right]$ where

$$\Lambda\left[t;\boldsymbol{w}\right] = \int_0^t \exp[\boldsymbol{\beta}_0^{\mathrm{T}}\boldsymbol{w}(s)]d\Lambda_0(s),$$

which can be estimated by

$$\begin{aligned}\widehat{\Lambda}(t;\boldsymbol{w}) &= \int_0^t \exp\big[\widehat{\boldsymbol{\beta}}^{\mathrm{T}}\boldsymbol{w}(s)\big]d\widehat{\Lambda}_0(s;\widehat{\boldsymbol{\beta}}) \\ &= \sum_{i=1}^n \int_0^t \frac{\exp\big[\widehat{\boldsymbol{\beta}}^{\mathrm{T}}\boldsymbol{w}(s)\big]dN_i(s)}{nS^{(0)}(\widehat{\boldsymbol{\beta}},s)} \\ &= \sum_{i=1}^n \frac{\delta_i\exp\big[\widehat{\boldsymbol{\beta}}^{\mathrm{T}}\boldsymbol{w}(X_i)\big]I(X_i\le t)}{nS^{(0)}(\widehat{\boldsymbol{\beta}},X_i)} \\ &= \sum_{i=1}^n \frac{\delta_i\exp\big[\widehat{\boldsymbol{\beta}}^{\mathrm{T}}\boldsymbol{w}(X_i)\big]I(X_i\le t)}{\sum_{m=1}^n Y_m(X_i)\exp\big[\widehat{\boldsymbol{\beta}}^{\mathrm{T}}\boldsymbol{W}_m(X_i)\big]}. \qquad (6.29)\end{aligned}$$

From this, $S(t;\boldsymbol{w})$ can be estimated by $\widehat{S}(t;\boldsymbol{w}) = \exp\big[-\widehat{\Lambda}(t;\boldsymbol{w})\big]$.

For large sample behavior of $\widehat{\Lambda}(t;\boldsymbol{w})$, let

$$\mathsf{A}(t;\boldsymbol{w}) = \sqrt{n}\big[\widehat{\Lambda}(t;\boldsymbol{w}) - \Lambda(t;\boldsymbol{w})\big].$$

An overview of convergence of a sequence of random variables or a sequence of stochastic processes is given in Appendices B and C. Analysis of $\mathsf{A}(t;\boldsymbol{w})$ is much simplified when it is approximated by an expression involving the martingales $M_1,\ldots,M_n$. From Andersen and Gill [8], $\mathsf{A}(t;\boldsymbol{w}) - \widetilde{\mathsf{A}}(t;\boldsymbol{w}) \xrightarrow{P} 0$, where

$$\widetilde{\mathsf{A}}(t;\boldsymbol{w}) = \frac{1}{\sqrt{n}}\sum_{i=1}^n\int_0^t \zeta(s;\boldsymbol{\beta}_0)dM_i(s) + \frac{\boldsymbol{\phi}(t;\boldsymbol{\beta}_0)}{\sqrt{n}}\sum_{i=1}^n\int_0^\infty \boldsymbol{\psi}_i(s;\boldsymbol{\beta}_0)dM_i(s) \qquad (6.30)$$

for certain scalar function $\zeta(t;\boldsymbol{\beta})$, $1\times p$ function $\boldsymbol{\phi}(t;\boldsymbol{\beta})$ and $p\times 1$ functions $\boldsymbol{\psi}_i(t;\boldsymbol{\beta})$. From this, it can be shown that $\widetilde{\mathsf{A}}(t;\boldsymbol{w})$, and therefore $\mathsf{A}(t;\boldsymbol{w})$, converges weakly to a Gaussian process with mean zero and variance $\sigma^2(t;\boldsymbol{w})$ that depends on $\boldsymbol{w},\boldsymbol{\beta}_0$ and the function $\Lambda_0(t)$, and that a consistent estimator $\widehat{\sigma}^2(t;\boldsymbol{w})$ of $\sigma^2(t;\boldsymbol{w})$ can obtained by the plug-in method, replacing $\boldsymbol{\beta}_0$ and $\Lambda_0(t)$ by their estimators $\widehat{\boldsymbol{\beta}}$ and $\widehat{\Lambda}_0(t,\widehat{\boldsymbol{\beta}})$, respectively. Therefore,

$$P\big(\sqrt{n}\big|\widehat{\Lambda}(t;\boldsymbol{w}) - \Lambda(t;\boldsymbol{w})\big| \le z(\alpha/2)\widehat{\sigma}(t;\boldsymbol{w})\big) \to 1-\alpha, \qquad (6.31)$$

and an asymptotic $100(1-\alpha)\%$ confidence interval for $\Lambda(t;\boldsymbol{w})$ is $\widehat{\Lambda}(t;\boldsymbol{w}) \mp z(\alpha/2)\widehat{\sigma}(t;\boldsymbol{w})$. From this and the monotone transformation $x \mapsto \exp(-x)$, confidence intervals for $S(t;\boldsymbol{w})$ can be obtained.

In (6.31), the coverage probability is only for one time point t. For two different time points t_1, t_2, we obtain

$$\lim_n P\big(\sqrt{n}\big|\widehat{\Lambda}(t_j;\boldsymbol{w}) - \Lambda(t_j;\boldsymbol{w})\big| \le z_{\alpha/2}\widehat{\sigma}(t_j;\boldsymbol{w})\big) = 1-\alpha, \quad j = 1,2.$$

By the Bonferroni inequality, for the joint coverage probability we can only be assured that

$$\lim_n P\big(\sqrt{n}\big|\widehat{\Lambda}(t_j;\boldsymbol{w}) - \Lambda(t_j;\boldsymbol{w})\big| \le z(\alpha/2)\widehat{\sigma}(t_j;\boldsymbol{w}),\quad j=1,2\big) \ge 1-2\alpha.$$

Often, it is desirable to have simultaneous confidence intervals such that

$$\lim_n P\big(\sqrt{n}\big|\widehat{\Lambda}(t;\boldsymbol{w}) - \Lambda(t;\boldsymbol{w})\big| \le c_\alpha\widehat{\sigma}(t;\boldsymbol{w}), t\in J\big) = 1-\alpha, \tag{6.32}$$

where J is an interval and c_α an appropriate critical value corresponding to the α level. For such purpose, Lin et al. [174] used a Monte Carlo method which was previously proposed for generating null distributions of statistics and processes in model checking by Lin et al. [178]. The basic idea is that for a process such as $\widetilde{\mathsf{A}}(t;\boldsymbol{w})$ in (6.30) that is expressed in terms of integrals with respect to the martingales $M_1,\ldots,M_n$, an approximation can be obtained by replacing $M_i(t)$ with $G_iN_i(t)$, where G_i, $i=1,\ldots,n$ are. *i.i.d.* standard normal variables that are independent from the data. This approximation is based on the fact that

$$EM_i(t)=0,\quad EM_i^2(t)=EN_i(t),\qquad i=1,\ldots,n.$$

Let

$$\begin{aligned}\widehat{\mathsf{A}}(t;\boldsymbol{w}) &= \frac{1}{\sqrt{n}}\sum_{i=1}^{n}\left\{\int_0^t G_i\widehat{\zeta}(s)dN_i(s) + \widehat{\boldsymbol{\phi}}(t)\int_0^\infty \widehat{\boldsymbol{\psi}}_i(s)G_i dN_i(s)\right\}\\ &= \frac{1}{\sqrt{n}}\sum_{i=1}^{n} G_i\delta_i\big[\widehat{\zeta}(X_i)I(X_i\le t) + \widehat{\boldsymbol{\phi}}(t))\widehat{\boldsymbol{\psi}}_i(X_i)\big],\end{aligned} \tag{6.33}$$

where $\widehat{\zeta}$, $\widehat{\boldsymbol{\phi}}$, $\widehat{\boldsymbol{\psi}}_i$ are estimators of ζ, $\boldsymbol{\phi}$, $\boldsymbol{\psi}_i$ from the plug-in method. Given data, $\widehat{\mathsf{A}}(t;\boldsymbol{w})$ is a sum of independent normal random variables. Lin et al. [174] showed that under certain regularity conditions, $\widehat{\mathsf{A}}(t;\boldsymbol{w})$ converges weakly to the same limiting zero-mean Gaussian process as that of $\mathsf{A}(t;\boldsymbol{w})$ for almost all realizations of the data $(X_i,\delta_i,\boldsymbol{W}_i), i\le n$. To approximate the limiting distribution, a large number of realizations from $\widehat{\mathsf{A}}(t;\boldsymbol{w})$ can be obtained by repeatedly generating normal variables $\{G_I : 1\le i\le n\}$ while fixing $(X_i,\delta_i,\boldsymbol{W}_i), i\le n$ at the observed values. From this, a procedure for obtaining c_α and a confidence band is as follows.

1. Use the data and independent standard normal variables G_i's that are independent of the data, to generate the process $\widehat{\mathsf{A}}(t,\boldsymbol{w})$, then evaluate

$$v = \max_{t\in J}\big|\widehat{\mathsf{A}}(t,\boldsymbol{w})/\widehat{\sigma}(t;\boldsymbol{w})\big|.$$

2. Repeat step 1 B times to obtain $v_1,\ldots,v_B$.

3. The sample $100(1-\alpha)$th percentile from the $v_1, \ldots, v_B$ in Step 2 is then the resampling approximation of c_α.

Instead of this Monte Carlo method, the bootstrap [70] can also be considered, which requires computation of $\widehat{\boldsymbol{\beta}}$ a large number of times. The Monte Carlo method above uses only the observed $\widehat{\boldsymbol{\beta}}$ and repeatedly sample normal variables a large number of times, thus has substantially reduced computing cost compared with the bootstrap. Because of this advantage, the Monte Carlo method is often used in other contexts as will be discussed in later chapters.

The choice of B is similar to the number of repetitions for bootstrap. It should be large enough to achieve stability or accuracy of a desired number of digits after the decimal point. Usually several hundreds or thousands are enough.

6.6 Model Adequacy Assessment

The Cox multiplicative hazards model and the partial likelihood inference procedures by now have been implemented in all major statistical software. With the computational ease, the model may sometimes be used when it does not fit the data well.

In certain specific situations, when the Cox model is misspecified, Lin and Wei [176] showed that a test of no treatment effect is still valid with an adjusted robust variance estimator. However, in those situations, the estimand, or the limit of the estimator under the misspecified Cox model, is a complicated functional that depends on censoring. Thus the use of the estimator as a measure of the treatment effect is questionable. In addition, even though the test of no treatment effect is valid, it may not be as powerful as tests obtained under a correctly specified model.

In general, estimation and testing results obtained under a misspecified Cox model may be biased or misleading. In this section, we discuss methods to assess if the model fits a given data set to an acceptable degree.

For an unadjusted analysis in a two-arm trial, a good and quick way to informally examine the model fit is to plot the Kaplan-Meier survival curves together with the model-based survival curve estimates. Good agreement between the model-based and Kaplan-Meier curves indicates an overall good fit by the model. Other functions derived from the survival curves, such as ratio or difference, can also be used for a visual inspection. However, generalizing this visual approach to regression setting is not easy. Furthermore, informal visual inspection needs to be verified by a formal testing procedure, which is usually known as lack-of-fit testing, also called goodness-of-fit testing.

6.6.1 The Two-Sample Case

To formally test adequacy of model (5.4), or equivalently, the condition of proportional hazards for the two groups, various options have been proposed in the literature. The test of Gill and Schumacher [100] has shown to have good power against monotone departures from the proportional hazards assumption, i.e., when the hazard ratio is increasing or decreasing over time. The test procedures are based on the relationship between generalized linear rank tests and estimates of the proportionality constant [6]. The key idea is that two nonparametric estimators of the hazard ratio should be close to each other under model (5.4), while they might be further apart from each other in non-proportional hazards situations.

Suppose that data are available under the two-sample setup described in Section 2.8.2, with hazard functions $\lambda_T(t)$, $\lambda_C(t)$ for the two groups, where the subscripts T and C refer to the treatment and control groups, respectively. Consider the hypothesis testing problem

$$H_0 : \lambda_T/\lambda_C = \theta \quad \text{for some} \quad \theta > 0, \qquad \text{vs.} \qquad H_a : \lambda_T/\lambda_C \text{ is not a constant.}$$

Recall the generalized rank estimator $\widehat{\theta}_\Phi$ discussed in Section 5.7. Let $\widehat{\theta}_\ell$ be the statistic from (5.40) corresponding to $\Psi = \Psi_\ell$, $\ell = 1,2$, respectively. Under H_0, $\widehat{\theta}_1$, $\widehat{\theta}_2$ are estimators of the same quantity θ, thus $\widehat{\theta}_2 - \widehat{\theta}_1 \approx 0$. Under H_a, suppose that $a_n\Psi_\ell$ approaches the limit ψ_ℓ, $\ell = 1,2$, where a_n is a proper scaling factor, and that both $\psi_2(t)/\psi_1(t)$ and $r(t) = \lambda_T(t)/\lambda_C(t)$ are monotone in t. Then it can be shown that $\widehat{\theta}_2 - \widehat{\theta}_1$ approaches a non-zero limit.

Instead of $\widehat{\theta}_2 - \widehat{\theta}_1$, a symmetrized statistic

$$Q_{12} = \int_0^\infty \Psi_2(t)d\widehat{\Lambda}_T(t)\int_0^\infty \Psi_1(t)d\widehat{\Lambda}_C(t) - \int_0^\infty \Psi_1(t)d\widehat{\Lambda}_T(t)\int_0^\infty \Psi_2(t)d\widehat{\Lambda}_C(t),$$

which is a multiple of $\widehat{\theta}_2 - \widehat{\theta}_1$, can be used. For a class of pairs Ψ_1, Ψ_2, a class of Q_{12} is obtained. This is the class of Gill and Schumacher test statistics. Using the counting process and martingale theory, which will be discussed in Chapter Eleven, a variance estimator $\widehat{v}_{12}$ can be obtained. Then the test of proportional hazards rejects H_0 at the $(1-\alpha)100\%$ level when

$$\frac{Q_{12}}{\sqrt{\widehat{v}_{12}}} > z(\alpha/2).$$

Gill and Schumacher recommend using the pair of weights Ψ_{LR}, Ψ_{PP} as the resulting test has certain optimality property. They also recommend against the pair Ψ_{GH}, Ψ_{PP}, where

$$\Psi_{GH} = K_T K_C$$

which corresponds to the Gehan test [87]. This is because such pairing yields a test with no power when there is no censoring.

6.6.2 Regression

If there are only a few baselines covariates in a covariate-adjusted regression analysis and the covariates only have a few levels each, to comparison between groups at different levels of the covariates, the Kaplan-Meier curves can be visually inspected to informally assess the proportionality condition. When some of the covariates are continuous, they are often discretized in order to apply this visual inspection strategy.

As in the two-sample case, visual inspection needs to be supplemented by a procedure for an overall goodness-of-fit assessment. Lin [169] extended the idea of Gill and Schumacher to general regression models. A class of estimation functions was proposed for the regression parameters by incorporating weight functions into the partial likelihood score function. The goodness-of-fit test statistic is the normalized difference between the partial likelihood estimator and an estimator using a proper weight function. Under model (6.16), the test statistic is asymptotically normal with mean zero and with a covariance matrix that can be consistently estimated. With a monotone weight function, the test is consistent against monotone departures from model (6.16). Versatile testing procedures with broad sensitivities can be developed based on simultaneous use of several weight functions.

To introduce Lin's test statistic, recall from (6.18) the score function

$$\boldsymbol{U}(\boldsymbol{\beta}) = \sum_{i=1}^{n} \delta_i [\boldsymbol{W}_i(X_i) - E(\boldsymbol{\beta}, X_i)] = \sum_{i=1}^{n} \int_0^\infty [\boldsymbol{W}_i(t) - E(\boldsymbol{\beta}, t)] dN_i(t).$$

It is the sum over event times (i.e., X_i with $\delta_i = 1,\ i = 1, \ldots, n$) of the difference between the observed value of $\boldsymbol{W}_i(X_i)$ at X_i and the conditional mean of $\boldsymbol{W}_i(X_i)$ on the risk set $\{X_j : X_j \geq X_i\}$, where the conditional mean is with respect to a probability distribution proportional to $\exp\left[\boldsymbol{W}_j(X_i)^{\mathrm{T}}\boldsymbol{\beta}\right]$. Furthermore, the sum assigns the same weight to all event times. Similar to weighted log-rank tests in Chapter Two, unequal weights may be assigned according to the event times. Define a class of weighted score functions

$$\begin{aligned} \boldsymbol{U}_\Phi(\boldsymbol{\beta}) &= \sum_{i=1}^{n} \delta_i \Phi(X_i) \left[\boldsymbol{W}_i(X_i) - E(\boldsymbol{\beta}, X_i)\right] \\ &= \sum_{i=1}^{n} \int_0^\infty \Phi(t) \left[\boldsymbol{W}_i(t) - E(\boldsymbol{\beta}, t)\right] dN_i(t), \end{aligned} \tag{6.34}$$

where Φ is nonnegative and satisfies certain regularity conditions. Let $\widehat{\boldsymbol{\beta}}_\Phi$ be the zero of $\boldsymbol{U}_\Phi(\boldsymbol{\beta})$. Then similar to the large sample theory for the partial likelihood estimator, it can be shown that under model (6.16), at the true parameter $\boldsymbol{\beta}_0$,

$$\sqrt{n}(\widehat{\boldsymbol{\beta}}_\Phi - \boldsymbol{\beta}_0) \xrightarrow{d} N(, \Sigma_\Phi),$$

where the limiting covariance matrix Σ_Φ can be consistently estimated by $\boldsymbol{C}_\Phi(\widehat{\boldsymbol{\beta}}) = \boldsymbol{A}_\Phi(\widehat{\boldsymbol{\beta}})^{-1}\boldsymbol{B}_\Phi(\widehat{\boldsymbol{\beta}}))^{-1}\boldsymbol{A}_\Phi(\widehat{\boldsymbol{\beta}})^{-1}$, where

$$\boldsymbol{A}_\Phi(\boldsymbol{\beta}) = n^{-1}\sum_{i=1}^{n}\delta_i\Phi(X_i)\mathbf{V}(\boldsymbol{\beta}, X_i), \tag{6.35}$$

$$\boldsymbol{B}_\Phi(\boldsymbol{\beta}) = n^{-1}\sum_{i=1}^{n}\delta_i\Phi^2(X_i)\mathbf{V}(\boldsymbol{\beta}, X_i), \tag{6.36}$$

with $\mathbf{V}(\boldsymbol{\beta}, t)$ in (6.24). Let $\widehat{\boldsymbol{\beta}}$ be the partial likelihood estimator under (6.16). Lin showed that under model (6.16), $\sqrt{n}(\widehat{\boldsymbol{\beta}}_\Phi - \widehat{\boldsymbol{\beta}})$ converges in distribution to the p-variate normal distribution with mean zero and variance that can be consistently estimated by $\boldsymbol{D}_\Phi(\widehat{\boldsymbol{\beta}}) = \boldsymbol{C}_\Phi(\widehat{\boldsymbol{\beta}}) - \boldsymbol{C}(\widehat{\boldsymbol{\beta}})$, where $\boldsymbol{C}$ is $\boldsymbol{C}_\Phi$ with $\Phi = 1$. Thus a goodness of-fit-test with weight Φ rejects model (6.16) when

$$Q_\Phi > \chi_p^2(\alpha), \tag{6.37}$$

where

$$Q_\Phi = n(\widehat{\boldsymbol{\beta}}_\Phi - \widehat{\boldsymbol{\beta}})^{\mathrm{T}}\boldsymbol{D}_\Phi^{-1}(\widehat{\boldsymbol{\beta}})(\widehat{\boldsymbol{\beta}}_\Phi - \widehat{\boldsymbol{\beta}}). \tag{6.38}$$

Under an alternative hypothesis of non-proportional hazards, an estimating function with an increasing weight leads to a $\widehat{\boldsymbol{\beta}}_\Phi$ that is more influenced by the hazards ratio at late event times than the hazard ratio at early event times. Thus $\widehat{\boldsymbol{\beta}}_\Phi$ will reflect a larger treatment effect than $\widehat{\boldsymbol{\beta}}$ when the hazard ratio is increasing. For $p = 1$, Lin showed that the test in (6.37) with a monotone Φ is consistent against monotone departures from model (6.16).

Since monotone departures from the proportionality are the most common and most important forms of model misspecification in applications, often the weight $\Phi = \widehat{S}_-$ is used, where $\widehat{S}_-$ is the left limit of the Kaplan-Meier estimator computed from the pooled sample. When the censoring is heavy, as in the example of the WHI E+P trial where the censoring rate is about 98%, the weight $\widehat{S}_-(t) \approx 1$ for all t. To better reflect monotone departures from the proportionality condition, an obvious modification is to use the weight function

$$\widehat{S}_-(t) - \widehat{S}_-(d^*),$$

where d^* is the duration of the trial. This weight is not quite the type of weight functions traditionally used which are required to be predictable. Buyske et al. [31] showed that the asymptotic normality and the variance formula are still valid for modified weights of the form $(\widehat{S}_-(t) - \widehat{S}_-(d^*))^\rho(1-\widehat{S}_-(t))^\gamma, \rho, \gamma \geq 0$. Since $\widehat{S}_-(d^*) = \widehat{S}_-(\max_i X_i)$, it is unnecessary to know d^* which may not be reported in some trials.

In addition to $\widehat{S}_-(t)$ or $\widehat{S}_-(t) - \widehat{S}_-(d^*)$, other weight functions may be supplemented to increase power against non-monotone alternatives. For example, the test with $\Phi(t) = (\widehat{S}_{-}(t) - \widehat{S}_{-}(d^*))(1 - \widehat{S}_{-}(t))$ is sensitive to quadratic trends. To preserve a given overall Type I error probability when several weight functions are used simultaneously, a global test can be obtained using several different weight functions.

When the test rejects model (6.16), the sources of model misspecification can be identified by inspecting component-wise differences between $\widehat{\boldsymbol{\beta}}_{\Phi}$ and $\widehat{\boldsymbol{\beta}}$. If a particular component of the covariate vector shows a significant P-value for the difference, options that could improve the model fit include transformation of the variable, stratified analysis, and inclusion of defined time-dependent covariates as exemplified by models (6.2), (6.4) and (6.6). Other possibilities will be discussed in Chapter Seven.

In the two-sample case, the test in (6.37) does not reduce to the test of Gill and Schumacher (1987). The is because the latter employs the generalized rank estimators rather than estimators using weighted score functions. Unlike the variance estimator used by Gill and Schumacher, the variance estimator for the test in (6.37) is always nonnegative.

Lin's test formalizes a graphical technique suggested by Schoenfeld (1982). Schoenfeld (1982) defined partial residuals for the proportional hazards model as the difference between the observed covariate value $\boldsymbol{W}_i(X_i)$ and its estimated conditional expectation $E(\widehat{\boldsymbol{\beta}}, t)$ in (6.19). These residuals can be plotted against the time axis to visually examine the fit of the model and detect outlying covariate values.

Example 6.2. For the TCD trial, consider model (5.4) for data on time to event, the minimum of relapse or death. Lin's lack-of-fit test with weight $\Phi_0(t) = \widehat{S}_{-}(t) - \widehat{S}_{-}(d^*)$ has a P-value of 0.02. This weight will be used in future applications of Lin's lack-of-fit test unless otherwise mentioned.

The test reveals strong evidence of non-proportional hazards. As illustrated in Figure 6.1, one consequence of model misspecification is the consistent underestimation of the group difference.

Since the non-proportionality is associated with the treatment indicator, there is no remedy via a stratified analysis. However, the model in Chapter Seven provides an alternative that fits the data well.

Example 6.3. For an unadjusted analysis of the TOPCAT trial's primary endpoint, consider the two-sample Cox model (5.4). Lin's lack-of-fit test with weight $\Phi_0(t)$ yields a P-value of 0.21. Visually, Figure 5.1 also shows good agreement with the Kaplan-Meier estimates.

Next, for the pre-specified covariate-adjusted analysis in TOPCAT mentioned in Example 5.2, let the covariates Z and $W_1 - W_3$ be as defined in Example 5.2, and let W_4 be the standardized age at the baseline. The covariate-adjusted model is

$$\lambda(t; \boldsymbol{W}) = \lambda_0(t) \exp\left(\beta_1 Z + \beta_2 W_1 + \beta_3 W_2 + \beta_4 W_3 + \beta_5 W_4\right). \tag{6.39}$$

For this model, Lin's lack-of-fit test with weight $\Phi_0(t)$ has a P-value of 0.03.

Let $\boldsymbol{z}_\Phi = (z_1, \ldots, z_5)^{\mathrm{T}}$, where

$$z_j = \sqrt{n}(\widehat{\beta}_j - \beta_j)/s_j,$$

with s_j being the square root of the (j, j) element of the estimated covariance matrix $\boldsymbol{D}_\Phi(\widehat{\boldsymbol{\beta}})$. The z_j's are the standardized component differences between $\widehat{\boldsymbol{\beta}}_\Phi$ and $\widehat{\boldsymbol{\beta}}$. They help identify which covariate components contribute to significance of the test in (6.37). For model (6.39), we have

$$\boldsymbol{z}_\Phi = (1.36, -0.22, 0.99, 0.82, -2.93)^{\mathrm{T}}.$$

This shows that the non-proportionality results from W_4, the standardized age at the baseline.

If the square of W_4 is added to the model, the lack-of-fit test remains significant with a P-value 0.01. Alternatively, if the standardized log(age) is used instead of the standardized age, the lack-of-fit test is also significant with a P-value 0.02. Furthermore, when fitting the Cox model to the single dichotomous covariate $W = I(age > 69)$, the lack-of-fit test is significant with a more extreme P-value of 0.005.

These results illustrate some of the drawbacks of pre-specifying a covariate-adjusted analysis in clinical trials. Related discussions can be found in Section 1.12. To minimize the risk of misspecifying a model, for the primary analysis of a clinical trial, it is advisable to use either an unadjusted analysis or a reliable and proven covariate-adjusted model.

In this example, the non-proportionality stems from a covariate. As shown in Example 5.2, a stratified analysis provides a simple remedy. It allows the log hazard ratio for the treatment variable to be a straightforward parameter for testing and describing the treatment effect, although this approach has several drawbacks as discussed in Section 5.4.

In Chapter Seven, an alternative approach will be discussed that addresses the non-proportionality of age. This approach retains the simplicity of testing and describing the treatment effect using the log hazard ratio of the treatment variable and does not require stratification.

6.7 Exercises and Complements

6.1 For model (6.2), derive the score vector and the information matrix.

6.2 For model (6.4), derive the score vector and the information matrix.

6.3 Consider the model

$$\lambda(t; Z_i) = \begin{cases} \lambda_0(t)e^{\beta_1 Z_i}, & \text{if } t < a \\ \lambda_0(t)e^{\beta_2 Z_i}, & \text{if } t \geq a \end{cases}$$

where $a > 0$ is a known constant. Derive the score function and the observed information matrix.

6.4 (a) Differentiate the partial likelihood $L(\boldsymbol{\beta})$ in (6.17) to obtain the score function.

(b) Use the counting process notation to show that the score function can be written in the form given in (6.18).

Hint: Remember that

$$\int_0^\infty g(t)dN_i(t) = g(X_i)\delta_i.$$

(c) Obtain the observed information matrix.

6.5 For the Breslow estimator in (6.25), extend the arguments for (5.19) and (5.20) to show that at the true parameter $\boldsymbol{\beta}_0$, $\widehat{\Lambda}(t; \boldsymbol{\beta}_0)$ is close to $\Lambda_0(t)$.

6.6 Suppose the conditional hazard function of T given $\boldsymbol{W}$ satisfies a piecewise proportional hazards model:

$$\lambda(t; Z) = \lambda_0(t)\exp\left[\beta_1 Z I(t < a) + \beta_2 Z I(t \geq a)\right],$$

where $a > 0$ is a known constant. That is, β_1 is the log hazard ratio on $t \in [0, a)$ and β_2 is the log hazard ratio on $t \in [a, \infty)$. Let $A(t)$ be a strictly increasing differentiable function on $[0, \infty)$, with inverse $B(t)$. Define the new random variable $\widetilde{T} = A(T)$. Prove that the conditional hazard function of $\widetilde{T}$ given $\boldsymbol{W}$, denoted by $\widetilde{\lambda}(t; Z)$, is also a piecewise proportional hazards model:

$$\widetilde{\lambda}(t; Z) = \widetilde{\lambda}_0(t)\exp\left[\beta_1 Z I\big(t < A(a)\big) + \beta_2 Z I\big(t \geq A(a)\big)\right],$$

where

$$\widetilde{\lambda}_0(t) = \lambda_0(B(t))\frac{dB(t)}{dt}.$$

Thus for the transformed variable $\widetilde{T}$, β_1 is the log hazard ratio on $t \in [0, A(a))$ and β_2 is the log hazard ratio on $t \in [A(a), \infty)$. Therefore, the interpretation of β_1 and β_2 depends on the transformation. This is different from the case in Chapter Five where a fixed covariate is considered.

6.7 For $M_i(t)$ in (6.26), show that $EM_i(t) = 0$ for any t under the random censorship model with time-dependent external covariates.

6.8 Note that $M_i(t)$ in (6.26) depends on the parameter $\boldsymbol{\beta}$ and the baseline function $\Lambda_0(t)$. To derive an estimator $\widetilde{\Lambda}_n(t)$ for $\Lambda_0(t)$, let

$$\widetilde{M}_i(t) = N_i(t) - \int_0^t Y_i(s)\exp(\boldsymbol{\beta}^{\mathrm{T}}\boldsymbol{W}_i(s))d\widetilde{\Lambda}(s).$$

Since $\sum_{i=1}^n EM_i(t) = 0$, it is reasonable to require $\widetilde{\Lambda}(t)$ to satisfy

$$\sum_{i=1}^n \widetilde{M}_i(t) = 0, \qquad t \geq 0.$$

That is, for any t,

$$\sum_{i=1}^n N_i(t) = n\int_0^t S^{(0)}(\boldsymbol{\beta}, s)d\widetilde{\Lambda}(s).$$

Taking the differential of both sides yields

$$\sum_{i=1}^n dN_i(t) = nS^{(0)}(\boldsymbol{\beta}, t)d\widetilde{\Lambda}(t).$$

Solving for $d\widetilde{\Lambda}(t)$ we get

$$d\widetilde{\Lambda}(t) = \frac{\sum_{i=1}^n dN_i(t)}{n\, S^{(0)}(\boldsymbol{\beta}, t)}.$$

Therefore,

$$\widetilde{\Lambda}(t) = \int_0^t d\widetilde{\Lambda}(s) = \int_0^t \frac{\sum_{i=1}^n dN_i(s)}{n\, S^{(0)}(\boldsymbol{\beta}, s)},$$

which is the Breslow estimator. Chen, Jin and Ying [38] used this type of argument, requiring the sum of martingale residuals to be identically zero, to propose an estimating equation for transformation models.

6.9 Suppose that $X_1, \ldots, X_n$ are i.i.d. with mean μ and variance σ^2. By the central limit theorem, we have

$$\sqrt{n}(\bar{X}_n - \mu) \xrightarrow{d} N(0, \sigma^2).$$

Thus a confidence interval for μ can be obtained as

$$\bar{X}_n \mp z(\alpha/2)\frac{\widehat{\sigma}}{\sqrt{n}},$$

where

$$\widehat{\sigma}^2 = \frac{1}{n-1}\sum_{i=1}^n (X_i - \bar{X}_n)^2.$$

Resampling methods, such as the bootstrap, can also be used.

Now consider a Monte Carlo method. Let

$$\widetilde{X}_n = \frac{1}{n}\sum_{i=1}^{n}(X_i - \bar{X}_n)G_i,$$

where G_i's are i.i.d. standard normal variables independent of the data.

(a) Show that given data, the mean of $\widetilde{X}_n$ is 0.

(b) Show that given data, the variance of $\widetilde{X}_n$ is $\sum_{i=1}^{n}(X_i - \bar{X}_n)^2/n^2$. which is a consistent estimator of the variance of $\bar{X}_n$. Therefore, the sample variance, v_n, from a large number of realizations of $\widetilde{X}_n$, can be used as an estimator of the variance of $\bar{X}_n$, σ^2/n. It follows that a confidence interval can be obtained as

$$\bar{X}_n \mp z(\alpha/2)\sqrt{v}_n.$$

6.10 Consider the weighted score function $\boldsymbol{U}_\Phi(\boldsymbol{\beta})$ in (6.34).

(a) Show that under model (6.16),

$$\boldsymbol{U}_\Phi(\boldsymbol{\beta}) = \sum_{i=1}^{n}\int_0^\infty \Phi(t)\left[\boldsymbol{W}_i(t) - E(\boldsymbol{\beta}, t)\right]\{dN_i(t) - Y_i(t)\exp\left[\boldsymbol{\beta}^{\mathrm{T}}\boldsymbol{W}_i(t)\right]d\Lambda_0(t)\}.$$

From this result and martingale theory in Chapter Eleven and Appendix B, it follows that if $\boldsymbol{W}_i(t)$'s and $\Phi(t)$ are predictable, then at the true parameter value $\boldsymbol{\beta}_0$,

$$E\boldsymbol{U}_\Phi(\boldsymbol{\beta}_0) = 0.$$

Hint: Let

$$J(t) = \sum_{i=1}^{n} Y_i(t)\exp[\boldsymbol{\beta}^{\mathrm{T}}\boldsymbol{W}_i(t)].$$

Then $J(t) > 0$ if and only if $\max_i X_i \le t$. Consider the ranges $J(t) > 0$ and $J(t) = 0$ separately and simplify.

(b) Let $\boldsymbol{W}_i(t) = (W_{i1}(t), \ldots, W_{ip}(t))^{\mathrm{T}}$ and $E(\boldsymbol{\beta}, t) = (e_1(t), \ldots, e_p(t))^{\mathrm{T}}$, for $E(\boldsymbol{\beta}, t)$ in (6.19). Define the matrix $\mathbf{V} = (v_{jk})$, where the (j,k) element is

$$\begin{aligned} v_{jk} &= \sum_{i=1}^{n}\int_0^\infty \Phi^2(t)\left\{W_{ij}(t) - e_j(t)\right\} \\ &\quad \cdot\left\{W_{ik}(t) - e_k(t)\right\} \\ &\quad \cdot Y_i(t)\exp\left[\boldsymbol{\beta}^{\mathrm{T}}\boldsymbol{W}_i(t)\right]d\Lambda_0(t). \end{aligned}$$

Show that

$$\mathbf{V} = n\int_0^\infty \Phi^2(t)\Big\{S^{(2)}(\boldsymbol{\beta},t) - \frac{S^{(1)}(\boldsymbol{\beta},t)\big[S^{(1)}(\boldsymbol{\beta},t)\big]^{\mathrm{T}}}{S^{(0)}(\boldsymbol{\beta},t)}\Big\}d\Lambda_0(t).$$

Replacing $\Lambda_0(t)$ by the Breslow estimator in (6.25), we obtain an estimator of $\mathbf{V}$. For $\Phi = 1$, show that this estimator coincides with the observed information matrix in (6.23).

(c) Show that the Jacobian matrix of $\boldsymbol{U}_\Phi(\boldsymbol{\beta})$ is

$$\frac{\partial \boldsymbol{U}_\Phi(\boldsymbol{\beta})}{\partial \boldsymbol{\beta}} = -\int_0^\infty \Phi(t)\mathbf{V}(\boldsymbol{\beta},t)dN_i(t).$$

(d) Consider model (6.16) with $\boldsymbol{\beta}^{\mathrm{T}}\boldsymbol{W} = \beta Z$. For this case, denote $\widehat{\boldsymbol{\beta}}$, $\widehat{\boldsymbol{\beta}}_\Phi$ and $\mathbf{V}(\boldsymbol{\beta},t)$ by $\widehat{\beta}, \widehat{\beta}_\Phi$ and $v(\beta,t)$, respectively. By the counting process and martingale theory, the variance in the limiting distribution of $\sqrt{n}(\widehat{\beta}_\Phi - \widehat{\beta})$ can be approximated by

$$v_\Phi = \frac{n\sum_{i=1}^n \int_0^\infty \Phi^2(t)v(\beta,t)dN_i(t)}{\Big[\sum_{i=1}^n \int_0^\infty \Phi(t)v(\beta,t)dN_i(t)\Big]^2}.$$

Use the Cauchy-Schwartz inequality to show that

$$v_\Phi \geq \frac{n}{\sum_{i=1}^n \int_0^\infty v(\beta,t)dN_i(t)},$$

with equality achieved when $\Phi(t) \equiv 1$.

6.11 Consider a general multiplicative hazards model

$$\lambda\big[t;\boldsymbol{W}(t)\big] = \lambda_0(t)h\big[t;\boldsymbol{W}(t),\boldsymbol{\beta}\big], \tag{6.40}$$

where $h\big[t;\boldsymbol{W}(t),\boldsymbol{\beta}\big] > 0$. Let

$$\widetilde{\boldsymbol{U}}(\boldsymbol{\beta}) = \sum_{m=1}^n \int_0^\infty \Big\{\boldsymbol{W}_m(t) - \frac{\sum_{i=1}^n Y_i(t)\boldsymbol{W}_i h\big[t;\boldsymbol{W}_i(t),\boldsymbol{\beta}\big]}{\sum_{i=1}^n Y_i(t)h\big[t;\boldsymbol{W}_i(t),\boldsymbol{\beta}\big]}\Big\}dN_m(t).$$

(a) Show that

$$\begin{aligned}\widetilde{\boldsymbol{U}}(\boldsymbol{\beta}) \quad &= \quad \sum_{m=1}^n \int_0^\infty \Big\{\boldsymbol{W}_m(t) - \frac{\sum_{i=1}^n Y_i(t)\boldsymbol{W}_i h\big[t;\boldsymbol{W}_i(t),\boldsymbol{\beta}\big]}{\sum_{i=1}^n Y_i(t)h\big[t;\boldsymbol{W}_i(t),\boldsymbol{\beta}\big]}\Big\} \\ &\quad\quad \big\{dN_m(t) - Y_m(t)h\big[t;\boldsymbol{W}_m(t),\boldsymbol{\beta}\big]d\Lambda_0(t)\big\}.\end{aligned}$$

From this result and martingale theory in Chapter Eleven and Appendix B, it follows that under model (6.40), at the true parameter value $\boldsymbol{\beta}_0$,

$$E\widetilde{\boldsymbol{U}}(\boldsymbol{\beta}_0) = 0.$$

7

The Model of Short-Term and Long-Term Hazard Ratios

7.1 Introduction

During exploratory data analysis, various parametric models from Chapter Three can be evaluated to arrive at the best model using criteria such as likelihood maximization, or minimization of AIC [4] or BIC [275]. One can also use spline models [272, 315] which typically involve more parameters or degrees of freedom [352]. However, confirmatory clinical trials necessitate pre-specification of objectives and analysis procedures before data collection or unblinding, which precludes exploring multiple models.

The hazard-focused Cox models discussed in the previous two chapters offer more robust options than parametric models. However, even these models may lack the flexibility to accommodate unexpected data patterns. For example, in the WHI E+P trial, careful planning based on prior studies led to the postulation that a full-compliance incidence-rate reduction of 30% would be achieved linearly over the first 3 years after randomization [296]. Nine years later, however, the data revealed crossing hazard functions, resulting in hazard ratio values close to 2 at the beginning of the trial and 0.7 near the end [249, 347].

Thus, flexible and robust models are necessary to accommodate diverse scenarios while maintaining efficiency. Although the proportional hazards model often provides a reasonable approximation, situations arise where the proportionality assumption is violated. A treatment may have long-term benefit but early adverse effects. Alternatively, for curable diseases, while the long-term survival rates in the treatment and control groups may be equal, deaths in the control group may occur earlier [28]. There are also situations where the treatment effect gradually increases or diminishes over time. In general, the longer the follow-up period is, the more likely it is for various non-proportional scenarios to develop, resulting in crossing hazard functions and, in extreme cases, crossing survival functions.

Even when deviations from proportionality are not severe, sub-optimal model fit may reduce test power or estimate precision. Therefore, alternative models allowing for non-proportional hazards are necessary.

DOI: 10.1201/9780429324437-7

In Chapter Six, defined time-dependent covariates are used in non-proportional situations. However, those convenient and ad hoc solutions have various limitations. Models (6.2) and (6.4) constrain the log hazard ratio to specific forms, while model (6.6) introduces higher degrees of freedom and discontinuous hazard ratios. The partition in (6.6) may be difficult to pre-specify, and different partitions can yield opposite log hazard ratio shapes [337]. Increasing number of parameters or degrees of freedom raises the risk of overfitting, potentially compromising generalizability. These models also imply fully parametric hazard ratios, which is less flexible than semiparametric alternatives. The limitations of these models and the challenges in utilizing them in clinical trials will be demonstrated through various real data applications later in this chapter.

Early literature on non-proportional hazards focused on stratification, with modeling attention primarily on the accelerated failure time and proportional odds models, These two models will be discussed in Chapter Eight. This chapter discusses a model closely connected to the Cox proportional hazards and multiplicative hazards models.

7.2 Formulation of the Model

Assume that the conditional distribution of T given the treatment indicator Z is absolutely continuous. Let the hazard and survival functions in the control and treatment groups be $\lambda_C(t)$, $S_C(t)$ and $\lambda_T(t)$, $S_T(t)$ respectively. Yang and Prentice [344] developed a model defined by

$$\lambda_T(t) = \frac{\theta_1\theta_2}{\theta_1 + (\theta_2 - \theta_1)S_C(t)}\lambda_C(t),\ t < \tau_0, \tag{7.1}$$

where $\tau_0 = \sup\{t : S_C(t) > 0\}$, and θ_1 and θ_2 are positive.

Under this model, the hazard ratio is determined semiparametrically by

$$\frac{\lambda_T(t)}{\lambda_C(t)} = \frac{\theta_1\theta_2}{\theta_1 + (\theta_2 - \theta_1)S_C(t)}. \tag{7.2}$$

This ratio is increasing if $\theta_2 > \theta_1$ and decreasing if $\theta_1 > \theta_2$. Also,

$$\theta_1 = \lim_{t\downarrow 0}\frac{\lambda_T(t)}{\lambda_C(t)},\ \theta_2 = \lim_{t\uparrow \tau_0}\frac{\lambda_T(t)}{\lambda_C(t)}. \tag{7.3}$$

Therefore, θ_1 and θ_2 can be interpreted as the short-term and long-term hazard ratios, respectively.

Let

$$R_C(t) = \frac{1 - S_C(t)}{S_C(t)},\ t < \tau_0. \tag{7.4}$$

Then

$$S_C(t) = \{1 + R_C(t)\}^{-1},\ S_T(t) = \left\{1 + \frac{\theta_1}{\theta_2} R_C(t)\right\}^{-\theta_2}. \tag{7.5}$$

It follows that S_C and S_T cross if either $\theta_1 < 1$ and $\theta_2 > 1$, or $\theta_1 > 1$ and $\theta_2 < 1$.

Let $\lambda_Z(t)$ be the conditional hazard function of T given Z. Then, an equivalent way to define the model of short-term and long-term hazard ratios is to specify that

$$\lambda_Z(t) = \frac{1}{\exp(-\beta_1 Z) + \exp(-\beta_2 Z) R(t)} \frac{dR(t)}{dt}. \tag{7.6}$$

for some scalar parameters β_1 and β_2 and an unknown increasing baseline function $R(t)$. This is exactly model (7.1) with

$$\beta_1 = \log\theta_1,\ \beta_2 = \log\theta_2,\ R(t) = R_C(t).$$

However, an advantage of the reformulated model (7.6) is that it does not involve the survival function of the control group. This facilitates easy extension to competing risks analysis, a topic that will be addressed in Chapter Thirteen. From (7.6),

$$R(t) = \exp[\Lambda_0(t)] - 1,$$

where $\Lambda_0(t) = \int_0^t \lambda_{Z=0}(x)dx$.

Model (7.6) is semiparametric with scalar parameters β_1, β_2 and infinite dimensional parameter $R(t)$. By leaving $R(t)$ unspecified, the model provides flexibility to accommodate a wide range of hazard ratio scenarios.

In comparison, the Cox model implies a constant hazard ratio, and the proportional odds model, to be discussed in Chapter Eight, implies a monotone hazard ratio that converges to unity as t increases. Model (7.1) contains the Cox model and the proportional odds model as two sub-models, corresponding to $\theta_1 = \theta_2$ and $\theta_2 = 1$, respectively. The case $\theta_1 = 1$ corresponds to the scenario when the effect progresses gradually, and the case $\theta_1 > 1, \theta_2 < 1$ describes a situation of long-term benefit with early adverse effect. Figure 7.1 illustrates the hazard ratio function for selected values of $\boldsymbol{\theta} = (\theta_1, \theta_2)$ when S_C follows the unit exponential distribution. Figure 7.2 displays the corresponding survival functions for the cases shown in Figure 7.1.

Model (7.6) is transformation-preserving in the sense that, if the conditional hazard of T given Z satisfies model (7.6), and A is smooth and strictly increasing with inverse B, then the conditional hazard of $\widetilde{T} = A(T)$ given Z is

$$\widetilde{\lambda}_Z(t) = \frac{1}{\exp(-\beta_1 Z) + \exp(-\beta_2 Z)\widetilde{R}(t)} \frac{d\widetilde{R}(t)}{dt}, \tag{7.7}$$

where $\widetilde{R}(t) = R(B(t))$. Hence model (7.6) still holds for the transformed variable, with the same short-term and long-term hazard ratio scalar parameters.

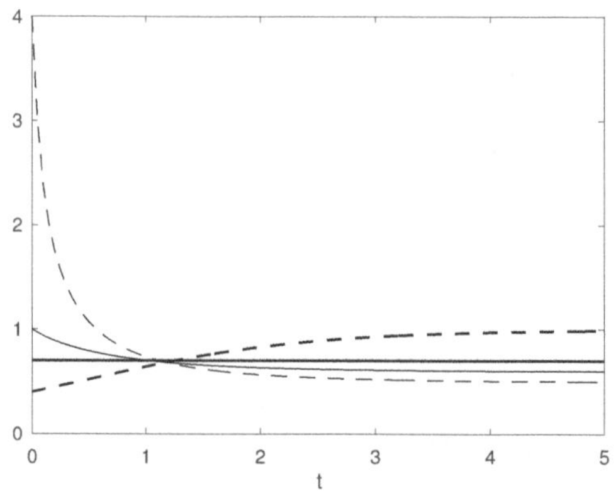

FIGURE 7.1
Hazard ratios for various treatment effect scenarios under model (7.1), with unit exponential $S_C(t)$. Thick solid—proportional hazards; thick dashed—proportional odds; thin solid—gradual effect progression; thin dashed—long-term benefit with early adverse effect.

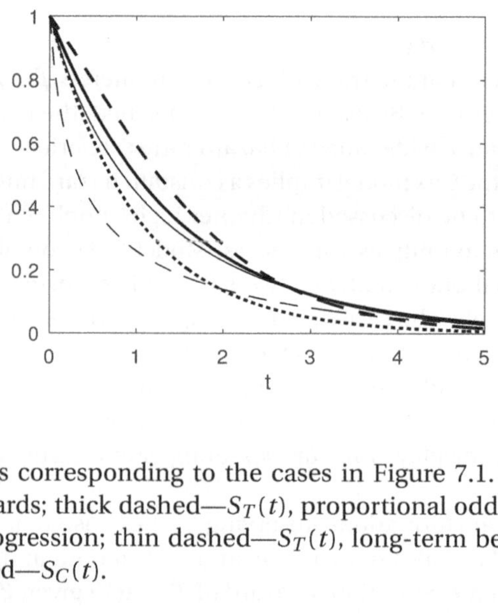

FIGURE 7.2
Survival functions corresponding to the cases in Figure 7.1. Thick solid—$S_T(t)$, proportional hazards; thick dashed—$S_T(t)$, proportional odds; thin solid—$S_T(t)$, gradual effect progression; thin dashed—$S_T(t)$, long-term benefit with early adverse effect; dotted—$S_C(t)$.

The Cox model with time-independent covariates has this transformation-preserving property, and the corresponding partial likelihood estimator is a rank estimator. Parallel to these results, model (7.6) continues to have this transformation-preserving property, and the pseudo likelihood estimator under (7.6), to be introduced in Section 7.4, remains a rank estimator. Rank estimators are typically more robust against the influence of outliers in data compared to other estimators. This robustness is a major motivation in deriving rank related tests and estimators in survival analysis and other statistical fields.

It's important to note, however, that when the Cox multiplicative hazards model contains time-dependent covariates, as in models (6.2), (6.4), and (6.6), the partial likelihood estimators are no longer rank estimators. This loss of robustness partly motivates the derivation of alternative models, such as (7.6), for situations involving possibly non-proportional hazards.

Under substantial censoring, there may be little or no data near τ_0. In this case, the parameters θ_1 and θ_2 remain identifiable. The parameter θ_1 still has the short-term hazard ratio interpretation, as the limit at 0 of the hazard ratio function, and θ_2 continues to determine the trend of the hazard ratio, increasing if $\theta_1 < \theta_2$ and decreasing if $\theta_1 > \theta_2$. Although θ_2 is no longer interpretable as the long-term hazard ratio due to heavy censoring, it continues to give an upper or lower bound of the hazard ratio within the observed data range.

7.3 Approximation of the Unspecified Function $R(t)^*$

This section is marked with an asterisk. Readers can focus on the resulting expression (7.14) for the approximation for $R(t)$ without fully exploring the details if they wish.

The unspecified $R(t)$ makes model (7.6) more flexible than the proportional hazards model, but it also poses considerable challenges in the analysis. To address this issue, Yang and Prentice [344] proposed a pseudo-likelihood inference procedure, using an approximation of the unknown $R(t)$ similar to the approach in Yang and Prentice [343] for the proportional odds model.

To motivate the approximation of $R(t)$, consider the conditional setup in Section 2.8.2 for the two sample comparison. In this setup, with $z_i = I(i \le n_1)$, model (7.1) or (7.6) can be expressed as

$$\lambda_i(t)dt = \frac{1}{h^*_{1i}(\boldsymbol{\beta}_0) + h^*_{2i}(\boldsymbol{\beta}_0)R(t)} dR(t), \qquad i = 1, \ldots, n, \tag{7.8}$$

where $\lambda_i(t)$ is the conditional hazard function of the ith individual, $h^*_{ji}(\boldsymbol{\beta}) = \exp(-\beta_j z_i)$ for $\boldsymbol{\beta} = (\beta_1, \beta_2)$, $j = 1, 2$, $i = 1, \ldots, n$, and $\boldsymbol{\beta}_0$ is the true parameter value.

Corresponding to $\lambda_i(t)$, let $F_i(t)$ and $G_i(t)$ be the CDFs of T_i and C_i respectively. Also, let $f_i(t)$ be the PDF of T_i, and denote $\overline{A}(x) = 1 - A(x)$ for a function $A(x)$. Note that $\overline{F}_i(t)\lambda_i(t)dt = f_i(t)dt = dF_i(t)$.

Multiplying both sides of (7.8) by

$$\overline{F}_{i-}(t)\overline{G}_{i-}(t)\left[h^*_{1i}(\boldsymbol{\beta}_0) + h^*_{2i}(\boldsymbol{\beta}_0)R(t)\right],$$

where $F_{i-}(t)$ and $G_{i-}(t)$ denote the left limit versions of $F_{i-}(t)$ and $G_{i-}(t)$, respectively. Adding up the n resulting equations, we obtain

$$\begin{aligned}
&\sum_{i=1}^{n} \overline{F}_{i-}(t)\overline{G}_{-}i(t)dR(t) \\
&= \sum_{i=1}^{n} h_{1i}^{*}(\boldsymbol{\beta}_0)\overline{G}_{i-}(t)dF_i(t) + R(t)\sum_{i=1}^{n} h_{2i}^{*}(\boldsymbol{\beta}_0)\overline{G}_{i-}(t)dF_i(t). \qquad (7.9)
\end{aligned}$$

For the counting process $N_i(t)$ and the at-risk process $Y_i(t)$ in (2.42). We have

$$\begin{aligned}
EN_i(t) &= \int_0^t \overline{G}_{i-}(s)dF_i(s), \\
EK_i(t) &= \overline{G}_{i-}(t)\overline{F}_{i-}(t).
\end{aligned}$$

Therefore, by the law of large numbers, under regularity conditions,

$$\begin{aligned}
\frac{1}{n}K(t) &\approx \frac{1}{n}\sum_{i=1}^{n} \overline{F}_{i-}(t)\overline{G}_{i-}(t), \\
\frac{1}{n}\sum_{i=1}^{n} h_{ji}^{*}(\boldsymbol{\beta}_0)dN_i(t) &\approx \frac{1}{n}\sum_{i=1}^{n} h_{ji}^{*}(\boldsymbol{\beta}_0)\overline{G}_{i-}(t)dF_i(t), \quad j=1,2, \qquad (7.10)
\end{aligned}$$

where $K(t)=\sum_{i=1}^{n} K_i(t)$ as in (2.43). Equations (7.9) and (7.10) suggest that

$$\begin{aligned}
&\frac{1}{n}K(t)(t)dR(t) \\
&\approx \frac{1}{n}\sum_{i=1}^{n} h_{1i}^{*}(\boldsymbol{\beta}_0)dN_i(t) + R(t)\sum_{i=1}^{n} h_{2i}^{*}(\boldsymbol{\beta}_0)dN_i(t),
\end{aligned}$$

or

$$R(t) \approx \int_0^t \frac{\sum_{i=1}^{n} h_{1i}^{*}(\boldsymbol{\beta}_0)dN_i(s)}{K(s)} + \int_0^t \frac{R(s)\sum_{i=1}^{n} h_{2i}^{*}(\boldsymbol{\beta}_0)dN_i(s)}{K(s)} \qquad (7.11)$$

Without the conditional setup simplification, $R(t)$ can also be approximated similarly under model (7.6). Suppose that data are available from the random censorship model with fixed covariates described in Section 4.1.1, with $\boldsymbol{W}_i = Z_i$. Assume that the conditional distribution of T given Z satisfies (7.6). Define the following equation in $\widehat{R}(t;\boldsymbol{\beta})$:

$$\widehat{R}(t;\boldsymbol{\beta}) = \int_0^t \widehat{R}(s;\boldsymbol{\beta})\widehat{\Lambda}_2(ds;\boldsymbol{\beta}) + \widehat{\Lambda}_1(t;\boldsymbol{\beta}), \qquad (7.12)$$

where

$$\widehat{\Lambda}_1(t;\boldsymbol{\beta}) = \int_0^t \frac{\sum_{i=1}^n h_{1i}(\boldsymbol{\beta})dN_i(s)}{K(s)},$$

$$\widehat{\Lambda}_2(t;\boldsymbol{\beta}) = \int_0^t \frac{\sum_{i=1}^n h_{2i}(\boldsymbol{\beta})dN_i(s)}{K(s)},$$

with $h_{ji}(\boldsymbol{\beta}) = \exp(-\beta_j Z_i)$, $j = 1,2, i = 1,\ldots,n$. The heuristics leading to (7.11) suggest that

$$\widehat{R}(t;\boldsymbol{\beta}_0) \approx R(t).$$

For $\widehat{\Lambda}_j(t;\boldsymbol{\beta})$, $j = 1,2$, to be well defined, we need to restrict $t \le \tau$, with τ satisfying

$$\lim_n K(\tau)/n > 0, \quad \text{with probability 1.} \tag{7.13}$$

Similarly to (22) of Yang [329], $\widehat{R}(t;\boldsymbol{\beta})$ has the expression

$$\widehat{R}(t;\boldsymbol{\beta}) = \frac{1}{\widehat{P}(t;\boldsymbol{\beta})}\int_0^t \widehat{P}_-(s;\boldsymbol{\beta})\widehat{\Lambda}_1(ds;\boldsymbol{\beta}), \tag{7.14}$$

with $\widehat{P}(t;\boldsymbol{\beta}) = \prod_{s\le t}\{1-\Delta\widehat{\Lambda}_2(s;\boldsymbol{\beta})\}$, where $\widehat{P}_-$ denotes the left-continuous, in t, version of $\widehat{P}$, and $\Delta\widehat{\Lambda}_2(s;\boldsymbol{\beta})$ is the jump of $\widehat{\Lambda}_2$ in s. See Exercise 7.8 for some algebraic and analytic details.

In real data applications, it is numerically more stable and convenient to use the asymptotically equivalent $\widetilde{P}(t;\boldsymbol{\beta}) = \exp[-\widehat{\Lambda}_2(s;\boldsymbol{\beta})]$ instead of $\widehat{P}$.

7.4 Pseudo-Likelihood Estimator

Using the function $\widehat{R}(t;\boldsymbol{\beta})$, Yang and Prentice derived a pseudo-likelihood estimator as follows. Let $L(\boldsymbol{\beta},R)$ be the likelihood function of $\boldsymbol{\beta}$ for model (7.6) when the function $R(t)$ is known, with the corresponding score vector $\boldsymbol{U}(\boldsymbol{\beta},R) = \frac{\partial}{\partial\boldsymbol{\beta}}\ln L(\boldsymbol{\beta},R)$. Then the pseudo-maximum likelihood estimator $\widehat{\boldsymbol{\beta}}$ is defined as the zero of $\boldsymbol{Q}(\boldsymbol{\beta})$, where

$$\boldsymbol{Q}(\boldsymbol{\beta}) = \boldsymbol{U}(\boldsymbol{\beta},R)|_{R(t)=\widehat{R}_n(t;\boldsymbol{\beta})}.$$

Specifically,

$$\boldsymbol{Q}(\boldsymbol{\beta}) = \left(Q_1(\boldsymbol{\beta}), Q_2(\boldsymbol{\beta})\right)^{\mathrm{T}},$$

$$Q_1(\boldsymbol{\beta}) = \sum_{i=1}^n \frac{Z_i\left[\delta_i h_{1i}(\boldsymbol{\beta}) - \widehat{R}(X_i;\boldsymbol{\beta})\right]}{h_{1i}(\boldsymbol{\beta}) + h_{2i}(\boldsymbol{\beta})\widehat{R}(X_i;\boldsymbol{\beta})},$$

$$
\begin{aligned}
Q_2(\boldsymbol{\beta}) &= \sum_{i=1}^{n} \frac{Z_i \widehat{R}(X_i;\boldsymbol{\beta})[\delta_i h_{2i}(\boldsymbol{\beta})+1]}{h_{1i}(\boldsymbol{\beta})+h_{2i}(\boldsymbol{\beta})\widehat{R}(X_i;\boldsymbol{\beta})} \\
&\quad -\sum_{i=1}^{n} \frac{Z_i}{h_{2i}(\boldsymbol{\beta})} \ln\left\{1+\frac{h_{2i}(\boldsymbol{\beta})}{h_{1i}(\boldsymbol{\beta})}\widehat{R}(X_i;\boldsymbol{\beta})\right\}. \qquad (7.15)
\end{aligned}
$$

After $\widehat{\boldsymbol{\beta}}$ is obtained, the baseline function $R(t)$ is estimated by $\widehat{R}(t;\widehat{\boldsymbol{\beta}})$.

For asymptotic analysis, it helps to connect the pseudo-maximum likelihood estimator with the martingale theory. Let

$$
M_i(t) = \delta_i I(X_i \le t) - \int_0^t I(X_i \ge s) \frac{dR(s)}{h_{1i}(\boldsymbol{\beta}_0)+h_{2i}(\boldsymbol{\beta}_0)R(s)}, \qquad (7.16)
$$

which is the martingale associated with the ith individual under (7.6), $1 \le i \le n$. Define the martingale residual

$$
\widehat{M}_i(t;\boldsymbol{\beta}) = \delta_i I(X_i \le t) - \int_0^t I(X_i \ge s) \frac{\widehat{R}(ds;\boldsymbol{\beta})}{h_{1i}(\boldsymbol{\beta})+h_{2i}(\boldsymbol{\beta})\widehat{R}(s;\boldsymbol{\beta})}, \qquad (7.17)
$$

for $1 \le i \le n$. It can be shown that at the true parameter value $\boldsymbol{\beta}_0$,

$$
n^{-1/2}\mathbf{Q}(\boldsymbol{\beta}_0) = n^{-1/2}\sum_{i=1}^{n}\int_0^{\tau} \boldsymbol{\Phi}_i(t;\boldsymbol{\beta}_0)\widehat{M}_i(dt;\boldsymbol{\beta}_0) + o_p(1), \qquad (7.18)
$$

where

$$
\begin{aligned}
\boldsymbol{\Phi}_i &= (\Phi_{1i}, \Phi_{2i})^{\mathrm{T}}, \\
\Phi_{1i}(t;\boldsymbol{\beta}) &= Z_i \frac{h_{1i}(\boldsymbol{\beta})}{h_{1i}(\boldsymbol{\beta})+h_{2i}(\boldsymbol{\beta})\widehat{R}(t;\boldsymbol{\beta})}, \\
\Phi_{2i}(t;\boldsymbol{\beta}) &= Z_i \frac{h_{2i}(\boldsymbol{\beta})\widehat{R}(t;\boldsymbol{\beta})}{h_{1i}(\boldsymbol{\beta})+h_{2i}(\boldsymbol{\beta})\widehat{R}(t;\boldsymbol{\beta})}. \qquad (7.19)
\end{aligned}
$$

Thus, the martingale residuals-based estimating function

$$
\sum_{i=1}^{n}\int_0^{\tau} \boldsymbol{\Phi}_i(t;\boldsymbol{\beta})\widehat{M}_i(dt;\boldsymbol{\beta}) \qquad (7.20)
$$

yields an estimator that is asymptotically equivalent to the pseudo-likelihood estimator. As shown in Chapter Six, the partial likelihood estimator under the Cox model is the zero of a martingale residuals-based estimating function.

From (7.19), $\Phi_{1i}(t;\boldsymbol{\beta})$ and $\Phi_{2i}(t;\boldsymbol{\beta})$ are monotone functions in t giving more weight to early and late observations, respectively. This seems intuitively sensible, as β_1 and β_2 are, respectively, the logarithms of the short-term and long-term hazard ratios.

The difference between estimating functions in (7.15) and (7.20) is due to the discreteness of $\widehat{R}(t;\boldsymbol{\beta})$. If $\widehat{R}(t;\boldsymbol{\beta})$ were continuous in t, then (7.15) and (7.20) coincide, because by the change of variable formula (A.11) in Section A.4 of Appendix A, for a continuous and increasing function Γ with $\Gamma(0) = 0$.

$$\int_0^t \frac{1}{[1+\Gamma(s)]^2} d\Gamma(s) = \frac{\Gamma(t)}{1+\Gamma(t)}.$$

Under certain regularity conditions, $\widehat{R}(t;\boldsymbol{\beta})$ can be shown to approach a continuous limit function in some uniform sense, thus (7.18) follows.

Due to the asymptotic equivalence, the pseudo-likelihood estimator of $\boldsymbol{\beta}$ can be obtained as either zero of the function in (7.15) or that in (7.20). Computationally (7.15) is slightly easier to work with. Also, various simulations and data applications suggest that the estimator from (7.15) often has better agreement with the Kaplan-Meier estimator in capturing difference between the treatment and control groups.

By (7.5) and the plug-in method, the model-based estimators for the survival functions $S_C(t)$ and $S_T(t)$ are given by

$$\begin{aligned} \widehat{S}_{CM}(t) &= \frac{1}{1+\widehat{R}(t;\widehat{\boldsymbol{\beta}})(t)}, \\ \widehat{S}_{TM}(t) &= \left[1+\exp(\widehat{\beta}_1-\widehat{\beta}_2)\widehat{R}(t;\widehat{\boldsymbol{\beta}})(t)\right]^{-\exp(\widehat{\beta}_2)}, \end{aligned} \tag{7.21}$$

respectively. Other quantities can be estimated analogously.

To apply the pseudo-likelihood estimator in practice, the value τ needs to be determined. Through various exploratory analysis with simulation studies and data applications, it was found that the choice $\tau = d^*$, the duration of the trial, yields stable results for the estimators. This choice of τ corresponds to using all data in the estimating function.

7.5 Asymptotic analysis of the Pseudo-Likelihood Estimator

From (7.11) and (7.12) we have, at the true parameter $\boldsymbol{\beta}_0$,

$$\begin{aligned} &\widehat{R}(t;\boldsymbol{\beta}_0) - R(t) \\ = &\int_0^t \left[\widehat{R}(s;\boldsymbol{\beta}_0) - R(s)\right] d\widehat{\Lambda}_2(s;\boldsymbol{\beta}_0) \\ &+ \int_0^t R(s) d\left[\widehat{\Lambda}_2(s;\boldsymbol{\beta}_0) - \widetilde{\Lambda}_2(s;\boldsymbol{\beta}_0)\right] + \widehat{\Lambda}_1(t;\boldsymbol{\beta}_0) - \widetilde{\Lambda}_1(t;\boldsymbol{\beta}_0). \end{aligned}$$

With some algebra this can be rewritten as

$$\widehat{R}(t;\boldsymbol{\beta}_0) - R(t) = \int_0^t [\widehat{R}(s;\boldsymbol{\beta}_0) - R(s)]\,d\widehat{\Lambda}_2(s;\boldsymbol{\beta}_0) + \mathcal{M}(t), \tag{7.22}$$

where

$$\mathcal{M}(t) = \int_0^t \frac{1}{K(s)} \sum_{i=1}^n [h_{1i}(\boldsymbol{\beta}_0) + h_{2i}(\boldsymbol{\beta}_0)R(s)]\,dM_i(s), \quad t \le \tau. \tag{7.23}$$

Thus similarly to solving (7.12), from (7.22) we obtain

$$\widehat{R}(t;\boldsymbol{\beta}_0) - R(t) = \frac{1}{\widehat{P}(t;\boldsymbol{\beta}_0)} \int_0^t \widehat{P}_-(t;\boldsymbol{\beta}_0)\,d\mathcal{M}(t), \tag{7.24}$$

for $\widehat{P}$ in (7.14). This is useful in asymptotic analysis where quantities of interest are expressed as sums of integrals with respect to the martingales $M_i(t)$, $1 \le i \le n$.

In particular, by using $\widehat{M}_i = \widehat{M}_i - M_i + M_i$ and (7.24), it can be shown that, under certain regularity conditions, at the true parameter value $\boldsymbol{\beta}_0$, $n^{-1/2}\boldsymbol{Q}(\boldsymbol{\beta}_0) = \mathsf{B} + o_p(1)$, where

$$\mathsf{B} = \frac{1}{\sqrt{n}} \sum_{i=1}^n \int_0^\tau \boldsymbol{\xi}_i(t)\,dM_i(t), \tag{7.25}$$

with $\boldsymbol{\xi}_1(t),\ldots,\boldsymbol{\xi}_n(t)$ being 2×1 functions that depend on $\boldsymbol{\beta}_0$ and $R(t)$. From this, Yang and Prentice [344] showed that $n^{-1/2}\boldsymbol{Q}(\boldsymbol{\beta}_0)$ converges in distribution to a bivariate normal vector with mean zero and a covariance matrix $\boldsymbol{A}(\boldsymbol{\beta}_0)$, where

$$\boldsymbol{A}(\boldsymbol{\beta}) = \lim_n \frac{1}{\sqrt{n}} \sum_{i=1}^n \int_0^\tau \boldsymbol{\xi}_i(t)\boldsymbol{\xi}_i^{\mathrm{T}}(t) I(X_i \ge t) \frac{dR(t)}{h_{1i}(\boldsymbol{\beta}) + h_{2i}(\boldsymbol{\beta})R(t)}. \tag{7.26}$$

Let $\boldsymbol{J_Q}$ be the Jacobian matrix of $\boldsymbol{Q}(\boldsymbol{\beta})$, with (i,j) element $\partial Q_i(\boldsymbol{\beta})/\partial \beta_j$, $i,\ j = 1,2$, and $\Omega(\boldsymbol{\beta}) = \boldsymbol{J_Q}(\boldsymbol{\beta})/n$. Then by the mean value theorem and smoothness of $\Omega(\boldsymbol{\beta})$,

$$-n^{-1/2}\boldsymbol{Q}(\boldsymbol{\beta}_0) = n^{-1/2}\left[\boldsymbol{Q}(\widehat{\boldsymbol{\beta}}) - \boldsymbol{Q}(\boldsymbol{\beta}_0)\right] \approx \Omega(\boldsymbol{\beta}_0)\sqrt{n}(\widehat{\boldsymbol{\beta}} - \boldsymbol{\beta}_0).$$

Thus if $\Omega(\boldsymbol{\beta}_0)$ has inverse $\Omega^{-1}(\boldsymbol{\beta}_0)$ that converges to the limit $\mathbf{V}_0(\boldsymbol{\beta}_0)$ as $n \to \infty$, then

$$\sqrt{n}(\widehat{\boldsymbol{\beta}} - \boldsymbol{\beta}_0) \approx -\mathbf{V}_0(\boldsymbol{\beta}_0) n^{-1/2}\boldsymbol{Q}(\boldsymbol{\beta}_0). \tag{7.27}$$

It follows that $\sqrt{n}(\widehat{\boldsymbol{\beta}} - \boldsymbol{\beta}_0)$ converges in distribution to the bivariate normal distribution with mean zero and the covariance matrix $\boldsymbol{B}(\boldsymbol{\beta}_0) = \mathbf{V}_0(\boldsymbol{\beta}_0)\boldsymbol{A}(\boldsymbol{\beta}_0)\mathbf{V}_0^{\mathrm{T}}(\boldsymbol{\beta}_0)$.

To obtain consistent estimators of the covariance matrices $\boldsymbol{A}(\boldsymbol{\beta}_0)$ and $\boldsymbol{B}(\boldsymbol{\beta}_0)$, an approximation of $\mathbf{V}_0$ is needed. Although the exact form of $\mathbf{V}_0$ can be obtained through some tedious algebra, numerical derivatives provide a simple and reliable way to approximate $\mathbf{V}_0$. The numerical derivative is typically very stable since $\boldsymbol{Q}(\boldsymbol{\beta})$ is a smooth function of $\boldsymbol{\beta}$. With the numerical derivatives, a covariance estimator can be obtained by the plug-in method in which $\widehat{\boldsymbol{\beta}}, \widehat{R}(t;\widehat{\boldsymbol{\beta}})$ are used to replace $\boldsymbol{\beta}_0$, $R(t)$, respectively.

Alternatively, the Monte Carlo method described in Section 6.5 of Chapter Six can be used to estimate $\boldsymbol{A}(\boldsymbol{\beta}_0)$. Let G_i, $i = 1,\ldots,n$ be *i.i.d.* standard normal variables that are independent from the data, and define

$$\begin{aligned}\widehat{\mathsf{B}} &= \frac{1}{\sqrt{n}}\sum_{i=1}^{n}\int_0^{\tau} G_i\widehat{\boldsymbol{\xi}}(t)dN_i(t) \\ &= \frac{1}{\sqrt{n}}\sum_{i=1}^{n} G_i\delta_i\widehat{\boldsymbol{\xi}}(X_i)I(X_i \le \tau), \qquad (7.28)\end{aligned}$$

where $\widehat{\boldsymbol{\xi}}_i(t)$ is obtained from $\boldsymbol{\xi}_i(t)$ using numerical derivatives and the plug-in method. It can be shown that under certain regularity conditions, $\widehat{\mathsf{B}}$ converges in distribution to the same zero-mean normal distribution as B in (7.25). To estimate the limiting covariance matrix $\boldsymbol{A}(\boldsymbol{\beta}_0)$ of $n^{-1/2}\boldsymbol{Q}(\boldsymbol{\beta}_0)$, a large number of realizations from $\widehat{\mathsf{B}}$ can be obtained by repeatedly generating normal variables $\{G_I : 1 \le i \le n\}$ a large number B times while fixing $(X_i, \delta_i, \boldsymbol{W}_i), i \le n$ at the observed values. The Monte Carlo estimator $\widehat{\boldsymbol{A}}$ of $\boldsymbol{A}(\boldsymbol{\beta}_0)$ is the sample variance from those B realizations. From this, an estimator $\boldsymbol{B}(\widehat{\boldsymbol{\beta}})$ of $\boldsymbol{B}(\boldsymbol{\beta}_0)$ can be obtained using numerical derivatives and the plug-in method.

For testing the null hypothesis of no treatment effect, or $\boldsymbol{\beta} = \boldsymbol{c}_0$ with $\boldsymbol{c}_0 = (0,0)^{\mathrm{T}}$, note that $\widehat{R}(t;\boldsymbol{c}_0)$ in (7.14) reduces to $1/\widehat{S}_-(t) - 1$, where $\widehat{S}(t)$ is the left limit version of the Kaplan-Meier survival function estimator based on the pooled sample. For brevity, denote $\boldsymbol{Q}((0,0)^{\mathrm{T}})$ by $\boldsymbol{Q}(0)$. With some algebra, it can be shown that $n^{-1/2}\boldsymbol{Q}(0) = n^{-1/2}\boldsymbol{\Gamma} + o_p(1)$, where

$$\begin{aligned}\boldsymbol{\Gamma} &= (\Gamma_1,\Gamma_2)^{\mathrm{T}}, \\ \Gamma_1 &= \int_0^{\tau}\frac{\widehat{S}_-(t)K_C(t)K_T(t)}{K_C(t)+K_T(t)}d\big(\widehat{\Lambda}_T(t)-\widehat{\Lambda}_C(t)\big), \\ \Gamma_2 &= \int_0^{\tau}\frac{\big[1-\widehat{S}_-(t)\big]K_C(t)K_T(t)}{K_C(t)+K_T(t)}d\big(\widehat{\Lambda}_T(t)-\widehat{\Lambda}_C(t)\big),\end{aligned}$$

with K_T, K_C the at-risk processes in (2.48) and $\widehat{\Lambda}_T(t)$, $\widehat{\Lambda}_C(t)$ the Nelson-Aalen estimators of the cumulative hazard functions of the two groups, respectively. Therefore,

$$n^{-1}\boldsymbol{Q}(0)^{\mathrm{T}}\widehat{\boldsymbol{A}}_0^{-1}\boldsymbol{Q}(0) = \xi + o_p(1), \qquad (7.29)$$

where $\widehat{\boldsymbol{A}}_0$ is obtained similarly to $\widehat{\boldsymbol{A}}$, but using $\boldsymbol{c}_0$ instead of $\widehat{\boldsymbol{\beta}}$, and ξ is the χ^2 test statistic based on two weighted log-rank statistics, with the PP weight $\widehat{S}_-$ and the CPP weight $1-\widehat{S}_-$, respectively.

The Wald statistic $n^{-1}\widehat{\boldsymbol{\beta}}^{\mathrm{T}}\big[\widehat{\boldsymbol{B}}(\widehat{\boldsymbol{\beta}})\big]^{-1}\widehat{\boldsymbol{\beta}}$. can also be used to test the hypothesis $\boldsymbol{\beta} = (0,0)^{\mathrm{T}}$. When substantial censoring is present, which is usually the case

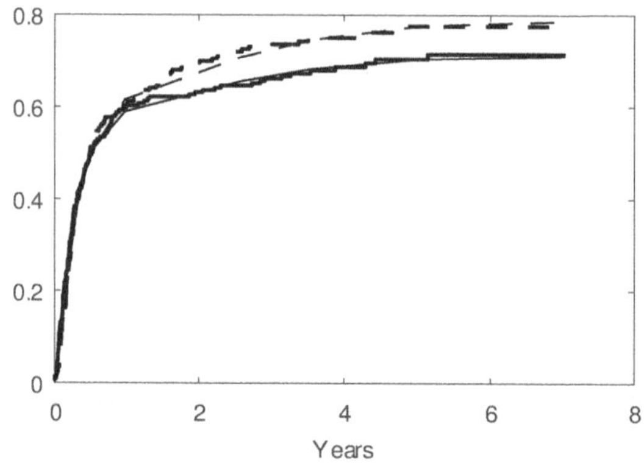

FIGURE 7.3
Estimated CDF for the TCD trial. Thick solid: control group, Kaplan-Meier; thick dashed: treatment group, Kaplan-Meier; thin solid: control group, model (7.6); thin dashed: treatment group, model (7.6).

in cardiology trials, there is less information on β_2. Thus the test based on $n^{-1}\boldsymbol{Q}(0)^{\mathrm{T}}\widehat{\boldsymbol{A}}_0^{-1}\boldsymbol{Q}(0)$, which will be referred to as the score test for simplicity, is generally preferred. Note that there is no simple analog of the likelihood ratio test using the pseudo-likelihood estimator $\widehat{\boldsymbol{\beta}}$.

Example 7.1. Consider model (7.6) for the TCD trial, with data on time to the minimum of relapse or death. From the pseudo-likelihood estimate, we obtain $e^{\widehat{\boldsymbol{\beta}}} = (0.73, 5.13)^{\mathrm{T}}$. Figure 7.3 displays the Kaplan-Meier and model-based CDF estimates. Compared with Figure 6.2 for model (6.2), the agreement with the Kaplan-Meier estimates is improved.

For testing the hypothesis of no treatment effect, $H_0 : \boldsymbol{\beta} = (0,0)^{\mathrm{T}}$, the score test statistic $n^{-1}\boldsymbol{Q}(0)^{\mathrm{T}}\widehat{\boldsymbol{A}}_0^{-1}\boldsymbol{Q}(0)$ gives a P-value of 0.04, the same as that from the asymptotically equivalent χ^2 test statistic ξ in (7.29). For the two component weighted log-rank test statistics of ξ, with PP and CPP weights, the standardized statistics are 0.04 and 1.90, respectively. The corresponding P-values are 0.96 and 0.06 respectively. The Wald test statistic $n^{-1}\widehat{\boldsymbol{\beta}}^{\mathrm{T}}[\widehat{\boldsymbol{B}}(\widehat{\boldsymbol{\beta}})]^{-1}\widehat{\boldsymbol{\beta}}$ yields a P-value of 0.30.

In non-proportional hazards situations, as illustrated in Examples 6.1 and 7.1, there is often less agreement among P-values from different methods. As noted before, the score test is generally more stable and robust than the Wald test. For model (7.6), due to censoring, there is often little information on β_2. Thus it is recommended that the score test be used for testing H_0 instead of the Wald test.

Neither the score test nor the Wald test, due to the χ^2 test nature, corresponds to a summary measure of the treatment effect. A rejection of the null hypothesis does not indicate whether the treatment has a beneficial or adverse effect. The rejection may occur because one group has a larger variance, while the means in the two groups are similar.

Therefore, such χ^2 test is adequate in situations where the interest is only in determining whether there is a difference between the two comparison groups. However, it is often also of interest to know if a treatment works and to quantify the effect. A separate chapter, Chapter Nine, will be devoted to discussions on testing and describing treatment effects.

7.6 Temporal Patterns

Traditionally, Kaplan-Meier curves for the control and treatment groups are plotted to show changes in the survival probability over time. While this provides a detailed description of the survival experience throughout the duration of a trial, it does not directly offer a quantitative value at time t to indicate the group difference at that specific time. In the literature, under the widely used Cox model, the treatment effect is typically summarized by the hazard ratio which is a constant, and there is little interest in going beyond the Kaplan-Meier curves.

Since this chapter focuses on possibly non-proportional hazards, it is important to explore visual tools that depict how relevant quantities change over time. This is especially important when model (7.6) is applied to heavily censored data, as such data can result in an estimate of β_2 that no longer maintains the long-term hazard ratio interpretation. This section discusses various quantities useful for displaying time trends in the treatment effect. All the curves to be discussed are estimates of underlying quantities that are functionals of the two survival distributions and do not depend on censoring.

7.6.1 The Hazard Ratio

As model (7.6) is motivated by relaxing the constant hazard ratio assumption of the Cox model (5.4), it is of particular interest to assess how the hazard ratio changes over time within the data range. The hazard ratio at t is

$$h(t) = \frac{\lambda_T(t)}{\lambda_C(t)} = \frac{1 + R(t)}{\exp(-\beta_1) + \exp(-\beta_2)R(t)}, \tag{7.30}$$

which can be estimated by

$$\widehat{h}(t) = \frac{1 + \widehat{R}(t; \widehat{\boldsymbol{\beta}})}{\exp(-\widehat{\beta}_1) + \exp(-\widehat{\beta}_2)\widehat{R}(t; \widehat{\boldsymbol{\beta}})}. \tag{7.31}$$

Since this estimator does not involve estimating the derivative $dR(t)/dt$, it is more stable and robust than those that rely on derivative estimators, such as the hazard ratio estimator under the semiparametric accelerated failure time model that will be discussed in Chapter Eight.

To visually display the hazard ratio and its variation over time, point-wise and simultaneous confidence intervals can be used. Let

$$\mathsf{C}(t) = \sqrt{n}\big[\widehat{h}(t) - h(t)\big].$$

To obtain critical values for a confidence interval at a fixed t or for simultaneous confidence intervals for t in an interval J, Yang and Prentice [346] showed that the process $\mathsf{C}(t) = \widetilde{\mathsf{C}}(t) + o_p(1)$, where

$$\widetilde{\mathsf{C}}(t) = \frac{a(t)}{\sqrt{n}} \sum_{i=1}^{n} \int_0^t b_i(s)dM_i(s) + \frac{\boldsymbol{\phi}(t)}{\sqrt{n}} \int_0^\infty \boldsymbol{\psi}_i(s)dM_i(s) \tag{7.32}$$

for certain scalar functions $a(t)$, $b_i(t)$, $1\times p$ function $\boldsymbol{\phi}(t)$ and $p\times 1$ functions $\boldsymbol{\psi}_i(t)$ that depend on $\boldsymbol{\beta}_0$ and the function $R(t)$. Loosely speaking, the condition $A_n(t) = B_n(t) + o_p(1)$ for two sequences of processes requires approximations in a proper uniform sense. An overview of related concepts and results is given in Appendix C.

From the asymptotic analysis of $\widetilde{\mathsf{C}}(t)$ and the approximation of $\mathsf{C}(t)$ by $\widetilde{\mathsf{C}}(t)$, it was shown that $\mathsf{C}(t)$ converges weakly to a Gaussian process with mean zero and variance $\sigma^2(t)$ that depends on $\boldsymbol{\beta}_0$ and the function $R(t)$. Using the martingale structure, a consistent estimator $\widehat{\sigma}(t)$ of $\sigma^2(t)$ was obtained, from which the point-wise and simultaneous confidence intervals over for t in a range J can be obtained.

Alternatively, the Monte Carlo method described in Section 6.5 can be used to obtain an estimator $\widetilde{\sigma}(t)$ of $\sigma^2(t)$ which often leads to more robust results. Let

$$\widehat{\mathsf{C}}(t) = \frac{\widehat{a}(t)}{\sqrt{n}} \sum_{i=1}^{n} \int_0^t G_i\widehat{b}_i(s)dN_i(s) + \frac{\widehat{\boldsymbol{\phi}}(t)}{\sqrt{n}} \int_0^\infty \widehat{\boldsymbol{\psi}}_i(s)G_i dN_i(s),$$

where G_i, $i = 1,\ldots,n$ are i.i.d. standard normal variables that are independent from the data, and $\widehat{a}$, $\widehat{b}_i$, $\widehat{\boldsymbol{\phi}}$, $\widehat{\boldsymbol{\psi}}_i$ are estimators of $a(t)$, $b_i(t)$, $\boldsymbol{\phi}(t)$, $\boldsymbol{\psi}_i(t)$ with $\widehat{\boldsymbol{\beta}}$ and $\widehat{R}(t;\widehat{\boldsymbol{\beta}})$ replacing $\boldsymbol{\beta}_0$ and $R(t)$, respectively, and with numerical derivatives replacing involved partial derivatives with respect to $\boldsymbol{\beta}$. It can be shown that $\widehat{\mathsf{C}}(t)$ converges weakly to the same limiting zero-mean Gaussian process as that of $\mathsf{C}(t)$ for almost all realizations of the data (X_i, δ_i, Z_i), $i \le n$.

At a single time point t,

$$\lim_n P\big(\sqrt{n}\big|\widehat{h}(t) - h(t)\big| \le z(\alpha/2)\widetilde{\sigma}(t)\big) = 1 - \alpha. \tag{7.33}$$

From this, point-wise confidence intervals of $h(t)$ over the interval $t \in J$ can be obtained. For better small sample behavior and assurance that the confidence intervals avoid negative values, a conventional method is to make a logarithmic transformation, resulting in the asymptotic $100(1-\alpha)\%$ confidence interval of $h(t)$

$$\widehat{h}(t)\exp\left(\mp z(\alpha/2)\frac{\sqrt{\widetilde{\sigma}(t)}}{\sqrt{n}\widehat{h}(t)}\right). \tag{7.34}$$

To obtain simultaneous confidence intervals, a critical value c_α is needed such that

$$\lim_n P\left(\sqrt{n}\left|\widehat{h}(t)-h(t)\right| \le c_\alpha \widehat{w}(t),\ t\in J\right)=1-\alpha, \tag{7.35}$$

where $\widehat{w}(t)$ is a scaling function depending on $\widetilde{\sigma}(t)$. The choice $\widehat{w}(t)=\widetilde{\sigma}(t)$ gives an equal-precision confidence band. Under certain regularity conditions, it can be shown that $\widehat{\mathrm{C}}(t)/\widehat{w}(t)$ converges weakly to the same limiting zero-mean Gaussian process as that of $\mathrm{C}(t)/w(t)$ for almost all realizations of the data $(X_i,\delta_i,Z_i), i\le n$, where $w(t)$ is the limit of $\widehat{w}(t)$. To approximate the distribution of the limiting Gaussian process, a large number of realizations from $\widehat{\mathrm{C}}(t)/\widehat{w}(t)$ can be obtained by repeatedly generating normal variables $\{G_i : 1\le i\le n\}$ while fixing $(X_i,\delta_i,Z_i), i\le n$ at the observed values. The procedure for approximating c_α is as follows.

1. Use the data and independent standard normal variables G_i's that are independent of the data as well as the G_i's used in obtaining $\widetilde{\sigma}(t)$, to generate the process $A(t)=\widehat{\mathrm{C}}/\widehat{w}(t)$ a large number B times to obtain $A_1(t),\ldots,A_B(t)$.

2. The estimator of c_α is then the sample upper αth percentile of $\sup_{t\in J}|A_1(t)|,\ldots,\sup_{t\in J}|A_B(t)|$.

As usual, a logarithmic transformation can be used which results in the $100(1-\alpha)\%$ simultaneous confidence intervals of $h(t)$ for $t\in J$:

$$\widehat{h}(t)\exp\left(\mp c_\alpha\frac{\widehat{w}(t)}{\sqrt{n}\widehat{h}(t)}\right), t\in J. \tag{7.36}$$

The asymptotic validity of the Monte Carlo method for simultaneous confidence intervals in (7.36) can be justified similar to the case in Yang and Prentice [347] which deals with a regression extension of the model (7.6) that will be discussed later in Section 7.8.

To avoid potential instability of estimators near the boundaries of data range, A strategy similar to Yang and Prentice [347] can be used when constructing the simultaneous confidence intervals. Specifically, a good choice for the weight function $\widehat{w}(t)$ is $\widehat{w}_0(t)$, which is obtained by interpolating the values of $\widetilde{\sigma}(t)$ at, for example, 50 equally spaced points across the data range. Furthermore, the range for the simultaneous confidence intervals is restricted to $[\min K, \max K]$, where K consists of those data points for which $\widehat{w}_0(t)$ does not exceed the 95th percentile of the set $\{\widehat{w}_0(t_j) : j=1,\ldots,m\}$, with t_j denoting the uncensored observations.

Example 7.2. First, consider the WHI E+P trial described in Section 1.20.3. The primary endpoint was time to coronary heart disease, defined as the time to the

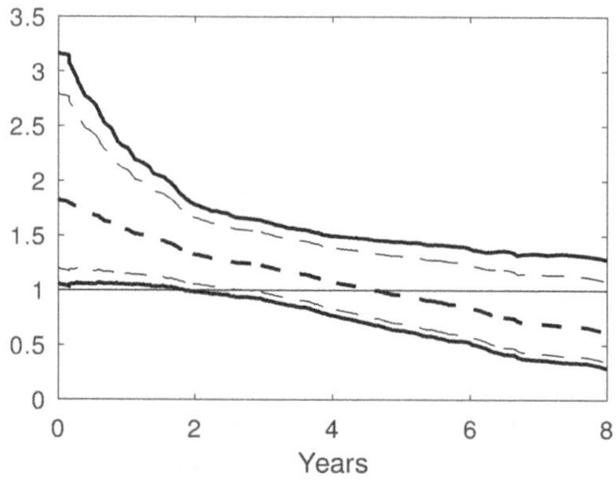

FIGURE 7.4
Estimated hazard ratio, with 95% point-wise and simultaneous confidence intervals, under model (7.6), for the primary endpoint in the WHI E+P trial. Thick solid: simultaneous confidence intervals; thick dashed: hazard ratio; thin dashed: point-wise confidence intervals.

first occurrence of non-fatal myocardial infarction or CHD death. The sample size was 16,608, with 8,102 in the control group. There were 147 and 188 events in the control and treatment group, respectively.

For model (5.4), Lin's lack-of-fit test with weight $\Phi_0(t)$ has a P-value of 0.02. Thus, there is strong evidence of non-proportional hazards. After fitting model (7.6), we obtain $e^{\hat{\beta}} = (1.84, 0.03)^T$. Due to heavy censoring, the value 0.03 does not have the long-term hazard ratio interpretation anymore, and confidence intervals of the hazard ratio function are needed for a more complete and visual assessment of the treatment effect. Figure 7.4 displays the 95% point-wise and simultaneous confidence intervals of the hazard ratio, based on the Monte Carlo method with repetition number $B = 2{,}000$. It shows that for most of the period from years 0 to 2, the simultaneous confidence intervals exclude the value 1. This indicate an early adverse effect of the treatment.

Even when the hazards are reasonably proportional, confidence intervals of the hazard ratio can provide insight into whether the treatment effect strengthens or weakens over time. Figure 7.5 displays the 95% point-wise and simultaneous confidence intervals of the hazard ratio for the TOPCAT primary endpoint. Both the hazard ratio and its confidence intervals gradually increase over time, suggesting that the treatment effect is reduced as time progresses.

From Figure 7.5, the estimated hazard ratio increases to above 1 around three and half years. To investigate whether this pattern reflects a genuine time trend or is an artifact of the model assumption, it is helpful to consider nonparametric

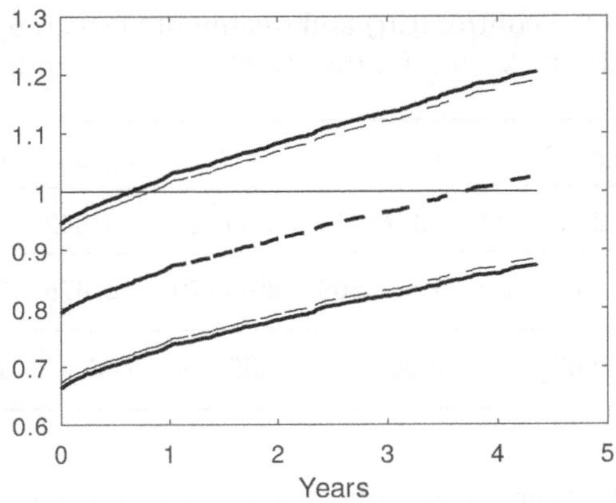

FIGURE 7.5
Estimated hazard ratio, with 95% point-wise and simultaneous confidence intervals, under model (7.6), for the primary endpoint in the TOPCAT trial. Thick solid: simultaneous confidence intervals; thick dashed: hazard ratio; thin dashed: point-wise confidence intervals.

quantities that capture the time-varying behavior of the hazard ratio without the model assumption (7.6).

Within each treatment group, assume that the event time T and censoring time C are independent. Let G be the survival function of C, and let F, f and λ be the CDF, density, and hazard function of T, respectively. Define $X = T \wedge C$ and $\delta = I(X = T)$. Fix a time t and a small interval length $\Delta > 0$. Define

$$A(t,\Delta) = \frac{P(X \in [t, t+\Delta), \delta = 1)}{P(X \geq t)}.$$

By the law of iterated expectations (B.6) in Appendix B, we have

$$\begin{aligned} A(t,\Delta) &= \frac{\int_t^{t+\Delta} G(x)dF(x)}{P(T \geq t)P(C \geq t)} \\ &\approx \frac{\Delta G(t) f(t)}{P(T \geq t)G(t)} \\ &= \Delta\lambda(t). \end{aligned}$$

Note that $A(t,\Delta)$ can be estimated empirically by

$$\widetilde{A}(t,\Delta) = \frac{\sum I(X_i \in [t, t+\Delta), \delta_i = 1)}{\sum I(X_i \geq t)},$$

TABLE 7.1
Values of $\widetilde{A}(t,\Delta)$ in the control (Ctr) and treatment (Txt) groups, and $\widetilde{h}(t)$, at $t = 0,1,2,3,4$ years and with $\Delta = 0.5$, for the TOPCAT primary endpoint.

	$t=0$	$t=1$	$t=2$	$t=3$	$t=4$
Ctr	238/1723	128/1479	89/1159	56/842	24/587
Txt	202/1722	125/1509	86/1179	62/875	32/617
$\widetilde{h}(t)$	0.85	0.96	0.95	1.07	1.27

where the summations are taken within each group. The ratio of $\widetilde{A}(t,\Delta)$ treatment over control gives a nonparametric quantity $\widetilde{h}(t)$ that approximates the hazard ratio at t.

For the TOPCAT primary endpoint, the quantities $\widetilde{A}(t,\Delta)$ and $\widetilde{h}(t)$ at $t = 0,1,2,3,4$ years and $\Delta = 0.5$ are provided in Table 7.1.

From Table 7.1, the data from TOPCAT provide evidence of a hazard ratio transitioning from below 1 to above 1 as time progresses. This nonparametric trend agrees with the estimated hazard ratio function depicted in Figure 7.5. These findings support the conclusion that the mild time-varying nature of the hazard ratio, as shown in Figure 7.5, represents a real feature of the data rather than an artifact of the model assumptions.

7.6.2 Absolute Risk Reduction

In non-proportional hazards situations, the hazard ratio is useful for assessing the temporal trend of the treatment effect, but it may not directly translate to the survival experience. For example, the hazard ratio may be less than 1 in a region where there is no improvement in the survival probability. Conversely, the hazard ratio may be greater than 1 in a region where the survival probability in the treatment group exceeds that in the control group, as illustrated in Figure 7.5.

Another more important consideration is that the hazard ratio is typically derived under an assumed model, thus different models yield different hazard ratio functions, which may display somewhat conflicting patterns, as shown for the WHI E+P trial [337]. Comparing and assessing different hazard ratio estimators is complex, because there is no simple nonparametric estimator to serve as a benchmark.

The absolute risk reduction at time t by the treatment is

$$\eta(t) = S_T(t) - S_C(t).$$

Without assuming a particular model, $\eta(t)$ can be estimated nonparametrically using the Kaplan-Meier estimators. This estimator will be denoted by $\hat{\eta}_N(t)$.

Under model (7.6), $\eta(t)$ can be estimated by

$$\hat{\eta}_M(t) = \hat{S}_{TM}(t) - \hat{S}_{CM}(t) \tag{7.37}$$

for $\hat{S}_{TM}(t)$, $\hat{S}_{CM}(t)$ in (7.21). Plots of the nonparametric estimator together with different model-based estimators provides a simple and quick visual assessment of how well different models fit the data.

Under model (7.6), for the absolute risk reduction, again point-wise and simultaneous confidence intervals of $\eta(t)$ can be derived. Let

$$\mathsf{F}(t) = \sqrt{n}\left[\hat{\eta}_M(t) - \eta(t)\right].$$

It was shown in Yang [337] that the process $\mathsf{F}(t)$ converges weakly to a Gaussian process with mean zero and variation process $\sigma_d^2(t)$. Analogously to the procedure described in Section 7.6.1, the Monte Carlo method can be used to obtain an estimator $\hat{\sigma}_d(t)$ of $\sigma_d(t)$. Point-wise confidence intervals can then be obtained.

For simultaneous confidence intervals, an estimator of c_α can also be obtained such that

$$\lim_n P\left(\sqrt{n}\left|\hat{h}(t) - h(t)\right| \leq c_\alpha \hat{\sigma}_d(t), t \in J\right) = 1 - \alpha. \tag{7.38}$$

for an interval J. From this, simultaneous confidence intervals of $\eta(t)$ over $t \in J$ can be obtained.

Example 7.3. Consider again the time to the minimum of relapse or death in the TCD trial. Figure (7.3) shows that model (7.6) provides a better fit than model (6.2). Now, consider the piecewise Cox model (6.6). Since the largest observation is 8.19, the partition $[0, 2.7) \cup [2.7, 5.4) \cup [5.4, \infty)$ is reasonable. Due to concerns about non-proportionality with the first 6 months, and data sparsity in the tail, the partition $[0, 0.5) \cup [0.5, 2.5) \cup [2.5, \infty)$ also warrants consideration. Figure 7.6 displays estimators of the absolute risk reduction derived under these two models and model (7.6), and the Kaplan-Meier-based estimator. It shows that the partition $[0, 0.5) \cup [0.5, 2.5) \cup [2.5, \infty)$ yields better agreement with the nonparametric estimator between the two piecewise Cox models, and model (7.6) overall has a closer agreement with the nonparametric estimator than the piecewise Cox models, particularly on $[0, 4]$ which contains 85% of all data.

This example highlights an issue with the piecewise Cox model, that the results heavily depend on the partition chosen. Since the analysis model must be pre-specified in the protocol before data unblinding, selecting an appropriate partition can be challenging. A similar dependence on partitions was also observed by Yang [337] in a discussion of the WHI E+P trial data, where it was shown that

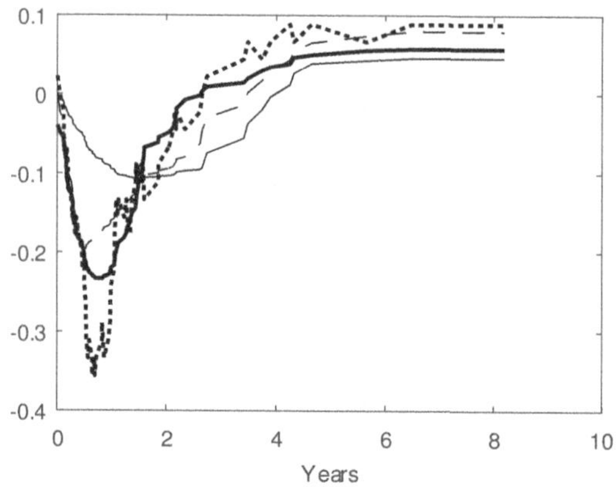

FIGURE 7.6
Nonparametric and model-based estimates of the absolute risk reduction for the TCD trial. Thick solid: model (7.6); Thick dotted: nonparametric; thin solid: piece-wise Cox model with cut-off points 2.7 and 5.4; thin dashed: piece-wise Cox model with cut-off points 0.5 and 2.5.

the estimator based on model (7.6) provided a better overall fit than the piecewise Cox models.

Example 7.4. Figure 7.7 displays the estimates and the 95% point-wise and simultaneous confidence intervals for the absolute risk reduction based on model (7.6), alongside the nonparametric estimates for the TOPCAT primary endpoint. According to Yang [337], to avoid instability near both extreme parts of the data range, the time interval is from the 25th percentile of the uncensored data to the 5th largest uncensored observation. Figure 7.7 shows good agreement between the model-based and nonparametric estimates. Furthermore, both point-wise and simultaneous confidence intervals exclude 1 only for a small portion of t early on. From year 3 onward, although the point estimate of the risk reduction only shows a slight downward trend, the variance steadily increases.

7.6.3 Restricted Mean Survival Difference

In diagnostic testing and machine learning, the receiver operating characteristic (ROC) curve is a foundational concept [108]. The area under the ROC curve, often simply referred to as area under the curve (AUC), is a single scalar value that summarizes the overall diagnostic ability of a test or the discriminating power of a classification model. Hanley and McNeil [108] provided an intuitive interpretation of the AUC and helped popularize its use in medical and diagnostic contexts.

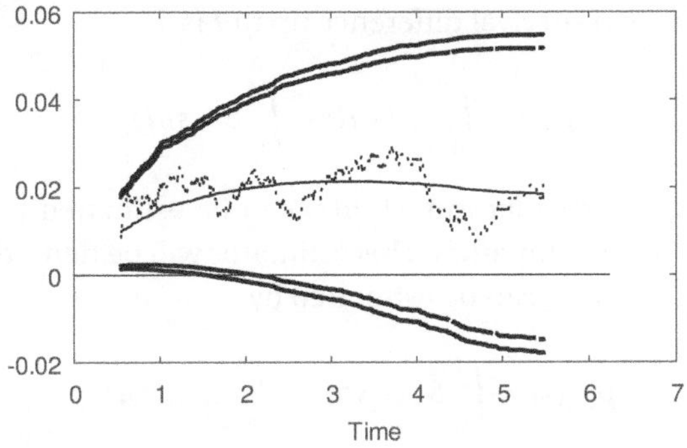

FIGURE 7.7
Estimates and 95% point-wise and simultaneous confidence intervals for the absolute risk reduction based on model (7.6), along with the nonparametric estimates, for the TOPCAT primary endpoint.

The Kaplan-Meier survival curves for the two treatment groups provide survival probability information during the trial. The area under the curve over the time interval $[0, t]$ is a reasonable summary of the survival experience within $[0, t]$ for the corresponding group. Thus, difference of the areas for the two groups serves as a measure of the treatment effect for time up to t. The area under the Kaplan-Meier survival curve is called the *restricted mean survival time* (RMST). This is because if a nonnegative random variable X has the survival function S, then

$$\int_0^\tau S(t)dt = E(X \wedge \tau). \tag{7.39}$$

Verification of this is left as Exercise 7.10. This quantity was first proposed by Irwin [121]. Over the last decade or so, it has received renewed interest, with many developments in the literature advocating its use in describing the treatment effect [370, 267, 298, 363].

Let T_C and T_T be the time-to-event variables in the control and treatment groups, respectively. Assume that the survival functions $S_C(t)$ and $S_T(t)$ are continuous. Define

$$A_C(t) = \int_0^t S_C(x)dx, \quad A_T(t) = \int_0^t S_T(x)dx.$$

Then, T_T is stochastically greater than T_C if and only if

$$A_T(t) \geq A_C(t)$$

for all t. Thus RMST has the important property that stochastic ordering can be equivalently expressed in terms of $A_C(t)$ and $A_T(t)$.

The restricted mean survival difference up to t is

$$\mu(t) = \int_0^t S_T(s)ds - \int_0^t S_C(s)ds.$$

Without assuming a particular model, $\mu(t)$ can be estimated nonparametrically using the Kaplan-Meier estimators. This estimator will be denoted by $\widehat{\mu}_N(t)$.

Under model (7.6), $\mu(t)$ can be estimated by

$$\widehat{\mu}_M(t) = \int_0^t \widehat{S}_{TM}(s)ds - \int_0^t \widehat{S}_{CM}(s)ds. \tag{7.40}$$

To display how the restricted mean survival difference changes over time, point-wise and simultaneous confidence bands for $\mu(t)$ over an interval $t \in J$ can be obtained using th Monte Carlo method. Details can be found in Yang [337].

Example 7.5. For the TOPCAT primary endpoint, Figure 7.8 displays the estimates and the 95% point-wise confidence intervals of the restricted mean survival difference based on model (7.6), alongside the nonparametric estimates. It shows that there is little difference between the model-based and nonparametric estimates. Since the restricted mean difference is an accumulative measure—meaning that the value at time t depends on the survival probabilities at all points prior to t—the nonparametric point estimate curve is much smoother than the one in Figure 7.7 for the absolute risk reduction. The intervals also exhibit a pattern similar to that in Figure 7.7: they exclude 1 for small values of t, and the variance gradually increases, leading to wider intervals that contain 1. Due to the accumulative nature of the measure, the time interval during which the confidence intervals exclude 1 is larger than the corresponding time interval in Figure 7.7.

7.6.4 Event Probability Ratio and the Ratio of Cumulative Hazards

The absolute risk reduction and restricted mean survival difference directly relate to the survival probability, The former is instantaneous at t, while the latter measures the cumulative or integrated survival difference up to time t. These measures can also be estimated nonparametrically without relying on an assumed model. However, they are difference measures, which can be heavily influenced by baseline characteristics of the population and censoring. Furthermore, a substantial amount of censoring can cause their values to become extremely small.

Define the event probability ratio and the ratio of cumulative hazards as

$$EPR(t) = \frac{F_T(t)}{F_C(t)}, \qquad RCH(t) = \frac{\Lambda_T(t)}{\Lambda_C(t)},$$

where $F_T(t) = 1 - S_T(t)$ and $F_C(t) = 1 - S_C(t)$. They are instantaneous measures of the relative treatment effect at t, in terms of the event probability and cumulative

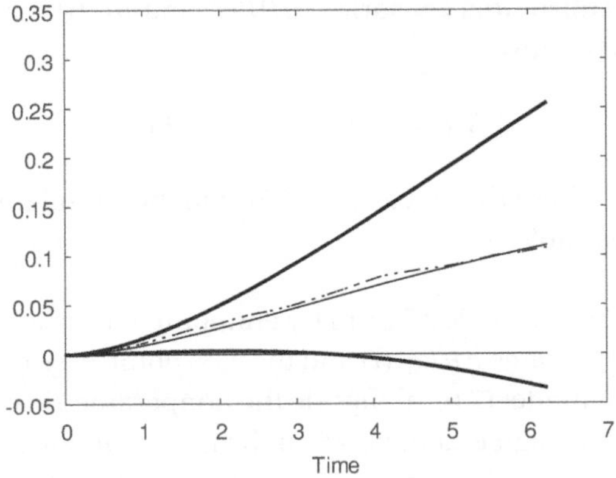

FIGURE 7.8
Estimates and 95% point-wise confidence intervals of the restricted mean survival difference based on model (7.6), alongside the nonparametric estimates. Thick solid: 95% point-wise confidence intervals based on model (7.6); thin solid: point estimates based on model (7.6); thin dotted: nonparametric estimates.

hazard, respectively. The event probability ratio relates to the probability directly, while the cumulative hazard is a log transformation of the survival probability. An appealing property of the ratio of cumulative hazards is that it reduces to the hazard ratio when the two sample Cox model (5.4) holds.

Both measures can be estimated nonparametrically, using the Kaplan-Meier estimators and the Nelson-Aalen estimators of the two groups, respectively. Denote the nonparametric estimators by

$$\widehat{EPR}_N(t), \quad \widehat{RCH}_N(t),$$

at t where the respective denominator does not vanish. These estimators can be unstable, especially near the two extremes of the data range. Yang [327] proposed to estimate $EPR(t)$ and $RCH(t)$ based on model (7.6). Let

$$\begin{aligned} \widehat{\Lambda}_{CM}(t) &= \log\left[1+\widehat{R}(t;\widehat{\boldsymbol{\beta}})(t)\right], \\ \widehat{\Lambda}_{TM}(t) &= \exp(\widehat{\beta}_2)\log\left[1+\exp(\widehat{\beta}_1-\widehat{\beta}_2)\widehat{R}(t;\widehat{\boldsymbol{\beta}})(t)\right]. \end{aligned} \tag{7.41}$$

Then the model-based estimators are

$$\widehat{EPR}_M(t) = \frac{1-\widehat{S}_{TM}(t)}{1-\widehat{S}_{CM}(t)}, \quad \widehat{RCH}_M(t) = \frac{\widehat{\Lambda}_{TM}(t)}{\widehat{\Lambda}_{CM}(t)}.$$

Yang obtained point-wise and simultaneous confidence intervals for $EPR(t)$ and $RCH(t)$ based on $\widehat{EPR}_M(t)$ and $\widehat{RCH}_M(t)$, respectively.

When there is substantial censoring, $EPR(t)$ and $RCH(t)$ will be very close to each other. This is because

$$\Lambda(t) = -\log[1 - F(t)] \approx F(t)$$

when $F(t)$ is small, where F and Λ are the CDF and the cumulative hazard function of a nonnegative variable.

Example 7.6. For the TOPCAT primary endpoint, Figure 7.9 displays the semiparametric point estimates $\widehat{EPR}_M(t)$ and the 95% point-wise confidence intervals of $EPR(t)$ based on model (7.6), alongside the nonparametric estimates $\widehat{EPR}_N(t)$. The figure shows good agreement between the nonparametric and semiparametric point estimates, except for very small values of t, where the ratios are unstable due to the denominator being near zero. The semiparametric curve smooths out the fluctuations of the nonparametric curve, suggesting a good model fit.

For the same data, Figure 7.10 displays the semiparametric point estimates $\widehat{RCH}_M(t)$ and 95% point-wise confidence intervals of $RCH(t)$ based on model (7.6), alongside the nonparametric estimates $\widehat{RCH}_N(t)$. The figure is almost identical to Figure 7.9 due to heavy censoring. Figure 7.10 also suggests that the proportional hazards assumption is reasonable, with $\widehat{RCH}_M(t)$ remaining nearly constant.

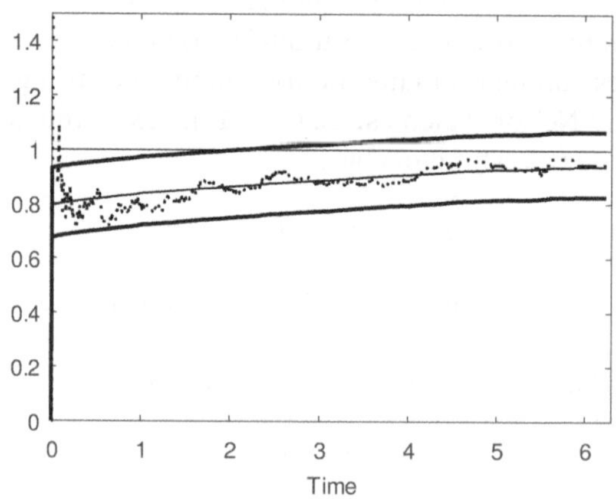

FIGURE 7.9
Estimates and the 95% point-wise confidence intervals of $EPR(t)$ based on model (7.6), alongside the nonparametric estimates, for the TOPCAT primary endpoint. Thick solid: 95% point-wise confidence intervals based on model (7.6); thin solid: semiparametric estimates based on model (7.6); dotted: nonparametric estimates.

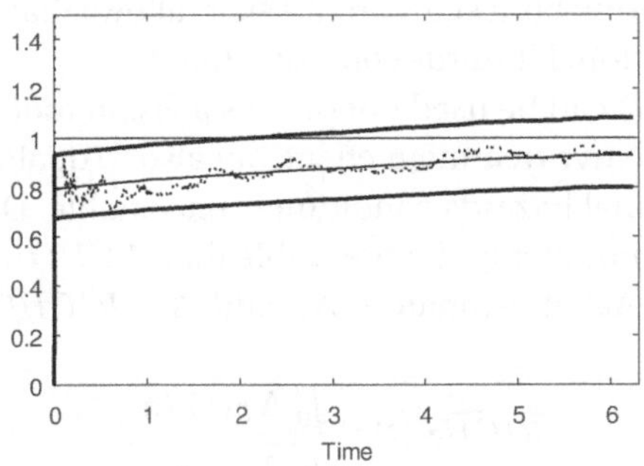

FIGURE 7.10
Estimates and the 95% point-wise confidence intervals of $RCH(t)$ based on model (7.6), alongside the nonparametric estimates, for the TOPCAT primary endpoint. Thick solid: 95% point-wise confidence intervals based on model (7.6); thin solid: semiparametric estimates based on model (7.6); dotted: nonparametric estimates.

7.6.5 Ratio of Areas Under the Nelson-Aalen Curves

The event probability ratio and the ratio of cumulative hazards provide instantaneous measures of the relative treatment effect at t, in terms of the event probability and cumulative hazard, respectively. They depend solely on the survival probabilities at t in the two groups.

For a cumulative effect measure reflecting all survival probabilities up to time t, we can consider

$$RICH(t) = \frac{\int_0^t \Lambda_T(x)dx}{\int_0^t \Lambda_C(x)dx}$$

This concept was originally proposed by Yang [340] in the analysis of terminal and non-terminal events, a topic that will be discussed in Chapter Fourteen. However, it is also applicable in the current setting.

Similar to the discussion in Section 7.6.3, T_T is stochastically greater than T_C if and only if

$$\int_0^t \Lambda_T(x)dx \leq \int_0^t \Lambda_C(x)dx$$

for all t.

Suppose that

$$\Lambda_T(t) = \theta\Lambda_C(t), \quad \text{for} \quad t \leq c, \tag{7.42}$$

where θ and c are fixed positive values. Then

$$\int_0^t \Lambda_T(x)dx = \theta \int_0^t \Lambda_C(x)dx, \quad \text{for} \quad t \leq c. \tag{7.43}$$

Conversely, if (7.43) holds, and Λ_T and Λ_C are continuous on $[0, c]$, then (7.42) holds upon differentiating both sides on (7.43). It follows that $RICH(t)$ is constant if and only the proportional hazards condition holds.

Therefore, $RICH(t)$ can be used not only as a visual tool to assess the change over time of the cumulative treatment effect, but also to qualitatively demonstrate whether the proportional hazards condition is reasonable. Due to the accumulative nature, it is also smoother and more stable than $RCH(t)$.

Using the Nelson-Aalen estimators $\widehat{\Lambda}_T$ and $\widehat{\Lambda}_C$, $RICH(t)$ can be estimated nonparametrically by

$$\widehat{RICH}_N(t) = \frac{\int_0^t \widehat{\Lambda}_T(x)dx}{\int_0^t \widehat{\Lambda}_C(x)dx}.$$

More discussion on $RICH(t)$ and the variance estimator for $\widehat{RICH}_N(t)$ can be found in Section 9.3.4 of Chapter Nine. A model-based estimator can also be obtained using $\widehat{\Lambda}_{CM}(x)$ and $\widehat{\Lambda}_{TM}(x)$.

Example 7.7. For the TOPCAT primary endpoint, Figure 7.11 displays nonparametric estimates $\widehat{RICH}_N(t)$ for $RICH(t)$, along with the 95% point-wise confidence intervals. It can be seen that $\widehat{RICH}_N(t)$ is much smoother than $\widehat{RCH}_N(t)$, and that $\widehat{RICH}_N(t)$, apart from the first 6 months where random variation is high, increases gradually from 0.8 to 0.89. The confidence intervals remain nearly constant in width from year 2 onward and eventually contain 1 from year 4.5 onward. This suggests a gradually decreasing cumulative treatment effect, although the slight variation in $\widehat{RICH}_N(t)$ is not large enough to discredit the two-sample Cox model as discussed in Example 6.3.

For the SPRINT trial primary endpoint, Figure 7.12 displays nonparametric estimates $\widehat{RICH}_N(t)$ for $RICH(t)$, along with the 95% point-wise confidence intervals. It can be seen that the confidence intervals contain 1 for most of the first 3 years. However, starting from year 1, the estimates steadily decrease from 1 to 0.78, and the confidence intervals also decrease slightly but steadily in width from year 1 onward, eventually excluding 1 from year 3 onward. This suggests a gradually increasing cumulative treatment effect.

From Figures 7.11 and 7.12, TOPCAT and SPRINT represent two opposite scenarios. While the proportional hazards assumption appear reasonable in both cases, the cumulative treatment effect gradually increases in SPRINT and gradually decreases in TOPCAT.

For a scenario with non-proportional hazards, Figure 7.13 displays the results of the nonparametric point and interval estimates of $RICH(t)$ for the time to death in the gastric cancer trial in Section 1.20.5. From year 1 onward, the estimated $RICH(t)$ gradually decreases from 3.5 to 0.9.

All the curves discussed above reflect change over time in a difference or ratio between relevant quantities of the two groups. They provide useful visual

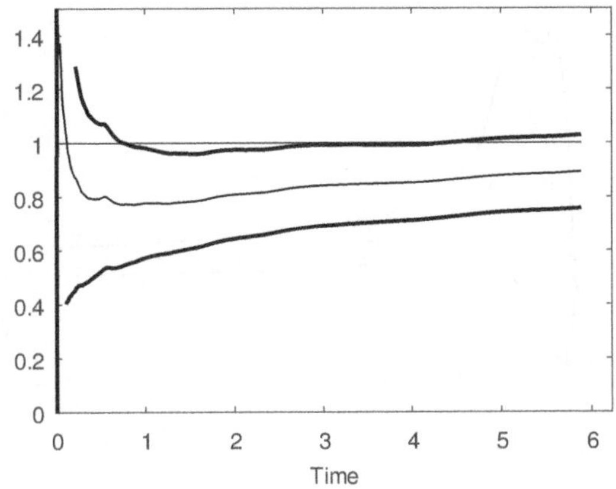

FIGURE 7.11
Nonparametric estimates and 95% point-wise confidence intervals of $RICH(t)$ for the TOPCAT primary endpoint. Thick solid: 95% point-wise confidence intervals; thin solid: point estimates.

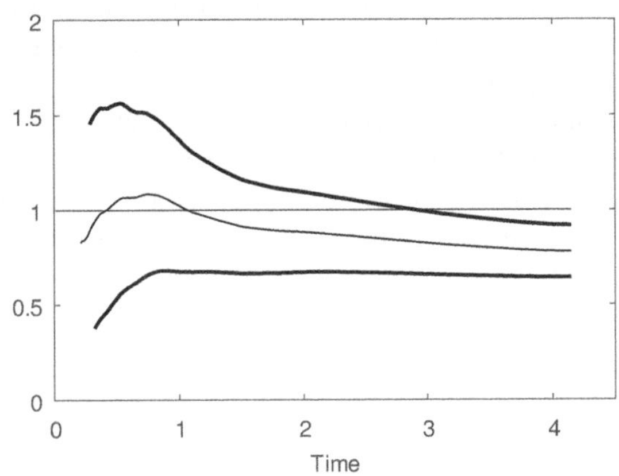

FIGURE 7.12
Nonparametric estimates and 95% point-wise confidence intervals of $RICH(t)$ for the SPRINT primary endpoint. Thick solid: 95% point-wise confidence intervals; thin solid: point estimates.

information on the trend of the treatment effect. Except for the hazard ratio, they all can be estimated nonparametrically. For smoother plots and more stable results, they can be estimated using model (7.6) when it fits.

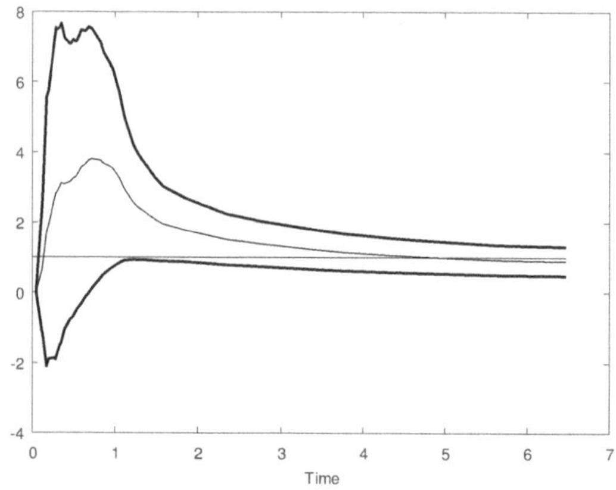

FIGURE 7.13
Nonparametric estimates and 95% point-wise confidence intervals of $RICH(t)$ for the gastric cancer trial data. Thick solid: 95% point-wise confidence intervals; thin solid: point estimates.

Some of the quantities used in plotting the curves are also related to various summary measures of the treatment effect, for which a more detailed discussion will be provided in Chapter Nine.

Due to its accumulative, model-free nature, more stable behavior, and connection with the proportional hazards assumption, $RICH(t)$ may be one of the most informative curves discussed. An additional crucial property is that it is derived from the hazard functions. Therefore, it allows an easy extension to competing risks problems. In fact, the concept was originally proposed in Yang [340] to handle competing risks.

7.7 Checking the Model of Short-Term and Long-Term Hazard Ratios

The model of short-term and long-term hazard ratios (7.6) includes the proportional hazards model and the proportional odds model as sub-models, and allows a wider range of hazard ratio patterns compared with some of the more traditional models. Nevertheless, it is still important to check model adequacy. Yang and Zhao [351] proposed two omnibus tests for model checking using, respectively, martingale residuals and contrast between the nonparametric and model-based estimators of the survival function. Under certain regularity conditions, these tests were shown to be consistent against any departure from the model.

Suppose that data are available from the two-sample random censorship model. To develop tests for model (7.6), an estimator for $\boldsymbol{\beta}$ is needed. Although it is possible to use the pseudo likelihood estimator in Section 7.4, Yang and Zhao used a simpler estimator. If the baseline function $R(t)$ were known, the log-likelihood of model (7.6) would be proportional to

$$-\sum_{i=1}^{n}\{\delta_i \log[h_{1i}(\boldsymbol{\beta})+h_{2i}(\boldsymbol{\beta})R(X_i)]+\log[1+h_{2i}(\boldsymbol{\beta})R(X_i)/h_{1i}(\boldsymbol{\beta})]/h_{2i}(\boldsymbol{\beta})\}.$$

This motivates the following estimator for $\boldsymbol{\beta}$. Let $\widehat{R}(t)$ be the odds function of the control group, based on the Kaplan-Meier estimator of S_C. Then $\widehat{R}(t)$ is a consistent estimator of $R(t)$. Define

$$p(\boldsymbol{\beta})=\sum_{i=1}^{n}\{\delta_i \log[h_{1i}(\boldsymbol{\beta})+h_{2i}(\boldsymbol{\beta})\widehat{R}(X_i)]+\log[1+h_{2i}(\boldsymbol{\beta})\widehat{R}(X_i)/h_{1i}(\boldsymbol{\beta})]/h_{2i}(\boldsymbol{\beta})\}.$$

Then the minimizer $\widetilde{\boldsymbol{\beta}}$ of $p(\boldsymbol{\beta})$ is a reasonable estimator of $\boldsymbol{\beta}$. Equivalently, $\widetilde{\boldsymbol{\beta}}$ is the zero of the gradient $\nabla p(\boldsymbol{\beta})$ of $p(\boldsymbol{\beta})$.

Let

$$\widetilde{M}_i(t)=\delta_i I(X_i\le t)-\int_0^t I(X_i\ge s)\frac{d\widehat{R}(s)}{h_{1i}(\widetilde{\boldsymbol{\beta}})+h_{2i}(\widetilde{\boldsymbol{\beta}})\widehat{R}(s)},\quad 1\le i\le n.$$

Note that $\widetilde{M}_i(t)$ does not involve $\widetilde{\boldsymbol{\beta}}$ when $Z_i=0$. Under model (7.6), $\widetilde{\boldsymbol{\beta}}$ is close to $\boldsymbol{\beta}$ and $\widehat{R}(t)$ close to $R(t)$, thus

$$\sum_{Z_i=1}\widetilde{M}_i(t)\approx\sum_{Z_i=1}M_i(t),$$

for martingales $M_1,\ldots,M_n$ in (7.16), which fluctuates around zero. This led Yang and Zhao to define a test using the martingale residuals. It rejects model (7.6) for large values of

$$\sup_{t\le\widetilde{\tau}}\Big|\sum_{Z_i=1}\int_0^t \Phi_r(s)d\widetilde{M}_i(s)\Big|/\sqrt{n}, \tag{7.44}$$

where Φ_r is a data-dependent nonnegative function and $\widetilde{\tau}\le\tau$ for τ in (7.11).

Under model (7.6) and certain regularity conditions, Yang and Zhao showed that the process

$$\sum_{Z_i=1}\int_0^t \Phi_r(s)d\widetilde{M}_i(s)/\sqrt{n},\quad t\in[0,\widetilde{\tau}],$$

converges weakly to a zero mean Gaussian process whose covariance process can be consistently estimated using $\widetilde{\boldsymbol{\beta}}$, $\widehat{R}(t)$ to replace $\boldsymbol{\beta}$, $R(t)$, respectively, in the limiting covariance process.

Let r_o be the observed value of the statistic in (7.44). Then the P-value

$$P\Big[\sup_{t\in[0,\widetilde{\tau}]}\Big|\sum_{Z_i=1}\int_0^t \Phi_r(s)d\widetilde{M}_i(s)\Big|/\sqrt{n} > r_o\Big]$$

can be approximated by the Monte Carlo method in Section 6.5. Yang and Zhao showed that under model (7.6) and certain regularity conditions, the martingale residual-based test is consistent against a general departure from model (7.6) on $t \in [0, \widetilde{\tau}]$.

In the literature, martingale residuals have been used quite extensively to detect departures from the assumed models [297, 178]. Lin et al. [178] studied various partial-sum processes of the martingale residuals, and used simulated Gaussian processes to approximate the distributions of those processes under the multiplicative hazards model. Note that the test based on martingale residuals here is slightly different from the test for checking the multiplicative hazards model in Lin et al. [178] in that integrals of the martingale residuals are used.

One advantage of the test based on martingale residuals is that it can be naturally extended from the two-sample case to regression settings. In fact, major use of martingale residuals in the literature so far relates to regression models. On the other hand, the partial-sum processes of martingale residuals themselves do not have a simple interpretation. The two-sample nature of model (7.6) makes it possible to consider a contrast-based test which has a very simple and direct interpretation as the difference between nonparametric and model-based estimators of the survival function for the treatment group. Intuitively, model (7.6) holds if the nonparametric and model-based estimators are close to each other.

Using $\widetilde{\boldsymbol{\beta}}$, a model-based estimator for S_T is

$$\widetilde{S}(t) = \{1 + \exp(\widetilde{\beta}_1 - \widetilde{\beta}_2)\widehat{R}(t)\}^{-\exp(\widetilde{\beta}_2)}.$$

On the other hand, a nonparametric estimator of S_T is $\widehat{S}_N = \exp(-\widehat{\Lambda}_T)$, where $\widehat{\Lambda}_T$ is the Nelson-Aalen estimator for the cumulative hazard function Λ_T. Yang and Zhao defined a contrast-based test using $\widehat{S}_N(t) - \widetilde{S}(t)$. It was noted that, although the Kaplan-Meier estimator could also be used in the contrast-based test, $\widetilde{S}$ showed better performance for small samples in various simulations.

Under model (7.6) and certain regularity conditions, it can be shown that the process $\sqrt{n}\{\widehat{S}_N(t) - \widetilde{S}(t)\}$, $0 \le t \le \widetilde{\tau}$, converges weakly to a zero mean Gaussian process whose variation process $\sigma_c^2(t)$ has a consistent estimator $\widehat{\sigma}_c^2(t)$ which is obtained by replacing $\boldsymbol{\beta}$, $R(t)$, with $\widetilde{\boldsymbol{\beta}}$, $\widehat{R}(t)$, respectively. The contrast-based rejects model (7.6) for large values of

$$\sqrt{n}\sup_{t\le\widetilde{\tau}}\Big\{\Phi_c(t)\big|\widehat{S}_T(t) - \widetilde{S}(t)\big|/\widehat{\sigma}_c(t)\Big\}, \tag{7.45}$$

where Φ_c is a data-dependent nonnegative function.

Let c_o be the observed value of the statistic in (7.45). Then the P-value

$$P\Big[\sup_{t\in[0,\widetilde{\tau}]}\Big\{\sqrt{n}\Phi_c(t)\big|\widehat{S}_T(t)-\widetilde{S}(t)\big|/\widehat{\sigma}_c(t)\Big\}>c_o\Big]$$

can be approximated by the Monte Carlo method in Section 6.5. Yang and Zhao showed that the standardized contrast-based test is consistent against a general departure from model (7.6) on $t\in[0,\widetilde{\tau}]$, except for the degenerate case where $\sigma_c(t)$ is zero for some $t\in[0,\widetilde{\tau}]$.

For the functions Φ_r, Φ_c in the two tests, based on exploration with various simulation studies and data applications, Yang and Zhao recommended the choice

$$\Phi_c(t)=1+\frac{4\big[K_C(t)+K_T(t)\big]}{n}\Big\{1-\frac{K_C(t)+K_T(t)}{n}\Big\}$$

and

$$\Phi_r(t)=\frac{K_C(t)}{K_C(t)+K_T(t)}\Phi_c(t),$$

where K_C, K_T are the at-risk processes of the two groups defined in (2.48). The first factor in $\Phi_r(t)$ is used to help stabilize the integral near the upper tail, and $\Phi_c(t)$ assigns weights between 1 and 2 to all data points, with more weight in the central region and less weight toward the boundaries of data range. As for $\widetilde{\tau}$, it was recommended to take

$$\widetilde{\tau}=(\max_i X_i Z_i)\wedge\big(\max_i X_i(1-Z_i)\big).$$

Furthermore, when using the Monte Carlo method to obtain the critical value for the contrast-based test, it was recommended to apply the multiplier $(1+1/\sqrt{n})$ to the i.i.d. standard normal G_i's for improved small sample behavior.

Example 7.8. For the TCD trial, Example 6.2 shows strong evidence of model violation for the two-sample Cox model (5.4). Now consider model (7.6). The martingale residual test in (7.41) and the contrast-based test in (7.42) have P-values 0.99 and 0.83, respectively. Figure 7.3 also shows good agreement between the Kaplan-Meier and model-based CDF estimates.

For the TOPCAT trial, Example 6.3 shows strong evidence of non-proportional effect of the covariate age. In particular, when the Cox model is fit to the single dichotomous covariate $W=I(age>69)$, the lack-of-fit test has an extreme P-value of 0.005.

Note that, although model (7.6) is motivated by comparison between the control and treatment groups, the model can be used for the general two-sample comparison problem. Now if we apply model (7.6) to the comparison of $W=0$ vs $W=1$, the martingale residual test and the contrast-based test have P-values 0.39 and 0.44, respectively. Figure 7.14 also shows good agreement between the Kaplan-Meier and model-based CDF estimates.

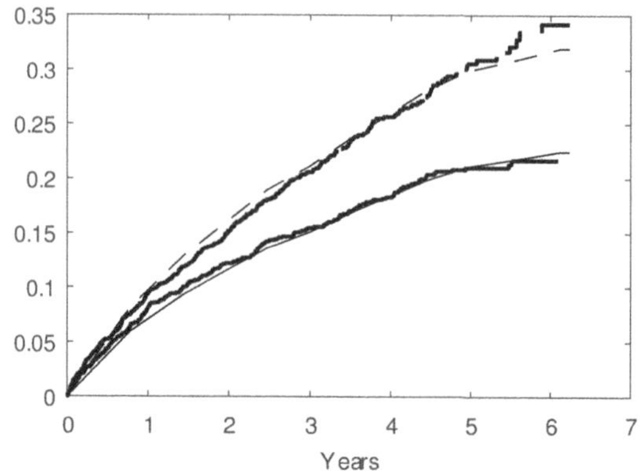

FIGURE 7.14
Estimated CDF for the TOPCAT primary endpoint for comparison between group 1, with $age \leq 69$, and group 2, with $age > 69$. Thick solid: group 1, Kaplan-Meier; thick dashed: group 2, Kaplan-Meier; thin solid: group 1, model (7.6); thin dashed: group 2, model (7.6).

For the primary outcome of time to coronary heart disease in the WHI E+P trial discussed in Examples 7.2, the martingale residual test in (7.41) and the contrast-based test in (7.42) have P-values 0.44 and 0.43, respectively, for model (7.6). For time to stroke discussed in Examples 7.3, the martingale residual test and the contrast-based test have P-values 0.82 and 0.97, respectively.

To implement some of the procedures, the R package YPModel is available at the Comprehensive R Archive Network [291]. Functions in the package include a function for obtaining the pseudo-likelihood estimator $\widehat{\boldsymbol{\beta}}$, a function for drawing point-wise and simultaneous confidence intervals for the hard ratio, and a function for implementing the two model-checking tests.

7.8 Adjustment for Covariates with Proportional Effects

Although the focused is on the two-sample case in Yang and Prentice [344], formulation (7.6) of the model allows natural extensions to the regression setting. One option is to include covariates which are assumed to have proportional effects on the hazard function. Let $\boldsymbol{W} = (Z, \boldsymbol{B})^{\mathrm{T}}$, where $\boldsymbol{B}$ is a $p \times 1$ vector of baseline characteristics of the individual. Then the model postulates that the conditional hazard function of T given $\boldsymbol{W}$ is

$$\lambda[t; \boldsymbol{W}] = \frac{\exp(\boldsymbol{\gamma}^{\mathrm{T}} \boldsymbol{B})}{\exp(-\beta_1 Z) + \exp(-\beta_2 Z) R(t)} \frac{dR(t)}{dt}. \tag{7.46}$$

where $\boldsymbol{\gamma}$ is a $p \times 1$ parameter vector and $R(t)$ is the unknown baseline odds function which is increasing with $R(0) = 0$.

Under this model, the hazard ratio of the treatment group over the control group at level $\boldsymbol{B} = \boldsymbol{b}$ is

$$h(t) = \frac{\lambda_{Z=1,\boldsymbol{B}=\boldsymbol{b}}(t)}{\lambda_{Z=0,\boldsymbol{B}=\boldsymbol{b}}(t)} = \frac{1 + R(t)}{\exp(-\beta_1 Z) + \exp(-\beta_2 Z)R(t)}. \quad (7.47)$$

Similarly to the Cox proportional hazards model, the hazard ratio is the same for different levels of baseline characteristics of individuals. However, the hazard ratio for the treatment effect in general is time-dependent, instead of being a constant as in the Cox proportional hazards model. As in the two-sample case, the hazard ratio approaches the values $\exp(\beta_1)$ and $\exp(\beta_2)$, respectively, as t tends to zero or ∞. Thus $\exp(\beta_1)$ and $\exp(\beta_2)$ retain the interpretations as short-term and long-term hazard ratios, respectively, and different values of β_1, β_2 correspond to various scenarios of the treatment effect, including constant hazard ratio, no initial effect, disappearing effect, and crossing hazards.

In Yang and Prentice [344], two methods were briefly discussed to extend the two-sample model to regression settings. The first method gives model (7.46), where the short-term and long-term effects of Z are separated, but components of $\boldsymbol{B}$ have constant effects on the hazard ratio over time. The second method is more general and separates short-term and long-term effects for all components of $\boldsymbol{W}$. It assumes that

$$\lambda[t; \boldsymbol{W}] = \frac{1}{\exp(-\boldsymbol{\theta}_1^{\mathrm{T}}\boldsymbol{W}) + \exp(-\boldsymbol{\theta}_2^{\mathrm{T}}\boldsymbol{W})R(t)} \frac{dR(t)}{dt}, \quad (7.48)$$

where $\boldsymbol{\theta}_1$, $\boldsymbol{\theta}_2$ are both $(p+1) \times 1$ parameter vectors. This model contains the proportional odds model in addition to the Cox proportional hazards model as sub-models. It can also be further extended to allow time-dependent covariates as in Diao, Zeng and Yang [62].

Note that there are $2(p+1)$ scalar parameters in addition to the unknown baseline $R(t)$ in model (7.48). Thus, the general degrees of freedom in (7.48) is larger than that of the Cox proportional hazards model by $p+1$ which can be substantial as p increases. While this may be acceptable for exploratory variable selection analyses, it is usually desirable to limit the general degrees of freedom. Often the covariates used for adjustment have proportional effects on survival, Therefore, model (7.46) is an important sub-model of the more general model (7.48).

Yang and Prentice [347] studied model (7.46) and used it to compare results from the WHI E+P trial and a companion observational study. They extended to model (7.46) the pseudo-likelihood estimation procedure of the two-sample case in Section 7.3.

Let $\boldsymbol{\theta}$ be the $(p+2)\times 1$ parameter vector in model (7.46) consisting of β_1, β_2 and $\boldsymbol{\gamma}$, and define $h_j(\boldsymbol{\theta}, \boldsymbol{W}_i) = \exp(-\beta_j - \boldsymbol{\gamma}^{\mathrm{T}}\boldsymbol{W}_i)$. For $t \le \max_i\{X_i\}$, let

$$\begin{aligned}
\widehat{P}(t;\boldsymbol{\theta}) &= \exp\left(-\int_0^t \frac{\sum_{i=1}^n \delta_i h_2(\theta, \boldsymbol{W}_i)dN_i(s)}{K(s)}\right), \\
\widehat{R}(t;\boldsymbol{\theta}) &= \frac{1}{\widehat{P}(t;\boldsymbol{\theta})}\int_0^t \frac{\widehat{P}_-(s;\boldsymbol{\theta})}{K(s)} \sum_{i=1}^n \delta_i h_1(\theta, \boldsymbol{W}_i)dN_i(s), \qquad (7.49)
\end{aligned}$$

where $\widehat{P}_-(s;\boldsymbol{\theta})$ denotes the left continuous version (in s) of $\widehat{P}(s;\boldsymbol{\theta})$. For t beyond $\max_i\{X_i\}$, similarly to the case for the Kaplan-Meier estimator, $\widehat{P}(t;\boldsymbol{\theta})$ and $\widehat{R}(t;\boldsymbol{\theta})$ are defined by using their respective values at $\max_i X_i$. Then the pseudo-likelihood estimator $\widehat{\boldsymbol{\theta}}$ is the zero of $\boldsymbol{Q}(\boldsymbol{\theta})$, where

$$\begin{aligned}
\boldsymbol{Q}(\boldsymbol{\theta}) &= \left(Q_1(\boldsymbol{\theta}), Q_2(\boldsymbol{\theta}), \boldsymbol{Q}_3(\boldsymbol{\theta})^{\mathrm{T}}\right)^{\mathrm{T}}, \\
Q_1(\boldsymbol{\theta}) &= \sum_{i=1}^n \frac{Z_i[\delta_i h_1(\boldsymbol{\theta}, \boldsymbol{W}_i) - \widehat{R}(X_i;\boldsymbol{\theta})]}{h_1(\boldsymbol{\theta}, \boldsymbol{W}_i) + h_2(\boldsymbol{\theta}, \boldsymbol{W}_i)\widehat{R}(X_i;\boldsymbol{\theta})}, \\
Q_2(\boldsymbol{\theta}) &= \sum_{i=1}^n \left\{\frac{Z_i\widehat{R}(X_i;\boldsymbol{\theta})[\delta_i h_2(\boldsymbol{\theta}, \boldsymbol{W}_i) + 1]}{h_1(\boldsymbol{\theta}, \boldsymbol{W}_i) + h_2(\boldsymbol{\theta}, \boldsymbol{W}_i)\widehat{R}(X_i;\boldsymbol{\theta})}\right. \\
&\quad \left. - \frac{Z_i}{h_2(\boldsymbol{\theta}, \boldsymbol{W}_i)}\ln\left(1 + \frac{h_2(\boldsymbol{\theta}, \boldsymbol{W}_i)}{h_1(\boldsymbol{\theta}, \boldsymbol{W}_i)}\widehat{R}(X_i;\boldsymbol{\theta})\right)\right\}, \\
\boldsymbol{Q}_3(\boldsymbol{\theta}) &= \sum_{i=1}^n \left\{\delta_i \boldsymbol{W}_i - \frac{\boldsymbol{W}_i}{h_2(\boldsymbol{\theta}, \boldsymbol{W}_i)}\ln\left(1 + \frac{h_2(\boldsymbol{\theta}, \boldsymbol{W}_i)}{h_1(\boldsymbol{\theta}, \boldsymbol{W}_i)}\widehat{R}(X_i;\boldsymbol{\theta})\right)\right\}. \qquad (7.50)
\end{aligned}$$

Similar to (7.27), under certain regularity conditions, the estimator $\widehat{\boldsymbol{\theta}}$ can be shown to be asymptotically normal, with an asymptotic covariance matrix $\boldsymbol{D}(\boldsymbol{\theta})$ that can be consistently estimated by an estimator $\widehat{\boldsymbol{D}}$.

Once $\widehat{\boldsymbol{\theta}}$ is obtained, $R(t)$ can be estimated by $\hat{R}(t;\widehat{\boldsymbol{\theta}})$. For the hazard ratio $h(t)$ under model (7.46), the estimator is

$$\widehat{h}(t) = \frac{1 + \widehat{R}(t;\widehat{\boldsymbol{\theta}})}{\exp(-\widehat{\beta}_1) + \exp(-\widehat{\beta}_2)\widehat{R}(t;\widehat{\boldsymbol{\theta}})}.$$

Applying the Monte Carlo method described in Section 7.6.1, point-wise and simultaneous confidence intervals of $h(t)$ can be obtained. Again, for better small sample behavior and assurance that the confidence intervals do not contain negative values, a logarithmic transformation can be used which results in the asymptotic $100(1-\alpha)\%$ confidence interval

$$\widehat{h}(t)\exp\left(\mp z(\alpha/2)\frac{\widehat{\sigma}(t)}{\sqrt{n}\widehat{h}(t)}\right) \tag{7.51}$$

for $h(t)$ at a fixed t, where $\widehat{\sigma}(t)$ is the Monte Carlo estimator for the variance of the limiting distribution of $\sqrt{n}\left[\widehat{h}(t)-h(t)\right]$. Furthermore, simultaneous confidence intervals can be constructed, replacing $z(\alpha/2)$ in (7.51) by an appropriate critical value c_α that is obtained by the Monte Carlo method.

To summarize the treatment effect over time period $[0,a]$, Yang and Prentice [347] considered the average hazard ratio on $(0,a]$:

$$\mu_a = \frac{1}{a}\int_{t\le a} h(t)dt,$$

which can be estimated by $\hat{\mu}_a = \int_{t\le a}\hat{h}(t)dt/a$. They showed that $\hat{\mu}_a$ is strongly consistent and asymptotically normal, and that a consistent estimator $\hat{\sigma}^2_\mu(a)$ of the limiting variance $\sigma^2_\mu(a)$ can be obtained by a Monte Carlo method. From these results, an asymptotic $100(1-\alpha)\%$ confidence interval for μ_a is

$$\hat{\mu}_a \exp\left(\mp z_{\alpha/2}\frac{\hat{\sigma}_\mu(a)}{\sqrt{n}\hat{\mu}_a}\right). \tag{7.52}$$

Simultaneous confidence intervals over $t \in J$ was also considered.

Example 7.9. Although model (7.43) is motivated by extending model (7.6) to adjust for covariates with proportional effects on the hazard, mathematically, it is a model in which one of the explanatory variables has separate short- and long-term effects while the other variables have proportional effects. For the TOPCT trial, consider the model

$$\lambda[t;\boldsymbol{W}] = \frac{\exp(\gamma_1 W_1+\gamma_2 W_2+\gamma_3 W_3+\gamma_4 Z)}{\exp(-\beta_1 W_4)+\exp(-\beta_2 W_4)R(t)}\frac{dR(t)}{dt}. \tag{7.53}$$

where W_1—W_3 are defined in Example 5.2, and W_4 is the standardized age.

Under model (7.53), the hazard ratio of the treatment group over the control group at level $\boldsymbol{B}=\boldsymbol{b}$, where $\boldsymbol{B}=(W_1,W_2,W_3,W_4)^{\mathrm{T}}$, is

$$\frac{\lambda_{Z=1,\boldsymbol{B}=\boldsymbol{b}}}{\lambda_{Z=0,\boldsymbol{B}=\boldsymbol{b}}} = \exp(\gamma_4). \tag{7.54}$$

Therefore, although one covariate, W_4, has a non-proportional effect on the hazard, the parameter γ_4 in the covariate-adjusted model (7.53) is the log hazard ratio for the treatment effect, holding $\boldsymbol{B}$ fixed at the same level. Thus e^{γ_4} is a simple summary measure of the treatment effect. This is somewhat reminiscent of the stratified model (5.24), in which the hazard ratio for the treatment effect gives a

TABLE 7.2
Point estimate ($\hat{\boldsymbol{\theta}}$), 95% confidence interval (CI), standardized z-score and P-value for β_1, β_2 and γ_1 through γ_4 in model (7.53).

	$\hat{\boldsymbol{\theta}}$	CI	z-score	P-value
$\beta_1(W_4)$	1.26	1.14–1.40	4.56	< 0.0001
$\beta_2(W_4)$	2.38	1.57–3.62	4.06	< 0.0001
$\gamma_1(W_1)$	1.55	1.24–1.93	3.91	0.0001
$\gamma_2(W_2)$	1.24	1.02–1.50	2.14	0.03
$\gamma_3(W_3)$	1.06	0.90–1.24	0.66	0.51
$\gamma_4(Z)$	0.89	0.76–1.03	-1.56	0.12

simple summary effect measure in the presence of different baseline hazard functions in the strata. The approach of using model (7.53) provides an alternative to a stratified analysis in dealing with a covariate with non-proportional effect. It avoids the need to discretization of a continuous covariate.

From the pseudo-likelihood estimator and the Monte Carlo variance estimator with 2,000 repetitions, point and interval estimates, and the P-value for the Wald test of $\gamma_j = 0,\ j = 1,\ldots,4$ or $\beta_k = 0, k = 1,2$, are obtained and presented in Table 7.2.

From Table 7.2, the estimated hazard ratio for treatment effect is 0.89, and the P-value for the test of no treatment effect hypothesis $H_0 : \gamma_4 = 0$ is 0.12. Due to heavy censoring, there is less precision in estimation of β_2, as reflected by the wider confidence interval. For γ_1—γ_4, the estimates are close to the stratified analysis results in Table 5.1.

If W_3 is dropped, the model becomes

$$\lambda[t;\boldsymbol{W}] = \frac{\exp(\gamma_1 W_1 + \gamma_2 W_2 + \gamma_3 Z)}{\exp(-\beta_1 W_4) + \exp(-\beta_2 W_4)R(t)} \frac{dR(t)}{dt}. \tag{7.55}$$

Table 7.3 provides results for model (7.55) parallel to those in Table 7.2. The results for models (7.53) and (7.55) on parameter estimates and P-values for coefficients of W_4, W_1, W_2, and Z, with or without the covariate W_3, are very close to each other. In particular, the estimated hazard ratio for the treatment effect and the P-value for the test of no treatment effect remain unchanged when rounding to two decimal places. These P-values for the test of no treatment effect are also smaller than those from other methods as shown in previous chapters. One reason is that

TABLE 7.3
Point estimate ($\widehat{\boldsymbol{\theta}}$), 95% confidence interval (CI), standardized z-score and P-value for β_1, β_2 and γ_1 through γ_3 in model (7.55).

	$\widehat{\boldsymbol{\theta}}$	CI	z-score	P-value
$\beta_1(W_4)$	1.26	1.14–1.39	4.67	< 0.0001
$\beta_2(W_4)$	2.36	1.55–3.58	4.01	< 0.0001
$\gamma_1(W_1)$	1.54	1.24–1.92	3.90	0.0001
$\gamma_2(W_2)$	1.24	1.02–1.50	2.18	0.03
$\gamma_3(Z)$	0.89	0.77–1.03	-1.56	0.12

the models used here account for the non-proportional effect of age without dichotomization and stratification, both of which can result in information loss.

To implement inference procedures under morel (7.46), the R package YPmodelPhreg is available at the Comprehensive R Archive Network [220]. The package provides point estimates and confidence intervals for model parameters, point estimate and confidence interval of the average hazard ratio, and plots of estimated hazard ratio function with point-wise and simultaneous confidence bands.

7.9 Nonparametric Likelihood Estimation and Profile Likelihood

As mentioned in Section 5.6, for a wide variety of semiparametric models, under appropriate regularity conditions, the method of nonparametric maximum likelihood estimation yields estimators that are consistent and asymptotically normal, and the asymptotic covariance matrix of the finite-dimensional parameter achieves the efficiency lower bound.

For model (7.6), (7.46) and (7.48), the conditional hazard function is semiparametrically determined by the scalar parameters and the baseline function $R(t)$, in expressions very similar to the case for the proportional odds regression model studied by Murphy, Rossini and van der Vaart [209]. Thus NPMLE can be obtained similarly.

As discussed in Chapter Six, time-dependent covariates may often be encountered. A natural extension of model (7.48) to allow time-dependent covariate $\boldsymbol{W}(t)$ is the following model:

$$\lambda[t;\boldsymbol{W}(t)] = \frac{1}{\exp(-\boldsymbol{\theta}_1^{\mathrm{T}}\boldsymbol{W}(t)) + \exp(-\boldsymbol{\theta}_2^{\mathrm{T}}\boldsymbol{W}(t))R(t)} \frac{dR(t)}{dt}. \tag{7.56}$$

Let $\lambda_0(t)$, $\Lambda_0(t)$ and $S_0(t)$ be the hazard, cumulative hazard and survival functions corresponding to the odds function $R(t)$, and $F_0(t)$ the associated CDF. Then model (7.56) can be re-expressed as

$$\lambda[t;\boldsymbol{W}(t)] = \frac{\lambda_0(t)}{\exp(-\boldsymbol{\theta}_1^{\mathrm{T}}\boldsymbol{W}(t))S_0(t) + \exp(-\boldsymbol{\theta}_2^{\mathrm{T}}\boldsymbol{W}(t))F_0(t)}. \tag{7.57}$$

Suppose data are obtained from the random censorship model with time-dependent external covariates as described in Section 6.3. Under (7.57), Diao, Zeng, and Yang [62] showed that the nonparametric MLE $\widehat{\boldsymbol{\theta}}$ and $\widehat{\Lambda}$ for $\boldsymbol{\theta} = (\boldsymbol{\theta}_1, \boldsymbol{\theta}_2)^{\mathrm{T}}$ and $\Lambda_0(t)$ are consistent and asymptotically normal, and that the asymptotic covariance matrix $\Sigma_{\boldsymbol{\theta}}$ of $\widehat{\boldsymbol{\theta}}$ achieves the efficiency lower bound. Furthermore, $\Sigma_{\boldsymbol{\theta}}$ can be consistently estimated by inverting the observed Fisher information matrix for $\boldsymbol{\theta}$.

As mentioned in Section 5.6, when the interest is only in $\boldsymbol{\theta}$, the profile likelihood approach proceeds very much as in the case for ordinary parametric inference. However, models such as (7.57) are often used to accommodate non-proportional hazards situations, where the parameter $\boldsymbol{\theta}$ alone may be inadequate in treatment effect assessment as will be discussed in Chapter Nine.

When a smooth function of both $\boldsymbol{\theta}$ and $\Lambda_0(t)$ is of interest, the limiting covariance matrix of $(\widehat{\boldsymbol{\theta}}, \widehat{\Lambda})$ can be estimated by inverting the observed Fisher information matrix for both $\boldsymbol{\theta}$ and Λ_0. The matrix is $q \times q$, where q is the dimension of $\boldsymbol{W}$ plus the number of uncensored times in data. Inverting such high dimensional matrix may present a challenge in implementing NPMLE procedures for large clinical trials, in terms of algorithm stability as well as computing cost as has been observed before [305, 361]. Regarding the computing cost and efficiency, Yang and Prentice [347] compared the nonparametric maximum likelihood estimator and the pseudo-likelihood estimator. Typically, when the number of events is of the magnitude observed in large clinical trials, both methods have virtually the same efficiency. On the other hand, efficiency gain of the NPMLE is more obvious for more moderate samples.

For competing risks to be discussed in Chapter Thirteen, the pseudo-likelihood procedure can be applied to event of interest without having to model other competing event types simultaneously. On the other hand, the NPMLE for competing risks data requires model specification for all event types. More related discussion can be found in Chapter Thirteen.

Example 7.10. For the TCD trial, the NPMLE for model (7.6) yields $e^{\widehat{\beta}} = (0.71, 7.33)^{\mathrm{T}}$. Figure 7.15 shows the Kaplan-Meier and NPMLE CDF estimates.

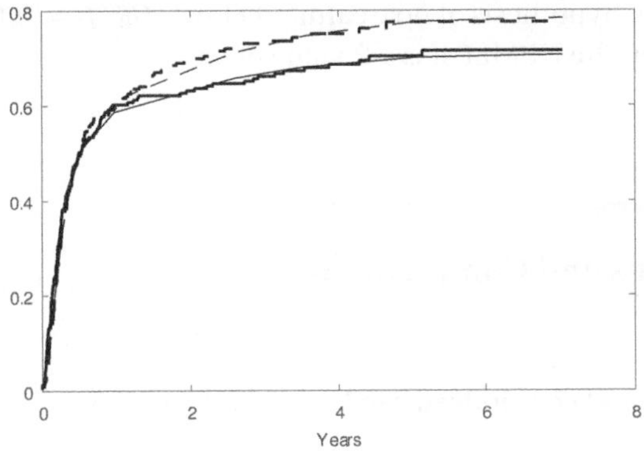

FIGURE 7.15
Estimated CDF for the TCD trial. Thick solid: control group, Kaplan-Meier; thick dashed: treatment group, Kaplan-Meier; thin solid: control group, NPMLE in model (7.6); thin dashed: treatment group, NPMLE in model (7.6).

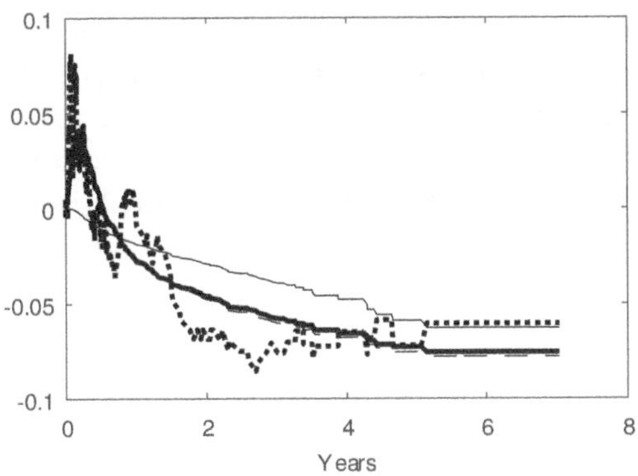

FIGURE 7.16
Estimated absolute risk reduction for the TCD trial data based on various methods and models. Thick solid: pseudo-likelihood, model (7.6); thick dotted: Kaplan-Meier; thin dashed: NPMLE, model (7.6); thin solid: model (6.2).

To compare with the pseudo-likelihood estimator and the with model (6.2), estimates of the absolute risk reduction from these different methods are plotted in Figure 7.16. The curves based on the NPMLE and the pseudo-likelihood estimator are virtually identical in the first two years, and hardly distinguishable afterwards. In comparison, the curve based on model (6.2) shows less than ideal agreement with the Kaplan-Meir method in most part of the data range, except for the region beyond 5.14 years where no event are observed.

For testing the hypothesis of no treatment effect, $H_0 : \boldsymbol{\beta} = (0,0)^T$, the likelihood ratio test based on the NPMLE has a P-value of 0.07.

7.10 Exercises and Complements

7.1 Verify (7.5).

7.2 Verify that model (7.1) indeed can be rewritten as (7.6).

7.3 Verify (7.7).

7.4 Derive the score function for model (7.6) with $R(t)$ a known function to confirm that the pseudo-likelihood estimating function is given by (7.15).

7.5 Verify that at $\boldsymbol{\beta} = 0$, $\widehat{R}(t;\boldsymbol{\beta})$ in (7.14) reduces to $1/\widehat{S}_p(t) - 1$, where $\widehat{S}(t)$ is the Kaplan-Meier survival function estimator based on the pooled sample.

7.6 $\widehat{R}(t;\boldsymbol{\beta})$ is obtained as the solution of an equation which closely resembles an identity for the underlying distribution. Similar idea can be applied to obtain the Kaplan-Meier estimator from the Nelson-Aalen estimator. Assume that data are available from the random censorship model and $\widehat{\Lambda}(t)$ is the Nelson-Aalen estimator of the cumulative hazard function $\Lambda(t)$ of T. From (2.17),

$$\Lambda(t) = \int_0^t \frac{dF(s)}{1 - F_-(s)}.$$

Thus it is reasonable to define an estimator $\widetilde{F}(t)$ by requiring

$$\widehat{\Lambda}(t) = \int_0^t \frac{d\widetilde{F}(s)}{1 - \widetilde{F}_-(s)}. \tag{7.58}$$

Furthermore, since $\widehat{\Lambda}(t)$ has jumps only at the uncensored data points, we require $\widetilde{F}(t)$ to have the same property. Let $t_1 < \cdots < t_k$ be the observed distinct event times. Let l_j and f_j be the jumps of $\widehat{\Lambda}$ and $\widetilde{F}$ at t_j, respectively, and $F_j = f_1 + \cdots + f_j$, $F_{j-} = F_j - f_j$, $j = 1, \ldots, k$.

From (7.58),

$$d\widehat{\Lambda}(t) = \frac{d\widetilde{F}(t)}{1 - \widetilde{F}_-(t)}.$$

That is,

$$l_j = \frac{f_j}{1 - F_{j-}} \qquad j = 1, \ldots, k$$

It follows that

$$1 - l_j = \frac{1 - F_j}{1 - F_{j-}} \qquad j = 1, \ldots, k,$$

and, for any m between 1 and k,

$$1 - F_m = \prod_{j=1}^{m} \frac{1 - F_j}{1 - F_{j-}} = \prod_{j=1}^{m} (1 - l_j).$$

Therefore, $\widetilde{F}$ is precisely the Kaplan-Meier estimator of the CDF F of T.

7.7 Similarly, the Nelson-Aalen estimator can be obtained by approximating population quantities by their sample versions from the definition of $\Lambda(t)$. Assume again that data are available from the random censorship model. Let the CDF of the censoring variable C_i be $G_i(t)$, $i = 1, \ldots, n$. Since

$$EN_i(t) = \int_0^t \overline{G}_{i-}(s) dF(s), \qquad EK_i(t) = \overline{G}_{i-}(s) \overline{F}_{i-}(s),$$

we have

$$\begin{aligned} \Lambda(t) &= \int_0^t \frac{dF(s)}{1 - F_-(s)} \\ &= \int_0^t \frac{\sum_{i=1}^n [1 - G_{i-}(s)] dF(s)}{\sum_{i=1}^n [1 - G_{i-}(s)][1 - F_-(s)]} \\ &= \int_0^t \frac{dE \sum_{i=1}^n N_i(s)}{EK(s)}. \end{aligned}$$

Therefore, it is reasonable to estimate $\Lambda(t)$ by

$$\int_0^t \frac{d \sum_{i=1}^n N_i(s)}{K(s)}.$$

This is precisely the Nelson-Aalen estimator of $\Lambda(t)$.

7.8 Suppose that $A(t)$ is a bounded right-continuous increasing function on $[0, \tau]$ for some $\tau > 0$, and that $B(t)$ is a right-continuous function of bounded variation on $[0, \tau]$, with $A(0) = B(0) = 0$. Consider the following integral equation in $X(t)$:

$$X(t) = \int_0^t X(s) dA(s) + B(t). \tag{7.59}$$

From this we obtain

$$dX(t) = X(t) dA(t) + dB(t).$$

Define the product integral

$$\Phi(t) = \mathcal{P}_{(0,t]}(1 - dA).$$

Note that since $A(t)$ is a bounded increasing function, $|\Delta A(t)| < 1$ except for finitely many points in $[0, \tau]$. From (2.20),

$$\Phi_-(t)dA(t) = -d\Phi(t).$$

(a) Use these results to show that

$$\Phi_-(t)dX(t) + X(t)d\Phi(t) = \Phi_-(t)dB(t).$$

From the integration by parts formula (A.10) in Appendix A, the above equality can be rewritten as

$$d\left[\Phi(t)X(t)\right] = \Phi_-(t)dB(t).$$

(b) Use the result in (a) and the fact that $X(0) = 0$ to show that the solution to (7.59) is

$$X(t) = \frac{1}{\Phi(t)} \int_0^t \Phi_-(s)dB(s).$$

This proves that $\widehat{R}(t; \boldsymbol{\beta})$ in (7.14) is indeed the solution to (7.12). It also proves that (7.24) follows from (7.22).

This form of solution to (7.59), which was provided by Yang [329], is an important part of the pseudo-likelihood estimation procedures for the proportional odds model and models (7.6), (7.46) and (7.48) [343, 344, 347].

(c) Consider a variation of the integral equation in (7.59), in the form of

$$X(t) = \int_0^t X_-(s)dA(s) + B(t). \tag{7.60}$$

It follows that

$$dX(t) = X_-(t)dA(t) + dB(t).$$

Define the product integral

$$\Psi(t) = \mathcal{P}_{(0,t]}(1 + dA).$$

It can be seen that

$$\Psi(t) = \Psi_-(t)(1 + \Delta A(t)).$$

This suggests that

$$d\Psi(t) = \Psi_-(t)dA(t),$$

which is indeed the case. $\Psi(t)$ is explicitly the product of the continuous part and the discrete part, as in part (d) of Exercise 2.6, if $A(t)$ is decomposed analogously to (2.21). Show that

$$dX(t) = \frac{X_-(t)}{\Psi_-(t)} d\Psi(t) + dB(t).$$

Then use $X = (X/\Psi)\Psi$ to show that

$$\Psi(t) d\left[\frac{X(t)}{\Psi(t)}\right] = dB(t).$$

Conclude that the solution to (7.60) is

$$X(t) = \Psi(t) \int_0^t \frac{dB(s)}{\Psi(s)}.$$

7.9 By the change of variable formula (A.11) in Appendix A,

$$\int_0^t h'(G(x)) dG(x) = h(G(t)) - h(G(0)) \tag{7.61}$$

for continuous G and differentiable h.

(a) The cumulative hazard function of a positive time-to-event variable T is defined as

$$\Lambda(t) = \int_0^t \frac{dF(s)}{1 - F_-(s)},$$

where $F(t)$ is the CDF of T. Show that when $F(t)$ is continuous,

$$\Lambda(t) = \int_0^t \frac{dF(s)}{1 - F(s)} = \log(1 - F(t)).$$

(b) Show that when $\Gamma(t)$ is continuous and increasing,

$$\int_0^t \frac{1}{[1 + \Gamma(s)]^2} d\Gamma(s) = \frac{\Gamma(t)}{1 + \Gamma(t)}.$$

7.10 (a) Verify (7.39).

Hint: $S(t) = P(T \geq t) = EI(T \geq t)$. Assume that the order of integration and expectation can be interchanged.

(b) Suppose the survival function $S_j(t)$ of T_j is continuous, $j = 1, 2$, and

$$A_j(t) = \int_0^t S_j(x) dx, \quad j = 1, 2.$$

Prove that

$$A_2(t) \geq A_1(t), \quad t \geq 0$$

if and only if

$$S_2(t) \geq S_1(t), \quad t \geq 0.$$

Hint: Let

$$D(t) = \int_0^t [S_2(x) - S_1(x)].$$

Then $D(0) = 0$ and $D'(t) = S_2(t) - S_1(t)$.

7.11 Verify (7.50).

7.12 (a) Assume that a nonnegative random variable T has a continuous distribution and has a finite mean ET. By (2.61), $\int_0^\infty S(t)dt < \infty$. Thus $S(t)$ should converge to 0 at a certain rate. In particular, it can be shown that

$$\lim_{t\to\infty} tS(t) = 0.$$

We have

$$tS(2t) \leq \int_t^{2t} S(x)dx \leq \int_t^\infty S(x)dx,$$

where the first inequality follows from the monotonicity of S. Thus

$$\lim_{t\to\infty} tS(2t) \leq \lim_{t\to\infty} \int_t^\infty S(x)dx = 0,$$

where the last equality follows from the existence of $\int_0^\infty S(t)dt$. Consequently,

$$\lim_{t\to\infty} 2tS(2t) = 0,$$

or

$$\lim_{t\to\infty} tS(t) = 0.$$

Use this result and integration by parts to show that

$$\int_t^\infty (x-t)dF(x) = \int_t^\infty S(x)dx.$$

Hint: Since $F = 1 - S$, we have $dF(x) = -dS(x)$.

(b) The expected residual life $L(t)$ at time t is defined by

$$L(t) = E(T - t | T \geq t).$$

Show that

$$L(t) = \frac{\int_t^\infty S(x)dx}{S(t)}. \tag{7.62}$$

(c) Taking derivative in (7.62), show that

$$L'(t) = \lambda(t)L(t) - 1,$$

where $\lambda(t)$ is the hazard function of T. It follows that

$$\lambda(t) = \frac{L'(t)+1}{L(t)},$$

and

$$\Lambda(t) = \int_0^t \frac{L'(x)+1}{L(x)} dx = \log\big(L(t)/L(0)\big) + \int_0^t \frac{dx}{L(x)},$$

$$S(t) = \frac{L(0)}{L(t)} \exp\left(-\int_0^t \frac{dx}{L(x)}\right).$$

Therefore, $L(t)$ determines the distribution of T.

7.13 Show that

$$ET \wedge \tau = E\big[TI(T \le \tau)\big] + \tau S(\tau).$$

In applications to heavily censored data, the above result shows that $ET \wedge \tau$ is primarily determined by the second term $\tau S(\tau)$. It then may be tempting to consider

$$B(t) = E\big[TI(T \le t)\big].$$

Assume that the distribution is continuous. Then

$$E\big[TI(T \le t)\big] = \int_0^t x dF(x) = tF(t) - \int_0^t F(x)dx = \int_0^t [F(t) - F(x)]dx.$$

Thus $E\big[TI(T \le t)\big]$ shares with the expected residual life the property that the stochastic ordering is not preserved.

7.14 Consider

$$C(t) = E\big(T \big| T \le t\big)$$

the conditional mean of T given $T \le t$. Assume that the distribution is continuous.

(a) Show that

$$C(t) = \frac{\int_0^t x dF(x)}{F(t)}. \tag{7.63}$$

Also show that $C(t) \le t$ for any t.

(b) From (7.63),

$$C(t)F(t) = \int_0^t x dF(x).$$

Taking derivative on both sides, we get

$$C'(t)F(t) + C(t)f(t) = tf(t).$$

It follows that

$$\frac{f(t)}{F(t)} = \frac{C'(t)}{t - C(t)}. \tag{7.64}$$

Since the function on the left has a non-integrable singularity at $t = 0$ and the function on the right side often has a non-integrable singularity at $t = \infty$, we can only integrate both sides of (7.64) on $t \in [a, x]$ for $0 < a < x < \infty$. This yields

$$\log \frac{F(x)}{F(a)} = \int_a^x \frac{C'(t)dt}{t - C(t)}.$$

It follows that there is no one-to-one relationship between $C(t)$ and $F(t)$. For example, if $F(t) = aF_0(t)$ for $t \in (0, x]$, then a has no impact on $C(t)$.

8

Other Semiparametric Models

8.1 Introduction

For semiparametric analysis of time-to-event data, the Cox proportional hazards model is by far the most frequently used. When an explanatory variable has non-proportional effect on the hazard, stratified analysis or a model with a defined time-dependent covariate can be used, though these approaches may be ad hoc. The model of short-term and long-term hazard ratios in Chapter Seven offer a more systematic approach to accommodate potential monotone departures from the proportional hazards condition, and yield more flexible and robust inference. In this chapter, we discuss some other semiparametric models.

Traditionally, the accelerated failure time (AFT) model and the proportional odds model are among the most recognized alternatives to the Cox model. Additive hazard model and transformation models have also gained attention in the last thirty years or so. These models not only can be used for non-proportional hazards situations, they also provide different perspectives on the probabilistic behavior of the time-to-event variable. Some of the models have important properties and offer more intuitive interpretations of treatment effects in certain scenarios. Therefore, even in situations where the hazards are reasonably proportional, they can also be used in addition to or instead of the Cox models.

8.2 The Two-Sample Semiparametric Scale Change/AFT Model

Before discussing the general AFT regression model, we study the two-sample case in this section. By a log transformation, the model also corresponds to the classical two-sample location model that is an important topic in standard statistics textbooks.

Suppose that data are available under the two-sample setup described in Section 2.8.2. The two-sample AFT model assumes that, for some $\theta > 0$,

$$\Lambda_T(t) = \Lambda_C(t/\theta), \quad t > 0. \tag{8.1}$$

DOI: 10.1201/9780429324437-8

Let F_C, and F_T be the CDFs corresponding to Λ_C and Λ_T, respectively. Then model (8.1) is equivalent to $F_T(t) = F_C(t/\theta)$. Let T_T, T_C be time-to-event variables of the two groups. Under (8.1), T_T/θ and T_C have the same distribution. That is, the treatment accelerates ($\theta < 1$) or decelerates ($\theta > 1$) the time to event, respectively. When the means of $\boldsymbol{T}_T$ and $\boldsymbol{T}_C$ exist,

$$\frac{ET_T}{ET_C} = \theta. \tag{8.2}$$

Therefore, θ is the multiplicative factor by which the expected survival time is prolonged or shortened by the treatment.

Model (8.1) is an important alternative to the Cox proportional hazards model discussed in Chapter Five. Instead of specifying the treatment effect or group difference through the hazard function, the AFT model directly relates the parameter to the time-to-event variable. Cox noted that the AFT models are in many ways more appealing than the proportional hazards model because of their quite direct physical interpretation [259].

Under model (8.1), the distributions of the two groups are stochastically ordered. In other words, the survival function of one group is always greater than or equal to that of the other group. It follows that the two survival curves will never cross each other. Furthermore, the hazard functions of the two groups will often not cross each other as well. Thus model (8.1) does not accommodate as many non-proportional hazards scenarios as the model of short-term and long-term hazard ratios can.

8.2.1 Estimating Functions Based on Statistics of Class K

Motivated by Gill's statistics of class $\mathcal{K}$ in (5.39), Wei and Gail [318] proposed the estimating function

$$U_\Psi(\theta) = \int_0^\infty \Psi(t;\theta)d\big[\widehat{\Lambda}_T(\theta t) - \widehat{\Lambda}_C(t)\big], \tag{8.3}$$

where $\Psi(t;\theta)$ is obtained from $\Psi(t)$ by replacing $X_{n_1+1},\ldots,X_n$ with $X_{n_1+1}/\theta,\ldots,$ X_n/θ, and satisfies certain monotonicity condition. In particular, for

$$\Psi(t;\theta) = \frac{K_C(t)K_T(\theta t)}{K_C(t) + K_T(\theta t)},$$

the corresponding function is called the log-rank estimating function and will be denoted by U_{LR}.

At the true parameter value θ_0, $\Lambda_T(\theta_0 t) = \Lambda_C(t)$. Therefore, the zero of $U_\Psi(\theta)$ is a reasonable estimator of θ_0. Due to discontinuity of $U_\Psi(\theta)$, it is simpler to define the estimator $\widehat{\theta}$ as a minimizer of $U_{\Psi}^2(\theta)$. Under certain regularity conditions,

$$U_{\Psi}(\theta_0) \sim N\big(0, V_{\Psi}(\theta_0)\big), \tag{8.4}$$

where

$$V_{\Psi}(\theta) = \int_0^{\infty} \Psi^2(t;\theta)\frac{K_C(t)+K_T(\theta t)}{K_C(t)K_T(\theta t)}d\widehat{\Lambda}(t;\theta),$$

with $\widehat{\Lambda}(t;\theta)$ being the pooled estimator of Λ_C based on $X,\ldots,X_{n_1},X_{n_1+1}/\theta,\ldots,X_n/\theta$. From this and a local linearity result of Hodges and Lehmann [113], Wei and Gail established the asymptotic normality of $\widehat{\theta}$.

However, the limiting variance of $\widehat{\theta}$ is difficult to estimate well with censored data, as it contains the hazard function of Λ_C and its derivative. To circumvent this difficulty, test inversion can be used to construct an asymptotic $100(1-\alpha)\%$ confidence interval. One option is the interval

$$\left\{\theta : U_{\Psi}^2(\theta)/V_{\Psi}(\theta) \le \chi_1^2(\alpha)\right\}. \tag{8.5}$$

However, this set may not be an interval. A different confidence interval is given by

$$\left\{\theta : U_{\Psi}^2(\theta)/V_{\Psi}(\widehat{\theta}) \le \chi_1^2(\alpha)\right\}. \tag{8.6}$$

By the monotonicity condition in Wei and Gail [318], the set in (8.6) is an interval. Alternatively, Bootstrap and other re-sampling methods can be used.

For the hypothesis of no group difference, $H_0 : \theta = 1$, based on the estimating function, an asymptotically valid test at significance level α is to reject H_0 when

$$U_{\Psi}^2(1)/V_{\Psi}(1) > \chi_1^2(\alpha). \tag{8.7}$$

8.2.2 Estimating Functions Based on Weighted Cumulative Hazards and Lack-of-Fit Tests

The confidence interval (8.5) cannot be guaranteed to be an interval. On the other hand, the confidence interval (8.6) sacrifices the usual duality property between hypothesis testing and interval estimation—the principle that a test rejects the null hypothesis if and only if the confidence interval excludes the null value. Consequently, the test in (8.7) may yield conclusions inconsistent with the interval produced by (8.6). Additionally, obtaining the interval in (8.6) requires plotting the interval-generating function, which can be tedious.

Note that loss of the duality property also exists for the score test in parametric models discussed in Chapter Four. However, the Wald test can avoid this problem. In Section 8.2.1 above, the absence of the Wald test is due to the difficulty in estimating the limiting variance of $\widehat{\theta}$.

Yang [335] developed a class of estimators using weighted differences of the Nelson-Aalen estimators of the two groups. This approach avoids numerically unstable density estimation and allows for reliable estimation of the limiting variance. The estimator $\widehat{\theta}_w$ is defined as a zero of $D(\theta)$, or, for simpler computation, a minimizer of $D^2(\theta)$, where

$$D(\theta) = \int_a^b W(t;\theta)\left[\widehat{\Lambda}_T(\theta t) - \widehat{\Lambda}_C(t)\right]dt, \tag{8.8}$$

with $a, b > 0$ and nonnegative $W(t;\theta)$. Under certain regularity conditions, $\sqrt{n}(\widehat{\theta}_w/\theta_0 - 1)$ is asymptotically normal with mean zero and variance σ_w^2, which can be consistently estimated by $\widehat{\sigma}_w^2 = \widehat{\gamma}^{-2}(\widehat{\theta})\widehat{V}(\widehat{\theta})$, where

$$\begin{aligned}
\widehat{\gamma}(\theta) &= \int_a^b tW(t;\theta)d\widehat{\Lambda}(t;\theta), \\
\widehat{V}(\theta) &= 2n\int_a^b\int_a^t W(t;\theta)W(s;\theta)\int_0^s\left[\frac{K_C(x)+K_T(\theta x)}{K_C(x)K_T(\theta x)}\right]d\widehat{\Lambda}(x;\theta)dsdt,
\end{aligned}$$

Based on the above results, an asymptotic $100(1-\alpha)\%$ confidence interval for θ_0 is

$$\left[\widehat{\theta}/(1+\eta), \widehat{\theta}/(1-\eta\right],$$

where $\eta = n^{-1/2}\widehat{\sigma}_w z(\alpha/2)$. This interval may contain negative values, or even undefined when $\eta = 1$. The usual log transformation avoids these problems and gives the interval

$$\left[\widehat{\theta}\exp(-\eta), \widehat{\theta}\exp(\eta)\right]. \tag{8.9}$$

This confidence interval often agrees better with the interval obtained from test inversion. Furthermore, the interval has a length not exceeding that of the untransformed interval (see Exercise 8.4).

Based on asymptotic efficiency considerations and various simulation studies, a good choice of the weight function in $D(\theta)$ is $W_1(t;\theta) = \left[1-\widehat{F}(t;\theta)\right]^{1+p}\widehat{F}(t;\theta)/t$, where $\widehat{F}(t;\theta)$ is the Kaplan-Meier CDF estimator corresponding to $\widehat{\Lambda}(t;\theta)$, and

$$p = \frac{\pi}{1-\pi},$$

with $\pi = \sum_{i=1}^n \delta_i/n$. Simulations and applications to real trial data show that a good choice of the integration range $[a, b]$ is

$$a = \max\left(\min_{i\le n_1} X_i, \min_{i>n_1} X_i\right), \ \ b = \min\left(\max_{i\le n_1} X_i, \max_{i>n_1} X_i\right).$$

To assess model adequacy, consider the null hypothesis

$$H_{m0}: \lambda_T(t) = \Lambda_C(t/\theta), \ t > 0, \ \ \text{for some} \ \ \theta > 0.$$

Let D_1 and D_2 be estimating functions corresponding to two weights $W_1(t;\theta)$ and $W_2(t;\theta)$, respectively. Let $\widehat{\theta}_j$ and $\widehat{\gamma}_j(\theta)$ be the corresponding parameter estimator and the asymptotic slope estimator, respectively, for $j = 1,2$. Similar to the Gill-Schumacker test for the two-sample Cox model [100], the estimators $\widehat{\theta}_1$ and $\widehat{\theta}_2$ should be close to each other when H_{m0} is true. Let

$$L_{W_1,W_2}(\theta) = D_2(\theta) - \frac{\widehat{\gamma}_2(\theta)}{\widehat{\gamma}_1(\theta)} D_1(\theta). \tag{8.10}$$

Under H_{m0}, it can be shown that, $\sqrt{n}(\widehat{\theta}_2/\widehat{\theta}_1 - 1)$ is asymptotically equivalent to

$$\sqrt{n}L_{W_1,W_2}(\widehat{\theta}_1)/\widehat{\gamma}_2(\widehat{\theta}_1), \tag{8.11}$$

and that $\sqrt{n}L_{W_1,W_2}(\widehat{\theta}_1)$ is asymptotically normal with mean zero and variance that has a consistent estimator V_L, where V_L is obtained from $\widehat{V}(\widehat{\theta}_1)$ by replacing $W_1(t;\widehat{\theta}_1)$ with

$$W_2(t;\widehat{\theta}_1) - \widehat{\gamma}_2(\widehat{\theta}_1)W_1(t,\widehat{\theta}_1)/\widehat{\gamma}_1(\widehat{\theta}_1).$$

Yang's lack-of-fit test rejects H_{m0} if

$$nL^2_{W_1,W_2}(\widehat{\theta}_1) > z(\alpha/2)V_L. \tag{8.12}$$

Note that this test only requires numerical root-finding for $\widehat{\theta}_1$, while the asymptotically equivalent test using $\sqrt{n}(\widehat{\theta}_2/\widehat{\theta}_1 - 1)$ requires both $\widehat{\theta}_1$ and $\widehat{\theta}_2$. The asymptotically ignorable second term $\widehat{\gamma}_2(\widehat{\theta}_1)D_1(\widehat{\theta}_1)/\widehat{\gamma}_1(\widehat{\theta}_1)$ in $L_{W_1,W_2}(\widehat{\theta}_1)$ can improve the test performance for small samples, where $D_1(\widehat{\theta}_1)$ may deviate more from zero than when the sample size is large.

Under the alternative hypothesis $H_a : \Lambda_T(t) = \Lambda_C(t/\theta(t))$, $t > 0$, for a bounded non-constant monotone function $\theta(t)$, it was shown that the lack-of-fit test (8.12) is consistent if $W_2(t;\theta)/W_1(t;\theta)$ is monotone. Similarly, if $\theta(t)$ is convex or concave, the test is consistent if $W_2(t;\theta)/W_1(t;\theta) = \theta(t)$.

In addition to the results discussed above, works on the two-sample AFT model include rank-based estimation [245, 190], minimum distance estimation [216, 144], weighted Kaplan-Meier statistics [225], and Monte Carlo methods for model checking [163], among others. Since the two-sample model is a special case of the general AFT regression models, the works described in the next section are also applicable.

Example 8.1. For an unadjusted analysis of the TOPCAT trial primary endpoint, the log-rank estimating function U_{LR} yields $\widehat{\theta} = 1.19$. Figure 8.1 displays the interval-generating function $U_{LR}(\theta)/V_{LR}(\widehat{\theta})$ in (8.6), where $V_{LR}(\theta)$ is the variance estimator for $U_{LR}(\theta)$. The plot shows that the 95% confidence interval of θ_0 is approximately 0.93–1.49.

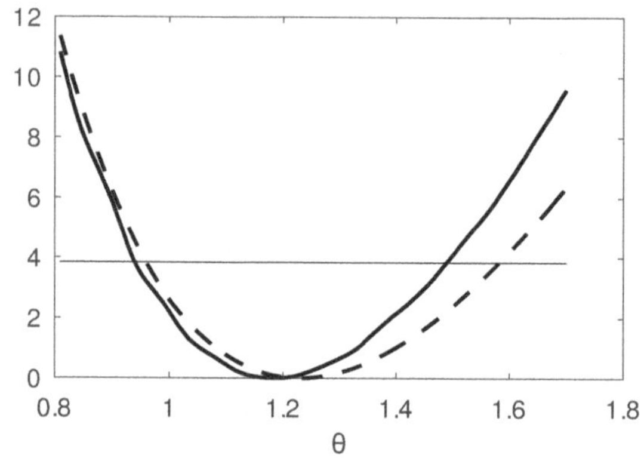

FIGURE 8.1
The interval-generating functions of θ for the TOPCAT primary endpoint based on model (8.1). Thick solid: log-rank estimating function; thick dashed: estimating function in (8.13). The thin horizontal line is at level 3.84.

Because the sample size is large and the curve is obtained by interpolation with values at 100 grid points, the plot does not show the discontinuity points of the estimating function. If needed, greater precision in the interval can be achieved by evaluating the function at more finely defined grid points near 0.93 or 1.49. However, this process is cumbersome, and it is desirable to have a more easily computed and clearly defined confidence interval, such as the one given in (8.9).

Figure 8.2 displays Kaplan-Meier and model-based CDF estimates of the two groups. It shows good agreement between the two methods. For testing $H_0 : \theta = 1$, the test statistic $\boldsymbol{U}^2_{LR}(1)/V_{LR}(1)$ is exactly the standardized log-rank statistic which has a P-value of 0.14.

Next, consider the estimating function D_1, with weight $W_1 = \left[1 - \widehat{F}(t;\theta)\right]^{1+p}$ $\widehat{F}(t;\theta)/t$. It yields $\widehat{\theta}_1 = 1.23$. Based on $\widehat{\theta}_1$ and with the log transformation, the 95% confidence interval in (8.9) for θ_0 is 0.98–1.55.

Note that by inverting the estimating function D_1, a 95% confidence interval is

$$\{\theta : D_1^2(\theta)/\widehat{V}_1(\widehat{\theta}_1) \leq 3.84\}, \tag{8.13}$$

where $\widehat{V}_1(\theta)$ denotes the variance estimator corresponding $D_1(\theta)$. Plot of the function $D_1^2(\theta)/\widehat{V}_1(\widehat{\theta}_1)$ is also included in Figure 8.1.

From Figure 8.1, the confidence interval from (8.9) using the estimating function D_1 is in good agreement with the interval based on test inversion.

The Kaplan-Meier CDF estimates and those using model (8.1) and $\widehat{\theta} = 1.23$ are plotted in Figure 8.3. It also shows good agreement between the two methods.

For testing $H_0 : \theta = 1$, the Wald test based on $\widehat{\theta}_1$ has a P-value of 0.07. For the lack-of-fit test, the pair of weights $W_1, W_2 = W_1\widehat{F}(t;\theta)$ results in a P-value of

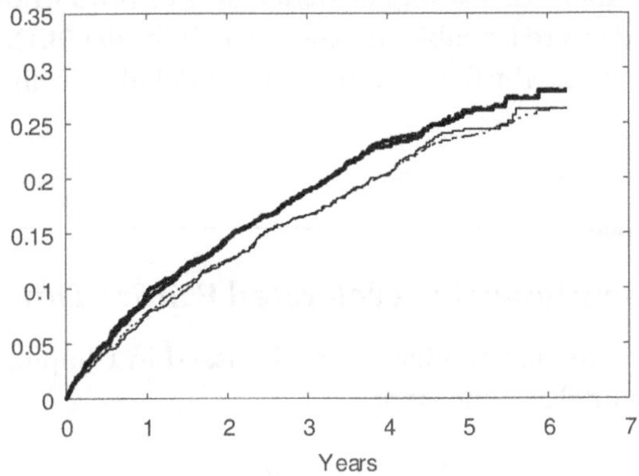

FIGURE 8.2
CDF estimates for the TOPCAT primary endpoint. Thick solid: Kaplan-Meier, control group; thick dashed: model (8.1) with U_{LR}-based $\widehat{\theta}$, control group; thin solid: Kaplan-Meier, treatment group; thin dashed: model (8.1) with U_{LR}-based $\widehat{\theta}$, treatment group.

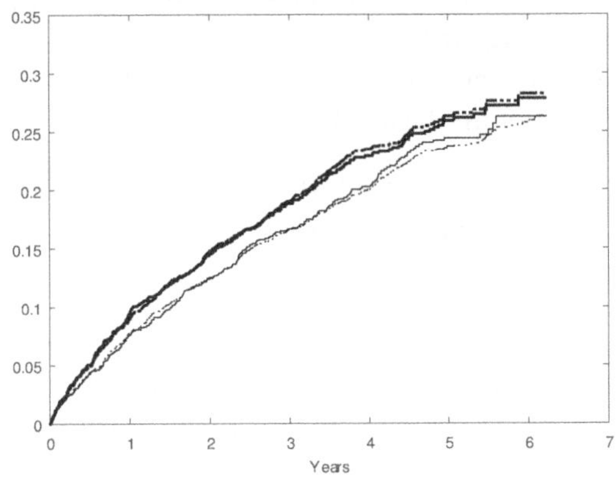

FIGURE 8.3
CDF estimates for the TOPCAT primary endpoint. Thick solid: Kaplan-Meier, control group; thick dashed: model (8.1) with D_1-based $\widehat{\theta}_1$, control group; thin solid: Kaplan-Meier, treatment group; thin dashed: model (8.1) with D_1-based $\widehat{\theta}_1$, treatment group.

0.59. This is consistent with the good agreement between the nonparametric and model-based CDF estimates shown in Figure 8.2 and 8.3.

Example 8.2. In Example 7.4, it was shown that, with the TOPCAT trial primary endpoint for the two groups formed by the single dichotomous covariate

$W = I(age > 69)$, there was strong evidence of non-proportional hazards, while model (7.6) provides a reasonable fit. Now if we fit model (8.1), the lack-of-fit test in (8.12) has an extreme P-value of 0.01. Thus model (8.1) is discredited.

8.3 The Semiparametric Accelerated Failure Time Model

Parametric AFT regression models were discussed in Chapter Three. The semiparametric AFT model assumes that

$$\log(T_i) = \boldsymbol{\beta}^{\mathrm{T}} \boldsymbol{W}_i + \varepsilon_i, \tag{8.14}$$

where ε_i is independent of $\boldsymbol{W}_i$ and has an unspecified CDF F_0.

Compared with the parametric versions, model (8.14) provides more flexibility. The logarithm in (8.14) may also be replaced by another known strictly increasing transformation from $(0, \infty)$ to $(-\infty, \infty)$. F_0 may not have a finite mean. Even when the mean of F_0 does exist, it may not necessarily be zero since the intercept parameter is often absorbed into ε_i. This is because the intercept cannot be reliably estimated due to censoring [317].

Let T be the time-to-event variable and $\boldsymbol{W}^{\mathrm{T}} = (Z, \boldsymbol{B}^{\mathrm{T}})$ where $\boldsymbol{B}$ is the vector of baseline covariates. Under model (8.14),

$$\frac{E(T|Z=1, \boldsymbol{B})}{E(T|Z=0, \boldsymbol{B})} = \exp(\beta_1), \tag{8.15}$$

where β_1 is the coefficient of Z in $\boldsymbol{\beta}^{\mathrm{T}} \boldsymbol{W}$. Thus, the treatment prolongs or shortens the conditional expected time to event by a multiplicative factor of $\exp(\beta_1)$, holding the baseline covariates fixed at the same level.

In spite of the appealing interpretation of the AFT model, censoring and the fact that relevant estimating functions are often discontinuous and nonmonotonic in parameters present challenges in computations and rigorous justifications of inference procedures. There have been many significant developments in analysis of the semiparametric AFT model, including works on least squares estimation [29, 143, 207, 147, 128], rank estimation [87, 245, 261, 302, 321, 148, 357, 355, 85, 333, 127], least absolute deviations estimation [244], M-estimation [366, 125], minimum distance estimation [334], extension to time-dependent covariates [264, 185], lack of fit testing [333, 335, 163], counting process formulation [179], empirical likelihood analysis [367, 368] and Kernel-smoothed profile likelihood estimation [360]. More thorough literature can be found in the review articles of Wei [317] and Jin [126]. Together with the increase in computing power, advances over the last forty years in research on the AFT model make it a more accessible alternative to the Cox proportional hazards model.

8.3.1 Inference Based on Rank Test Statistics

Suppose that data $(X_i, \delta_i, \boldsymbol{W}_i), i = 1, \ldots, n$ are available from the random censorship model with covariates that was introduced in Section 4.1.1. Suppose furthermore that T_i is given by (8.14), where the ε_i's are i.i.d. and independent of the $\boldsymbol{W}_i$'s, and that T_i's and C_i's are positive. Let

$$e_i(\boldsymbol{\beta}) = \log X_i - \boldsymbol{\beta}^{\mathrm{T}} \boldsymbol{W}_i,\ i = 1, \ldots, n.$$

In the case of $\boldsymbol{W}_i = Z_i$, similar to the equivalence of expressions in (2.51) and (2.55), the log-rank estimating function U_{LR} in Section 8.2.1 can be rewritten as

$$\sum_{i=1}^{n} \delta_i \left[Z_i - \frac{\sum_{m=1}^{n} Z_m I\left(e_m(\beta) \geq e_i(\beta)\right)}{\sum_{m=1}^{n} I\left(e_m(\beta) \geq e_i(\beta)\right)} \right], \tag{8.16}$$

where $\exp(\beta) = \theta$.

For the general case where $\boldsymbol{W}_i$ is a $p \times 1$ vector of baseline variables, and with additional weight function, the weighted log-rank estimating function is

$$\begin{aligned} \boldsymbol{U}_{\Phi}(\boldsymbol{\beta}) &= \sum_{i=1}^{n} \delta_i \Phi\left(e_i(\boldsymbol{\beta}); \boldsymbol{\beta}\right) \left[\boldsymbol{W}_i - \frac{\sum_{m=1}^{n} \boldsymbol{W}_m I\left(e_m(\boldsymbol{\beta}) \geq e_i(\boldsymbol{\beta})\right)}{\sum_{m=1}^{n} I\left(\left(e_m(\boldsymbol{\beta}) \geq e_i(\boldsymbol{\beta})\right)\right.} \right] \\ &= \sum_{i=1}^{n} \int_{-\infty}^{\infty} \Phi\left(t; \boldsymbol{\beta}\right) \left[\boldsymbol{W}_i - \frac{\sum_{m=1}^{n} \boldsymbol{W}_m I\left(e_m(\boldsymbol{\beta}) \geq t\right)}{\sum_{m=1}^{n} I\left(\left(e_m(\boldsymbol{\beta}) \geq t\right)\right.} \right] dN_i(t; \boldsymbol{\beta}), \end{aligned} \tag{8.17}$$

where $\Phi\left(t; \boldsymbol{\beta}\right)$ is nonnegative and possibly data-dependent, and $N_i(t; \boldsymbol{\beta}) = \delta_i I\left(e_i(\boldsymbol{\beta}) \leq t\right), i = 1, \ldots, n$. The zero $\widehat{\boldsymbol{\beta}}_{\Phi}$ of $\boldsymbol{U}_{\Phi}(\boldsymbol{\beta})$ is the rank estimator of $\boldsymbol{\beta}$ corresponding to the weight Φ.

Let $\lambda_0(t)$ be the hazard function corresponding to the error term CDF $F_0(t)$. Denote by $\dot{\lambda}_0(t)$ the derivative of $\lambda_0(t)$. Under certain regularity conditions, at the true parameter value $\boldsymbol{\beta}_0$, $\boldsymbol{U}_{\Phi}(\boldsymbol{\beta}_0)/\sqrt{n}$ converges weakly to the p-variate normal distribution with mean zero and covariance matrix $\boldsymbol{B}_{\Phi}(\boldsymbol{\beta}_0)$ that can be consistently estimated by $\widehat{\boldsymbol{B}}_{\Phi}(\widehat{\boldsymbol{\beta}})$, where

$$\widehat{\boldsymbol{B}}_{\Phi}(\boldsymbol{\beta}) = \frac{1}{n} \sum_{i=1}^{n} \int_{-\infty}^{\infty} \Phi^2\left(t; \boldsymbol{\beta}\right) \left[\boldsymbol{W}_i - \frac{\sum_{m=1}^{n} \boldsymbol{W}_m I\left(e_m(\boldsymbol{\beta}) \geq t\right)}{\sum_{m=1}^{n} I\left(\left(e_m(\boldsymbol{\beta}) \geq t\right)\right.} \right]^{\otimes 2} dN_i(t; \boldsymbol{\beta}), \tag{8.18}$$

with $\mathbf{V}^{\otimes 2} = \mathbf{V}\mathbf{V}^{\mathrm{T}}$ for a vector $\mathbf{V}$ as in (5.13). Moreover, $\sqrt{n}(\widehat{\boldsymbol{\beta}}_{\Phi} - \boldsymbol{\beta}_0)$ converges weakly to the p-variate normal distribution with mean zero and covariance matrix $\boldsymbol{A}_{\Phi}^{-1}(\boldsymbol{\beta}_0)\boldsymbol{B}_{\Phi}(\boldsymbol{\beta}_0)\boldsymbol{A}_{\Phi}^{-1}(\boldsymbol{\beta}_0)$, where

$$\boldsymbol{A}_{\Phi}(\boldsymbol{\beta}) = \lim \frac{1}{n} \sum_{i=1}^{n} \int_{-\infty}^{\infty} \Phi\left(t; \boldsymbol{\beta}\right) \left[\boldsymbol{W}_i - \frac{\sum_{m=1}^{n} \boldsymbol{W}_m I\left(e_m(\boldsymbol{\beta}) \geq t\right)}{\sum_{m=1}^{n} I\left(\left(e_m(\boldsymbol{\beta}) \geq t\right)\right.} \right]^{\otimes 2} \frac{\dot{\lambda}_0(t)}{\lambda_0(t)} dN_i(t; \boldsymbol{\beta}). \tag{8.19}$$

Rigorous justifications and applications of these asymptotic results were the fruits of active research in the early 1990s by various authors [261, 302, 321, 148, 357, 355, 85].

For $\Phi \equiv 1$, the resulting $\boldsymbol{U}_\Phi$ corresponds to the log-rank statistic. For $\Phi(t;\boldsymbol{\beta}) = \sum_{i=1}^n I(e_i(\boldsymbol{\beta}) \geq t)/n$, the resulting $\boldsymbol{U}_\Phi$ corresponds to the Gehan statistic [87], which is component-wise monotone in a sense that will be made clear later.

For an unadjusted analysis, with $\boldsymbol{\beta}^{\mathrm{T}}\boldsymbol{W}_i = \beta Z_i$, the matrix $\boldsymbol{A}_\Phi^{-1}\boldsymbol{B}_\Phi\boldsymbol{A}_\Phi^{-1}$ reduces to a positive number which, by the Cauchy-Schwartz inequality, is no less than the limiting variance corresponding to $\Phi = \dot{\lambda}_0(t)/\lambda_0(t)$. Thus this particular choice of Φ has a nice asymptotic optimality property. However, this result is mainly of theoretical value since in practice, the density function and the hazard function in general cannot be reliably estimated with censored data.

The estimating function $\boldsymbol{U}_\Phi$ is not a smooth function of $\boldsymbol{\beta}$. Instead, it is a discontinuous step function that in general is not component-wise monotone except for the Gehan weight function. This may be the main source of difficulty in analyzing and implementing the semiparametric AFT model for real data. The proposal by Jin et al. [127] is an important development in overcoming the challenge, with the idea of utilizing the Gehan statistic in an iterative way.

The estimating function with the Gehan weight is

$$\boldsymbol{U}_G(\boldsymbol{\beta}) = \frac{1}{n}\sum_{i=1}^{n}\sum_{m=1}^{n}\delta_i(\boldsymbol{W}_i - \boldsymbol{W}_m)I\big(\log(X_i) - \log(X_m) - \boldsymbol{\beta}^{\mathrm{T}}(\boldsymbol{W}_i - \boldsymbol{W}_m) \leq 0\big). \quad (8.20)$$

It is component-wise monotone in the sense that, for any $p \times 1$ vectors $\boldsymbol{a}, \boldsymbol{b}$, $\boldsymbol{a}^{\mathrm{T}}\boldsymbol{U}_G(\boldsymbol{b} + x\boldsymbol{a})$ is a nondecreasing function in x [85]. $\boldsymbol{v}$ is called a general solution of $\boldsymbol{A}(\boldsymbol{v}) = 0$ for a vector function $\boldsymbol{A}$ if a slight change in any of its components changes the sign of $\boldsymbol{A}$. The component-wise monotonicity ensures that all general solutions of $\boldsymbol{U}_G(\boldsymbol{\beta}) = 0$ belongs to a convex set whose diameter is of order n^{-1} as $n \to \infty$ [85]. It can be shown that the function $\boldsymbol{U}_G(\boldsymbol{\beta})$ is the gradient of the convex function

$$\boldsymbol{Q}_G(\boldsymbol{\beta}) = \frac{1}{n}\sum_{i=1}^{n}\sum_{m=1}^{n}\delta_i\big(e_i(\boldsymbol{\beta}) - e_m(\boldsymbol{\beta})\big)^{-}, \quad (8.21)$$

where $x^{-} = |x|I(x < 0)$ for a real x. Thus finding zero $\widehat{\boldsymbol{\beta}}_G$ of $\boldsymbol{U}_G$ is equivalent to minimizing $\boldsymbol{Q}_G(\boldsymbol{\beta})$.

For the general rank estimating function, Jin et al. [127] proposed to find $\widehat{\boldsymbol{\beta}}_G$ first, and then use the modified estimating function

$$\begin{aligned}\boldsymbol{U}^*(\boldsymbol{\beta};\widehat{\boldsymbol{\beta}}) &= \sum_{i=1}^{n}\int_{-\infty}^{\infty}\Psi\big(t + (\boldsymbol{\beta} - \widehat{\boldsymbol{\beta}})^{\mathrm{T}}\boldsymbol{W}_i;\widehat{\boldsymbol{\beta}}\big)S^{(0)}(t;\boldsymbol{\beta}) \\ &\quad \cdot \left[\boldsymbol{W}_i - \frac{\sum_{m=1}^n \boldsymbol{W}_m I\big(e_m(\boldsymbol{\beta}) \geq t\big)}{\sum_{m=1}^n I\big(e_m(\boldsymbol{\beta}) \geq t\big)}\right] dN_i(t;\boldsymbol{\beta}), \quad (8.22)\end{aligned}$$

where $\Psi(t;\boldsymbol{\beta}) = \Phi(t;\boldsymbol{\beta})/S^{(0)}(t;\boldsymbol{\beta})$, $S^{(0)}(t;\boldsymbol{\beta}) = \sum_{i=1}^n I(e_i(\boldsymbol{\beta}) \geq t)/n$, and $\widehat{\boldsymbol{\beta}}$ is an initial estimator such as $\widehat{\boldsymbol{\beta}}_G$. This modified estimating function can be written as

$$\frac{1}{n}\sum_{i=1}^n \sum_{m=1}^n \Psi\big(e_i(\widehat{\boldsymbol{\beta}});\widehat{\boldsymbol{\beta}}\big)\delta_i(\boldsymbol{W}_i - \boldsymbol{W}_m)I\big(e_i(\boldsymbol{\beta}) \leq e_m(\boldsymbol{\beta})\big),$$

which is component-wise monotone and the gradient of

$$\boldsymbol{Q}^*(\boldsymbol{\beta};\widehat{\boldsymbol{\beta}}) = \frac{1}{n}\sum_{i=1}^n \sum_{m=1}^n \Psi\big(e_i(\widehat{\boldsymbol{\beta}});\widehat{\boldsymbol{\beta}}\big)\delta_i\big(e_i(\boldsymbol{\beta}) - e_m(\boldsymbol{\beta})\big)^-.$$

The iterative algorithm of Jin et al. is to find an estimator of $\boldsymbol{\beta}$ by the iteration

$$\widehat{\boldsymbol{\beta}}_{(0)} = \widehat{\boldsymbol{\beta}}_G, \quad \widehat{\boldsymbol{\beta}}_{(k)} = \arg\min_{\boldsymbol{\beta}} \boldsymbol{Q}^*\big(\boldsymbol{\beta};\widehat{\boldsymbol{\beta}}_{(k-1)}\big), \quad k \geq 1.$$

Under certain regularity conditions, it was shown that each estimator $\widehat{\boldsymbol{\beta}}_{(k)}$ in the iteration is consistent and asymptotically normal, and if $\widehat{\boldsymbol{\beta}}_{(k)}$ converges as $k \to \infty$, then the limit is the zero of $\boldsymbol{U}_\Phi$.

8.3.2 Inference Based on Least-Squares Estimation

When there is no censoring, least-squares estimation is often used in standard statistics textbooks. Let β_0 be the mean of ε_i's in (8.14). An estimator of $\boldsymbol{\beta}$ and β_0 can be obtained by minimizing $\sum_{i=1}^n \big(\log(T_i) - \boldsymbol{\beta}^{\mathrm{T}}\boldsymbol{W}_i - \beta_0\big)^2$ as a function of $\boldsymbol{\beta}, \beta_0$. Taking partial derivative in $\boldsymbol{\beta}$ and β_0, respectively, we obtain

$$\begin{aligned}\sum_{i=1}^n \boldsymbol{W}_i\big[\log(T_i) - \boldsymbol{\beta}^{\mathrm{T}}\boldsymbol{W}_i - \beta_0\big] &= 0,\\ \sum_{i=1}^n \big[\log(T_i) - \boldsymbol{\beta}^{\mathrm{T}}\boldsymbol{W}_i - \beta_0\big] &= 0.\end{aligned} \tag{8.23}$$

Eliminating β_0, the least squares estimator of $\boldsymbol{\beta}$ is the zero of the estimating function

$$\sum_{i=1}^n (\boldsymbol{W}_i - \overline{\boldsymbol{W}})\big[\log(T_i) - \boldsymbol{\beta}^{\mathrm{T}}\boldsymbol{W}_i\big], \tag{8.24}$$

where $\overline{\boldsymbol{W}} = \sum_{i=1}^n \boldsymbol{W}_i/n$. Verification of this is left to Exercise 8.5.

In the random censorship model setup, not all time-to-event variables are observed. Koul, Susarla, and van Ryzin [143] proposed least-squares estimation using only the uncensored times, with the adjustment that they are weighted with inverse of the probability of being uncensored.

To describe the basic idea of inverse probability weighting, suppose a function $h(T)$ of a survival time T has mean μ:

$$Eh(T) = \mu.$$

Assume that T is censored by an independent variable C, and only $X = T \wedge C$ and $\delta = I(T \wedge C)$ are observed. Let the survival functions of T and C be $S(t)$ and $G(t)$, respectively. A naive estimator of μ is $\delta h(X)$. However, it is a biased estimator:

$$E\delta h(X) = EI(T \le C)h(T) = EG_{-}(T)h(T). \tag{8.25}$$

where the last equality follows from (B.6). Verification of this is left to Exercise 8.6. However, (8.25) suggests an unbiased "estimator" $\delta h(X)\left[G_{-}(X)\right]^{-1}$:

$$E\frac{\delta h(X)}{G_{-}(X)} = Eh(T) = \mu. \tag{8.26}$$

Verification of (8.26) is left to Exercise 8.7.

Since G is typically unknown, an estimator is needed. Suppose $P(T = C) = 0$. Then the censored data problem is symmetric in T and C and they censor each other. Therefore, the survival function G of C can be estimated by the Kaplan-Meier estimator $\widehat{G}$.

Suppose a sample of data (X_i, δ_i), $1 \le i \le n$ is available, where $X_i = T_i \wedge C_i$ and $\delta_i = I(T_i \le C_i)$, with the C_i's being i.i.d. and T_i's being independent (and also independent of the C_i's). Analogous to (2.45), $\widehat{G}$ is given by

$$\widehat{G}(t) = \mathcal{P}_{(0,t]}(1 - d\widehat{\Lambda}_G), \tag{8.27}$$

where

$$\widehat{\Lambda}_G(t) = \int_0^t \frac{\sum_{i=1}^n d\left[(1-\delta_i)I(X_i \le s)\right]}{K(s)} \tag{8.28}$$

for $K(t)$ in (2.43). Then μ can be estimated by

$$\delta h(X)\left[\widehat{G}_{-}(X)\right]^{-1}.$$

Note that, just as in Chapter Two, the "censoring" variables T_i's can have different distributions.

Using inverse probability weighting, Koul et al. derived a modified least squares estimator and established its asymptotic normality. Over the years, the idea of inverse probability weighting has also become useful in many other contexts [263, 42, 172, 175, 298].

However, the inverse probability weighting method implicitly requires a strong assumption that the support of $G(t)$ contains that of $S(t)$. In a clinical trial that ends at time τ_0, $G(\tau_0) = 0$. Therefore, we must restrict the analysis to an interval over which $G_{-}(t) > 0$.

Suppose $[0,\tau]$ is such an interval. Then the corrected version of (8.26) is

$$E\frac{\delta h(X)}{G_{-}(X)}I(X \le \tau) = E\frac{h(T)}{G_{-}(T)}I(T \le \tau)I(T \le C) = Eh(T)I(T \le \tau). \tag{8.29}$$

Verification of (8.29) is left to Exercise 8.8. This result shows that the corrected estimator,

$$\widehat{\mu} = \delta h(X)I(X \le \tau)\left[\widehat{G}_{-}(X)\right]^{-1},$$

is estimating $Eh(T)I(T \le \tau)$, which equals μ only if $[0,\tau]$ contains the support of $h(T)$. Furthermore, because the Kaplan-Meier estimator is known to be unstable near the upper end of the data range, $\widehat{\mu}$ may be unstable or may have large variance.

A more efficient adaptation of least-squares estimation to censored data was given by Buckley and James [29], who proposed to replace Y_i by its conditional expectation given data. Specifically, let

$$\widetilde{Y}_i = \delta_i \log(X_i) + (1-\delta_i)\left[\frac{\int_{e_i(\boldsymbol{\beta})}^{\infty} x d\widehat{F}(x;\boldsymbol{\beta})}{1-\widehat{F}\left(e_i(\boldsymbol{\beta});\boldsymbol{\beta}\right)} + \boldsymbol{\beta}^{\mathrm{T}}\boldsymbol{W}_i\right], \tag{8.30}$$

where $\widehat{F}(x;\boldsymbol{\beta})$ is the Kaplan-Meier estimator based on $\left(e_i(\boldsymbol{\beta}),\delta_i\right)$, $i = 1,\ldots,n$. The Buckley-James estimator $\widehat{\boldsymbol{\beta}}_{BJ}$ is the zero of the function

$$\sum_{i=1}^{n}(\boldsymbol{W}_i - \overline{\boldsymbol{W}})\left(\widetilde{Y}_i - \boldsymbol{\beta}^{\mathrm{T}}\boldsymbol{W}_i\right). \tag{8.31}$$

Again, discontinuity and non-monotonicity of the function in (8.31) makes the computation challenging. Jin et al. [128] proposed an iterative algorithm similar to the rank estimation case in Section 8.3.1.

8.4 Odds-Related Models

8.4.1 The Proportional Odds Model

The semiparametric AFT model (8.14) and the proportional odds model are two traditional alternatives to the Cox model (5.1). The odds of an outcome is the ratio of the probability of that outcome over the probability of the complement of the outcome. Thus the odds of observing event T within time window $[0, t]$ is

$$\frac{F(t)}{1-F(t)} = \frac{1-S(t)}{S(t)},$$

if T has the CDF $F(t)$ and survival function $S(t)$. In the two sample case with S_T, S_C being the survival functions of the two groups, the proportional odds model specifies that

$$\frac{1-S_T(t)}{S_T(t)} = \theta\frac{1-S_C(t)}{S_C(t)}, \tag{8.32}$$

for t such that $S_C(t) > 0$, where $\theta > 0$. Therefore the parameter θ is the odds ratio of the two groups. It is left to Exercise 8.10 to verify that model (8.32) can be rewritten as

$$\lambda_T(t) = \frac{\theta\lambda_C(t)}{S_C(t) + \theta F_C(t)}. \tag{8.33}$$

It follows that (8.32) is a sub-model of model (7.1) with $\theta_2 = 1, \theta_1 = \theta$.

In general, with a covariate vector $\boldsymbol{W}$, the proportional odds model assumes that

$$\frac{1-S(t;\boldsymbol{W})}{S(t;\boldsymbol{W})} = \exp(\boldsymbol{\beta}^{\mathrm{T}}\boldsymbol{W})R(t),\ t < \tau_0, \tag{8.34}$$

where $S(t;\boldsymbol{W})$ is the conditional survival function of T given $\boldsymbol{W}$, $R(t)$ is an unspecified baseline odds function, and $\tau_0 = \sup\{t : R(t) \in [0,\infty)\}$. Therefore, the proportional odds model specifies that the covariate effect is through a multiplicative factor on the conditional odds function.

For an unadjusted analysis in a two-arm trial, $\boldsymbol{\beta}^{\mathrm{T}}\boldsymbol{W}$ reduces to βZ. From (8.34), $\exp(\beta)$ is the multiplicative factor by which the odds of having the event in $[0,t]$ is modified by the treatment, with a negative β indicating beneficial effect. In a covariate-adjusted analysis with $\boldsymbol{W}^{\mathrm{T}} = (Z, \boldsymbol{B}^{\mathrm{T}})$ where $\boldsymbol{B}$ is the vector of baseline covariates, it can be shown that

$$\frac{O(t;Z=1,\boldsymbol{B})}{O(t;Z=0,\boldsymbol{B})} = \exp(\beta_1), \tag{8.35}$$

where $O(t;Z,\boldsymbol{B})$ is the conditional odds of having the event in $[0,t]$ given Z and $\boldsymbol{B}$, and β_1 is the coefficient of Z in $\boldsymbol{\beta}^{\mathrm{T}}\boldsymbol{W}$. Thus $\exp(\beta_1)$ is the odds ratio of treatment over control, holding the covariates fixed at the same level.

Since $R(t)$ is an odds function, it is increasing and $R(0) = 0$. It is left to Exercise 8.10 to verify that model (8.34) can be rewritten as

$$\lambda[t;\boldsymbol{W}] = \frac{1}{\exp(-\boldsymbol{\beta}^{\mathrm{T}}\boldsymbol{W}) + R(t)}\frac{dR(t)}{dt}. \tag{8.36}$$

Therefore, (8.34) is a sub-model of model (7.48) with $\boldsymbol{\theta}_2 = 0, \boldsymbol{\theta}_1 = \boldsymbol{\beta}$.

From (8.36), for two different levels $\boldsymbol{W}$, $\widetilde{\boldsymbol{W}}$ of the covariate,

$$\frac{\lambda[t;\boldsymbol{W}]}{\lambda[t;\widetilde{\boldsymbol{W}}]} = \frac{\exp(-\boldsymbol{\beta}^{\mathrm{T}}\boldsymbol{W}) + R(t)}{\exp(-\boldsymbol{\beta}^{\mathrm{T}}\widetilde{\boldsymbol{W}}) + R(t)}.$$

Thus, the hazard ratio stays above 1 or below 1 all the time and

$$\lim_{t\to\infty}\frac{\lambda[t;\boldsymbol{W}]}{\lambda[t;\widetilde{\boldsymbol{W}}]}=1.$$

It follows that the proportional odds model can provide a good fit for data in situations where the treatment is beneficial or harmful at the beginning and the effect diminishes over time.

Bennett [19] generalized the proportional odds model to survival data and proposed, without proofs, an analysis using nonparametric maximum likelihood estimation. Early works on the proportional odds model include results for the two-sample case [58, 325] and estimation using ranks or generalized estimating equation in the linear transformation model [230, 57, 42], among others. The linear transformation model, which will be discussed in the next section, contains the proportional odds model as a sub-model.

Murphy, Rossini, and van der Vaart [209] provided rigorous justification of the nonparametric maximum likelihood estimation method. They considered the likelihood function

$$\begin{aligned} L(\boldsymbol{\beta},R) &= \prod_{i=1}^{n}\left[\frac{\exp(-\boldsymbol{\beta}^{\mathrm{T}}\boldsymbol{W}_i)\Delta R(X_i)}{[R(X_i)+\exp(-\boldsymbol{\beta}^{\mathrm{T}}\boldsymbol{W}_i)][R(X_i-)+\exp(-\boldsymbol{\beta}^{\mathrm{T}}\boldsymbol{W}_i)]}\right]^{\delta_i} \\ &\quad \cdot\prod_{i=1}^{n}\left[\frac{\exp(-\boldsymbol{\beta}^{\mathrm{T}}\boldsymbol{W}_i)}{R(X_i)+\exp(-\boldsymbol{\beta}^{\mathrm{T}}\boldsymbol{W}_i)}\right]^{1-\delta_i}, \end{aligned} \tag{8.37}$$

where $\Delta R(t)=R(t)-R(t-)$ is the jump of R at t. In calculating the nonparametric MLE $(\widehat{\boldsymbol{\beta}},\widehat{R})$, when the largest order statistic $X_{(n)}$ is uncensored, the mass of $\widehat{R}$ at $X_{(n)}$ is set to infinity. For obtaining remaining jumps of $\widehat{R}$, all observed event times equal to $X_{(n)}$ are treated in the likelihood as if they are censored. One fact that helps explain this delicacy is that, from $R=1/S-1$, for t such that $S(t)=1$, $S(t)$ is well defined but $R(t)=\infty$.

Murphy, Rossini, and van der Vaart showed that the nonparametric MLE that maximizes (8.37) is consistent and asymptotically normal, and that the asymptotic covariance matrix of $\widehat{\boldsymbol{\beta}}$ achieves the efficiency lower bound and has a consistent estimator from inverting the observed Fisher information matrix for $\boldsymbol{\beta}$.

Similarly to the re-expression of (7.56) by (7.57), model (8.36) can be re-expressed as

$$\lambda[t;\boldsymbol{W}(t)]=\frac{\lambda_0(t)}{\exp(-\boldsymbol{\beta}_1^{\mathrm{T}}\boldsymbol{W}(t))S_0(t)+F_0(t)}, \tag{8.38}$$

where $\lambda_0(t)$, $S_0(t)$ are the hazard and survival functions corresponding to the odds function $R(t)$, respectively, and $F_0(t)$ is the associated CDF. Thus an alternative form of the nonparametric likelihood, as a function of $(\boldsymbol{\beta},\Lambda_0)$, where Λ_0 is the cumulative hazard function corresponding to R, is

$$L(\boldsymbol{\theta},\Lambda_0) = \prod_{i=1}^{n}\Big[\frac{\Delta L_0(X_i)}{\exp(-\boldsymbol{\beta}^{\mathrm{T}}\boldsymbol{W}_i)S_0(X_i)+F_0(X_i)}\Big]^{\delta_i} \cdot\prod_{i=1}^{n}\exp\{-\Lambda[X_i;\boldsymbol{W}_i]\}, \tag{8.39}$$

where

$$\Lambda[t;\boldsymbol{W}_i(t)] = \int_0^t \frac{d\Lambda_0(s)}{\exp[-\boldsymbol{\beta}^{\mathrm{T}}\boldsymbol{W}_i]S_0(s)+F_0(s)}. \tag{8.40}$$

Yang and Prentice [343] introduced some weighted empirical odds functions obtained from certain self-consistency equations that have a nice martingale representation. They proposed several classes of regression parameter estimators, including pseudo-likelihood estimation, martingale residual-based estimation, and minimum distance estimation. Similar to discussion in Section 7.9, these parameter estimators and estimators of their limiting covariance matrices make the inference procedures much easier to implement than the nonparametric MLE procedures. Extensive numerical studies showed that the minimum distance estimators have high finite-sample efficiency. The weighted odds function-based approach also provides some measures for lack-of-fit analysis. Additionally, the pseudo-likelihood method inspired extensions to short-term and long-term hazard ratio models (7.6) and (7.46).

8.4.2 The Proportional ρ-Odds Model

Consider the Box-Cox [26] class of transformations

$$h(s,\rho) = \rho^{-1}(s^{-\rho}-1), \tag{8.41}$$

for $\rho \ge 0$, where at $\rho = 0$, the expression is defined as its limit $-\log(s)$ as $\rho \downarrow 0$ (for $s > 0$). The proportional ρ-odds model, sometimes referred to as the generalized odds-rate model, specifies that

$$h\big(S(t;\boldsymbol{W}),\rho\big) = h\big(S_0(t),\rho\big)\exp(\boldsymbol{\beta}^{\mathrm{T}}\boldsymbol{W}),\ t < \tau_0, \tag{8.42}$$

where $S_0(t)$ is an unspecified baseline survival distribution function. This model includes both the proportional odds model and the proportional hazards model as sub-models, corresponding to $\rho = 1$ and $\rho = 0$, respectively.

For model (8.42), the conditional hazard function given the covariate is

$$\lambda[t;\boldsymbol{W}] = \frac{1}{\exp(-\boldsymbol{\beta}^{\mathrm{T}}\boldsymbol{W})+\rho R(t)}\frac{dR(t)}{dt}, \tag{8.43}$$

where

$$R(t) = \rho^{-1}\left[S_0(t)^{-\rho} - 1\right].$$

Verification of this is left to Exercise 8.12. Note that for a fixed ρ, $R(0) = 0$ and $R(t)$ increases to infinity as $t \to \infty$.

For two different levels $\boldsymbol{W}$, $\widetilde{\boldsymbol{W}}$ of the covariate,

$$\frac{\lambda[t; \boldsymbol{W}]}{\lambda[t; \widetilde{\boldsymbol{W}}]} = \frac{\exp(-\boldsymbol{\beta}^{\mathrm{T}}\boldsymbol{W}) + \rho R(t)}{\exp(-\boldsymbol{\beta}^{\mathrm{T}}\widetilde{\boldsymbol{W}}) + \rho R(t)}. \tag{8.44}$$

It follows that the hazard ratio is approximately $\exp\left[-\boldsymbol{\beta}^{\mathrm{T}}(\boldsymbol{W} - \widetilde{\boldsymbol{W}})\right]$ for small t. Furthermore, if $\rho > 0$, then the hazard ratio approaches 1 as $t \to \infty$. Therefore, similarly to model (8.36), model (8.43) is also a converging hazard model for $\rho > 0$. The difference between the two models is that model (8.43) has an additional fine-tuning parameter ρ to modulate the rate at which the hazard ratio approaches 1. Under either model, between the conditional hazard functions for two different covariate levels $\boldsymbol{W}$, $\widetilde{\boldsymbol{W}}$, one always stays above or below the other, hence they do not cross each other.

Model (8.43) has been discussed previously in the two-sample setting by Dabrowska and Doksum [58], in which the model is equivalent to the family of models discussed by Harrington and Fleming [109] which led to the G^{ρ} family of weighted log-rank statistics. Dabrowska and Doksum provided interpretations of this model in terms of failure models for multi-component systems. Clayton and Cuzick [45] discussed an equivalent form of the model. They showed that it has an interpretation as a proportional hazards model with the hazard function multiplied by a random frailty factor having a gamma distribution with mean 1 and variance ρ. Scharfstein, Tsiatis, and Gilbert [269] considered the nonparametric MLE and showed that they are consistent and asymptotically normal, and that the estimator for $\boldsymbol{\beta}$ is semiparametric efficient in the sense that it attains the efficiency lower bound.

Most works on model (8.43) take ρ as a known constant. Zucker and Yang [372] extended to model (8.43) the pseudo-likelihood and martingale residuals methods in Yang and Prentice [343]. Both the case of known and unknown ρ were studied. Kosorok, Lee, and Fine [140] considered a proportional hazards model with the hazard function multiplied by a random frailty factor, which includes model (8.43) with unknown ρ as a special case when the frailty has a gamma distribution. Their estimation procedure uses the profile likelihood approach discussed in Sections 5.6 and 7.9, and employs on an iterative algorithm to compute the estimator of the cumulative hazard function. The approach in Zucker and Yang can be much more easily implemented, while the approach in Kosorok, Lee, and Fine may lead to improved efficiency.

8.5 Transformation Models

For a random variable X with cumulative hazard function Λ,

$$P(X > x) = \exp[-\Lambda(x)].$$

If Λ is continuous and strictly increasing over $[0,\infty)$, with $\Lambda(0) = 0$ and $\Lambda(x) \to \infty$ as $x \to \infty$, then its inverse Λ^{-1} is well defined. By (2.8),

$$P(\Lambda(X) > x) = P(X > \Lambda^{-1}(x)) = \exp[-\Lambda(\Lambda^{-1}(x))] = \exp(-x), \; x \geq 0.$$

That is, the transformed variable $\Lambda(X)$ has a standard exponential distribution. In particular, if the conditional cumulative hazard function of T given $\boldsymbol{W}$ is $\exp(\boldsymbol{\beta}^{\mathrm{T}}\boldsymbol{W})\Lambda_0(t)$, then $\exp(\boldsymbol{\beta}^{\mathrm{T}}\boldsymbol{W})\Lambda_0(T)$ has a standard exponential distribution. Thus

$$\log \Lambda_0(T) = -\boldsymbol{\beta}^{\mathrm{T}}\boldsymbol{W} + \log\eta, \tag{8.45}$$

where η is a standard exponential random variable. That is, a transformation of T can be represented as $-\boldsymbol{\beta}^{\mathrm{T}}\boldsymbol{W}$ plus a variable that has a known distribution, which in the case here is the extreme value distribution.

Similarly, if the conditional cumulative hazard function of T given $\boldsymbol{W}$ follows that proportional ρ-odds model, then the variable $\eta = \ln\left[1 + \rho\exp(\boldsymbol{\beta}^{\mathrm{T}}\boldsymbol{W})R(T)\right]/\rho$ has a standard exponential distribution. We have

$$\log R(T) = -\boldsymbol{\beta}^{\mathrm{T}}\boldsymbol{W} + \log\left[\frac{\exp(\rho\eta) - 1}{\rho}\right]. \tag{8.46}$$

Verification of this is left to Exercise 8.13.

The semiparametric linear transformation model postulates that there exists an unknown strictly monotone function H such that the transformed variable $H(T)$ has the representation

$$H(T) = -\boldsymbol{\beta}^{\mathrm{T}}\boldsymbol{W} + \varepsilon, \tag{8.47}$$

where ε has a known distribution and is independent of $\boldsymbol{W}$. It follows that the proportional hazards model, the proportional odds model and the proportional ρ- odds model all belong to the class of linear transformation models.

Similar to the case for the AFT model, under the linear transformation model, the conditional distributions at two different levels of the covariates are also stochastically ordered.

In the special cases of the proportional hazards model and the proportional odds model, as shown before, the regression parameter $\boldsymbol{\beta}$ has the interpretation of log hazard ratio or log odds ratio, respectively. As noted in Kalbfleisch and Prentice [131], for the general case, model (8.47) suffers from a lack of ready interpretation for the regression parameter $\boldsymbol{\beta}$. Thus, although a test of $\beta = 0$ in the unadjusted analysis for a two-arm trial can be used to test the existence of treatment effect, β is not an easily interpretable effect measure. This is because, in general, $\exp(\beta)$ is the gain or loss in the expected value of $H(T)$ due to treatment, which does not offer a clear understanding since H is an unknown monotone function.

For model (8.47), among the works mentioned in Section 8.4, Cheng, Wei, and Ying [42] derived inference procedures from a class of generalized estimating equations using inverse probability weighting. Validity of their procedures relies on the assumptions that the censoring variable is independent of the covariates and that the support of the censoring variable contains that of the time-to-event variable. Both of these assumptions may be violated in many clinical trials, and consequently the estimators may be asymptotically biased. To relax the latter assumption, Fine, Ying, and Wei [78] provided a simple modification to yield consistent estimators.

Chen, Jin, and Ying [38] proposed an estimator using a martingale-based estimating function. In the special case of the proportional hazards model, their estimator reduces to the partial likelihood estimator. Their approach does not require the two restrictive assumptions mentioned in the previous paragraph.

Zeng and Lin [359] worked with a counting process formulation of model (8.47) to accommodate time-dependent covariates and considered the nonparametric MLE for the resulting model. The estimators are consistent and asymptotically normal, with limiting variances for the regression parameter estimators achieving the efficient lower bounds and being consistently estimated.

Since the linear transformation model (8.47) encompasses various important models such as the proportional hazards model and the proportional odds model, it might seem analogous to model (7.48), which also contains these sub-models. This analogy holds if the index of the sub-models is part of the parameter to be estimated. However, most of existing works treat the index as a known constant, as in the case of the proportional ρ-odds model with known ρ. Two of the exceptions are the works of Zucker and Yang [372] and Kosorok, Lee, and Fine [140], in which ρ is part of the parameter. For an exploratory analysis, it may be acceptable to fit data with various models corresponding to different values of ρ in the proportional ρ-odds model, to arrive at the best model under a specific criterion. For clinical trials, however, the model, the covariates and the analysis plan need to be pre-specified to prevent selection bias from data-dredging.

8.6 Additive Hazards Model

The proportional hazards model (5.1) assumes that the effect of covariate is a multiplicative factor on the hazard function. Alternative to that, the additive hazards model assumes that

$$\lambda[t;\boldsymbol{W}] = \lambda_0(t) + \boldsymbol{\beta}^{\mathrm{T}}\boldsymbol{W}. \tag{8.48}$$

The model has been discussed by Cox and Oakes [54], Breslow and Day [27], Lin and Ying [183, 184], among others. Lin and Ying [183] proposed an estimating function that results in an explicit expression for the estimator, and showed that the estimator is consistent and asymptotically normal. Lin and Ying [184] considered the general additive-multiplicative hazard models for counting processes, and developed a class of simple estimating functions that contains the estimating function for the partial likelihood estimator in the special case of proportional hazards model. Consistency and asymptotic normality were established for both parameter estimator and the estimator of baseline cumulative hazard function.

Under model (8.48), covariate effects are additive on the hazard. As an absolute effect measure, the regression coefficient is more sensitive to censoring than the relative effect measured in model (5.1). In particular, in two-arm unadjusted analyses with heavily censored data, the regression coefficient estimates may be extremely small or exhibit large variation across trials.

8.7 Location-Scale Type Extensions of the Transformation Model

The linear transformation model (8.47) can be viewed as a semiparametric extension of the parametric location model. To accommodate heterogeneity in errors, the parametric location model can be extended to the location-scale model. Following this framework, Zeng and Lin [361] extended (8.47) to

$$H(T) = -\boldsymbol{\beta}^{\mathrm{T}}\boldsymbol{W} + \exp(-\boldsymbol{\gamma}^{\mathrm{T}}\widetilde{\boldsymbol{W}})\varepsilon, \tag{8.49}$$

where H is an unknown monotone function, $\widetilde{\boldsymbol{W}}$ is a subset of $\boldsymbol{W}$, and ε has a known distribution and is independent of $\boldsymbol{W}$. They further extended (8.49) to allow time-dependent covariates, to prevent the hazard function from being infinite at time 0, and to accommodate random effects.

For univariate survival data, a resulting model postulates that given time-dependent $\boldsymbol{W}$, the conditional cumulative hazard function of T is

$$\exp\left[\boldsymbol{\beta}^{\mathrm{T}}\boldsymbol{W}(t) + \boldsymbol{\gamma}^{\mathrm{T}}\widetilde{\boldsymbol{W}}\right]\{1 + \int_0^t \exp[\boldsymbol{\beta}^{\mathrm{T}}\boldsymbol{W}(s)]d\Lambda(s)\}^{\exp(\boldsymbol{\gamma}^{\mathrm{T}}\widetilde{\boldsymbol{W}})-1}\lambda(t). \tag{8.50}$$

In particular, for an unadjusted analysis in a two-arm trial, with $\boldsymbol{W} = \widetilde{\boldsymbol{W}} = Z$, under model (8.50) the hazard ratio is

$$\frac{\lambda_T(t)}{\lambda_C(t)} = \exp(\beta+\gamma)\left[1 + \exp(\beta)\Lambda(t)\right]^{\exp(\gamma)-1}, \tag{8.51}$$

where λ_C, λ_T are the hazard functions of the control and treatment groups, respectively. This hazard ratio is monotone in general, and contains the proportional hazards model as a sub-model at $\gamma = 0$. Furthermore,

$$\lim_{t \downarrow 0} \frac{\lambda_T(t)}{\lambda_C(t)} = \exp(\beta + \gamma).$$

and

$$\lim_{t \to \infty} \frac{\lambda_T(t)}{\lambda_C(t)} = \begin{cases} 0, & \text{if } \gamma < 0; \\ \infty, & \text{if } \gamma > 0; \\ \exp(\beta + \gamma), & \text{if } \gamma = 0. \end{cases}$$

Therefore, $\exp(\beta + \gamma)$ is the short-term hazard ratio. However, $\exp(\beta)$ or $\exp(\gamma)$ alone is not easy to interpret. This model is useful in situations where the treatment effect, beneficial or harmful, increases without bound over time.

8.8 Other Models

Since the seminal work of Cox [51], semiparametric modeling and analysis has been a major research area in survival analysis. It is impossible to provide an exhaustive list for this vast field. In addition to the models previously discussed, a few more will be briefly mentioned here. Chen and Wang [41] considered a model which assumes that the conditional hazard function of T given $\boldsymbol{W}$ is

$$\lambda(t; \boldsymbol{W}) = \lambda_0\left[t \exp(\boldsymbol{\beta}^{\mathrm{T}} \boldsymbol{W})\right]. \tag{8.52}$$

The model is termed the accelerated hazards model. It accommodates a range of non-proportional hazards scenarios including crossing hazards or survival functions.

Chen and Jewell [40] considered a class of models

$$\lambda(t; \boldsymbol{W}) = \lambda_0\left[t \exp(\boldsymbol{\beta}_1^{\mathrm{T}} \boldsymbol{W})\right] \exp(\boldsymbol{\beta}_2^{\mathrm{T}} \boldsymbol{W}). \tag{8.53}$$

This contains the proportional hazards model with $\boldsymbol{\beta}_1 = 0$, the accelerated failure time model with $\boldsymbol{\beta}_1 = \boldsymbol{\beta}_2$, and the accelerated hazards model with $\boldsymbol{\beta}_2 = 0$. Thus model (8.53) can be used in discriminating the three models. It has an identifiability problem if and only if the baseline hazard function corresponds to the Weibull distribution, at which the three models coincide. Chen and Jewell proposed a rank-based procedure for parameter estimation and provided the asymptotic distribution theory.

8.9 Exercises and Complements

8.1 Verify (8.2).

8.2 For the two-sample AFT model, consider the one-sided hypothesis testing problem

$$H_0 : \theta = 1 \quad vs. \quad H_a' : \theta > 1.$$

By (8.2), H_a' corresponds to a beneficial treatment effect.

(a) Parallel to (8.7), obtain an asymptotically valid test for this one-sided testing problem.

(b) Obtain an asymptotically valid test for the one-sided testing problem

$$H_0 : \theta = 1 \quad vs. \quad H_a'' : \theta < 1.$$

8.3 Verify (8.15).

8.4 For $x \in [0,1)$, use Taylor series expansions of relevant functions to show that

$$\frac{1}{1-x} - \frac{1}{1+x} \geq e^x - e^{-x}.$$

8.5 Obtain the estimating equation (8.24) by eliminating β_0 in equation (8.23).

8.6 Let T, C be independent random variables with CDF F and G, respectively. Let $X = T \wedge C$ and $\delta = I(T \leq C)$. Then the mean of T is ET. When the observation is not T but (X, δ), it is natural to estimate the mean of T by the conditional expectation $E(T|X, \delta)$ given available data. The general definition of conditional expectation and its properties are given in Section B.2 of Appendix B. It turns out that $E(a(T)|X, \delta)$ is given by

$$m(X, \delta) = \delta a(X) + (1-\delta) \frac{\int_X^\infty a(t)dF(t)}{1-F(X)}. \tag{8.54}$$

(a) Show that , for function b defined on $(0, \infty) \times \{0, 1\}$,

$$E\big(a(T)b(X, \delta)\big) = E\big(m(X, \delta)b(X, \delta)\big).$$

Hint: Use the law of iterated expectations (B.6) in Appendix B.

(b) Use (8.54) to show that $\widetilde{Y}_i$ in (8.30) is the conditional expectation of $\log(T_i)$ given (X_i, δ_i).

8.7 Assume that $G_-(t) > 0$ on the support of the distribution of T. Verify (8.26).

8.8 Assume that $G_-(t) > 0$ on an interval $[0, \tau]$. Verify (8.29).

8.9 Suppose that $(T_i, C_i, \boldsymbol{W}_i)$ are i.i.d., where the survival time T_i has conditional median $\boldsymbol{\beta}^{\mathrm{T}}\boldsymbol{W}_i$ given $\boldsymbol{W}_i$, and C_i is independent of $(T_i, \boldsymbol{W}_i)$. It follows that

$$E\big[I(T_i - \boldsymbol{\beta}^{\mathrm{T}}\boldsymbol{W}_i \geq 0)\big|\boldsymbol{W}_i\big] = E\big[I(T_i \geq \boldsymbol{\beta}^{\mathrm{T}}\boldsymbol{W}_i)\big|\boldsymbol{W}_i\big] = \frac{1}{2}.$$

(a) Let $X_i = T_i \wedge C_i$, $\delta_i = I(X_i = T_i)$, and $G(t) = P(C_i \geq t)$. Show that

$$E\Big[\frac{I(X_i - \boldsymbol{\beta}^{\mathrm{T}}\boldsymbol{W}_i \geq 0)}{G(\boldsymbol{\beta}^{\mathrm{T}}\boldsymbol{W}_i)}\Big|\boldsymbol{W}_i\Big] = \frac{1}{2}.$$

Ying, Jung and Wei [356] used this property to derive an estimating function for a censored median regression model (note, however, the implicit assumption that $G(\boldsymbol{\beta}^{\mathrm{T}}\boldsymbol{W}_i) > 0$).

(b) Show that

$$E\Big\{\frac{\delta_i}{G(X_i)}\Big[I(X_i - \boldsymbol{\beta}^{\mathrm{T}}\boldsymbol{W}_i \geq 0) - \frac{1}{2}\Big]\Big\} = 0.$$

Bang and Tsiatis [14] and Zhou [365] used this property to derive alternative estimating functions for the censored median regression model (note, however, the implicit assumption that $G(X_i) > 0$).

8.10 (a) Verify that model (8.32) can be rewritten in the form in (8.33), and that it is a sub-model of (7.1).

(b) Verify that model (8.34) can be rewritten in the form in (8.36).

8.11 Verify that as $\rho \downarrow 0$, the expression in (8.41) converges to $-\log s$ for $s > 0$.

8.12 Verify that model (8.42) can be re-expressed as model (8.43).

8.13 (a) Find the survival function and PDF of $\log \eta$ in (8.45).

(b) Derive the expression (8.46), then find the survival function and PDF of $\log\{[\exp(\rho\eta) - 1]/\rho\}$.

8.14 Consider the random censorship model with fixed covariates described in Section 4.1.1, with the additional assumption that the censoring variables C_i's are i.i.d. Suppose that $(T, \boldsymbol{W})$ satisfies the transformation model (8.47). Then for $i \neq j$,

$$E\big[I(T_i \geq T_j\big|\boldsymbol{W}_i, \boldsymbol{W}_j\big] = E\big[I(H(T_i) \geq H(T_j)\big|\boldsymbol{W}_i, \boldsymbol{W}_j\big].$$

(a) Show that the latter conditional expectation is given by $A\big(\boldsymbol{\beta}^{\mathrm{T}}(\boldsymbol{W}_i - \boldsymbol{W}_j)\big)$, where

$$A(x) = \int_{-\infty}^{\infty} \big[1 - F_0(x + y)\big]\,dF_0(y),$$

with F_0 the known CDF of ε in (8.47).

(b) Show that for any function $B(t) > 0$,

$$\frac{\delta_j I(X_i \geq X_j)}{B(X_j)} = \frac{I(T_i \geq T_j)I(C_i \wedge C_j \geq T_j)}{B(T_j)}.$$

(c) Let $S_0(x) = 1 - F_0(x)$ and $S(t; \boldsymbol{w})$ the conditional survival function of T_i given $\boldsymbol{W}_i = \boldsymbol{w}$. Show that

$$S(t; \boldsymbol{w}) = S_0(H(t) + \boldsymbol{\beta}^{\mathrm{T}}\boldsymbol{w}).$$

(d) Let $G(x)$ be the survival function of the censoring variable C. Show that

$$\begin{aligned} & E\Big[\frac{I(T_i \geq T_j)I(C_i \wedge C_j \geq T_j)}{G^2(T_j)}\Big|T_j, \boldsymbol{W}_i, \boldsymbol{W}_j\Big] \\ = \;& S(T_j; \boldsymbol{W}_i) \\ = \;& S_0(H(T_j) + \boldsymbol{\beta}^{\mathrm{T}}\boldsymbol{W}_i). \end{aligned}$$

Note that the above result requires the implicit assumption that $G(T_i) > 0$.

(e) By (a) and the law of iterated expectations (B.4) in Appendix B,

$$\begin{aligned} & E\Big[\frac{\delta_j I(X_i \geq X_j)}{G^2(X_j)}\Big|\boldsymbol{W}_i, \boldsymbol{W}_j\Big] \\ = \;& E\Big\{E\Big[\frac{I(T_i \geq T_j)I(C_i \wedge C_j \geq T_j)}{G^2(T_j)}\Big|T_j, \boldsymbol{W}_i, \boldsymbol{W}_j\Big]\Big|\boldsymbol{W}_i, \boldsymbol{W}_j\Big\} \\ = \;& E\big[S_0(H(T_j) + \boldsymbol{\beta}^{\mathrm{T}}\boldsymbol{W}_i)\big|\boldsymbol{W}_i, \boldsymbol{W}_j\big]. \end{aligned}$$

Show that the latter reduces to $A\big(\boldsymbol{\beta}^{\mathrm{T}}(\boldsymbol{W}_i - \boldsymbol{W}_j)\big)$. Cheng, Wei and Ying [42] used such applications of inverse probability weighting to derive an estimating function for the transformation model (8.47).

8.15 For the additive model in (8.48), obtain the cumulative hazard and survival functions $\Lambda(t; \boldsymbol{W})$ and $S(t; \boldsymbol{W})$.

8.16 For the two-sample case of model (8.49), obtain the hazard, survival and cumulative hazard functions.

8.17 For the two-sample model that yields (8.51), verify the limits at 0 and ∞ of the hazard ratio are as given in Section 8.7.

8.18 (a) Obtain the cumulative and survival functions for model (8.52).

(b) Obtain the cumulative and survival functions for model (8.53).

9

Testing and Summarizing Differences Between Comparison Groups

9.1 Introduction

The log-rank test is one of the most widely used methods for comparing two groups of survival data, particularly for assessing treatment effects. It is asymptotically the optimal test under proportional hazards alternatives when censoring patterns in the two groups are equal [95, 82]. In many situations, the proportional hazards assumption provides an adequate approximation, and the log-rank test yields good power.

As discussed in Chapters Six and Seven, there are important situations in which the proportionality condition is not met, leading to a reduced power of the log-rank test, sometimes substantially. In this chapter, we explore methods to improve the log-rank test.

In addition to testing the hypothesis of equal distributions in the two groups, another important aspect of two-group comparison is to define appropriate measures that quantify the group difference, particularly the magnitude of the treatment effect. Various model-based and nonparametric measures of treatment effects and their estimators will also be discussed.

9.2 Weighted Log-Rank Tests and Their Combinations

Among various attempts to improve the power to detect treatment effects in nonproportional situations, weighted log-rank tests may be the most studied approach. For the two-sample random censorship model described in Section 2.8.2, consider the hypothesis testing problem

$$H_0 : S_T = S_C \qquad vs. \qquad H_a : S_T \neq S_C. \tag{9.1}$$

The censoring variables $C_1, \dots, C_n$ are not required to be identically distributed to allow different censoring patterns in the control and treatment groups. From

DOI: 10.1201/9780429324437-9

(2.51) and (2.53) in Section 2.8.2, the weighted log-rank statistic is

$$U_\Phi = \sum_{i=1}^{n} \int_0^\infty \Phi(t)\Big[Z_i - \frac{K_T(t)}{K(t)}\Big] dN_i(t),$$

and its estimated variance is

$$V_\Phi = \sum_{i=1}^{n} \int_0^\infty \Phi^2(t) \frac{K_C(t)K_T(t)}{K^2(t)} dN_i(t).$$

The standardized test statistic is then

$$W_\Phi = U_\Phi / \sqrt{V_\Phi}. \tag{9.2}$$

In particular, the standardized log-rank test statistic corresponds to $\Phi \equiv 1$.

As shown in Chapter Two, with appropriately chosen weights, the weighted log-rank tests can lead to improved power over the log-rank test for specific non-proportional hazards situations. For example, when the treatment effect diminishes over time, the difference between the two groups is primarily reflected in early event times. Consequently a function $\Phi(t)$ that puts more weight on small t would yield a test more sensitive to the group differences in this case.

In particular, it will be shown in Chapter Eleven that the Peto-Prentice test [228, 245], which corresponds to $\Phi = \widehat{S}_-$, has the maximal power under the alternative hypothesis that data follow the proportional odds model. Conversely, when there is a delayed treatment effect or when the effect is gradually realized to its full extent, the choice $\Phi(t) = 1 - \widehat{S}_-(t)$, which puts more weight on large t, would have higher power than the log-rank test. In general, weights from the $G^{\rho,\gamma}$ family [82] can be considered for situations in which a specific combination of ρ and γ results in more weight on a region where the group difference is more pronounced.

As discussed in Chapter Seven, actual data patterns may deviate from expectations, even with a well-designed statistical analysis plan. For confirmatory clinical trials, it's essential to pre-specify a test with robust power for various non-proportional hazards scenarios. While a specific weighted log-rank test (e.g., Peto-Prentice) can enhance power over the standard log-rank test for a targeted alternative, it often has reduced power for other alternatives. To address this, combinations of weighted log-rank tests are frequently used, including linear combinations [86, 371], the maximum of standardized tests [293, 95, 28, 83, 82, 161, 141, 162], χ^2 tests based on component tests, and the empirical likelihood methods [350, 16]. These approaches generally outperform the log-rank test under a range of non-proportional hazards alternatives. However, they are typically no longer optimal under the proportional hazards alternative, the most important and widely considered alternative hypothesis.

Yang and Prentice [345] proposed an adaptively weighted log-rank test that maintains asymptotic optimality under proportional hazards while improving power over the log-rank test in non-proportional hazards scenarios. The test uses weight functions Φ_1 and $\Phi_2 = 1/\Phi_1$, where Φ_1 is the estimated hazard ratio when fitting model (7.6) to the data. Using notations from Chapter Seven, we have

$$\Phi_1(t) = \frac{1 + \widehat{R}(t;\widehat{\beta})}{\exp(-\widehat{\beta}_1) + \exp(-\widehat{\beta}_2)\widehat{R}(t;\widehat{\beta})}. \tag{9.3}$$

Φ_2 simply switches the numerator and denominator. The asymptotic optimality was initially argued intuitively in Yang and Prentice [345] and later formally proved [339].

The adaptively weighted log-rank test uses the test statistic

$$\max(|W_1|, |W_2|), \tag{9.4}$$

where W_1 and W_2 are standardized versions of weighted log-rank test statistics U_1 and U_2 corresponding to weights Φ_1 and Φ_2.

Due to the dependence on $\widehat{\boldsymbol{\beta}}$, the weights Φ_1, Φ_2 are no longer predictable, a property that holds true for traditional weighted log-rank tests. Nevertheless, Yang and Prentice showed that under certain regularity conditions, the weights approach non-random and continuous limits and the variance estimator in (2.53) is still consistent, and that $(W_1, W_2)^{\mathrm{T}}$ converges in distribution to a bivariate normal distribution with standard normal marginals. Their argument uses the empirical process theory, an overview of which is given in Appendix C.

Under the null hypothesis H_0, Φ_1 and Φ_2 converge to the function that is identically 1. Thus asymptotically, the test statistic (9.4) has the same limiting distribution as the log-rank test statistic. An asymptotically valid test for H_0 rejects H_0 when

$$\max(|W_1|, |W_2|) > z(\alpha/2). \tag{9.5}$$

However, for finite samples, under H_0, W_1 and W_2 will not be have perfect correlation with probability one. Thus the test in (9.5) may inflate the size or type one error rate in small samples. To control the size, a modification is to reject H_0 if

$$\max(|W_1|, |W_2|) > c_\rho(\alpha), \tag{9.6}$$

where ρ is the correlation coefficient between W_1 and W_2, and the critical value $c_\rho(\alpha)$ is derived from the asymptotic bivariate normal distribution of W_1 and W_2. Specifically, $c_\rho(\alpha)$ satisfies

$$P\big[\max(|V_1|, |V_2|) > c_\rho(\alpha)\big] = \alpha, \tag{9.7}$$

where $\mathbf{V} = (V_1, V_2)^{\mathrm{T}}$ is a bivariate normal random vector with standard normal marginals and correlation ρ.

For a given data set, the P-value of the test in (9.6) is determined by

$$1-p=\int_{-t}^{t}\left\{F\left(\frac{t-\rho w}{\sqrt{1-\rho^2}}\right)-F\left(\frac{-t-\rho w}{\sqrt{1-\rho^2}}\right)\right\}f(w)dw, \tag{9.8}$$

where t is the observed value of $\max(|W_1|,|W_2|)$, and f, F the density and cumulative distribution functions of the standard normal distribution, respectively.

It has been noted that for small samples, the test in (9.6) may still have inflated size. Yang [339] showed that the Monte Carlo method described in Section 7.4 can effectively control the size of the test. Alternatively, a finite-sample correction can be applied to deal with the issue. Simulation studies have shown that a suitable correction is to reject H_0 when

$$\frac{\max(|W_1|,|W_2|)}{1+\frac{1}{2\sqrt{n}}} > c_\rho(\alpha). \tag{9.9}$$

Similar correction has also been used in the construction of confidence bands for the hazard ratio under model (7.6) [346]. This adjustment ensures better control of type I error rates in finite samples while maintaining the asymptotic properties of the test.

For one-sided alternative hypotheses, the adaptively weighted test can be modified accordingly. Assume that the survival distributions of the two groups are absolutely contentious, with hazard functions λ_C, λ_T, respectively. Consider the alternative $H_a' : \lambda_T \le \lambda_C$, where the strict inequality holds over an interval in the real line. Note that H_0 is equivalent to the hypothesis of $\lambda_T \equiv \lambda_C$, and that H_a' implies the stochastic ordering $S_T \ge S_C$. A test analogous to (9.9) is to reject H_0 when

$$\frac{\max(-W_1,-W_2)}{1+\frac{1}{2\sqrt{n}}} > \tilde{c}_\rho(\alpha).$$

where $\tilde{c}_\rho(\alpha)$ is the one-sided analogue of $c_\rho(\alpha)$. Similarly, the alternative $H_a'' : \lambda_T \ge \lambda_C$, where the strict inequality holds over an interval in the real line, can be considered. The details are left to Exercise 9.2.

There have been advocates for certain maximum test with specific members of the $G^{\rho,\gamma}$ family, such as $\max(G^{1,0},G^{0,1})$ [162], $\max(G^{1,0},G^{0,1},G^{0,0})$ [133], and $\max(G^{1,0},G^{0,1},G^{0,0},G^{1,1})$ [186], where $\max(G^{1,0},G^{0,1})$ is the abbreviation for maximum of the absolute value of standardized test statistics $\widehat{S}_-^\rho(1-\widehat{S}_-)^\gamma,(\rho,\gamma) = (1,0),(0,1)$. The other two abbreviations are defined similarly. For ease of reference, the three maximum tests will be denoted by MAX_1, MAX_2 and MAX_3, respectively. The adaptively weighted log-rank tests (9.6) and (9.9) will be denoted by LRAD and LRAD_c, respectively. The log-rank test is denoted by *LR*.

Example 9.1. To illustrate the effect of the finite-sample correction in (9.9) and to compare the size for various tests, a simulation study with 1,000 repetitions

TABLE 9.1
Empirical type I error rate for various tests, based on 1,000 repetitions.

Test	LR	MAX_1	MAX_2	MAX_3	LRAD	$LRAD_c$
$n = 60$	0.051	0.041	0.040	0.036	0.067	0.049
$n = 100$	0.064	0.056	0.060	0.058	0.078	0.062
$n = 200$	0.044	0.045	0.045	0.040	0.053	0.049

was conducted. The time-to-event variables follow the standard exponential. The censoring variables are exponential, with the parameter chosen to achieve 50% censoring. The results are reported in Table 9.2.

From Table 9.1, it can be seen that $LRAD_c$ effectively controls the type I error rate.

Example 9.2. To compare $LRAD_c$ and other tests in applications to real trial data, Table 9.2 summarizes the P-values of various tests for the primary endpoints of the TOPCAT, SPRINT, WHI E+P, and gastric cancer trials, described in Section 1.20.

For the TOPCAT and SPRINT trials, the proportional hazards model fits well [234, 341]. Therefore, the log-rank test should perform well. The $LRAD_c$ test yields results very close to those for the log-rank test, while MAX_1, MAX_2 and MAX_3 produce slightly larger P-vales.

For the WHI E+P and gastric cancer trials, there is strong evidence of non-proportional hazards [338]. Notably, the $LRAD_c$ test is the only one showing significant P-values for these trials. These results, together with additional simulations and applications to trial data, suggest that the $LRAD_c$ test generally demonstrates better overall performance compared to other tests.

9.3 Summary Measures for the Group Difference

A summary measure quantifies the group difference or the magnitude of the treatment effect by describing how data differ between the comparison groups with respect to a specific metric. For survival data, the proportional hazards assumption provides a reasonable approximation in many situations. Under this assumption, the hazard ratio offers an interpretable summary measure of the treatment effect,

TABLE 9.2
P-values for primary endpoints in TOPCAT, SPRINT, WHI E+P, and gastric cancer trials.

Test	LR	MAX_1	MAX_2	MAX_3	$LRAD_c$
TOPCAT	0.143	0.177	0.178	0.180	0.137
SPRINT	< 0.001	< 0.001	< 0.001	< 0.001	< 0.001
WHI E+P	0.099	0.143	0.143	0.143	0.044
Gastric	0.637	0.083	0.087	0.096	0.042

even when the model is applied to a situation where the hazard ratio is moderately time-dependent [250].

However, in situations where the proportional hazards assumption does not hold, the hazard ratio estimate derived from the Cox model generally converges to a limit that depends on censoring in complex ways [290]. As a result, it loses its interpretation as a summary measure of the treatment effect. Thus, alternative summary measures are necessary. Yang [338] provided an overview of several summary measures that do not rely on the proportional hazards assumption. Those measures, along with a few additional ones, will be discussed in this section.

Even when the proportional hazards assumption is reasonable, other measures can describe different aspects of the treatment effect and provide useful information.

First, the hazard ratio is a relative measure. As such, the same hazard ratio of 0.8 implies different improvements in survival probability depending on the control group survival function at the specific time points. In some cases, absolutely measures may be more informative.

Additionally, while the hazard ratio gives an overall effect measure, it can be beneficial to report more specific metrics, such as the chance of 5-year survival or a qth quantile. Note that the population median can be reliably estimated by the median of Kaplan-Meier estimator when censoring is light, such as in many oncology trials. For cardiovascular trials, where the censoring can be quite heavy, only lower quantiles (qth quantile for a very small q) can be reliably estimated.

As we transition from proportional hazards to non-proportional situations, it becomes evident that no single summary measure can fully describe the entire survival profile for a treatment group. It has been noted that the choice of measures used to report trial results may influence the acceptance of different treatments [25]. Therefore, it is crucial to have a clear understanding of how various measures complement each other in describing the treatment effect.

Several summary measures, in both absolute and relative terms, are discussed below. These measures provide different perspectives on the group difference, allowing for a more comprehensive understanding of the treatment effect. By considering both absolute and relative measures, researchers and clinicians can gain a more nuanced perspective on the impact of a treatment across various time points and subgroups of patients.

Note that with relative measures, effect sizes are usually more consistent across different studies or sub-populations. Thus, they are more advantageous for summarizing the treatment effect over several studies. This is one reason why the hazard ratio has been the most used measure to describe treatment effect. However, the hazard ratio does not demonstrate absolute improvement in survival-related quantities.

In some situations, absolute measures can inform individual decisions in clinical practice more accurately than relative measures [369]. On the other hand, effect sizes under absolute measures generally have larger variations, even within the same study but with different follow-up durations.

Under heavy censoring, effect sizes from absolute measures may be very small, which makes them less sensible. This limitation of absolute measures in heavily censored data should be considered when choosing appropriate summary statistics for survival analysis.

It is worthy pointing out that while t-year survival probability and qth quantile are simple and useful measures of the treatment effect, they are not quite "summary" measures as they consider only a specific time point or quantile. This characteristic also results in less efficient use of data and larger variance. On the other hand, the most obvious summary measure that utilizes the entire distribution function, the mean, can rarely be estimated reliably due to censoring. These considerations highlight the importance of carefully selecting and interpreting summary measures in survival analysis. Often, it is necessary to use multiple measures to provide a more comprehensive understanding of the treatment effect.

9.3.1 Average Hazard Ratios

When the hazard ratio is time-dependent, it is natural to use an average of the hazard ratio function as a summary measure. Under the model of short-term and long-term hazard ratios (7.6), the average hazard ratio over an interval $[0, \tau]$ is

$$AHR_\tau = \frac{1}{\tau}\int_0^\tau \frac{1+R(t)}{\exp(-\beta_1)+\exp(-\beta_2)R(t)}dt, \tag{9.10}$$

where $\tau \le d^*$, the duration of the trial. Under model (5.4), this summary measure reduces to the usual hazard ratio.

AHR can be estimated by replacing the model parameters with the pseudo-likelihood estimators. The asymptotic normality of the average hazard ratio estimators was established in Yang and Prentice [346].

The average hazard ratio depends on the range $[0,\tau]$, which can also be replaced by $[L,U]$ for some $0 < L < U$, if it is of interest to consider the effect in that specific range. Regardless of the choice, it needs to be pre-specified in the protocol. The importance of pre-specifying the range in the protocol has been noted in the literature [249]. Pre-specifying these parameters ensures analytical integrity and prevents the post-hoc selection of ranges that could artificially inflate the treatment effect. A weighted version of the average hazard ratio can also be considered:

$$AHR_{w,\tau} = \int_0^{\tau} h(t)dw(t), \tag{9.11}$$

where $\int_0^{\tau} dw(t) = 1$. When model (5.4) holds, the weighted average hazard ratios with different weights are usually close to each other and to the unweighted version in (9.10). When the hazards are severely non-proportional, different weights can yield very different results, analogous to the case for weighted log-rank tests.

The integral in (9.10) allows equal contribution from time points in $[0,\tau]$. To reflect the data distribution over $[0,\tau]$, one option is to choose $w(t)$ in (9.11) to be $F_C(t)/F_C(\tau)$. Let $AHR_{F,\tau}$ be the resulting weighted average hazard ratio. Then

$$AHR_{F,\tau} = \frac{1+R(\tau)}{\{\exp(-\beta_1)-\exp(-\beta_2)\}R(\tau)} \log \frac{\exp(-\beta_1)(1+R(\tau))}{\exp(-\beta_1)+\exp(-\beta_2)R(\tau)}, \tag{9.12}$$

where the measure is defined at $\beta_1 = \beta_2$ as the limit when $\beta_1 - \beta_2 \to 0$, namely $\exp(\beta_1)$. Estimators of $AHR_{F,\tau}$ can be obtained by the plug-in method as before.

In various simulations and real data applications, the weighted average hazard ratio in (9.12) performed well compared with other choices of the weight. Under certain regularity conditions, it was shown that the estimator is asymptotically normal [338].

9.3.2 Superiority Probability Ratio

The average hazard ratio depends on an assumed model. Although the model of short-term and long-term hazard ratios (7.6) is quite flexible, there are no simple nonparametric estimators to serve as a gold standard. The kernel-based hazard ratio estimator may yield wide and unstable confidence intervals near both extremes of the data range, in addition to the challenge of bandwidth selection [346].

The probability of superiority $P(T_T > T_C)$ is an intuitive measure for comparing two groups, where T_C and T_T denote independent time-to-event variables in the control and treatment groups, respectively. It is the expectation of a scaled Wilcoxon rank sum statistic. More precisely, if $\xi_1,\ldots,\xi_{n_1}$ and $\zeta_1,\ldots,\zeta_{n_2}$ are i.i.d. copies of T_T and T_C, respectively, then

$$E\sum_{i=1}^{n_1}\sum_{j=1}^{n_2} I(\xi_i > \zeta_j) = n_1 n_2 P(T_T > T_C).$$

The probability of superiority is also known as concordance probability or probabilistic index. It can be expressed as $\int_0^\infty S_T dF_C$, where S_T is survival function of the treatment group and F_C is the CDF of the control group.

However, due to censoring, S_T and F_C are not estimable on the entire real line. Suppose subjects have uniform entry into a clinical trial which ends after τ years. Then comparison between T_T and T_C can be made if and only if one of T_C, T_T is no greater than τ. Thus it is natural to consider the conditional probabilities $P(T_C > T_T|\mathscr{F}_\tau), P(T_T > T_C|\mathscr{F}_\tau)$, where

$$\mathscr{F}_\tau = \{T_C \le \tau \text{ or } T_T \le \tau\}.$$

The superiority probability ratio, sometimes referred to as the win ratio, is

$$RSP_\tau = \frac{P(T_C > T_T|\mathscr{F}_\tau)}{P(T_T > T_C|\mathscr{F}_\tau)}. \tag{9.13}$$

It can be shown that

$$RSP_\tau = \frac{\int_0^\tau S_C dF_T}{\int_0^\tau S_T dF_C}, \tag{9.14}$$

where $S_C = 1 - F_C$ and F_T is the CDF of the treatment group. Thus RSP_τ is free of the conditioning event $\mathscr{F}_\tau$.

In general, RSP_τ is well defined for any $\tau \le d^*$. Note that

$$RSP_\tau = \frac{\int_0^\tau S_C S_T d\Lambda_T}{\int_0^\tau S_C S_T d\Lambda_C}. \tag{9.15}$$

Therefore, under model (5.4), the win ratio or superiority probability ratio reduces to the hazard ratio for any $\tau \le d^*$.

Conversely, assume that the distributions are continuous and that

$$\frac{\int_0^t S_C S_T d\Lambda_T}{\int_0^t S_C S_T d\Lambda_C} = c,$$

for a constant $c > 0$ and t in an interval (a, b), $0 \le a < b \le \infty$. Then

$$\int_0^t S_C S_T d\Lambda_T = c \int_0^t S_C S_T d\Lambda_C, \quad t \in (a, b)$$

and

$$S_C(t) S_T(t) \lambda_T(t) = c S_C(t) S_T(t) \lambda_C(t), \quad t \in (a, b)$$

upon taking derivatives. It follows that

$$\lambda_T(t) = c\lambda_C(t), \quad t \in (a, b).$$

That is, the proportional hazards condition holds on the interval (a, b).

In the literature, it is sometimes proposed to use the difference

$$\int_0^\tau S_C dF_T - \int_0^\tau S_T dF_C \tag{9.16}$$

as a summary measure of the treatment effect. This quantity is more influenced by the censoring level and the value of τ, even under the proportional hazards condition. Also, under heavy censoring, the difference is extremely small, making interpretation difficult. If there is no censoring and τ can be taken to be ∞, then $\int_0^\infty S_C dF_T - \int_0^\infty S_T dF_C$ makes more sense as a summary measure. It is called the net benefit or the net chance of a longer survival [227]. Note that the difference is 0 if there is no treatment effect. A positive value indicates a beneficial treatment effect.

Kalbfleisch and Prentice [130] proposed a class of weighted average hazard ratios

$$\frac{\int_0^\tau S_C^\alpha dS_T^\alpha}{\int_0^\tau S_T^\alpha dS_C^\alpha}, \quad \alpha > 0. \tag{9.17}$$

This contains RSP_τ with $\alpha = 1$. These weighted hazard ratios are related to a truncated version of the Wilcoxon-type test statistic studied by Efron [68]. Note that they can also be rewritten in the form in (9.11), with weights

$$dw(t) = \frac{S_T^\alpha(t) S_C^\alpha(t) d\Lambda_C(t)}{\int_0^\tau S_T^\alpha(x) S_C^\alpha(x) d\Lambda_C(x)}, \quad \alpha > 0. \tag{9.18}$$

They can be estimated nonparametrically using Kaplan-Meier estimators.

Yang [338] proposed to estimate the win ratio under the model of short-term and long-term hazard ratios (7.6). Under certain regularity conditions, it was shown that the model-based estimator is asymptotically normal. Compared with the nonparametric version, the model-based estimator is more stable and often leads to some power improvement in the corresponding Wald test for the null hypothesis of no treatment effect.

Note that the weighted average hazard ratios in (9.17) with $\alpha \neq 1$ do not have the interpretation in terms of the superiority probability. Furthermore, prespecifying α is challenging and fixed values of α other than 1 may result in counter-intuitive summary measures and lower power in various simulations [338].

9.3.3 Restricted Mean Survival Related Measures

In Section 7.6.3, the restricted mean survival difference $\mu(t)$ was studied to display the change of treatment effect over time. Now for a summary measure, fix a τ that is close to d^*, the duration of the trial, and let

$$RMSD_\tau = \int_0^\tau S_T(t)dt - \int_0^\tau S_C(t)dt. \tag{9.19}$$

This provides a summary measure for the absolute treatment effect over the range $[0,\tau]$, with a positive value of $RMSD_\tau$ indicating a beneficial treatment effect. For a relative measure of the treatment effect, the ratio of the restricted mean survival times can be used. However, when the event rate is low, which is typically the case for cardiovascular trials, this ratio may give values extremely close to 1 and therefore is not very informative. Instead, the ratio of restricted mean times lost or $RRMTL_\tau$, can be used, where

$$RRMTL_\tau = \frac{\tau - \int_0^\tau S_T(t)dt}{\tau - \int_0^\tau S_C(t)dt} = \frac{\int_0^\tau F_T(t)dt}{\int_0^\tau F_C(t)dt}. \tag{9.20}$$

For consistency with the other ratios measures, $RRMTL_\tau$ is defined such that a value < 1 indicates a beneficial treatment effect.

Under the proportional hazards model (5.4), $RRMTL_\tau$ does not reduce to the hazard ratio, though typically the two ratios are close. Note that $RRMTL_\tau$ can also be viewed as the ratio of average event rates of the two groups. In the literature, $RMSD_\tau$ and $RRMTL_\tau$ are often estimated nonparametrically with the Kaplan-Meier estimators. Yang proposed to estimate them under the model of short-term and long-term hazard ratios (7.6) [337, 338]. Under certain regularity conditions, the model-based estimators are consistent for the respective parameters they target and asymptotic normality also holds. Similar to the case for the superiority probability ratio, the model-based estimators are more stable and often leads to power improvement over the nonparametric estimators.

9.3.4 Measures Based on the Area Under the Nelson-Aalen Curve

The restricted mean survival time, $\int_0^\tau S(t)dt$, and the restricted mean time lost, $\int_0^\tau F(t)dt$, where S and F are survival function and CDF of a time-to-event variable, are both area-under-the-curve summary measures. In a study of terminal and non-terminal events, which will be discussed in Chapter Fourteen, Yang [340] proposed summary measures based on area under the cumulative hazard function.

Although the idea was originally developed in association with analysis of terminal and non-terminal events, it can be used in the context here. Specifically, the ratio of the integrated cumulative hazards for treatment over control is

$$RICH_\tau = \frac{\int_0^\tau \Lambda_T(t)dt}{\int_0^\tau \Lambda_C(t)dt}. \tag{9.21}$$

The ratio is defined such that a beneficial treatment corresponds to a value less than 1.

As argued in Yang [340], the integrated cumulative hazard provides a summary measure for the risk profile of an individual over the time interval $[0,\tau]$. The concept of cumulative hazard function is just as fundamental as the CDF in survival analysis, and it also lends itself to more straightforward modeling, analysis, and interpretation, especially in more intriguing situations such as competing risks analysis that will be discussed in Chapter Thirteen.

Similar to the restricted mean survival related measures discussed in Section 9.3.3, $RICH_\tau$ is a nonparametric measure and allows simple estimation using the Nelson-Aalen estimators. An appealing property of this measure is that, when the proportional hazards condition holds, it reduces to the hazard ratio.

Note that

$$\begin{aligned} RICH_\tau &= \frac{\int_0^\tau \Lambda_T(t)/\Lambda_C(t)\Lambda_C(t)dt}{\int_0^\tau \Lambda_C(t)dt} \\ &= \int_0^\tau \frac{\Lambda_T(t)}{\Lambda_C(t)} dw(t), \end{aligned} \tag{9.22}$$

where

$$dw(t) = \frac{\Lambda_C(t)dt}{\int_0^\tau \Lambda_C(t)dt}.$$

Since $\int_0^\tau dw(t) = 1$, $RICH_\tau$ is an average of the ratio of cumulative hazards over $[0,\tau]$. Assuming continuity of Λ_T and Λ_C on $[0,\tau]$, by the weighted mean value theorem (Exercise 9.14), there exists a point $\xi \in [0,\tau]$ such that

$$RICH_\tau = \frac{\Lambda_T(\xi)}{\Lambda_C(\xi)}.$$

Thus, $RICH_\tau$ is the ratio of cumulative hazard functions at a representative point. It offers advantages over the ratio of cumulative hazards at a fixed point t_0 or percentile in that it reflects the hazard profile over an entire interval and allows a more stable estimator due to the integration.

Integration by parts yields (Exercise 9.15(a))

$$RICH_\tau = \frac{\int_0^\tau (\tau - t)d\Lambda_T(t)}{\int_0^\tau (\tau - t)d\Lambda_C(t)}. \tag{9.23}$$

Therefore, $RICH_\tau$ is in the form of a GRE in (5.40), with $\Psi(t) = (\tau - t)T(t \le \tau)$. However, it is important to note that there is no assumption of the proportional hazards condition (5.38). Let $r = RICH_\tau$ and $\hat{r}$ be the estimator of r using $\widehat{\Lambda}_C$ and $\widehat{\Lambda}_T$. Similar to (5.43), it can be shown that $\sqrt{n}(\hat{r} - r)$ converges in distribution to a mean zero normal distribution whose variance v_r can be estimated by

$$\widehat{v}_r = n\Big[\int_0^\tau (\tau-t)^2 \frac{d\widehat{\Lambda}_T(t)}{K_T(t)} + r^2 \int_0^\tau (\tau-t)^2 \frac{d\widehat{\Lambda}_C(t)}{K_C(t)}\Big] \cdot \Big[\int_0^\tau (\tau-t) d\widehat{\Lambda}_C(t)\Big]^{-2}. \quad (9.24)$$

Confidence intervals and test of the hypothesis $H_0 : r = r_0$, where r_0 is a known constant, can be obtained. $r_0 = 1$ corresponds to the hypothesis that there is no difference between the integrated cumulative hazards of two groups.

Instead of the ratio, the difference can be considered:

$$DICH_\tau = \int_0^\tau \Lambda_C(t)dt - \int_0^\tau \Lambda_T(t)dt. \quad (9.25)$$

Note that $DICH_\tau$ is defined such that a beneficial treatment corresponds to a positive value, consistent with $RMSD_\tau$.

From (9.23),

$$DICH_\tau = \int_0^\tau (\tau-t)\lambda_C(t)dt - \int_0^\tau (\tau-t)\lambda_T(t)dt. \quad (9.26)$$

Define

$$DAH_\tau = \tau^2 DICH_\tau / 2. \quad (9.27)$$

It follows that DAH_τ is an average of hazard difference between the two groups in the interval $[0,\tau]$ (Exercise 9.15(b)). Assume that λ_C and λ_T are continuous in $[0,\tau]$. By the weighted mean value theorem again, there exists a $\eta \in [0,\tau]$ such that

$$DAH_\tau = \lambda_C(\eta) - \lambda_T(\eta).$$

Therefore, DAH_τ is the difference of hazard functions at a representative point η.

Similar to $RICH_\tau$, DAH_τ can be estimated nonparametrically using the Nelson-Aalen estimators. Let $d = RICH_\tau$ and $\widehat{d}$ be the estimator of d using $\widehat{\Lambda}_C$ and $\widehat{\Lambda}_T$. It can be shown that $\sqrt{n}(\widehat{d} - d)$ converges in distribution to a mean zero normal distribution whose variance v_d can be estimated by

$$\widehat{v}_d = n\Big[\int_0^\tau (\tau-t)^2 \frac{d\widehat{\Lambda}_T(t)}{K_T(t)} + \int_0^\tau (\tau-t)^2 \frac{d\widehat{\Lambda}_C(t)}{K_C(t)}\Big]. \quad (9.28)$$

Confidence intervals and test of the hypothesis $H_0 : d = d_0$, where d_0 is a known constant, can be obtained. $d_0 = 0$ corresponds to the hypothesis that there is no difference between the integrated cumulative hazards of the two groups. Confidence intervals and tests regarding DAH_τ can be obtained using (9.27).

For all measures discussed in Sections 9.3.1 through 9.3.4, the integration range $[0,\tau]$ needs to be pre-specified. Since the Kaplan-Meier estimator and Nelson-Aalen estimator are known to be unstable near the upper end of the data range, τ needs to be smaller than d^*, the trial's duration. Based on various simulations and real trial data applications, the choice $\tau = .9d^*$ provides a good compromise between the stability requirement and the need to be representative for a summary measure. For trials with exceptionally long follow-up, a smaller value of τ, say 80% of the trial duration, may be more appropriate. For consistency across different methods, the same choice of τ can be used in the model based measures discussed in Sections 9.3.1 through 9.3.3. In applications to data from previous trials where d^* is unknown, it can be approximated by $\max X_i$.

Example 9.3. In Example 6.3, the proportional hazards model (5.4) was shown to be reasonable for the primary endpoint of the TOPCAT trial. For the SPRINT trial described in Section 1.20.1, the primary endpoint was the composite of myocardial infarction, other acute coronary syndromes, stroke, heart failure, or death from cardiovascular causes. As discussed in Yang [338], model (5.4) is also reasonable for the SPRINT primary outcome, with Lin's lack-of-fit test yielding a P-value of 0.16.

Table 9.3 displays results for estimation and testing with various effect measures for both TOPCAT and SPRINT. The model-based and nonparametric estimates of the measures discussed in Sections 9.3.1 through 9.3.3 are denoted by subscripts M and N, respectively. τ in the integration range is set to 6.15 for TOPCAT and 4.30 for SPRINT, with each value representing 90% of the respective trial duration.

Example 9.4. Consider the primary endpoint of the WHI E+P trial and the survival data from the gastric cancer trial described in sections 1.20.3 and 1.20.5. As discussed in Yang [338], model (5.4) is questionable, while model (7.6) is reasonable for both of these two datasets. Table 9.4 provides results for estimation and testing with various effect measures for these two trials. τ in the integration range is set to 7.91 for WHI E+P and 8.19 for the gastric cancer trial.

From Tables 9.3 and 9.4, as well as additional simulations and applications to trial data, in general, results from different methods are generally close to each other when the proportional hazards model (5.4) is reasonable and the difference in the two comparison groups is highly significant. However, large differences, sometimes in opposite directions, can occur when the hazards are non-proportional. When model (7.6) provides a reasonable fit, the model-based results are generally more stable and often lead to improved precision of estimators or greater power in tests.

When non-proportionality is substantial, certain methods will outperform others for any given dataset. However, it remains challenging to formulate broad

TABLE 9.3
Point estimates, 95% confidence intervals, and P-values for the Wald test of no treatment effect based on various summary measures, for primary endpoints of the TOPCAT and SPRINT trials. Results on SPRINT, except for HR, $RICH$, and DAH, are from Tables 2 and 3 in Yang [338].

Measure	TOPCAT	SPRINT
HR	0.893, 0.767–1.039,0.142	0.755, 0.639–0.892, < 0.001
AHR	0.963, 0.8269–1.118, 0.617	0.720, 0.598–0.865, < 0.001
AHR_F	0.921, 0.792–1.071, 0.285	0.721, 0.594–0.876, < 0.001
RSP_M	0.914, 0.786–1.063, 0.241	0.723, 0.597–0.877, < 0.001
RSP_N	0.919, 0.776–1.088, 0.325	0.791, 0.653–0.958, 0.016
$RRMTL_M$	0.902, 0.787–1.032, 0.133	0.785, 0.659–0.934, 0.006
$RRMTL_N$	0.904, 0.790–1.034, 0.141	0.788, 0.666–0.933, 0.006
$RMSD_M$	0.109, -0.033–0.251, 0.133	0.042, 0.011–0.074, 0.009
$RMSD_N$	0.107, -0.035–0.248, 0.141	0.041, 0.012–0.077, 0.005
RICH	0.896, 0.760–1.031, 0.132	0.782, 0.647–0.917, 0.002
DAH	0.007, -0.003–0.016, 0.154	0.005, 0.001–0.008, 0.005

generalizations or definitive conclusions about which measures are superior for a specific scenario. More research is needed to better understand non-proportional effects and how the measures react to them.

Whether the hazards are proportional or not, overall, the adaptively weighted log-rank test $LRAD_c$ is generally more sensitive to the group differences than tests based summary measures. However, as noted before, a summary measure-based test maintains a one-to-one correspondence between the test and the confidence interval. Thus, depending on the research objectives, clinical trialists can decide whether to focus on testing using $LRAD_c$ or to maintain the test-estimation coherency with a summary measure. More detailed discussions and comparison among various methods can be found in and Yang [338] and Yang et al. [341].

For model-based inference with these summary measures, the R package ClinicalTrialSummary is available at the Comprehensive R Archive Network [217]. The package provides point estimates, confidence intervals, standardized test statistics, and P-values for estimation and testing with AHR, AHR_F, RSP, RRMTL and RMSD based on model (7.6).

TABLE 9.4
Point estimates, 95% confidence intervals, and P-values for the Wald test of no treatment effect based on various summary measures, for the primary endpoint of the WHI E+P trial and the survival data from the gastric cancer trial. Except for $RICH$ and DAH, the results are from Tables 2 and 3 in Yang [338].

Measure	WHI E+P	Gastric
AHR	1.118, 0.893–1.400, 0.329	0.730, 0.454–1.175, 0.194
AHR_F	1.027, 0.775–1.359, 0.855	1.154, 0.777–1.713, 0.479
RSP_M	1.029, 0.779–1.361, 0.840	1.578, 0.974–2.556, 0.064
RSP_N	1.042, 0.752–1.444, 0.804	1.622, 0.975–2.696, 0.062
$RRMTL_M$	1.251, 1.005–1.558, 0.045	1.011, 0.857–1.192, 0.897
$RRMTL_N$	1.234, 0.991–1.537, 0.061	0.997, 0.846–1.175, 0.970
$RMSD_M$	-0.025, -0.049– -0.001, 0.042	-0.067, -1.076–0.942, 0.897
$RMSD_N$	-0.024, -0.048–0.001, 0.060	0.019, -0.988–1.025, 0.971
RICH	1.235, 0.962–1.509, 0.092	0.820, 0.432–1.209, 0.364
DAH	-0.0008, -0.0016–0.00003, 0.061	0.082, -0.116–0.279, 0.416

9.3.5 Other Measures

In addition to the measures discussed above, many other measures have also been proposed. A couple of them will be briefly mentioned below.

Uno and Horiguchi [306] proposed ratio and difference measures of treatment effect based on a particular average of the hazard function. Let h_C and h_T be the hazard functions in the control and treatment groups, respectively. Then the average hazard in the two groups over a range $[0,\tau]$ are

$$\eta_C(\tau) = \frac{\int_0^\tau h_C(t)S_C(t)dt}{\int_0^\tau S_C(t)dt}, \qquad \eta_T(\tau) = \frac{\int_0^\tau h_T(t)S_T(t)dt}{\int_0^\tau S_T(t)dt}, \tag{9.29}$$

where S_C and S_T are the survival functions of the two groups, respectively. When the treatment group event time is stochastically greater than the control group event time over $[0,\tau]$, $\eta_T \le \eta_C$. The measure can also be interpreted as the person-years event rate when general random censoring would not exist. The constant τ needs to be pre-specified before data unblinding.

Paukner and Chappell [222] extended the restricted mean survival time to the window mean survival time. For an event time variable with survival function $S(t)$, the measure is defined as

$$\mu(a,\tau) = \int_a^\tau S(t)dt. \tag{9.30}$$

Then difference in the window mean survival times between the treatment and control groups can be used as a treatment effect measure. The constants a and τ need to be pre-specified before data unblinding, analogous to the case for other measures.

9.4 Exercises and Complements

9.1 Verify that the variance estimator in (2.52) for the weighted log-rank test statistic with weight Φ reduces to (2.53) when the survival distribution functions of the two groups are continuous.

9.2 Formulate the one-sided hypothesis testing problem for the alternative $H_a'' : \lambda_T \geq \lambda_C$. Then describe the appropriate testing procedure using the adaptively weighted test.

9.3 Suppose (X,Y) has a bivariate normal distribution with standard normal marginals and correlation coefficient ρ. That is, the joint density is

$$f(x,y) = \frac{1}{2\pi\sqrt{1-\rho^2}} \exp\left[-\frac{1}{2(1-\rho^2)}(x^2+y^2-2\rho xy)\right].$$

Let

$$m(x) = \frac{1}{\sqrt{2\pi}} \exp\left(-\frac{x^2}{2}\right),$$

the marginal PDF of X. Let $c(y|x)$ be the conditional PDF of Y given $X = x$.

(a) Use the identity

$$f(x,y) = m(x)c(y|x)$$

to show that

$$c(y|x) = \frac{1}{\sqrt{2\pi(1-\rho^2)}} \exp\left[-\frac{1}{2(1-\rho^2)}(y-\rho x)^2\right].$$

That is, the conditional distribution of Y given $X = x$ is normal with mean ρx and variance $1-\rho^2$.

(b) Use the result of part (a) to show that

$$\begin{aligned} EI[|Y| \le c_\alpha)|X] &= E[I(-c_\alpha \le Y \le c_\alpha)|X] \\ &= \Phi\Big(\frac{c_\alpha - \rho X}{\sqrt{1-\rho^2}}\Big) - \Phi\Big(\frac{-c_\alpha - \rho X}{\sqrt{1-\rho^2}}\Big), \end{aligned}$$

where Φ is the standard normal CDF.

(c) The critical value c_α of the maximum test $\max(|X|,|Y|)$ satisfies

$$P\big(\max(|X|,|Y|) > c_\alpha\big) = \alpha,$$

or

$$\begin{aligned} 1-\alpha &= P\big(\max(|X|,|Y|) \le c_\alpha\big) \\ &= E\big(I(|X| \le c_\alpha)I(|Y| \le c_\alpha)\big). \end{aligned}$$

By the law of iterated expectations (B.6) in Appendix B,

$$\begin{aligned} E\big(I(|X| \le c_\alpha)I(|Y| \le c_\alpha)\big) &= EE\big(I(|X| \le c_\alpha)I(|Y| \le c_\alpha)\big|X\big) \\ &= E\big[I(|X| \le c_\alpha)E\big(I(|Y| \le c_\alpha)\big|X\big)\big]. \end{aligned}$$

Use this result and the result of part (b) to show that

$$1-\alpha = \int_{-c_\alpha}^{c_\alpha} \Big\{\Phi\Big(\frac{c_\alpha - \rho x}{\sqrt{1-\rho^2}}\Big) - \Phi\Big(\frac{-c_\alpha - \rho x}{\sqrt{1-\rho^2}}\Big)\Big\}\phi(x)dx,$$

where ϕ is the standard normal PDF. Note that this implies (9.8).

9.4 For a serial system where the system works if and only if each of the two components works, it makes sense to use the minimum test. Let (X, Y) be as in Exercise 9.3. The critical value ξ_α of the minimum test $\min(|X|,|Y|)$ satisfies

$$P\big(\min(|X|,|Y|) > \xi_\alpha\big) = \alpha,$$

or

$$\alpha = E\big(I(|X| > \xi_\alpha)I(|Y| > \xi_\alpha)\big).$$

Show that

$$\alpha = \int_{-\infty}^{\infty} I(|x| > a\xi\alpha)\Big\{\Phi\Big(\frac{-\xi_\alpha - \rho x}{\sqrt{1-\rho^2}}\Big) - \Phi\Big(\frac{\xi_\alpha - \rho x}{\sqrt{1-\rho^2}}\Big) + 1\Big\}\phi(x)dx,$$

9.5 Yang, Hsu and Zhao [342] studied the power behavior of the absolute value average test as well as that of the maximum, χ^2 and average tests. The critical value η_α of the absolute value average test $(|X|+|Y|)/2$ satisfies

$$P\Big(\frac{|X|+|Y|}{2} > \eta_\alpha\Big) = \alpha.$$

Show that

$$1-\alpha = \int_{-\eta_\alpha}^{\eta_\alpha} \Big\{\Phi\Big(\frac{2\eta_\alpha - |x| - \rho x}{\sqrt{1-\rho^2}}\Big) - \Phi\Big(\frac{|x| - 2\eta_\alpha - \rho x}{\sqrt{1-\rho^2}}\Big)\Big\}\phi(x)dx.$$

9.6 Suppose that the component test statistics X and Y are independent and standard normal.

(a) Show that the maximum test critical value is

$$c_\alpha = z\big([1-\sqrt{1-\alpha}]/2\big).$$

(b) Show that the minimum test critical value is

$$\xi_\alpha = z\big(\sqrt{\alpha}/2\big).$$

9.7 Verify the formula (9.12).

9.8 Formula (9.12) is for the weighted average hazard ratio based on model (7.6). Simplify the corresponding nonparametric version

$$\frac{\int_0^\tau h(t)dF_C(t)}{F_C(\tau)},$$

where h is the hazard ratio function, to express it in terms of F_C and F_T.

9.9 Verify that when the proportional hazards condition holds, the ratios in (9.17) reduce to the hazard ratio for any $\alpha > 0$.

9.10 Verify (9.18). That is, the class of weighted average hazard ratios of Kalbfleisch and Prentice can be written in the form in (9.11) with the specified measure $dw(t)$.

9.11 Consider the setting in Section 9.3.2 for motivating the superiority probability ratio. As mentioned there, it makes sense to compare T_C and T_T given $\mathscr{F}_\tau$, i.e., given that the comparison is possible (the trial ends after τ years, so T_C and T_T can't be compared if both are greater than τ).

Let $\mathscr{G}_\tau = \{T_C \le \tau, T_T \le \tau\}$. Then $\mathscr{G}_\tau \subset \mathscr{F}_\tau$. Thus T_C and T_T can also be compared given $\mathscr{G}_\tau$. Although it makes sense to use the weaker condition that $\mathscr{F}_\tau$ holds, it is interesting to consider the comparison problem given $\mathscr{G}_\tau$.

(a) Show that

$$P(T_T > T_C | \mathcal{G}_\tau) = \frac{\int_0^\tau F_C(x) dF_T(x)}{F_C(\tau) F_T(\tau)}.$$

(b) Show that

$$\frac{P(T_T > T_C | \mathcal{G}_\tau)}{P(T_C > T_T | \mathcal{G}_\tau)} = H(\tau),$$

where

$$H(t) = \frac{\int_0^t F_C dF_T}{\int_0^t F_T dF_C}.$$

(c) Assume that the distributions are continuous and that

$$\frac{\int_0^t F_C dF_T}{\int_0^t F_T dF_C} = c,$$

for t in the interval (a, b), $0 \le a < b \le \infty$. Show that

$$F_C(t) f_T(t) = c F_T(t) f_C(t), \qquad t \in (a, b),$$

where f_C and f_T are the PDFs corresponding to F_C and F_T. It follows that

$$\frac{f_T(t)}{F_T(t)} = c \frac{f_C(t)}{F_C(t)}, \qquad t \in (a, b).$$

This resembles the two-sample proportional hazards model, with the distinction that the CDFs are used in the denominators instead of the survival functions.

(d) If $a = 0$ and $b = \infty$, Show that

$$F_T(t) = \left[F_C(t)\right]^c.$$

9.12 The restricted mean survival time is the mean of $T \wedge \tau$, where the restriction τ is at the upper end. Consider the double-restricted mean survival time (DRMST)

$$DRMST(a, \tau) = E(T \wedge \tau \vee a),$$

where $0 < a < \tau$ and $x \vee y$ denotes the maximum between x and y. This quantity can be useful when the interest is in an interval within the data range. Show that

$$DRMST(a, \tau) = a + \int_a^\tau S(t) dt.$$

The integral in the expression above is the window mean survival time proposed by Paukner and Chappell [222]. Note that if two event times are stochastically ordered, then their DRMSTs are ordered correspondingly.

9.13 Consider the double-truncated mean survival time

$$DTMST(a,\tau) = ETI(T \in [a,\tau]).$$

Show that

$$DTMST(a,\tau) = \int_a^\tau S(t)dt - [tS(t)]|_a^\tau.$$

Therefore, when two event times are stochastically ordered, their DTMSTs may not be ordered correspondingly.

9.14 (*Weighted mean value theorem*) Suppose that $A(t)$ is a continuous function on $[0,\tau]$, with $\tau < \infty$, and $w(t)$ is a nonnegative and integrable function on $[0,\tau]$, such that

$$\int_0^\tau w(t)dt = 1.$$

(a) By the Weierstrass extreme value theorem, A attains both its minimum a and maximum b in $[0,\tau]$. Show that

$$a \le \int_0^\tau A(t)w(t)dt \le b. \tag{9.31}$$

(b) The intermediate value theorem guarantees that A takes on all values between a and b. Therefore, from (9.31), there exists a point $\xi \in [0,\tau]$ such that

$$\int_0^\tau A(t)w(t)dt = A(\xi). \tag{9.32}$$

(c) Note that if $A \ge 0$, then $\int_0^x A(t)w(t)dt$ is an increasing function in x. Therefore, if ξ in (9.32) is not unique, there will be a sub-interval of $[0,\tau]$ over which the values of A are identically $\int_0^\tau A(t)w(t)dt$. On the other hand, if A can take positive and negative values, there may be a union of disconnected sub-intervals over which the values of A are identically $\int_0^\tau A(t)w(t)dt$.

9.15 (a) Verify (9.23).

(b) Verify that DAH_τ in (9.27) is the difference of average hazard functions between the two groups in the interval $[0,\tau]$.

9.16 Verify that when the treatment group event time is stochastically greater than the control group event time over $[0,\tau]$, $\eta_T \le \eta_C$ for η_C and η_T in (9.29).

10

Sample Size, Power, and Interim Monitoring

10.1 Introduction

Sample size calculation is essential in clinical studies, surveys, psychological research, market research, and education research—any empirical study aiming to make inferences about a population based on a sample. In clinical trials, it determines the number of participants required to meet the specified type I and II error rates for testing the primary hypothesis. Sample size depends on the hypotheses, test statistics, and assumptions on relevant factors and quantities. It should be appropriate, neither too large nor too small. Too small a sample may result in a large type II error rate, or low power, while too large a sample increases cost and may lead to rejection of the null hypothesis when the difference between the comparison groups is too small to have any clinical or meaningful significance.

Interim monitoring is a critical part of trial management to ensure that the trial is progressing on the right track. If necessary, the trial may be stopped early for efficacy, harm, or futility, when the interim data show strong evidence. Due to repeated testing, the critical values need to be adjusted so that the overall type I error rate does not exceed the specified significance level.

There have been numerous methods proposed for sample size calculation/estimation. Results on the log-rank test include the works by Schoenfeld [274], Lachin [146], and Lakatos [149] in early literature, and Yung and Liu [358] recently. More works can be found in references of those articles. For interim monitoring, books on basic concepts, statistical analysis methods, and related issues in clinical trials include Jennison and Turnbull [123], Proschan, Lan and Wittes [253], and Ellenberg, Fleming and DeMets [71].

10.2 Sample Size for Testing a Normal Mean

Before the heuristic derivation of the sample size formula for weighted log-rank tests, it is helpful to first look at the simplest case where no asymptotic theory is involved. Let $\bar{X}_n$ be the mean of a random sample of independent observations from

DOI: 10.1201/9780429324437-10

the $N(\mu, \sigma^2)$ distribution with known σ. Consider the hypothesis testing problem

$$H_0 : \mu = 0 \quad \text{vs.} \quad H_a : \mu \neq 0,$$

with the test statistic $\sqrt{n}\bar{X}_n/\sigma$. Under H_0, $\sqrt{n}\bar{X}_n/\sigma$ has the $N(0,1)$ distribution and

$$P(|\sqrt{n}\bar{X}_n/\sigma| > z(\alpha/2)) = \alpha.$$

Thus if the test rejects the hypothesis H_0 when $|\sqrt{n}\bar{X}_n/\sigma| > z(\alpha/2)$, then it has the exact significance level α.

For a sample size n to yield power $1-\beta$ at $H_{a1} : \mu = \mu_1$, where β is the type II error rate and $\mu_1 < 0$, we need

$$\begin{aligned} & 1-\beta \\ = \; & P(|\sqrt{n}\bar{X}_n/\sigma| > z(\alpha/2)|H_{a1}) \\ = \; & P(\sqrt{n}\bar{X}_n/\sigma > z(\alpha/2)|H_{a1}) + P(\sqrt{n}\bar{X}_n/\sigma < -z(\alpha/2)|H_{a1}). \end{aligned} \tag{10.1}$$

Note that under H_{a1}, $\sqrt{n}\bar{X}_n/\sigma$ is close to its mean $\sqrt{n}\mu_1/\sigma$ which is negative and has the factor $\sqrt{n}$. For practical scenarios, the term

$$P(\sqrt{n}\bar{X}_n/\sigma > z(\alpha/2)|H_{a1}),$$

is negligibly small. Thus the sample size requirement of (10.1) can be approximated by the simper condition that

$$1-\beta = P(\sqrt{n}\bar{X}_n/\sigma < -z(\alpha/2)|H_{a1}). \tag{10.2}$$

This approximation also gives a conservative result, that is, the power will be at least $1-\beta$. This is because the quantity on the right-hand side in (10.2) is less than the last expression in (10.1).

Since $\sqrt{n}\bar{X}_n/\sigma$ has the $N(\sqrt{n}\mu_1/\sigma, 1)$ distribution under H_{a1}, condition (10.2) holds if and only if

$$-z(\alpha/2) - \sqrt{n}\mu_1/\sigma = z(\beta),$$

or

$$n = \left(\frac{z(\beta) + z(\alpha/2)}{\mu_1/\sigma}\right)^2. \tag{10.3}$$

This sample size, or more precisely, the integer part of the right-hand side of (10.3) plus one, ensures that the power is $1-\beta$ at $\mu = \mu_1$ (up to a negligible term). It is left to Exercise 10.2 to show that, when the intent is to have power $1-\beta$ at $\mu = \mu_2 > 0$, then n satisfies an equation parallel to (10.3) with μ_1 replaced by μ_2.

Suppose instead that the interest is in the one-sided hypothesis testing problem

$$H_0 : \mu = 0 \quad \text{vs.} \quad H_a : \mu < 0,$$

and the same test statistic $\sqrt{n}\bar{X}_n/\sigma$ is used. As discussed in Section 1.11, normally the test is performed at half of the significance level used in the two-sided test. Now the test rejects H_0 when $\sqrt{n}\bar{X}_n/\sigma < z(\alpha/2)$. For a sample size n to yield power $1-\beta$ at $H_{a1} : \mu = \mu_1 < 0$, we need (10.2) to hold. Consequently, the sample size formal (10.3) still applies, being exact as opposed to being conservative for the tow-sided test.

When σ is unknown, it is natural to use a consistent estimator $\hat{\sigma}$ instead of σ in (10.3), and expect that the asymptotic normality of $\sqrt{n}\bar{X}_n/\hat{\sigma}$ can justify the validity of this substitution. However, note that under H_{a1}, $\bar{X}_n/\hat{\sigma} \to \mu_1/\sigma$, thus $\sqrt{n}\bar{X}_n/\hat{\sigma} \to -\infty$ and the power $P(|\sqrt{n}\bar{X}_n/\sigma| > z(\alpha/2)|H_{a1})$ approaches 1. More generally, by the law of large numbers, any reasonable test will have power that converges to 1 under a fixed alternative hypothesis.

Therefore, a more refined setup and analysis is needed for the study of power and sample size. This leads to the concept of a sequence of *local* alternative hypotheses that converges to H_0 at the rate $n^{-1/2}$. Let the sequence of local alternative hypotheses be

$$H_{na} : \mu = \mu_n$$

where μ_n converges to 0 at the $n^{-1/2}$ rate: $\lim \sqrt{n}\mu_n = \nu$ for a fixed $\nu < 0$. Under this setup, (10.2) is replaced by

$$1-\beta = \lim_n P(\sqrt{n}\bar{X}_n/\hat{\sigma} < -z(\alpha/2)|H_{na}), \tag{10.4}$$

It can be shown that, under H_{na}, $\sqrt{n}\bar{X}_n/\hat{\sigma}$ converges in distribution to $N(\nu/\sigma, 1)$. From this and (10.4), we obtain

$$-z(\alpha/2) - \nu/\sigma = z_\beta,$$

or

$$-\nu/\sigma = z(\beta) + z(\alpha/2). \tag{10.5}$$

Since $\nu/\sigma = \lim \sqrt{n}\mu_n/\hat{\sigma}$, it follows that $\sqrt{n}(-\mu_n)/\hat{\sigma} \simeq z(\beta) + z(\alpha/2)$, or

$$n \simeq \left(\frac{z(\beta) + z(\alpha/2)}{\mu_n/\hat{\sigma}}\right)^2. \tag{10.6}$$

This type of maneuver extends the sample size formula (10.3) to cases where the test statistic is asymptotically normal. A rigorous analysis of an asymptotically normal test under local alternatives can be based on the contiguity theory by Le Cam [157], as discussed in books such as van der Vaart [309] and Le Cam and Yang

[158], among others. In the survival analysis context, power analysis of weighted log-rank tests can be found in various sources such as Gill [95] and Fleming and Harrington [82]. In the next two sections, we will provide a simple heuristic presentation on sample size calculation and power for weighted log-rank tests.

10.3 Sample Size for Weighted Log-Rank Tests

For weighted log-rank tests, with notations in Section 2.8.2, assume that the survival functions S_C, S_T are absolutely continuous with corresponding hazard functions λ_C, λ_T, respectively. Consider the hypothesis testing problem

$$H_0 : \lambda_T = \lambda_C = \lambda_0 \quad \text{vs.} \quad H_{na} : \lambda_C = \lambda_0, \ \ \lambda_T = \exp(\theta_n)\lambda_0, \tag{10.7}$$

where λ_0 is a hazard function and θ_n converges to 0 at the $n^{-1/2}$ rate:

$$\lim \sqrt{n}\theta_n = \nu$$

for a fixed ν. Note that in the sequence of local alternatives in (10.7), the control group hazard function does not change with n. This results in a simpler presentation compared with a more complete setup where both λ_C and λ_T change with n at the $n^{-1/2}$ rate [82].

We first look at the case when $\nu < 0$. Assume that there are n_1 observations in the control group and the rest in the treatment group. For a clearer heuristic argument, assume in addition that the censoring variables have the same distribution within each group. The survival functions of the censoring distributions in the control and treatment groups will be denoted by Γ_C and Γ_T, respectively. Furthermore, assume that

$$p_C = \lim_n \frac{n_1}{n} \in (0,1).$$

Let $p_T = 1 - p_C$. Then we also have $p_T \in (0,1)$.

Consider the weighted log-rank statistic U_Φ in (9.2). From (2.55),

$$U_\Phi = \int_0^\infty \frac{\Phi(t)K_C(t)K_T(t)}{K_C(t)+K_T(t)} d\big(\widehat{\Lambda}_T(t) - \widehat{\Lambda}_C(t)\big).$$

Thus we have the decomposition $U_\Phi = A_n + B_n$, where

$$A_n = \int_0^\infty \frac{\Phi(t)K_C(t)K_T(t)}{K_C(t)+K_T(t)} d\big[\big(\widehat{\Lambda}_T(t) - \Lambda_T(t)\big) - \big(\widehat{\Lambda}_C(t) - \Lambda_C(t)\big)\big], \tag{10.8}$$

$$B_n = \int_0^\infty \frac{\Phi(t)K_C(t)K_T(t)}{K_C(t)+K_T(t)} d\big(\Lambda_T(t) - \Lambda_C(t)\big). \tag{10.9}$$

Assume that Φ is predictable. Then from the martingale theory in Appendix B, A_n has mean zero and variance

$$E\int_0^\infty \left\{\frac{\Phi(t)K_C(t)K_T(t)}{K_C(t)+K_T(t)}\right\}^2\left(\frac{d\Lambda_T(t)}{K_T(t)}+\frac{d\Lambda_C(t)}{K_C(t)}\right).$$

By the uniform strong law of large numbers [243], with probability 1,

$$\begin{aligned}\frac{K_C(t)}{n_1}-S_C(t)\Gamma_C(t) &\rightarrow 0,\\ \frac{K_T(t)}{n_2}-S_T(t)\Gamma_T(t) &\rightarrow 0,\end{aligned}$$

uniformly on any fixed bounded interval, where $n_2 = n - n_1$, and

$$\Gamma_C(t)=\lim\frac{1}{n_1}\sum_{i\le n_1}P(C_i\ge t),\quad \Gamma_T(t)=\lim\frac{1}{n_2}\sum_{i>n_1}P(C_i\ge t).$$

Furthermore, S_T is equal to S_C under H_0 and converges to S_C under H_{na}. Assume additional regularity conditions that ensure uniform convergence of $\Phi(t)$ to its limit $\phi(t)$. Then from the martingale convergence theory, $n^{-1/2}A_n$ converges in distribution to the normal distribution with mean zero and variance

$$\sigma^2=\int_0^\infty\frac{\phi^2(t)p_Cp_TS_0(t)\Gamma_C(t)\Gamma_T(t)}{p_C\Gamma_C(t)+p_T\Gamma_T(t)}d\Lambda_0(t), \tag{10.10}$$

where $S_0(t)$, $\Lambda_0(t)$ are the survival and cumulative hazard functions associated with $\lambda_0(t)$, respectively. In addition, V_Φ/n with V_Φ in (9.2) is an estimator consistent for σ^2 under both H_0 and H_{na}.

As for B_n, note that under H_{na},

$$d\Lambda_T(t)-d\Lambda_C(t)=\left[\exp(\theta_n)-1\right]d\Lambda_0(t).$$

Under H_0, $n^{-1/2}B_n=0$. Under H_{na}, it can be shown that

$$n^{-1/2}B_n\rightarrow \nu\xi,$$

where

$$\xi=\int_0^\infty\frac{\phi(t)p_Cp_TS_0(t)\Gamma_C(t)\Gamma_T(t)}{p_C\Gamma_C(t)+p_T\Gamma_T(t)}d\Lambda_0(t).$$

Combining these results, we have

$$U_\Phi/V_\Phi\xrightarrow{d}N(0,1) \tag{10.11}$$

under H_0, and

$$U_\Phi/V_\Phi \xrightarrow{d} N\Big(\frac{\nu\xi}{\sigma},1\Big) \tag{10.12}$$

under H_{na}. Thus, similarly to (10.5), we have

$$-\frac{\nu\xi}{\sigma} = z(\beta) + z(\alpha/2). \tag{10.13}$$

Note that

$$-\frac{\nu\xi}{\sigma} = -\frac{\lim\sqrt{n}\theta_n\xi}{\sigma} = -\lim\frac{\sqrt{n}\log(h)\xi}{\sigma}, \tag{10.14}$$

where $h = \lambda_T/\lambda_C$ is the hazard ratio of the two groups. From (10.13) and (10.14) we finally obtain

$$n \simeq \Big(\frac{\sigma}{\xi}\cdot\frac{z(\beta)+z(\alpha/2)}{\log(h)}\Big)^2. \tag{10.15}$$

When $\nu > 0$, a parallel argument shows that formula (10.15) still holds.

Note that from (10.15), the required sample size depends on the distributions of time-to-event and censoring variables through ξ and σ. When the censoring distributions in the two groups are the same, there is a very simple form for the required number of events to meet the specified type I and II error rates. Suppose

$$\Gamma_C = \Gamma_T = \Gamma,$$

it is left to Exercise 10.4 to verify that, for the log-rank test,

$$\sigma^2 = \xi = \int_0^\infty p_C p_T \Gamma(t) dF_0(t), \tag{10.16}$$

where $F_0(t)$ is the CDF associated with $\lambda_0(t)$. Let $D_n = \sum_{i=1}^n \delta_i$, the number of events in the sample. Note that

$$\begin{aligned} ED_n &= E\sum_{i\le n_1}\delta_i + E\sum_{i>n_1}\delta_i \\ &= n_1 P(T_i \le C_1) + n_2 P(T_n \le C_n) \\ &= n_1\int_0^\infty \Gamma_C(t)dF_C(t) + n_2\int_0^\infty \Gamma_T(t)dF_T(t), \end{aligned}$$

where F_C, F_T are the CDFs of the control and treatment groups, respectively. Thus

$$E\frac{D_n}{n} \to p_C\int_0^\infty \Gamma(t)dF_0(t) + p_T\int_0^\infty \Gamma(t)dF_0(t) = \int_0^\infty \Gamma(t)dF_0(t). \tag{10.17}$$

With all these results, (10.13) can be re-written as

TABLE 10.1
The number of events needed for the log-rank test to achieve 80%, 85%, or 90% power at a significance level of $\alpha = 0.05$ with a hazard ratio of 0.8.

Power	80%	85%	90%
#Events	630	723	844

$$-\lim \sqrt{p_C p_T ED_n} \log(h) = z(\beta) + z(\alpha/2). \tag{10.18}$$

Thus

$$D_n \simeq \frac{1}{p_C p_T} \cdot \left(\frac{z(\beta) + z(\alpha/2)}{\log(h)}\right)^2. \tag{10.19}$$

This recovers the well-known formula for number of events given in Schoenfeld [273]. This simple formula shows that for testing the treatment effect with the log-rank test, the number of events is determined by the type I and type II error rates and the hazard ratio. From this, along with the assumed censoring distribution and recruitment pattern, the corresponding sample size can be estimated.

Due to its appealing simplicity, formula (10.19) provides a basis for the idea of an event-driven trial, where the trial duration is flexible to accommodate censoring and recruitment patterns that may differ from those anticipated at the design stage, as long as the number of events determined by (10.19) is achieved. However, as indicated by the results here, this applies only when the proportional hazards condition holds, the censoring distributions in the two groups are equal, and the log-rank test is used. In general, for a weighted log-rank test, the sample size may depend on the assumed censoring and event time distributions.

The above heuristic derivation relies on working with local alternatives and on the technical analysis of tests statistics under those local alternatives. More general settings and related detailed technical justifications can be found in Chapter Five of Gill [95] and Chapter Seven of Fleming and Harrington [82]. Alternatively, relevant convergence results can also be established using empirical process theory [279, 310, 309].

Example 10.1. Suppose that the two arms have equal sample sizes, and that the hazard ratio is 0.8. Then, at the significance level of $\alpha = .05$, the number of events required for the log-rank test to achieve different power levels is shown in Table 10.1.

Note that in the case of an asymptotically normal test statistic, the sample size formula is only approximate, and different approaches may yield slightly different results. In particular, if the sequence of local alternatives in (10.7) is replaced by

$$H_{na} : \lambda_C = \lambda_0, \quad \lambda_T = (1 + \theta_n)\lambda_0,$$

then (10.12) holds with $\nu = \lim \sqrt{n}\theta_n = \lim \sqrt{n}(h-1)$, and the corresponding sample size formula is

$$n \simeq \left(\frac{\sigma}{\xi} \cdot \frac{z(\beta) + z(\alpha/2)}{h-1}\right)^2. \tag{10.20}$$

That is, the factor $\log(h)$ in (10.15) is replaced by $h-1$ in (10.20). For h close to 1 as required by the local alternative argument, these two factors should be close to each other. In applications, one of the two formulas may yield a more accurate result than the other in a given situation, but there is no established uniform superiority one way or the other. Some additional discussions on alternative formulas can be found in Yung and Liu [358].

More generally, the local alternative setup can be used to obtain asymptotic normality of the weighted log-rank test when the sequence of local alternatives is specified by a parametric model other than the proportional hazards model. From the asymptotic normality, sample size formulas can be obtained. Let $\{\lambda_\theta, \theta \in \Theta\}$ be a parametric family of hazard functions where θ is in an open interval containing 0. Consider the hypothesis testing problem

$$H_0 : \lambda_T = \lambda_C = \lambda_0 \quad \text{vs.} \quad H_{na} : \lambda_C = \lambda_0, \ \ \lambda_T = \lambda_{\theta_n}, \tag{10.21}$$

where θ_n converges to 0 at the $n^{-1/2}$ rate: $\lim \sqrt{n}\theta_n = \nu$ for a fixed ν. For the weighted log-rank test statistic U_Φ, the decomposition $U_\Phi = A_n + B_n$ for A_n, B_n in (10.8) and (10.9) is still valid. Let

$$\kappa_\theta(t) = \frac{\partial}{\partial\theta} \ln \lambda_\theta(t) = \frac{\partial \lambda_\theta(t)}{\partial\theta} \frac{1}{\lambda_\theta(t)}.$$

Under H_{na} and certain regularity conditions,

$$\begin{aligned}
\sqrt{n}[d\Lambda_T(t) - d\Lambda_C(t)] &= \sqrt{n}[\lambda_{\theta_n}(t) - \lambda_0(t)]dt \\
&\simeq \nu \frac{\partial}{\partial\theta} \lambda_\theta(t)\big|_{\theta=0} dt \\
&= \nu\kappa_0(t) d\Lambda_0(t).
\end{aligned}$$

From this, analogously to the derivation of (10.11) and (10.12), we have

$$U_\Phi / V_\Phi \xrightarrow{d} N(0,1) \tag{10.22}$$

under H_0, and

$$U_\Phi / V_\Phi \xrightarrow{d} N\left(\frac{\eta}{\sigma}, 1\right) \tag{10.23}$$

under H_{na}, where

$$\eta = \int_0^\infty \frac{\nu\kappa_0(t)\phi(t) p_C p_T S_0(t) \Gamma_C(t) \Gamma_T(t)}{p_C \Gamma_C(t) + p_T \Gamma_T(t)} d\Lambda_0(t). \tag{10.24}$$

Note that the factor ν that appears in (10.12) is now absorbed in η. Similarly to (10.13), when $\nu < 0$, we have

$$-\frac{\eta}{\sigma} = z(\beta) + z(\alpha/2). \tag{10.25}$$

Since $\ln \lambda_T(t) = \ln \lambda_{\theta_n}(t) \simeq \ln \lambda_0(t) + \theta_n \kappa_0(t)$, we get

$$\theta_n \simeq \frac{\ln \lambda_{\theta_n}(t) - \ln \lambda_0(t)}{\kappa_0(t)} = \frac{\ln[h(t)]}{\kappa_0(t)}, \tag{10.26}$$

where $h(t) = \lambda_T(t)/\lambda_C(t)$ is the hazard ratio function which may not be a constant in this general situation. From (10.24) through (10.26), and $\nu = \lim \sqrt{n}\theta_n$, similarly to (10.15) we obtain the sample size formula

$$n \simeq \left(\frac{\sigma[z(\beta) + z(\alpha/2)]}{\zeta}\right)^2. \tag{10.27}$$

where

$$\zeta = \int_0^\infty \frac{\ln[h(t)]\phi(t) p_C p_T S_0(t)\Gamma_C(t)\Gamma_T(t)}{p_C\Gamma_C(t) + p_T\Gamma_T(t)} d\Lambda_0(t).$$

Verification of this is left to Exercise 10.10 (a). When $\nu > 0$, a parallel argument shows that formula (10.26) still holds.

Instead of approximating $\ln \lambda_{\theta_n}(t)$, it is also possible to use the approximation

$$\lambda_T(t) = \lambda_{\theta_n}(t) \simeq \lambda_0(t) + \theta_n \partial\lambda_0(t)/\partial\theta = \lambda_0(t) + \theta_n \lambda_0(t)\kappa_0(t),$$

which yields

$$\theta_n \simeq \frac{\lambda_{\theta_n}(t) - \lambda_0(t)}{\lambda_0(t)\kappa_0(t)} = \frac{h(t) - 1}{\kappa_0(t)}, \tag{10.28}$$

Thus instead of (10.27), we get

$$n \simeq \left(\frac{\sigma[z(\beta) + z(\alpha/2)]}{\zeta^*}\right)^2. \tag{10.29}$$

where

$$\zeta^* = \int_0^\infty \frac{[h(t) - 1]\phi(t) p_C p_T S_0(t)\Gamma_C(t)\Gamma_T(t)}{p_C\Gamma_C(t) + p_T\Gamma_T(t)} d\Lambda_0(t).$$

Verification of this is left to Exercise 10.10(b).

10.4 Efficiencies of Weighted Log-Rank Tests

In the previous section, the focus was on obtaining appropriate sample size for a specific weighted log-rank test to achieve the given type I and type II error rates.

The local alternative setup was originally introduced to study power behavior of tests. From the asymptotic normality under both the null and local alternative hypotheses, tests can be compared and it is possible to establish conditions for maximal power. Let $\{\lambda_\theta, \theta \in \Theta\}$ be a parametric family of hazard functions where θ is in an open interval containing 0. For the hypothesis testing problem in (10.20), by (10.22) the asymptotic power is determined by η/σ, whose square is called the asymptotic efficacy of the test. A larger asymptotic efficacy corresponds to a higher power. Let e_A and e_B be the asymptotic efficacy of two tests A and B, respectively. The ratio e_B/e_A can be used to compare the tests. Under appropriate conditions, this ratio coincides with the Pitman asymptotic relative efficiency of test B with respect to test A, a classical measure used in comparing tests.

From (10.26), the sample size is proportional to the inverse of the asymptotic efficacy. Thus if $e_B/e_A = 1.3$, then the sample size needed for test B is only $1/1.3 \times 100\% = 77\%$ of the sample size needed for test A.

From expressions (10.10) and (10.24), by the Cauchy-Schwartz inequality,

$$\frac{\eta^2}{\sigma^2} \le \nu^2 \int_0^\infty \frac{\kappa_0^2(t) p_C p_T S_0(t) \Gamma_C(t) \Gamma_T(t)}{p_C \Gamma_C(t) + p_T \Gamma_T(t)} d\Lambda_0(t), \tag{10.30}$$

with equality achieved when

$$\phi(t) = \kappa_0(t) = \frac{\partial}{\partial\theta} \ln \lambda_\theta(t)\big|_{\theta=0}. \tag{10.31}$$

Thus, subject to necessary regularity conditions, given a particular parametric family for the sequence of local alternatives, the weighted log-rank test with this weight has the highest power among all weighted log-rank tests.

Besides weighted log-rank tests, many other tests are possible. Under certain regularity conditions, the likelihood ratio test is the most powerful test for the testing problem (10.20), with asymptotic efficacy

$$\int_0^\infty \left[\nu\kappa_0(t)\right]^2 S_0(t) \big(p_C \Gamma_C(t) + p_T \Gamma_T(t)\big) d\Lambda_0(t). \tag{10.32}$$

Rigorous justification for this is given in Gill [95]. From (10.30) and (10.32), the asymptotic efficacy of the weighted log-rank test with $\Phi(t) = \kappa_0(t)$ is equal to that of the most powerful test if and only if $\Gamma_C = \Gamma_T$.

Example 10.2. Suppose $\{\lambda_\theta, \theta \in \Theta\}$ follows the proportional hazards model: $\lambda_\theta(t) = \exp(\theta)\lambda(t)$ for a hazard function $\lambda(t)$. Then $\kappa_\theta = 1$. Thus the log-rank test, corresponding to $\Phi(t) \equiv 1$, is the optimal test among all weighted log-rank tests.

Example 10.3. Suppose $\{\lambda_\theta, \theta \in \Theta\}$ follows the proportional ρ-hazards model with a known $\rho > 0$. From (8.40), we have

$$\lambda_\theta(t) = \frac{1}{\exp(-\theta) + \rho R(t)} \frac{dR(t)}{dt},$$

for an odds function $R(t)$. Note that the corresponding cumulative hazard and survival functions are

$$\Lambda_\theta(t) = \frac{1}{\rho}\ln\left[1+\rho\exp(\theta)R(t)\right],\ S_\theta(t) = \left[1+\rho\exp(\theta)R(t)\right]^{-1/\rho}.$$

We have

$$\kappa_\theta = \frac{\exp(-\theta)}{\exp(-\theta)+\rho R(t)}.$$

Thus

$$\kappa_0 = \frac{1}{1+\rho R(t)} = S_0(t)^\rho.$$

It follows that the weighted log-rank test with $\Phi(t) = \widehat{S}_-^\rho(t)$, where $\widehat{S}_-(t)$ is the left continuous version of the Kaplan-Meier survival estimator based on the pooled sample, is the optimal test among all weighted log-rank tests. This result was first obtained by Harrington and Fleming [109]. Intuitively, since the hazard ratio converges to 1 under the proportional ρ-odds model, it makes sense to consider a weighted log-rank test with weight function such as $\widehat{S}_-^\rho(t)$ that puts more weight on early event times where there is more discrepancy between the two groups. The optimality result here confirms that such strategy is reasonable and goes a step further by establishing the asymptotic optimality for the specific weight function $\widehat{S}_-^\rho(t)$.

In particular, taking $\rho = 1$, we obtain that the Peto-Prentice weight $\widehat{S}_-(t)$ is the optimal weighted log-rank test for the proportional odds model.

Example 10.4. Recall that in the two-sample case, both proportional hazards model and proportional odds model are sub-models of the model of short-term and long-term hazard ratios (7.6) in Chapter Seven. In the previous two examples, the optimal weight for the weighted log-rank test was obtained under each of those two sub-models. Now consider one more sub-model of (7.6):

$$\lambda_\theta(t) = \frac{1}{1+\exp(-\theta)R(t)}\frac{dR(t)}{dt}. \tag{10.33}$$

That is, the parameter (β_1, β_1) in (7.6) is restricted to the sub-space where the first component is identically 0. The corresponding cumulative hazard and survival functions are

$$\Lambda_\theta(t) = \exp(\theta)\ln\left[1+\exp(-\theta)R(t)\right],\ S_\theta(t) = \left[1+\exp(-\theta)R(t)\right]^{-\exp(\theta)}.$$

We have

$$\kappa_\theta = \frac{\exp(-\theta)R(t)}{1+\exp(-\theta)R(t)}.$$

Thus

$$\kappa_0 = \frac{R(t)}{1+R(t)} = S_0(t). \tag{10.34}$$

It follows that the weighted log-rank test with $\Phi(t) = 1 - \widehat{S}_{-}(t)$, is the optimal test among all weighted log-rank tests. In model (10.33), the hazards ratio is 1 at time 0 and increases/decreases to $\exp(\theta)$ as $R(t) \to \infty$. Thus it makes sense to consider a weighted log-rank test with weight function such as $1 - \widehat{S}_{-}(t)$ that puts more weight on late event times where the discrepancy is larger between the two groups. The result (10.34) shows that the weight $1 - \widehat{S}_{-}(t)$ is not only reasonable, but also asymptotically optimal for this sub-model.

10.5 Interim Monitoring

Clinical trials typically span over several years, during which it is important to monitor accumulating data on a periodic basis to ensure that the trial is progressing as planned and address any emerging issues promptly. If compelling evidence of harm, efficacy or futility arises before the trial's planned completion, the DSMB may recommend stopping the trial early. A brief description of a DSMB is provided in Section 1.16.

The decision-making process to terminate a trial early due to evidence of harm, benefit or futility is complex. While statistical methods alone are not sufficient to determine whether the trial should be stopped early, they can provide very useful guidelines. The DSMB often uses pre-specified statistical stopping rules to guide their decisions. These rules help adjust the boundaries needed to declare treatment success at either an interim analysis or the final analysis, correcting for repeated significance testing to prevent inflation of the type I error rate.

The DSMB considers study-specific data as well as relevant background knowledge about the disease, intervention strategy, or patient population under study when making recommendations. Their primary responsibility is to safeguard the interests of study participants while preserving the scientific integrity of the trial.

Discussions on interim analysis and trial monitoring can be found in various sources, such as DeMets and Lan [60], Fleming and DeMets [81], and Pocock [237]. Jennison and Turnbull [124] provide a systematic exposition of group sequential methods. Proschan et al. [253] and Pocock et al. [239] contain many interesting clinical trial examples with practical insights on using interim analysis methods.

10.5.1 Group Sequential Designs

Suppose that $\widehat{T}$ is the test statistic and that accumulating data are analyzed at calendar times $x_1 < \cdots < x_K = d^*$, $K > 1$, where d^* denote the time when the trial ends. Note that in this notation, the final analysis is at $x_K = d^*$, and there are $K-1$

interim analyses. For group sequential designs, typically it is assumed that $\widehat{T}$ is obtained from standardizing an asymptotically normal test statistic $\widetilde{T}$. Let $\widetilde{T}_1,\ldots,\widetilde{T}_K$ be values of $\widetilde{T}$ at the analysis times and assume that $\left(\widetilde{T}_1,\ldots,\widetilde{T}_K\right)$ converges in distribution to a multivariate normal vector $(A(x_1),\ldots,A(x_K))^{\mathrm{T}}$. Assume that under the null hypothesis, the mean and covariance structure of the normal vector are such that

$$EA(x_j)=0, \quad Cov(A(x_j),A(x_\ell))=v(x_j), \quad 1\le j\le \ell\le K, \tag{10.35}$$

where $v(x)$ is an increasing function. Note that the covariance structure implies that $v(x)$ is the variance of $A(x)$, and $A(x)$ as a process in x has independent increments. $\widehat{T}_j$ is obtained from $\widetilde{T}_j$ as

$$\widehat{T}_j=\frac{\widetilde{T}_j}{\sqrt{\widehat{v}_j}}, \quad 1\le j\le K,$$

where $\widehat{v}_j$ is a consistent estimator of $v(x_j)$.

As x increases toward the trial's end, $v(x)$ increases to $v(d^*)$, the asymptotic variance of $\widetilde{T}$ using all data. The fraction $s(x)=v(x)/v(d^*)$ is called the *information fraction* which increases from 0 at the trial start to 1 at the trial end. The information fraction provides a natural time scale for the trial. Let $s_j=s(x_j)$. For completely observed continuous or binary outcomes, s_j is estimated by the fraction of sample size at time x out of the planned total sample size. For survival data, due to the widespread use of log-rank test and equations (10.15) and (10.16), s_j is estimated by the fraction of the number of events at time x relative to the targeted total number of events. Regardless of the data type, the estimator of s_j will be denoted by $\widehat{s}_j$.

From (10.35), under the null hypothesis, $(\widehat{T}_1,\ldots,\widehat{T}_K)$ converges in distribution to the K-variate normal distribution with standard normal marginals and correlation coefficients

$$\rho_{j\ell}=\sqrt{\frac{v(x_j)}{v(x_\ell)}}, \quad 1\le j<\ell\le K, \tag{10.36}$$

which can be estimated by

$$\widehat{\rho}_{j\ell}=\sqrt{\frac{\widehat{s}_j}{\widehat{s}_\ell}}, \quad 1\le j<\ell\le K. \tag{10.37}$$

Note that $\widehat{s}_K=1$. For $\widehat{\rho}_{j\ell}$, since the estimated total sample size/number of events appears in both $\widehat{s}_j$ and $\widehat{s}_\ell$, $1\le j<\ell\le K$, $\widehat{\rho}_{j\ell}$ only depends on sample sizes/number of events at times x_j, x_ℓ and not on future data.

Consider a two-sided test at significance level α. In a group sequential design, the null hypothesis of no treatment effect is rejected if $|\widehat{T}_j|$ exceeds an appropriate critical value c_j for some $j \leq K$. The critical values are often referred to as the stopping boundaries. The procedure is as follows:

1. At the jth look, if $|\widehat{T}_j| > c_j$, the trial is stopped and the null hypothesis rejected; otherwise, the trial continues to the next analysis, $j = 1, \ldots, K-1$.
2. If the trial continues after the $(K-1)$th look, then at the final (Kth) look, the null hypothesis is rejected if $|\widehat{T}_K| > c_K$.

Let

$$\begin{aligned} P_0\big(|\widehat{T}_1| > c_1\big) &= p_1 \\ P_0\big(|\widehat{T}_1| \leq c_1, |\widehat{T}_2| > c_2\big) &= p_2 \\ &\cdots \\ P_0\big(|\widehat{T}_1| \leq c_1, \ldots, |\widehat{T}_{K-1}| \leq c_{K-1}, |\widehat{T}_K| > c_K\big) &= p_K, \end{aligned} \tag{10.38}$$

where P_0 denotes the probability calculated under the null hypothesis of no treatment effect. Then p_j is the probability of stopping the trial at the jth look, and

$$P_0\Big(\bigcup_{j=1}^{K} \{|\widehat{T}_j| > c_j\}\Big) = \sum_{j=1}^{K} p_j.$$

To ensure that the overall type I error rate is α, we need

$$p_1 + \cdots + p_K = \alpha, \quad p_1, \ldots, p_K > 0. \tag{10.39}$$

Pocock [235] developed a boundary by requiring that the time points $x_1, \ldots, x_j$ are equally spaced in terms of the information fraction and that $c_1 = \cdots = c_K = c_P$, where the common value c_P satisfies

$$P_0\Big(\bigcup_{j=1}^{K} \{|\widehat{T}_j| > c_P\}\Big) = \alpha.$$

The Pocock boundary simplifies the general problem of finding K critical values to finding a single critical value c_P. However, it requires the same amount of evidence to stop the trial at all looks. This may not be desirable, since it is generally accepted that a higher level of evidence is required at early looks where the test statistics have larger variances. In other words, the Pocock boundary does not account for the varying precision of the estimates at different time points, which could potentially lead to premature termination of the trial.

Note that for the Pocock boundary, the number of looks K needs to be prespecified, as the critical value c_P implicitly depends on K. To determine c_P, numerical multivariate integration is typically required, which can be computationally intensive.

A proposal simpler than the Pocock boundary was given by Haybittle [110], who suggested, for the significance level 0.05, using the critical value of 3 at all interim looks and then the usual 1.96 at the last look. A variation is to use the critical value of 4 instead of 3 at all interim looks. Note that for any j,

$$P(|\widehat{T}_j| > 3) = 0.00270$$

$$P(|\widehat{T}_j| > 4) = 0.00006.$$

Thus the size inflation with 4 is negligible. The size inflation with 3 is also quite small if there is only one interim look. However, when the number of interim looks increases, the size inflation with 3 can be more noticeable.

At a given look, for a cut-off point that is either the observed value of the test statistic or a critical value, the corresponding *nominal P-value* is the P-value that is computed the usual way without considering behavior of the test statistic at other looks. Peto et al. [229] proposed a variation of the Haybittle method, setting a boundary corresponding to a nominal P-value of 0.001 (two-sided) at all interim analyses, and 0.05 at the final analysis. Note that the critical value of 3 corresponds to a nominal P-value of 0.0027.

Additional variations of these methods are possible. For instance, one could set the nominal P-value to be 0.0001 before reaching a certain information fraction (e.g., 0.5), and 0.001 afterwards but before the final analysis, where the nominal P-value is set at 0.05. The boundaries proposed by Haybittle, Peto, or their variants all result in slight inflation of the overall type I error rate.

To correct this error rate inflation in the Haybittle-Peto approaches, the Bonferroni method can be used. Let $c_1, \ldots, c_K$ be the critical values corresponding to nominal P-values $p_{0,1}, \ldots, p_{0,K}$, where $p_{0,K} = 0.05 - p_{0,1} - \cdots - p_{0,K-1}$. The corrected procedure rejects the null hypothesis if the nominal P-value at the jth look is less than $p_{0,j}$, $j = 1, \cdots, K$. By the Bonferroni inequality,

$$
\begin{aligned}
& P_0\Big(\bigcup_{j=1}^{K} \{|\widehat{T}_j| > c_j\}\Big) \\
\leq\ & \sum_{j=1}^{K-1} P_0(|\widehat{T}_j| > c_i) + P_0(|\widehat{T}_K| > c_K) \\
=\ & \sum_{j=1}^{K-1} p_{0,j} + 0.05 - \sum_{j=1}^{K-1} p_{0,j} = 0.05.
\end{aligned}
$$

Therefore, the overall type I error rate is controlled not to exceed 0.05.

For example, with one single interim look, the corrected Haybittle procedure rejects the null hypothesis at the interim look if $|\widehat{T}_1| > 3$, or at the final look if $|\widehat{T}_2| >$

1.984. This adjustment ensures rigorous control of type I error while only slightly increasing the critical value at the final look compared to the value of 1.96 when there are no interim looks.

O'Brien and Fleming [215] proposed a boundary that has a common critical value at all looks for a properly scaled $|\widehat{T}|$, again under the condition that the looks are equally spaced in terms of the information fraction. Let c_{OBF} be the common critical value for the scaled $|\widehat{T}|$, then the boundary for $|\widehat{T}|$ at time x_j is $c_{OBF}/\sqrt{\widehat{s}_j}$. The use of $\sqrt{\widehat{s}_j}$ in the formula means that the boundary is more stringent at earlier interim analyses where the boundary value $c_{OBF}/\sqrt{\widehat{s}_j}$ is large. Note that for the O'Brien-Fleming boundary, the number of looks K also needs to be pre-specified as the critical value c_{OBF} implicitly depends on K.

The boundaries of Pocock, Haybittle-Peto, and O'Brien-Fleming can also be properly modified to yield one-sided versions using $\widehat{T}$ instead of $|\widehat{T}|$. Additional boundaries and related discussions can be found in Kennison and Turnbull [124], among others.

10.5.2 The Alpha Spending Function

To address emerging issues and manage DSMB meeting scheduling, it is desirable to keep the timing and number of interim analyses flexible. While various group sequential methods were proposed during the early development stages, the alpha spending method proposed by Lan and DeMets [150] and later extended by Kim and DeMets [136] has become the most widely used and flexible approach.

The method uses a specified alpha spending function, which determines the maximum amount of type I error rate allocated at each interim analysis. Unlike other methods, such as those proposed by Pocock [235], O'Brien and Fleming [215], Slud and Wei [282], and Tsiatis [301], there is no need to pre-specify the number or timing of interim analyses. The alpha spending function method has gained widespread acceptance due to its flexibility and has been adopted by regulatory agencies such as the FDA and EMA.

To motivate the spending function approach, it helps to express the probabilities in (10.38) in alternative forms. Consider the case of one-sided test for benefit. Let α be the specified significance level, and suppose positive values of $\widehat{T}$ correspond to a beneficial treatment effect. Similar to the discussion in Section 10.5.1 for two-sided tests, in a group sequential design, the null hypothesis of no treatment effect is rejected and a benefit is claimed if $\widehat{T}_j$ exceeds certain critical value u_j for some $j \le K$. The procedure is as follows:

1. At the jth look, if $\widehat{T}_j > c_j$, the trial is stopped for benefit; otherwise, the trial continues, $j = 1, \dots, K-1$.

2. Suppose the trial continues after the $(K-1)$th look. Then at the final, Kth look, if $\widehat{T}_K > c_K$, the trial concludes with a claim of benefit; otherwise, there is insufficient evidence to reject the null hypothesis.

Let

$$\begin{aligned} P_0\left(\widehat{T}_1 > u_1\right) &= q_1 \\ P_0\left(\widehat{T}_1 \le u_1, \widehat{T}_2 > u_2\right) &= q_2 \\ &\cdots \\ P_0\left(\widehat{T}_1 \le u_1, \cdots, \widehat{T}_{K-1} \le u_{K-1}, \widehat{T}_K > u_K\right) &= q_K. \end{aligned} \tag{10.40}$$

To ensure that the overall type I error rate is α, similarly to (10.39) we need

$$q_1 + \cdots + q_K = \alpha, \quad q_1, \ldots, q_K > 0. \tag{10.41}$$

Note that if we let

$$\begin{aligned} \alpha_1 &= q_1 \\ \alpha_j &= q_1 + \cdots + q_j, \quad 1 < j \le K, \end{aligned}$$

then (10.40) can be equivalently expressed as

$$\begin{aligned} P_0\left(\widehat{T}_1 > u_1\right) &= \alpha_1 \\ P_0\left(\widehat{T}_{\ell-1} \le u_{\ell-1}, 1 < \ell \le j, \widehat{T}_j > u_j\right) &= \alpha_j - \alpha_{j-1}, \quad j = 2, \ldots, K. \end{aligned} \tag{10.42}$$

In these expressions, α_j is the probability of stopping the trial for benefit no later than the jth look. The sequence α_j increases up to $\alpha_K = \alpha$.

An *alpha spending function* $\alpha^*(s)$ is an increasing function over $[0,1]$ such that $\alpha^*(0) = 0$ and $\alpha^*(1) = \alpha$, where s is the information fraction. At each analysis, a portion of the overall alpha is "spent." Recall that the information fraction at the jth look is s_j, $j \le K$, with $s_K = 1$. The boundaries at $u_1, \cdots, u_K$ are chosen to satisfy:

$$\begin{aligned} P_0\left(\widehat{T}_1 > u_1\right) &= \alpha^*(s_1), \\ P_0\left(\widehat{T}_{\ell-1} \le u_{\ell-1}, 1 < \ell \le j, \widehat{T}_j > u_j\right) &= \left[\alpha^*(s_j) - \alpha^*(s_{j-1})\right], \end{aligned} \tag{10.43}$$

for $j = 2, \ldots, K$. Note that the probabilities on the left-hand side of (10.43) add up to $P_0\left(\bigcup_{j=1}^{K}\{\widehat{T}_j > u_j\}\right)$, and the probabilities on right-hand side in (10.43) add up to

$$\begin{aligned} & \alpha^*(s_1) + \left[\alpha^*(s_2) - \alpha^*(s_1)\right] + \cdots + \left[\alpha^*(s_K) - \alpha^*(s_{K-1})\right] \\ = \; & \alpha^*(s_K) = \alpha. \end{aligned} \tag{10.44}$$

Thus the overall type I error rate is α. To apply the spending function approach, the points where the function is evaluated, that is, the information fractions $s_1,\ldots,s_K$, are estimated by $\widehat{s}_1,\ldots,\widehat{s}_K$ in (10.43).

Next, consider the one-sided test for safety (negative values of $\widehat{T}_j$ indicating harm). By symmetry of the normal distributions, the boundary values are simply $-u_1,\cdots,-u_K$. In the associated group sequential design, the null hypothesis of no treatment effect is rejected with a claim of harm if $\widehat{T}_j < -u_j$ for some $j \le K$.

Recall from discussions in Section 1.11 that, for one-sided tests, it is common practice to use a significance level that is half of what is typically considered in the corresponding two-sided test. Thus usually an alpha level of 0.025 is used for a one-sided test.

Kim and DeMets [136] considered the case of two-sided tests. To allow asymmetric upper and lower boundaries, two alpha spending functions are used. For clarity, let's focus on the significance level of 0.05 as an example, but the approach can be adapted for other levels. Denote the two alpha spending functions by $\alpha_l^*(s)$ and $\alpha_u^*(s)$, with both increasing from 0 to 0.05. The upper and lower boundary values $a_j,\ b_j,\ j=1,\cdots,K$ are chosen to satisfy the following conditions:

$$\begin{aligned}
P_0\big(\widehat{T}_1 > b_1\big) &= \frac{1}{2}\alpha_u^*(s_1),\\
P_0\big(\widehat{T}_1 < a_1\big) &= \frac{1}{2}\alpha_l^*(s_1),\\
P_0\big(\widehat{T}_{\ell-1} \in [a_{\ell-1}, b_{\ell-1}], 1<\ell\le j, \widehat{T}_j > b_j\big) &= \frac{1}{2}\big[\alpha_u^*(s_j) - \alpha_u^*(s_{j-1})\big],\\
P_0\big(\widehat{T}_{\ell-1} \in [a_{\ell-1}, b_{\ell-1}], 1<\ell\le j, \widehat{T}_j < a_j\big) &= \frac{1}{2}\big[\alpha_l^*(s_j) - \alpha_l^*(s_{j-1})\big], \quad (10.45)
\end{aligned}$$

for $j=2,\ldots,K$. All probabilities in (10.45) add up to

$$\frac{1}{2}\alpha_u^*(s_K) + \frac{1}{2}\alpha_l^*(s_K) = 0.05.$$

Thus the overall type I error rate is maintained. Symmetric boundaries are generated by setting $\alpha_l^* = \alpha_u^*$ and $a_j = b_j,\ j \le K$.

Instead of the above procedure for a two-sided test with an exact overall type I error rate of 0.05, a conservative two-sided procedure can also be considered. It uses a spending function $\alpha^*(s)$ in (10.43) that increases from 0 to 0.025 to obtain upper boundaries $u_1,\cdots,u_K$, and then the lower boundaries are simply $-u_1,\cdots,-u_K$. This approach is valid because

$$\begin{aligned}
&P_0\big(\widehat{T}_{\ell-1} \in [-u_{\ell-1}, u_{\ell-1}], 1<\ell\le j, \widehat{T}_j > u_j\big)\\
\le\ &P_0\big(\widehat{T}_{\ell-1} \le u_{\ell-1}, 1<\ell\le j, \widehat{T}_j > u_j\big), \quad (10.46)
\end{aligned}$$

which implies that the overall type I error rate is controlled not to exceed 0.05. Verification of this statement is left to Exercise 10.15.

In practical interim monitoring scenarios, the probabilities on both sides of the inequality in (10.46) are close to each other and the conservatism is usually not much of a concern. The two-sided procedure in (10.45) is exact and has bounded ranges for looks prior to the jth look, avoiding numerical integration over infinite range involving those prior looks. On the other hand, using boundaries from the one-sided tests offers the flexibility of separately considering stopping for benefit and stopping for harm. The one-sided setup also results in a simpler iterative procedure for numerical integrals with multivariate normal distributions [253].

Before interim analysis, the alpha spending function needs to be specified. Let

$$\begin{aligned} \alpha_1^*(s) &= 2-2\Phi\left[\frac{z(\alpha/2)}{\sqrt{s}}\right], \\ \alpha_2^*(s) &= \alpha\ln\left[1+(e-1)s\right], \\ \alpha_3^*(s) &= \alpha s^{\kappa}, \end{aligned} \tag{10.47}$$

where $\Phi(x)$ is the CDF of the standard normal distribution and κ is often taken to be 1.5 or 2. The first two functions were proposed in Lan and DeMets [150] which produce boundaries similar to O'Brien-Fleming and Pocock boundaries, respectively. They are referred to as O'Brien-Fleming type and Pocock type boundaries, respectively. The third function was proposed by Kim and DeMets [136] who argued for the use of strictly convex spending functions. In addition to these alpha spending functions, other options are possible [124].

Figure 10.1 illustrates plots of the three functions with $\alpha = 0.025$. Note that α_1^* is very flat at the beginning and increases steeply at the end. It allocates very little of the total type I error rate to early interim looks, which results in critical values at the final look very close to that for a design with no interim looks. On the other hand, α_2^* is concave and allocates a considerable amount of the total type I error rate to early interim looks. This results in relatively larger penalties at the final look. Plots for the function α_3^* with $\kappa = 1,2$ are between α_1^* and α_2^*.

To demonstrate the effect of interim analysis on alpha allocation to the final analysis, consider the scenario when there is only one interim look at the information fraction of 0.5. In this case, for $\alpha = 0.025$, $\alpha_1^*(.5) = 0.0015$, and $\alpha_2^*(.5) = 0.0155$, thus the alpha allocated for the final analysis is 0.0235 and 0.0095, respectively.

Note that $\alpha_2^*(s)$ and $\alpha_3^*(s)$ are linear in α but $\alpha_1^*(s)$ is not. Therefore, the one-sided version in (10.43) with significance level 0.025,

$$2-2\Phi\left[\frac{z(0.025/2)}{\sqrt{s}}\right], \tag{10.48}$$

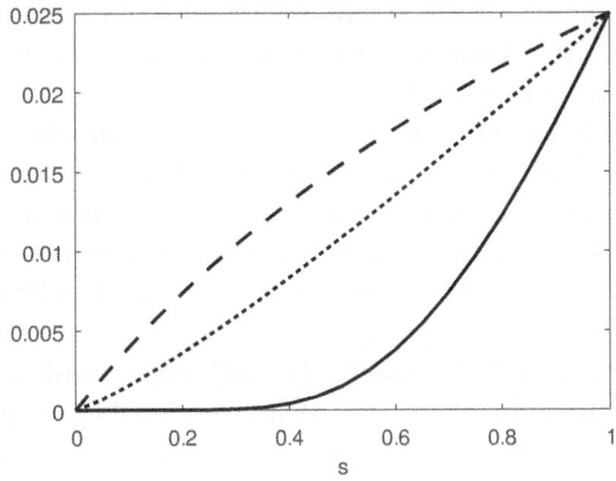

FIGURE 10.1
Plots of the three alpha spending functions in (10.47), for $\alpha = 0.025$. Solid—$\alpha_1^*(s)$; dashed—$\alpha_2^*(s)$; dotted—$\alpha_3^*(s)$ with $\kappa = 1.2$.

is different from what is used in (10.45) for symmetric boundaries, or

$$\frac{1}{2}\alpha^*(s) = \frac{1}{2}\left\{2 - 2\Phi\left[\frac{z(0.05/2)}{\sqrt{s}}\right]\right\}. \tag{10.49}$$

The function in (10.48) allocates smaller fractions of the total alpha to early looks than the one in (10.49).

For the calculation of the boundary values, a guideline on the number and timing of interim looks is typically specified in the protocol. However, the spending function approach provides flexibility to determine those factors during the trial should the need arise, as long as the spending function is pre-specified and decisions on future boundary locations and values are not data-dependent.

In applications, however, the placement of interim looks may sometimes be influenced by data due to ethical and practical reasons. For instance, the DSMB may decide to schedule the next look sooner than planned when the test statistic is near the boundary, or delay the next look if the test statistic is far from the boundary. Fortunately, the impact on type I error rate and power of such data-dependent timing and frequency of looks typically is negligible [151, 254].

For test statistics with the limiting mean and covariance structure specified by (10.35), the alpha spending function approach determines critical values in (10.43) and (10.45) using the asymptotic normality of the joint distribution of $(\widehat{T}_1, \ldots, \widehat{T}_K)$ and the information fractions at which the spending function is evaluated. Since each $\widehat{T}_j$ is asymptotically standard normal, the joint distribution is completely specified once the correlation coefficients are determined.

By (10.36), the correlation coefficients are determined by the information fractions. Therefore the critical values or boundaries are completely determined by the information fractions. These fractions serve two purposes: first, they indicate the points at which the spending function is evaluated; second, they are used to estimate the correlation coefficients.

For the log-rank test with time-to-event data, information fractions are estimated using the number of events at interim times. However, it is important to note that this estimation assumes equal censoring patterns in the two groups being compared. This assumption may be too strong in scenarios where maintaining or monitoring a treatment or intervention requires substantially more effort than managing a placebo or control group.

For interim testing with the adaptively weighted log-rank test, Yang [339] proposed using a Monte Carlo method to obtain the critical values given the spending function and interim data. This method utilizes the martingale structure [95] to simplify covariance estimation for the test statistics at different time points. Importantly, it does not require the assumption of equal censoring distributions in the two comparison groups. The R package *YPInterimTesting* is available for obtaining the interim monitoring bounds using the adaptively weighted log-rank test with the Monte Carlo method [219]. This approach can be applied more broadly to other test statistics. It provides a more robust way to determine critical values for interim analyses in time-to-event studies, particularly when there are differences in censoring patterns between groups.

Given an alpha spending function, the amount of type I error rate spent at a specific look is determined by the information fractions at that look and the previous look. For time-to-event outcomes, the information fraction at time t is estimated by the fraction of the number of events at time t relative to the targeted total number of events. If the actual number of events exceeds the targeted total, the estimated information fraction could reach or exceeds 1 at a look before the trial's end, and the total alpha would all be spent prior to trial's completion. To avoid this problem, an alternative time scale, such as the calendar time fraction [152], can be used instead of the information fraction.

For example, consider a trial planned with 2 years of recruitment and 4 years of minimum follow-up, totaling 6 years. At a look 2 years after the trial start, the calendar time fraction would be $2/6 = 1/3$. This approach ensures that the fraction will not reach 1 before the trial's conclusion.

In the calendar time fraction approach above, the fraction of $1/3$ at year 2 may seem high, as the trial has just completed its recruitment period. One could argue that the trial's average follow-up duration is 5 years, and at year 2, the average follow-up duration is 1 year. Thus the average follow-up duration fraction would provide a scale of $1/5$ for year 2. This would result in a smaller allocation of total alpha to the interim look at year 2 compared to an approach based on the calendar time fraction of $1/3$.

10.6 Stopping for Benefit vs. Stopping for Safety

When there are no particular safety concerns over the treatment, no known safety outcomes that need monitoring, or when both arms are active treatments, often a two-sided test with symmetric upper and lower boundaries for interim monitoring can be considered. However, since clinical trials are typically designed to show that a new treatment is superior to a placebo or standard treatment, a one-sided test with asymmetric upper boundary for benefit and lower boundary for safety can be used. It's also possible that safety monitoring is based on outcomes other than the primary outcome.

When separate monitoring plans for benefit and safety are used, early stopping for benefit usually requires a much higher level of evidence than early stopping for safety. With a one-sided test of benefit, it's more appropriate to use the O'Brien-Fleming type spending function or a corrected Haybittle-Peto method with nominal P-value < 0.0001 before 0.5 information fraction (or any other fraction) and < 0.001 afterwards.

The careful attention in a group sequential design to control the overall type I error rate, combined with the flexibility of the alpha spending function approach, may tempt researchers to zealously conduct frequent interim analyses. However, this is not advisable. Although the overall type I error rate is protected, conducting too many interim analyses can substantially reduce statistical power. It is good practice to avoid looking too early, too often, or too close to the end of the trial.

Some have argued that for benefit testing, 2 or 3 interim looks are sufficient and that there is little to be gained by conducting more than 4 or 5 interim analyses during a trial[239, 236, 202]. Note that a $(K-1)$th look (the second last look) closer to end of the trial not only makes little logistical sense but also results in a higher boundary for the final look compared to a scenario where the second last look is scheduled further away from the trial's conclusion.

On the other hand, having too many early looks offers little practical benefit. For example, at the information fraction of 0.20, for $\alpha = 0.025$, $\alpha_1^*(.2) = 5.39 \times 10^{-7}$. If this is where the first interim analysis occurs, then the allocated alpha is also 5.39×10^{-7} at that look, and the corresponding boundary is 4.877. It is highly unlikely that the test statistic will cross such a high boundary so early in the trial. Even if it does, the DSMB may recommend continuing the trial. This is because, in the early stages of a trial, there is often insufficient supporting evidence from other aspects of the study to justify early termination. Consequently, efficacy boundaries are typically set at an information fraction of 0.5 or later.

Although group sequential designs for efficacy or benefit monitoring are generally utilized in larger and long-term trials, safety must be monitored in all trials. A one-sided test of harm often uses a less stringent spending function such as the Pocock type or the linear function $\alpha^*(s) = \alpha s$, or a corrected Haybittle-Peto method with nominal P-value < 0.001 before 0.5 fraction and < 0.01 afterwards. Additionally, safety monitoring requires more frequent looks because, ethically, a trial must be stopped promptly if a new treatment is causing harm.

Furthermore, a significance level higher than the usual two-sided level of 0.05, such as 0.10, may be used for safety monitoring. In some cases, trials are stopped early for safety without formal stopping boundaries when ethical and safety concerns outweigh the formality of statistical analysis. Additionally, statistical stopping guidelines may not capture all potential safety issues in a trial. In such cases, the DSMB can incorporate additional safety reports and medical expertise to make a benefit-versus-harm judgment on whether to recommend early stopping for safety.

10.7 Stopping for Futility

Although clinical trials are designed to meet specified type I and II error rates (or equivalently, size and power), it may become apparent during the trial that a statistically significant result is unlikely. A futility stopping guideline helps decide whether the trial should be terminated for futility. Reviews on futility analysis can be found in Snapinn et al. [283], Lachin [145] and DeMets [59], among others.

There are two main approaches for futility analysis. The first is based on the probability of a statistically significant final result conditional on interim data. If a measure based on this conditional probability falls below a predefined threshold, the trial is stopped for futility. This approach can be further divided into stochastic curtailment, a frequentist method based on conditional power, and predictive power and predictive probability, which are partially and fully Bayesian methods.

The second approach defines group sequential futility stopping boundaries similarly to the alpha spending function approach for efficacy or safety stopping, but with the goal of stopping the trial with the conclusion that there is insufficient evidence to reject the null hypothesis.

In the frequentist conditional approach, the trial is stopped for futility if the conditional probability, calculated under the alternative hypothesis, is below a pre-specified threshold. This is called the *stochastic curtailment* approach. It can also be used for benefit testing, where the null hypothesis is rejected when the conditional power, calculated under the null hypothesis, exceeds a pre-specified threshold.

For futility analysis, the behavior of test statistics under alternative hypotheses needs to be considered. Using the notations and setup in Section 10.5.1, assume that under a sequence of local alternatives, $\left(\widehat{T}_1,\ldots,\widehat{T}_K\right)$ converges in distribution to a K-variate normal vector $\left(B(x_1),\ldots,B(x_j)\right)^{\mathrm{T}}$ whose mean and covariance are given by

$$EB(x_j) = \psi\sqrt{s_j}, \quad Cov(B(x_j), B(t_\ell)) = \sqrt{\frac{s_j}{s_\ell}}, \quad 1 \le j \le \ell \le K. \tag{10.50}$$

The parameter ψ is called the *drift parameter.* It is the asymptotic mean of $\widehat{T}_K$, or the test statistic at the trial's end, calculated under the sequence of local alternatives.

From the joint normal distribution of $B(x_j)$ and $B(x_j)$, conditional on $\widehat{T}_j$, the distribution of $\widehat{T}_K$ is approximately normal with mean

$$\psi + \sqrt{s_j}[\widehat{T}_j - \psi\sqrt{s_j}] = (1 - s_j)\psi + \sqrt{s_j}\widehat{T}_j$$

and variance $1 - s_j$. Thus for the one-sided test of benefit at significance level $\alpha/2$, where α is the significance level for a two-sided test, given $\widehat{T}_j$, the probability of rejecting the null hypothesis is

$$\begin{aligned} p_j(\psi) &= P(\widehat{T}_K > z(\alpha/2) | \widehat{T}_j) \\ &\simeq 1 - \Phi\Big(\frac{z(\alpha/2) - (1 - s_j)\psi - \sqrt{s_j}\widehat{T}_j}{\sqrt{1 - s_j}}\Big) \\ &= \Phi\Big(\frac{(1 - s_j)\psi + \sqrt{s_j}\widehat{T}_j - z(\alpha/2)}{\sqrt{1 - s_j}}\Big). \end{aligned} \tag{10.51}$$

This conditional probability $p_j(\psi)$ depends on the drift parameter ψ and the information fraction s_j, where the latter is estimated by $\widehat{s}_j$. $p_j(\psi)$ is usually calculated for specific choices of ψ.

One common choice is the value that corresponds to specifications in the trial design for hypothesis testing with a required sample size. Similarly to (10.5) and (10.12), this value of the drift parameter, denoted by ψ_D, can be shown to be $z(\beta) + z(\alpha/2)$. For the corresponding conditional power, the threshold for futility is typically 0.10 to 0.15.

Another option is to take ψ at the estimated value $\widehat{\psi}_j$ given the current data. By (10.50), this is given by $\widehat{\psi}_j = \widehat{T}_j / \sqrt{s}_j$. A third choice is $\psi = 0$, which gives the conditional probability of rejecting the null hypothesis when it is true. Usually the threshold for futility stopping is 0.20 or 0.15 for these conditional probabilities.

From (10.51), the condition $p_j(\psi) \le CP_L$ is approximated by the condition

$$\widehat{T}_j \le \frac{z(\alpha/2) + \sqrt{1 - s_j}\Phi^{-1}(CP_L) - (1 - s_j)\psi}{\sqrt{s_j}}. \tag{10.52}$$

Thus futility stopping based on the conditional power is equivalent to stopping based on a boundary for the test statistic $\widehat{T}_j$. Note that as $s_j \to 1$, condition (10.52) becomes

$$\widehat{T}_j \leq z(\alpha/2),$$

the condition of not rejecting the null hypothesis in cases where there is no interim analysis.

Let β_D be the type II error rate if no interim analysis is conducted. With futility stopping, the type II error rate exceeds β_D. However, if the stopping threshold on the conditional power is low, this inflation can be controlled. For a design that stops for futility when the conditional power, computed under the original design, is below a pre-specified value c_L, Lan et al. [153] showed that, regardless of the number of interim analyses, the type II error rate is bounded by $\beta_D/(1-c_L)$, with equality achieved if the trial is monitored continuously. For example, with $c_L = 0.15$, the type II error rate is bounded by 0.118 if $\beta_D = 0.10$ and by 0.176 if $\beta_D = 0.15$.

At the same time, futility stopping decreases the type I error rate, and methods exist to take advantage of this reduction. However, such methods are rarely used. This is because statistical boundaries are typically treated as guidelines rather than strict stopping rules, as mentioned earlier. Futility stopping often plays an even more advisory role compared to safety and efficacy stopping, which are driven by stronger ethical and scientific considerations. By adhering to the pre-specified type I error rate, trials ensure that they maintain the correct type I error rate even in scenarios where a futility boundary is crossed but the trial is not stopped for futility.

For time-to-event data, while group sequential methods have mostly focused on the log-rank test, Lin et al. [181] presented a general theory for assessing conditional power for weighted log-rank tests, with or without covariance adjustment. In particular, for the commonly considered case of a two-sample log-rank test without covariate adjustment, they shown that the conditional powers can be calculated analytically without stringent assumptions required in prior works.

In the conditional power approach above, there are various choices for the drift parameter, each representing different scenarios of treatment effect size. It may not always be clear which drift parameter should be used. In contrast, the predictive power approach averages the conditional power function using weights based on the posterior density of the treatment effect given the observed data [43, 285]. This approach can be viewed as a hybrid of frequentist and Bayesian concepts.

The predictive probability approach is fully Bayesian. In this framework, a trial's outcome is defined in terms of the posterior probability of achieving a clinically important treatment effect given both interim data and predicted values for subsequent unobserved data. The predicted values are derived from interim data and the prior distribution of the treatment effect parameter [88, 63]. If the predictive probability falls below a pre-specified threshold, stopping for futility can be considered.

For both partially and fully Bayesian approaches, it is recommended to calculate frequentist quantities such as type I and II error rates during trial design [283]. This ensures comparability with alternative designs and provides additional context for decision-making.

In the group sequential approach for futility analysis, stopping boundaries are obtained similarly to those in the alpha spending function approach for efficacy testing. The spending function used in this context is called the beta spending function and is designed to control the type II (or beta) error rate [304, 72].

10.8 Analysis of Survival Data in Trials with Staggered Entry

The interim analysis approaches outlined in the previous sections start with the basic assumptions that, asymptotically, the test statistics at various time points are jointly normal under both null and a sequence of local alternative hypotheses, with the limiting mean and covariance structure specified by (10.35) and (10.50). These assumptions are relatively straightforward to verify for continuous and dichotomous outcomes under general and mild conditions. For these types of outcomes, observations collected from time intervals $[0, x_1], \ldots, [x_{K-1}, x_K]$ are independent, and the corresponding test statistics have the independent increment property. This allows a simple multivariate analysis for problems such as obtaining critical values in (10.38) or (10.40).

For time-to-event outcomes, data collected from different time intervals in general are no longer independent. An individual contributes possibly censored observations at interim analysis times $x_1, \ldots, x_j$, which are clearly correlated. To further complicate matters, participants of a trial are typically enrolled in a staggered entry fashion rather than all at once as described in Section 2.1.

In this section, we describe the two-sample interim testing setup with staggered entry. Some related martingale and convergence results can also be found in Chapter Fifteen and Appendix B.

In the staggered entry set up, relevant variables are represented as n independent quadruplets $(\xi_i, T_i, \widetilde{C}_i, Z_i)$, $i = 1, \ldots, n$, where for the ith individual, ξ_i, T_i and $\widetilde{C}_i$ are the trial starting time (i.e., time of randomization), time to event, and time to loss to follow-up, respectively, and Z_i is the treatment assignment indicator taking value 1 for the treatment group and 0 otherwise. It is assumed that ξ_i is independent of all other variables. Given Z_i, T_i and $\widetilde{C}_i$ are assumed to be independent and the conditional cumulative hazard function of T_i is $\Lambda(s, Z_i)$, where

$$\Lambda(s, Z_i) = Z_i \Lambda_T + (1 - Z_i)\Lambda_C. \tag{10.53}$$

The survival functions corresponding to Λ_C, Λ_T, are denoted by S_C, S_T, respectively.

Let $a^+ = \max(a, 0)$ for a real number a. At calendar time x_j, $j = 1, \ldots, K$, due to loss to follow-up and the administrative censoring, the available data are $(X_{i,j}, \delta_{i,j}, Z_i)$, where

$$X_{i,j} = T_i \wedge \widetilde{C}_i \wedge (x_j - \xi_i)^+, \quad \delta_{i,j} = I(X_{i,j} = T_i), \quad i = 1, \ldots, n, \; j = 1, \ldots, K. \tag{10.54}$$

Note that in the set up here, individuals not yet in the trial are censored by 0. The censoring variables $\widetilde{C}_i \wedge (x_j - \xi_i)^+$, $i = 1, \ldots, n$, need not be identically distributed, and in particular the two treatment groups may have different censoring distributions.

Note also that we differentiate the censoring from loss to follow-up and the administrative censoring by the follow-up duration $x_j - \xi_i$ at calendar time x_j. This is necessary since joint distributions of test statistics at different interim analysis times are needed. If we are only interested in test statistics at just one time point x (i.e., there is no interim analysis), then we can combine both types of censoring into a single variable $C_i = \widetilde{C}_i \wedge (x - \xi_i)$, and all discussions on random censorship model and related topics from previous sections and chapters apply.

With data available at calendar time x_j, analogously to the at-risk processes in (2.48),define

$$K_{C,j}(t) = \sum_{Z_i=0} I(X_{i,j} \ge t), \quad K_{T,j}(t) = \sum_{Z_i=1} I(X_{i,j} \ge t), \quad K_j = K_{C,j} + K_{T,j}. \tag{10.55}$$

Then the log-rank test statistic at x_j is

$$U_j = \sum_{i=1}^{n} \int_0^\infty \left[Z_i - \frac{K_{T,j}(s)}{K_j(s)} \right] dN_{i,j}(s) = \sum_{i=1}^{n} \delta_{i,j} \left(Z_i - \frac{\sum_{m=1}^{n} Z_m I(X_{m,j} \ge X_{i,j})}{\sum_{m=1}^{n} I(X_{m,j} \ge X_{i,j})} \right), \tag{10.56}$$

where $N_{i,j}(t)$ is the number of events observed in $[0, t]$:

$$N_{i,j}(t) = \delta_{i,j} I(X_{i,j} \le t) = I\big(T_i \le \widetilde{C}_i \wedge (x_j - \xi_i)^+ \wedge t\big). \tag{10.57}$$

For the case of continuous survival distributions, from (2.53), the variance estimator of U_j is,

$$\sum_{i=1}^{n} \int_0^\infty \frac{K_{C,j}(s) K_{T,j}(s)}{K_j^2(s)} dN_{i,j}(s). \tag{10.58}$$

To perform interim analysis with the log-rank test, asymptotic joint distribution is needed for $U_1, \ldots, U_K$. Due to censoring by $\widetilde{C}_i \wedge (x_j - \xi_i)^+$ with different time points $x_1, \ldots, x_K$, from (10.56) the covariance structure may appear complex. The situation becomes even more intricate for a weighted log-rank test, which is defined similarly to U_j but with an extra factor $Q_j(s)$ inserted inside the integral in (10.56).

Early literature conjectured that both the log-rank test and certain weighted log-rank tests had the limiting covariance structure specified in (10.35) and

(10.50). However, subsequent rigorous analysis confirmed this conjecture for the log-rank test while disproving it for weighted log-rank tests.

Early works in the literature include Tsiatis [301], Sellke and Siegmund [276], and Slud [281], all of which focused on the asymptotic properties under the null hypothesis. More complete and general results were obtained by Gu and Lai [107], Bilias, Gu and Ying [22], and Lin, Yao and Ying [181]. The latter considered a broad class of weighted log-rank type statistics that includes two-sample weighted log-rank statistics and the partial likelihood score statistic with covariate adjustment under the proportional hazards model. They derived asymptotic joint distributions for these statistics, under both the null hypothesis and a sequence of local alternatives.

Based on these works, the asymptotic distribution structure specified by (10.35) and (10.50) holds for the log-rank type statistics, but not for the weighted log-rank type statistics in general. However, asymptotic normality of the joint distribution is still valid. Below, we give an outline of the proof that the asymptotic joint distribution of log-rank test statistics at different time points has the mean and covariance structure for specified by (10.35) and (10.50).

Let

$$\begin{aligned} M_{i,j}(t) &= N_{i,j}(t) - \int_0^t I(X_{i,j} \geq s)\, d\Lambda(s; Z_i), \\ &\qquad x \geq 0, \quad i = 1, \ldots, n, \quad j = 1, \ldots, K. \end{aligned} \tag{10.59}$$

From Section B.12 in Appendix B, $M_{i,j}$ is a martingale. It is the martingale associated with the ith individual and data at time x_j for the two-sample problem. Using $M_{i,j}$, we have the decomposition

$$U_j = \mathcal{M}_j(\infty) + \mu_j, \tag{10.60}$$

where

$$\begin{aligned} \mathcal{M}_j(t) &= \sum_{i=1}^n \int_0^t \left[Z_i - \frac{K_{T,j}(s)}{K_j(s)} \right] dM_{i,j}(s), \; t \geq 0, \\ \mu_j &= \int_0^\infty \frac{K_{C,j}(s) K_{T,j}(s)}{K_j(s)} \left[d\Lambda_T(s) - d\Lambda_C(s) \right]. \end{aligned} \tag{10.61}$$

From (10.61) and (B.75), it can be shown [82, Theorem 2.5.4] that, for $1 \leq j \leq \ell \leq K$,

$$E\mathcal{M}_j(\infty) = 0, \tag{10.62}$$

$$E\mathcal{M}_j(\infty)\mathcal{M}_\ell(\infty) = \int_0^\infty E\frac{K_{C,j}(s)K_{C,\ell}(s)}{K_j(s)K_\ell(s)}K_{T,j}(s)d\Lambda_T(s) \tag{10.63}$$

$$+\int_0^\infty E\frac{K_{T,j}(s)K_{T,\ell}(s)}{K_j(s)K_\ell(s)}K_{C,j}(s)d\Lambda_C(s). \tag{10.64}$$

Thus under the null hypothesis $H_0 : \Lambda_T = \Lambda_C = \Lambda_0$,

$$E\mathcal{M}_j(\infty)\mathcal{M}_\ell(\infty) = \int_0^\infty E\frac{K_{C,j}(s)K_{T,j}(s)}{K_j(s)K_\ell(s)}[K_{C,\ell}(s)+K_{T,\ell}(s)]d\Lambda_0(s)$$

$$= \int_0^\infty E\frac{K_{C,j}(s)K_{T,j}(s)}{K_j(s)}d\Lambda_0(s). \tag{10.65}$$

It is important to observe that in (10.64), the factors involving quantities at the ℓth look cancel out. As a result, $E\mathcal{M}_j(\infty)\mathcal{M}_\ell(\infty)$ depends only on Λ_0 and data at the jth look. Using the variance estimator in (10.58), the log-rank test statistic U_j can be standardized. Denote the resulting test statistic by W_j, $j = 1,\ldots,K$. Under certain regularity conditions, it can be shown that under H_0, the variance estimator in (10.58) converges to a positive limit σ_j^2, and the vector of test statistics $(W_1,\ldots,W_K)$ converges in distribution to a K- variate normal vector $(A_1,\ldots,A_K)$ with

$$EA_j = 0,\ 1 \le j \le K,\quad Cov(A_j, A_\ell) = \sigma_j^2,\quad 1 \le j \le \ell \le K. \tag{10.66}$$

Convergence results under the local alternatives can also be obtained. With these results, it can be shown that for the log-rank test, the asymptotic distribution has the properties specified in (10.35) and (10.50).

10.9 Exercises and Complements

10.1 Consider the setting in Section 10.2 that yields formula (10.3). Suppose $\sigma = 1$, $\mu_1 = -0.1$, $\alpha = 0.05$, and $n = 400$. Obtain $P\big(\sqrt{n}\bar{X}_n/\sigma > z(\alpha/2)\big|H_{a1}\big)$.

10.2 Derive a sample size formula analogous to (10.3) for the case where the alternative hypothesis specifies that $\mu = \mu_2$ with $\mu_2 > 0$.

10.3 (a) Fill the details of obtaining (10.5) from (10.4).

(b) Fill the details of obtaining (10.6).

10.4 (a) Verify that, for the log-rank test, when $\Gamma_C = \Gamma_T = \Gamma$, the quantities σ^2 and ξ in (10.12) both simplify to

$$\int_0^\infty p_C p_T \Gamma(t) dF_0(t).$$

(b) Use (a) to verify (10.17) and (10.18).

10.5 Verify the results in Table 10.1.

10.6 Consider the hypothesis testing problem

$$H_0 : \lambda_T = \lambda_C = \lambda_0 \quad vs.$$

$$H_{an} : \lambda_C = \lambda_0, \ \ \lambda_T(t) = \big[1 + \exp(\theta_n) I(t \geq a)\big]\lambda_0(t),$$

where $a > 0$ is a known fixed constant. Assume that

$$\lim \sqrt{n}\theta_n = \nu,$$

for a fixed ν. Consider the weighted log-rank test statistic U_{Φ_0} with

$$\Phi_0(t) = I(t \geq a).$$

(a) Use an argument similar to that for (10.8) through (10.15) to show that for U_{Φ_0}, the result analogous to (10.16) is

$$\int_a^\infty p_C p_T \Gamma(t) dF_0(t).$$

(b) Let

$$D_{na} = \sum_{i \leq n_1, X_i \geq a} \delta_i + \sum_{i > n_1, X_i \geq a} \delta_i,$$

the number of events greater than or equal to a. Modify (10.17) through (10.19) to show that

$$D_{na} \simeq \frac{1}{p_C p_T} \cdot \Big(\frac{z(\beta) + z(\alpha/2)}{\log(h)}\Big)^2. \tag{10.67}$$

10.7 Consider the problem of comparing two proportions. Let p_j and $\widehat{p}_j$ be the population and sample proportions, respectively, $j = 1, 2$. For the hypothesis

$$H_0 : p_2 = p_1,$$

the standardized test statistic is

$$\widehat{T} = \frac{\widehat{p}_2 - \widehat{p}_1}{\sqrt{(\frac{1}{n_1} + \frac{1}{n_2}) p^*(1 - p^*)}},$$

where n_j is the sample size from the jth population, $j = 1, 2$, and p^* is the pooled estimator of the common proportion under the null. Suppose $n_1 = n_2 = n/2$, where n is the size of the pooled sample. Define a sequence of local alternatives

$$H_{an} : p_2 - p_1 = \Delta_n$$

where Δ_n converges to 0 at the $n^{-1/2}$ rate: $\lim \sqrt{n}\Delta_n = \nu$ for a fixed $\nu < 0$. It can be shown that, under H_{an}, $\widehat{T}$ converges in distribution to

$$N\Big(\frac{\nu}{2\sqrt{p_0(1-p_0)}}, 1\Big)$$

where p_0 is the common value of p_1 and p_2 under H_0.

(a) Use an argument analogous to (10.5) to show that

$$-\frac{\nu}{2\sqrt{p_0(1-p_0)}} = z(\beta) + z(\alpha/2).$$

(b) Use an argument analogous to (10.6) to show that

$$n \approx 4\bar{p}(1-\bar{p})\Big(\frac{z(\beta)+z(\alpha/2)}{p_2 - p_1}\Big)^2,$$

where $\bar{p} = (p_1 + p_2)/2$.

10.8 Consider the problem of comparing two survival probabilities. Let $F_j(t)$ and $\widehat{F}_j(t)$ be the CDF and the Kaplan-Meier estimator for the two groups, respectively, $j = 1,2$. Let a be a given fixed time point. Suppose the control and treatment groups each has sample size $n/2$, where n is the total sample size. Let $\widehat{S}_j = 1 - \widehat{F}_j$, $j = 1,2$ and denote the Kaplan-Meier estimators of the censoring distribution survival functions of the two groups by $\widehat{S}_{C1}$ and $\widehat{S}_{C2}$. For the hypothesis

$$H_0 : F_2(a) = F_1(a),$$

the standardized test statistic is

$$\widehat{T} = \sqrt{\frac{n}{2}} \frac{\widehat{F}_2(a) - \widehat{F}_1(a)}{\sqrt{\widehat{v}}},$$

where

$$\widehat{v} = \widehat{S}_1^2(a)\int_0^a \frac{d\widehat{F}_1(t)}{\widehat{S}_{C1}(t)\widehat{S}_1^2(t)} + \widehat{S}_2^2(a)\int_0^a \frac{d\widehat{F}_2(t)}{\widehat{S}_{C2}(t)\widehat{S}_2^2(t)}.$$

Define a sequence of local alternatives

$$H_{an} : F_2(a) - F_1(a) = \Delta_n$$

where Δ_n converges to 0 at the $n^{-1/2}$ rate: $\lim \sqrt{n}\Delta_n = \nu$ for a fixed $\nu < 0$. It can be shown that, under H_{an}, $\widehat{T}$ converges in distribution to

$$N\Big(\frac{\nu}{\sqrt{2\sigma}}, 1\Big),$$

where σ is the limit of $\widehat{v}$.

(a) Use an argument analogous to (10.5) to show that

$$-\frac{\nu}{\sqrt{2}\sigma} = z(\beta) + z(\alpha/2).$$

(b) Use an argument analogous to (10.6) to show that

$$n \approx 2\hat{\sigma}^2 \Big(\frac{z(\beta) + z(\alpha/2)}{F_2(a) - F_1(a)}\Big)^2,$$

where $\hat{\sigma}$ is an estimator of σ.

10.9 Use an argument analogous to that for (10.15) to fill the details for obtaining (10.20).

10.10 (a) Verify that (10.27) follows from (10.24) through (10.26).

(b) Use (10.28) to derive (10.29).

10.11 Verify the expression for κ_0 in Example 10.3.

10.12 Verify the expression for κ_0 in Example 10.4.

10.13 Consider the setup for testing (10.21) with

$$\lambda_\theta(t) = e^\theta [1 + \Lambda_0(t)]^{e^\theta - 1} \lambda_0(t).$$

Calculate $\kappa_0(t)$ in (10.31) to show that the optimal weight is

$$1 + \log[1 + \Lambda_0(t)].$$

10.14 For model (10.33), fill out the details in deriving formula (10.34).

10.15 Verify that $\pm u_1, \cdots, \pm u_K$, where $u_1, \cdots, u_K$ are the boundaries for the one-sided test for benefit, form the upper and lower boundaries of a conservative two-sided test. That is, show that

$$P_0\Big(\bigcup_{j=1}^{K} \{\widehat{T}_j \notin [-u_j, u_j]\}\Big) \le \alpha.$$

10.16 Use the bivariate normality specified in (10.50) for $\widehat{T}_j$ and $\widehat{T}_K$, where $j < K$, to obtain the conditional distribution of $\widehat{T}_K$ given $\widehat{T}_j$ and verify (10.51).

10.17 Use (10.63) and algebraic simplification to verify (10.64).

11

Counting Processes and Martingales

11.1 Reformulation of the Hazard Function in Terms of the Observed Counting Process

To motivate the concepts of martingales and intensity models to be introduced later in this chapter, it helps to reformulate the hazard function in terms of the associated counting process. Suppose data are obtained from the random censorship model with an absolutely continuous survival distribution. Let the PDF, CDF, survival function, hazard function, and cumulative hazard function be denoted by f, F, S, λ, and Λ, respectively.

Fix one i that is between 1 and n. Let $S_{Ci}(t)$ be the survival function of C_i. Suppose that the right limit f_+ of f exists. Then

$$\lim_{x \downarrow t} S_{Ci-}(x) f(x) = S_{Ci}(t) f_+(t). \tag{11.1}$$

From this and the law of iterated expectations (B.6) in Appendix B,

$$\begin{aligned}
& P\big(t < T_i \le t+h, T_i \le C_i \big| T_i \wedge C_i > t\big) \\
= & \frac{P\big(t < T_i \le t+h, T_i \le C_i\big)}{P\big(T_i > t, C_i > t\big)} \\
= & \frac{E\big[I(t < T_i \le t+h) S_{Ci-}(T_i)\big]}{P\big(T_i > t\big) P\big(C_i > t\big)} \\
= & \frac{\int_{(t,t+h]} S_{Ci-}(x) f(x) dx}{S_{Ci}(t) S(t)} \\
\approx & \frac{S_{Ci}(t) f_+(t) h}{S_{Ci}(t) S(t)} = \lambda_+(t) h,
\end{aligned} \tag{11.2}$$

DOI: 10.1201/9780429324437-11

where λ_+ is the right limit of λ. It follows that

$$\lim_{h\downarrow 0} P\big(t < T_i \leq t+h, T_i \leq C_i \big| T_i > t, C_i > t\big)/h = \lambda_+(t), \tag{11.3}$$

when $P(T_i \wedge C_i > t) > 0$.

In terms of the counting process, the conditional probability $P\big(t < T_i \leq t + h, T_i \leq C_i \big| T_i \wedge C_i > t\big)$ can be re-written as

$$P\big(N_i \text{ jumps in } (t, t+h] \big| Y_{i+}(t) = 1\big) = P\big(\Delta_h N_i(t) = 1 \big| Y_{i+}(t) = 1\big),$$

where $Y_{i+}(t)$ is the right limit of $Y_i(t)$: $Y_{i+}(t) = I(X_i > t) = I(T_i \wedge C_i > t)$, and $\Delta_h \psi(t) = \psi(t+h) - \psi(t)$ for any function ψ. Thus (11.3) can be re-written as

$$\lambda_+(t) = \lim_{h\downarrow 0} P\big(\Delta_h N_i(t) = 1 \big| Y_{i+}(t) = 1\big)/h. \tag{11.4}$$

11.2 Martingales

In the previous section, for the absolutely continuous case, the hazard function was reformulated as a conditional probability of the observed counting process. The derivation helps motivate a particularly important class of stochastic processes called martingales. Here, an informal heuristic argument will be used to introduce the concept, with exact specifications delegated to Appendix B. Again the random censorship model with absolutely continuous survival distribution is assumed in the heuristic development.

Let $\mathscr{F}_t$ be the collection of information available up to time t on event and censoring for all n individuals. $\mathscr{F}_t$ is a collection of sets in the probability space known as a σ-algebra, a formal definition of which is given in Section A.2 of Appendix A. As time progresses, more information is available, so $\mathscr{F}_s \subset \mathscr{F}_t$ for $s < t$. Under the censored data setup, all information on event and censoring on $[0, t]$ for the ith individual is contained in the cadlag processes $N_i(s)$ and $Y_{i+}(s)$, $0 \leq s \leq t$. In probability language, these processes generate the σ-algebra $\mathscr{F}_t$.

Given $\mathscr{F}_t$, $\Delta_h N_i(t) = 0$ if $Y_{i+}(t) = 0$ (either event or censoring has occurred in $[0, t]$); and if $Y_i(t+) = 1$, $\Delta_h N_i(t) = 1$ with probability

$$\frac{P\big(t < T_i \leq t+h, T_i \leq C_i\big)}{P\big(T_i > t, C_i > t\big)}.$$

Since $\Delta_h N_i(t)$ takes values 0 or 1 only,

$$E\big(\Delta_h N_i(t) \big| \mathscr{F}_t\big) = E\big(\Delta_h N_i(t) \big| Y_{i+}(t)\big) = Y_{i+}(t) \frac{P\big(t < T_i \leq t+h, T_i \leq C_i\big)}{P\big(T_i > t, C_i > t\big)}. \tag{11.5}$$

Given $\mathscr{F}_t$, $Y_{i+}(t)$ is determined. From (11.3) and (11.5) it follows that

$$E\big(\Delta_h N_i(t) - Y_{i+}(t)\lambda_+(t)h \big| \mathscr{F}_t\big) = h\varepsilon \tag{11.6}$$

where ε tends to 0 as $h \downarrow 0$.

Because Y_i is caglad and f_+ exists, similarly to (11.1),

$$\lim_{h\downarrow 0} \int_{(t,t+h]} Y_i(s)\lambda(s)ds/h = Y_{i+}(t)\lambda_+(t). \tag{11.7}$$

If λ is bounded on an interval $[0,\tau]$ and $t < \tau$, then by the dominated convergence theorem (B.1) of Appendix B,

$$\lim_{h\downarrow 0} E\Big(\int_{(t,t+h]} Y_i(s)\lambda(s)ds/h \big| \mathscr{F}_t\Big) = E\big(Y_{i+}(t)\lambda_+(t)\big|\mathscr{F}_t\big) = Y_{i+}(t)\lambda_+(t). \tag{11.8}$$

From (11.6) and (11.8), it follows that

$$E\Big(\Delta_h N_i(t) - \int_t^{t+h} Y_i(s)\lambda(s)ds \big| \mathscr{F}_t\Big) = h\varepsilon, \tag{11.9}$$

where ε tends to 0 as $h \downarrow 0$.

Heuristically, letting $h \downarrow 0$ in (11.9) yields

$$E\Big(\mathfrak{D}N_i(t) - \mathfrak{D}\int_0^t Y_i(s)\lambda(s)ds \big| \mathscr{F}_t\Big) = 0, \tag{11.10}$$

where $\mathfrak{D}G$ denotes the differential of the Riemann-Stieltjes integral with respect to an increasing cadlag function G. An overview of the Riemann-Stieltjes integral is given in Section A.5 of Appendix A. Note that the notation $\mathfrak{D}G$ is used instead of dG, as the latter denotes the Lebesgue-Stieltjes differential. From (A.17) in Appendix A, if G is either absolutely continuous or discrete, and f satisfies certain regularity conditions, the Riemann-Stieltjes integrals coincide with Lebesgue-Stieltjes integrals:

$$\int_0^t f\mathfrak{D}G = \int_0^t f dG.$$

The Riemann-Stieltjes integral is similar to the Riemann integral, as both use Riemann sums with partitions of intervals over which the functions are defined. This approach is often referred to as the x-axis approach. In contrast, the measure theory approach for Lebesgue and Lebesgue-Stieltjes integrals is sometimes called the y-axis approach because it focuses on the range rather than the domain of a function. Although the y-axis approach is more advanced and general, the x-axis approach is useful for heuristic arguments and can provide valuable insights.

From (11.10), it appears plausible that the process $N_i(t) - \int_0^t Y_i(s)\lambda(s)ds$ may have conditional mean 0 in some sense. However, since t appears in both the differential and the conditioning σ-algebra, it is challenging to derive a precise interpretation from (11.10). Below, we present a heuristic derivation of an important property of $N_i(t) - \int_0^t Y_i(s)\lambda(s)ds$ using properties of conditional expectation.

For fixed $0 \le s < t$, let $s = s_0 < s_1 < \cdots < s_k = t$ be a partition of the interval $[s, t]$ with equally paced points so that each interval $[s_{j-1}, s_j]$ has length $h = (t-s)/k$, and let $\mathscr{F}_j = \mathscr{F}_{s_{j-1}}$, $j = 1, \ldots, k$. Then

$$
\begin{aligned}
E\big(N_i(t) - N_i(s)\big|\mathscr{F}_s\big) &= \sum_{j=1}^{k} E\big(N_i(s_j) - N_i(s_{j-1})\big|\mathscr{F}_s\big) \\
&= \sum_{j=1}^{k} E\big[E\big(N_i(s_j) - N_i(s_{j-1})\big|\mathscr{F}_j\big)\big|\mathscr{F}_s\big] \\
&= \sum_{j=1}^{k} E\big[E\big(\int_{s_{j-1}}^{s_j} Y_i(x)\lambda(x)dx\big|\mathscr{F}_j\big)\big|\mathscr{F}_s\big] + \sum_{j=1}^{k} E\big(h\varepsilon_j\big|\mathscr{F}_s\big) \\
&= \sum_{j=1}^{k} E\big(\int_{s_{j-1}}^{s_j} Y_i(x)\lambda(x)dx\big|\mathscr{F}_s\big) + \sum_{j=1}^{k} E\big(h\varepsilon_j\big|\mathscr{F}_s\big) \\
&= E\big(\int_{s}^{t} Y_i(s)\lambda(s)ds\big|\mathscr{F}_s\big) + \frac{t-s}{k}\sum_{j=1}^{k} E\big(\varepsilon_j\big|\mathscr{F}_s\big), \qquad (11.11)
\end{aligned}
$$

where each ε_j tends to 0 as $h \downarrow 0$ by (11.9), and where the law of iterated expectations (B.4) in Appendix B has been used in obtaining the second and fourth lines. If ε_j, $j = 1, \ldots, k$ tend to 0 uniformly in j as $h \downarrow 0$, then taking limit as $h \downarrow 0$ in (11.11) yields

$$
E\big(N_i(t) - N_i(s)\big|\mathscr{F}_s\big) = E\big(\int_{s}^{t} Y_i(s)\lambda(s)ds\big|\mathscr{F}_s\big). \qquad (11.12)
$$

It is possible to modify the argument leading to the above assertion and rigorously justify it, starting with using partitions with dyadic numbers in $[s, t]$ so that a sequence of nested σ-algebras can be obtained. However, surprisingly, it turns out that the assertion can be proved directly with relatively straightforward calculation of conditional expectations. Moreover, the proof is valid under broader and weaker conditions.

For observations (X_i, δ_i) with $X_i = T_i \wedge C_i$, $\delta_i = I(T_i \le C_i), 1 \le i \le n$, assume that T_i's are i.i.d. with cumulative hazard function Λ that is not necessarily absolutely continuous. There is no assumption of independence between T_i and C_i. Define

$$
M_i(t) = N_i(t) - A_i(t), \quad \text{where } A_i(t) = \int_0^t Y_i(s)d\Lambda(s), \ t \ge 0. \qquad (11.13)
$$

Note that $M_i(t)$ is determined given $\mathscr{F}_t$, for any $t \geq 0$. Similarly to (11.5),

$$E\big(N_i(t) - N_i(s)\big|\mathscr{F}_s\big) = Y_{i+}(s)\frac{P\big(s < T_i \leq t, T_i \leq C_i\big)}{P\big(T_i > s, C_i > s\big)}. \tag{11.14}$$

Note that the argument for (11.5) and (11.14) do not assume the random censorship model and only uses the basic censored data structure and the counting process definitions.

As for A_i,

$$E\big(A_i(t) - A_i(s)\big|\mathscr{F}_s\big) = E\Big(\int_{(s,t]} Y_i(x)d\Lambda(x)\big|\mathscr{F}_s\Big) = \int_{(s,t]} E\big(Y_i(x)\big|\mathscr{F}_s\big)d\Lambda(x).$$

For fixed $x \in (s,t]$, given $\mathscr{F}_s$, $Y_i(x) = 0$ if $Y_{i+}(s) = 0$; and if $Y_{i+}(s) = 1$, $Y_i(x) = 1$ with probability

$$P(T_i \geq x, C_i \geq x\big|T_i \wedge C_i > s) = \frac{P(T_i \wedge C_i \geq x)}{P(T_i \wedge C_i > s)}.$$

It follows that

$$E\big(Y_i(x)\big|\mathscr{F}_s\big) = Y_{i+}(s)\frac{P(T_i \wedge C_i \geq x)}{P(T_i \wedge C_i > s)},$$

and

$$E\big(A_i(t) - A_i(s)\big|\mathscr{F}_s\big) = \int_{(s,t]} Y_{i+}(s)\frac{P(T_i \wedge C_i \geq x)}{P(T_i \wedge C_i > s)}d\Lambda(x). \tag{11.15}$$

Thus

$$E\big(N_i(t) - N_i(s)\big|\mathscr{F}_s\big) = E\big(A_i(t) - A_i(s)\big|\mathscr{F}_s\big)$$

if and only if

$$P(s < T_i \leq t, T_i \leq C_i) = \int_{(s,t]} P(T_i \wedge C_i \geq x)d\Lambda(x),$$

on $\{X_i > s\}$. This holds for any $s < t$ on $\{X_i > s\}$ if and only if

$$\frac{dP(T_i \leq x, T_i \leq C_i)}{P(T_i \wedge C_i \geq x)} = d\Lambda(x), \tag{11.16}$$

for x with $P(T_i \wedge C_i \geq x) > 0$. This is exactly the independent censoring condition (2.39).

Under condition (11.16), for M_i defined in (11.13),

$$E\big(M_i(t)\big|\mathscr{F}_s\big) = M_i(s), \quad \text{for any } 0 \leq s < t. \tag{11.17}$$

A process which has the conditional expectation property (11.17) is called a martingale. The exact definition involves a list of technical preliminaries that are given in Section B.4 of Appendix B.

Now, under the random censorship model, by the assumed independence between T_i and C_i, $P(T_i \wedge C_i \geq x) = S_-(x)S_{Ci-}(x)$ and

$$P(T_i \leq t, T_i \leq C_i) = \int_{(0,t]} S_{Ci-}(x)dF(x).$$

It follows that
$$\frac{dP(T_i \leq x, T_i \leq C_i)}{P(T_i \wedge C_i \geq x)} = \frac{S_{Ci-}(x)dF(x)}{S_-(x)S_{Ci-}(x)} = d\Lambda(x),$$

for x with $P(T_i \wedge C_i \geq x) > 0$. Thus the random censorship model satisfies (11.16), and the martingale representation applies.

For type II censoring, the observations are (X_i, δ_i), $1 \leq i \leq n$ where $X_i = T_i \wedge C_i$, $\delta_i = I(T_i \leq C_i)$, and $C_i = T_{(k)}, 1 \leq i \leq n$, with $T_{(k)}$ the kth order statistic for a pre-determined k. Assume that the event times $T_i, 1 \leq i \leq n$ are independent and have a common hazard function $\lambda(t)$. It can be shown that the independent censoring condition (11.16) is satisfied.

For the random censorship model with absolutely continuous survival distribution, the martingale condition (11.17) can be directly verified as shown above. This might make the heuristic argument starting from (11.2) seem unnecessary. However, that argument serves several important purposes. It gives rise to the conjecture that (11.17) is true with the function $A_i(t)$ specified in (11.13). Much of the argument utilizes conditional expectation properties and conditioning reasoning, which are very important and useful for survival analysis in general. Derivations such as those from (11.2) to (11.11) offer opportunities for readers to become familiar with conditional expectation properties and how they are applied.

From the definition, M_i is drift-less. Assume that $EM_i^2(t) < \infty$ for any t. Then

$$\begin{aligned} E[(M_i(t) - M_i(s))M_i(s)] &= EE[(M_i(t) - M_i(s))M_i(s)|\mathscr{F}_s] \\ &= E\{M_i(s)E[(M_i(t) - M_i(s))|\mathscr{F}_s]\} \\ &= 0, \quad 0 \leq s < t. \end{aligned} \tag{11.18}$$

That is, M_i has uncorrelated increments.

Using the martingale $M_i(t)$, $N_i(t)$ can be re-written as

$$N_i(t) = M_i(t) + \int_0^t Y_i(s)d\Lambda_i(s). \tag{11.19}$$

It turns out that such a decomposition using a martingale is possible more generally. For a process Q and a family of increasing σ-algebras $\{\mathscr{G}_t\}$, Q is said to be adapted to $\{\mathscr{G}_t\}$, or to $\mathscr{G}_t$ for short, when $Q(t)$ is measurable with respect to $\mathscr{G}_t$ for each t. For a nonnegative $\mathscr{G}_t$-adapted process $Q(t)$ such that $EQ(t) < \infty$ for any t, if

$$E[Q(t)|\mathscr{G}_s] \geq Q(s), \quad 0 \leq s \leq t, \tag{11.20}$$

then there exists a martingale M such that

$$Q(t) = M(t) + A(t), \tag{11.21}$$

where for any t, $A(t)$ $EA(t) < \infty$ and $A(t)$ is predictable with respect to $\mathcal{G}_t$. $A(t)$ is called the compensator of Q. The decomposition (11.21) is unique if it is required that $A(0) = 0$ $a.s.$

Loosely speaking, $A(t)$ being predictable with respect to $\mathcal{G}_t$ means that $A(t)$ is determined given $\mathcal{G}_s$ for $s < t$. In particular, if a process is $\mathcal{G}_t$ -adapted and left continuous, then the process is predictable. Thus if the at-risk process Y_i is adapted to $\mathcal{G}_t$, then it is predictable (with respect to $\mathcal{G}_t$). The process $\int_0^t Y_i(s)d\Lambda(s)$ is also predictable. Note that N_i satisfies (11.20) since $N_i(t) \geq N_i(s)$ when $0 \leq s < t$. Also, $EN_i(t) \leq 1 < \infty$.

The decomposition of Q as the sum of a martingale and a predictable process is known as the Doob-Meyer decomposition. Details and technical assumptions needed for this decomposition are given in (B.12) and (B.13) of Appendix B.

For the martingale $M(t)$ in (11.21), we have

$$M(t) = Q(t) - A(t).$$

From (B.10) in Appendix B,

$$E\big[M(t)\big|\mathcal{G}_{t-}\big] = M_-(t),$$

where $M_-(t)$ is the left limit of $M(t)$ and $\mathcal{G}_{t-}$ is, loosely speaking, the σ-algebra generated by information in $\mathcal{G}_s$ for all $s < t$. Informally, the result can be re-written as

$$E\big[dM(t)\big|\mathcal{G}_{t-}\big] = 0. \tag{11.22}$$

That is, the conditional mean of the differential $dM(t)$ given $\mathcal{G}_{t-}$ is zero. Condition (11.22) can be used as an informal and compact way of stating that $M(t)$ is a martingale with respect to $\{\mathcal{G}_t\}$.

Since $dM(t) = dQ(t) - dA(t)$, from (11.22) and the property that a $\mathcal{G}_t$-predictable process is $\mathcal{G}_{t-}$-measurable,

$$E\big[dQ(t)\big|\mathcal{G}_{t-}\big] = dA(t). \tag{11.23}$$

This informal expression is a simple way to state that $A(t)$ is the compensator of $Q(t)$.

When the compensator $A(t)$ is absolutely continuous, it can be written as

$$A(t) = \int_0^t a(s)ds, \tag{11.24}$$

for a predictable process $a(t)$. The latter is called the intensity process of Q. The argument prior to (11.17) shows that for the random censorship model, the compensator of the counting process N_i is $A_i(t) = \int_0^t Y_i(s)d\Lambda(s)$, and the intensity process of N_i is $Y_i(t)\lambda(s)$ when Λ is absolutely continuous with hazard function $\lambda(t)$.

11.3 Variation Processes and Martingale Integrals

For the martingale in (11.21), if $EM^2(t) < \infty$ for any t, then by the uncorrelated increments property,

$$\begin{aligned} E[M^2(t)|\mathscr{F}_s] &= E\{[M(t) - M(s)]^2|\mathscr{F}_s\} + E[M^2(s)|\mathscr{F}_s] \\ &\geq E[M^2(s)|\mathscr{F}_s]. \end{aligned}$$

Thus $M^2(t)$ satisfies (11.20) and the Doob-Meyer decomposition applies. Let $\langle M, M\rangle$ be the compensator of M^2, then $M^2(t) - \langle M, M\rangle(t)$ is a martingale. $\langle M, M\rangle$ is called the *variation process of* M.

For a heuristic argument to determine $\langle M, M\rangle(t)$, we have

$$\begin{aligned} dM^2(t) &= M^2(t) - M_-^2(t) \\ &= [M_-(t) + dM(t)]^2 - M_-^2(t) \\ &= [dM(t)]^2 - 2M_-(t)dM(t). \end{aligned}$$

From (11.23), predictability of $M_-(t)$ and (11.22), it follows that

$$\begin{aligned} d\langle M, M\rangle(t) &= E[dM^2(t)|\mathscr{G}_{t-}] \\ &= E\{\{[dM(t)]^2 - 2M_-(t)dM(t)\}|\mathscr{G}_{t-}\} \\ &= E\{[dM(t)]^2|\mathscr{G}_{t-}\} \\ &= Var\{[dM(t)]|\mathscr{G}_{t-}\}, \end{aligned} \tag{11.25}$$

where (11.22) has been used to obtain the third equality. Thus the differential of $\langle M, M\rangle(t)$ is the conditional variance of $dM(t)$ given $\mathscr{G}_{t-}$.

In particular, when $Q(t)$ is a counting process, $dQ(t)$ is a Bernoulli variable. By (11.23), conditional on $\mathscr{G}_{t-}$, $dQ(t)$ has mean $dA(t)$ and variance $[1 - dA(t)]dA(t)$.

Thus from (11.25),

$$d\langle M,M\rangle(t) = Var\Big\{\big[dQ(t)-dA(t)\big]\big|\mathcal{G}_{t-}\Big\} = [1-dA(t)]dA(t). \quad (11.26)$$

This suggests that, when $A(t)$ is absolutely continuous, $\langle M,M\rangle(t) = A(t)$, which turns out to be true. Precise statements are given in Section B.8 of Appendix B, for either continuous or discontinuous compensators.

More generally, for two martingales M_1 and M_2, if $EM_j^2(t) < \infty$, $j = 1,2$, the product M_1M_2 has a compensator and it is denoted by $\langle M_1, M_2\rangle$. That is, $M_1(t)M_2(t) - \langle M_1, M_2\rangle(t)$ is a martingale. $\langle M_1, M_2\rangle$ is called the covariation process of M_1 and M_2.

Often, random quantities of interest can be written as integrals with respect to the process $Q(t)$. One of the most important results from the martingale theory is that if Q has the Doob-Meyer decomposition $Q = M+A$ and H is predictable, then

$$X(t) = \int_0^t H(s)dM(s) \text{ is a martingale with compensator } \int_0^t H(s)dA(s) \quad (11.27)$$

and

$$\langle X,X\rangle(t) = \int_0^t H^2(s)d\langle M\rangle(s), \quad (11.28)$$

assuming that proper integrability conditions hold. Moreover, if M_1 and M_2 are martingales and H_1, H_2 predictable, and X_1, X_2 are defined analogously to X in (11.27), then

$$\langle X_1, X_2\rangle(t) = \int_0^t H_1(s)H_2(s)d\langle M_1, M_2\rangle(s). \quad (11.29)$$

Precise statements are given in Section B.7 of Appendix B, These properties can be used to derive variance and covariance formulas in survival analysis where alternative methods can be quite messy.

To help understand the results (11.27)–(11.29), again the informal expressions (11.22), (11.23) and (11.25) can be used. By the definition of $X(t)$ and predictability of $H(t)$, we have

$$E\big[dX(t)\big|\mathcal{G}_{t-}\big] = E\big[H(t)dM(t)\big|\mathcal{G}_{t-}\big] = H(t)E\big[dM(t)\big|\mathcal{G}_{t-}\big] = 0. \quad (11.30)$$

This suggests that $X(t)$ is a martingale. Moreover, from (11.30),

$$\begin{aligned} E\big[H(t)dQ(t)\big|\mathscr{G}_{t-}\big] &= E\big[H(t)dA(t)\big|\mathscr{G}_{t-}\big] \\ &= H(t)dA(t), \end{aligned}$$

where the last equality follows from the predictability of $H(t)$ and $dA(t)$. This suggests that the compensator of $\int_0^t H(s)dQ(s)$ is $\int_0^t H(s)dA(s)$. Furthermore, by (11.25) and predictability of $H(t)$,

$$\begin{aligned} d\langle X,X\rangle(t) &= Var\Big\{[dX(t)]\big|\mathscr{G}_{t-}\Big\} \\ &= Var\Big\{[H(t)dM(t)]\big|\mathscr{G}_{t-}\Big\} \\ &= H^2(t)Var\Big\{[dM(t)]\big|\mathscr{G}_{t-}\Big\} \\ &= H^2(t)d\langle M,M\rangle(t). \end{aligned} \tag{11.31}$$

This suggests that the variation process of $X(t)$ is $\int_0^t H^2(s)dA(s)$.

Approximations (11.6) and (11.8) are established for the random censorship model with absolutely continuous survival distribution. This setting is most widely used in censored data analysis, and the approximations demonstrate the usual continuity argument or the x-axis approach.

The informal expressions (11.22) and (11.23) offer a more compact way to heuristically derive the results (11.25) through (11.31). However, rigorous proofs for more general situations often require the measure theory or y-axis approach. For example, to establish (11.27), the standard approach is to first verify it for simple functions such as the step functions with appropriate measurability properties, and then to establish the general result by passage to the limit, as demonstrated in Fleming and Harrington [82].

For linear combinations

$$X_\ell(t) = \sum_{i=1}^{n}\int_0^t H_{i,\ell}(s)dM_i(s),\ 1 \le i \le n,\ \ell = 1,2,$$

where the integrands $H_{i,j}$ are predictable, Section B.7 in Appendix B specifies conditions under which

$$EX_\ell(t)X_m(u) = E\sum_{i=1}^{n}\sum_{j=1}^{n}\int_0^t H_{i\ell}H_{jm}d\langle M_i,M_j\rangle.$$

Thus, once $\langle M_i,M_j\rangle,\ i,j = 1,\ldots,n$ are available, the variance and covariance of the martingale integrals can be obtained.

11.4 Regression with Fixed or External Covariates

Suppose that a regression analysis with a time-dependent external covariate vector $\boldsymbol{W}(t)$ is of interest. This includes the case when $\boldsymbol{W}(t)$ consists of only baseline covariates and the treatment group indicator. The Doob-Meyer decomposition holds with $\mathscr{F}_t$ being the collection of information on all n individuals up to time t on event, censoring, plus the entire covariate process history $\boldsymbol{W}_i^* = \{\boldsymbol{W}_i(t) : t \geq 0\}, i = 1, \ldots, n$.

Under this setup, all information on event, censoring and covariate history on $[0, t]$ for the ith individual is contained in the processes $N_i(s), Y_{i+}(s), 0 \leq s \leq t$ plus $\boldsymbol{W}_i^*$. Let $\lambda[t; \boldsymbol{W}_i(t)]$ be the conditional hazard function of T_i given $\boldsymbol{W}_i^*(t)$, and

$$\begin{aligned} A_i(t) &= \int_0^t Y_i(s)\lambda[s; \boldsymbol{W}_i(s)]ds = \int_0^t Y_i(s)\lambda(s; \boldsymbol{W}_i^*)ds, \\ M_i(t) &= N_i(t) - A_i(t). \end{aligned} \tag{11.32}$$

Similarly to (11.14),

$$E(N_i(t) - N_i(s)|\mathscr{F}_s) = Y_{i+}(s)\frac{P(s < T_i \leq t, T_i \leq C_i|\boldsymbol{W}_i^*)}{P(T_i > s, C_i > s|\boldsymbol{W}_i^*)}. \tag{11.33}$$

For A_i, similarly to (11.15),

$$E(A_i(t) - A_i(s)|\mathscr{F}_s) = \int_{(s,t]} Y_{i+}(s)\frac{P(T_i \wedge C_i \geq x|\boldsymbol{W}_i^*)}{P(T_i \wedge C_i > s|\boldsymbol{W}_i^*)}\lambda(x; \boldsymbol{W}_i^*)dx. \tag{11.34}$$

Therefore

$$E(N_i(t) - N_i(s)|\mathscr{F}_s) = E(A_i(t) - A_i(s)|\mathscr{F}_s)$$

if and only

$$\begin{aligned} & P(s < T_i \leq t, T_i \leq C_i|\boldsymbol{W}_i^*) \\ = & \int_{(s,t]} P(T_i \wedge C_i \geq x|\boldsymbol{W}_i^*)\lambda(x; \boldsymbol{W}_i^*)dx, \end{aligned}$$

on $\{X_i > s\}$. This holds for any $s < t$ on $\{X_i > s\}$ if and only if

$$\frac{dP(T_i \leq x, T_i \leq C_i|\boldsymbol{W}_i^*)}{P(T_i \wedge C_i \geq x|\boldsymbol{W}_i^*)} = \lambda(x; \boldsymbol{W}_i^*)dx, \tag{11.35}$$

for x with $P(T_i \wedge C_i \geq x|\boldsymbol{W}_i^*) > 0$.

Under (11.35), M_i in (11.32) is a martingale:

$$E\big(M_i(t)|\mathscr{F}_s\big) = M_i(s),$$

for any $0 \le s < t$. Equivalently, $N_i(t)$ has the intensity process $Y_i(t)\lambda(t; \boldsymbol{W}_i(t))$. Parallel to (11.16) for data without covariates, a censoring mechanism that satisfies the condition (11.35) is called independent censoring with external covariates.

Under the random censorship model with time-dependent external covariate as described in Section 6.3, part of the derivation for (11.2) shows that

$$P\big(T_i \le x, T_i \le C_i \big| \boldsymbol{W}_i^*\big) = \int_{(s,t]} P\big(C_i \ge x \big| \boldsymbol{W}_i^*\big) dF\big(x; \boldsymbol{W}_i^*\big),$$

where $F\big(x; \boldsymbol{W}_i^*\big) = P\big(T_i \le x \big| \boldsymbol{W}_i^*\big)$. In addition,

$$P\big(T_i \wedge C_i \ge x \big| \boldsymbol{W}_i^*\big) = P\big(T_i \ge x \big| \boldsymbol{W}_i^*\big) P\big(C_i \ge x \big| \boldsymbol{W}_i^*\big)$$

by the assumed conditional independence. Thus the condition (11.35) is satisfied.

11.5 Intensity Models for Counting Processes

Let $Q(t)$ be a counting process with $EQ(t) < \infty$ for any t, and assume that $Q(t)$ satisfies (11.20) for a family of increasing σ-algebras $\{\mathscr{G}_t\}$. The Doob-Meyer decomposition ensures existence of the compensator for the counting process and allows an analysis using the martingale theory.

In the case of $N_i(t)$ with no covariates or with external covariates, as shown in Sections 11.2 and 11.4, when the compensator is absolutely continuous, any model for the hazard or conditional hazard function of T_i gives rise to a corresponding model for the intensity process associated with $N_i(t)$. Thus, instead of the usual approach of working with random variables and their distributions, counting processes can be studied by modeling their intensity processes. This approach is pioneered by Aalen [2] for the nonparametric case and extended by Andersen and Gill [8] for the semiparametric Cox model.

Suppose it is of interest to study the behavior of $Q_i(t)$ in association with $\boldsymbol{W}_i(t)$, where $Q_i(t)$ and $\boldsymbol{W}_i(t)$ are the counting process and the covariate process for the ith individual, respectively. The covariate process $\boldsymbol{W}_i(t)$ may contain internal or external components. For the case with no covariates, it can be considered as a special case when $\boldsymbol{W}_i(t) \equiv 0$. For brevity, this special case will not be discussed separately. Assume that for each i, $Q_i(t)$ is $\mathscr{G}_t$-adapted and $\boldsymbol{W}_i(t)$ is $\mathscr{G}_t$-predictable. By the Doob-Meyer decomposition, $Q_i(t)$ has a predictable compensator. The intensity model assumes that $Q_i(t)$ has the intensity process

$$a_i(t) = \widetilde{Y}_i(t)\lambda_i\big[t; \boldsymbol{W}_i(t)\big], \tag{11.36}$$

where $\widetilde{Y}_i(t)$ is an observable and predictable process, and does not depend on $\boldsymbol{W}_i(t)$, while $\lambda_i\big[t; \boldsymbol{W}_i(t)\big]$ is predictable and a parametric, nonparametric or semiparametric function of the covariate history $\boldsymbol{W}_i^h(t) = \big\{\boldsymbol{W}_i(s), 0 \le s < t\big\}$, and

$$E\int_0^t \widetilde{Y}_i(x)\lambda_i\big[x; \boldsymbol{W}_i(x)\big]dx < \infty,$$

for any $t < \infty$.

Using (11.23) and (11.24), an informal and succinct way of stating the intensity model is to specify that

$$E\big[dQ_i(t)\big|\mathscr{G}_{t-}\big] = \widetilde{Y}_i(t)\lambda_i\big[t; \boldsymbol{W}_i(t)\big]dt. \tag{11.37}$$

For intensity models, an important requirement is that $Q_1(t), \ldots, Q_n(t)$ have distinct jump points. When $Q_i(t)$ is obtained from right censored data, this condition is satisfied when the underlying processes $Q_1^*(t), \ldots, Q_n^*(t)$ that generate the jumps for the n individuals (defined in the absence of censoring) are independent, and the jump point distributions are absolutely continuous. Under (11.37), the condition of absolute continuity is met. For compensators with discontinuities, results can be found in Appendix B. The relationship between the underlying process and the observed process is that

$$Q_i(t) = Q_i^*(t \wedge C_i),$$

where C_i is the censoring variable for the ith individual. More discussions on underlying and observed processes are given in Chapter Fifteen.

Typically, $\widetilde{Y}_i(t)$ is the at-risk process and $\lambda_i\big[t; \boldsymbol{W}_i(t)\big]$ can be interpreted as an individual hazard function conditional on the covariate history $\boldsymbol{W}_i^h(t)$. The multiplicative intensity model assumes that

$$\lambda_i\big[t; \boldsymbol{W}_i(t)\big] = \lambda_0(t)\exp\big[\boldsymbol{\beta}^{\mathrm{T}}\boldsymbol{W}_i(t)\big], \tag{11.38}$$

where $\boldsymbol{\beta}$ is the unknown regression parameter and $\lambda_0(t)$ is an unspecified deterministic baseline function. When there are no covariates, $\lambda_i\big[t; \boldsymbol{W}_i(t)\big]$ reduces to $\lambda_0(t)$. Other forms of the intensity model are also possible, such as the additive intensity model which specifies that

$$E\big[dQ_i(t)\big|\mathscr{G}_{t-}\big] = \widetilde{Y}_i(t)\big[\lambda_0(t) + \boldsymbol{\beta}^{\mathrm{T}}\boldsymbol{W}_i(t)\big]dt.$$

Intensity models can be obtained more generally for a counting process by dropping the requirement that $EQ_i(t) < \infty$ for any t, and working with the concept of local martingales [8, 7]. Some related definitions and properties can be found in Section B.6 in Appendix B.

From the results in Section 11.2 and 11.4, if each individual only experiences at most one event, then in both the case without covariates and the case with external covariates, the intensity model for $Q_i(t) = N_i(t)$ is simply another way of stating the corresponding distributional model under the appropriate independent censoring condition, in (11.16) and (11.35), respectively.

When $Q_i(t)$ is an observed counting process obtained from right censored data, as in the case of $Q_i(t) = N_i(t)$, the intensity model (11.36) is stated in terms of the observed process rather than the underlying process. Thus it has a built-in independent censoring condition that the censoring does not change the factor $\lambda_i[t; \boldsymbol{W}_i(t)]$. Alternatively, an intensity model can be stated in terms of the underlying process, and then an independent censoring condition is imposed such that the intensity process of the observed process has the form (11.36). This is done in Chapter Fifteen in the analysis of recurrent events. More discussions on censoring can be found in Section III.2 of the book by Andersen et al. [7].

To better understand the intensity model, in particular the relationship between the intensity process $a_i(t)$ and the counting process $Q_i(t)$, it helps to know that, under some technical conditions,

$$\lim_{h \downarrow 0} h^{-1} E\big(Q_i(t+h) - Q_i(t) \big| \mathcal{G}_t\big) = a_{i+}(t), \tag{11.39}$$

$$\lim_{h \downarrow 0} h^{-1} P\big(Q_i(t+h) - Q_i(t) = 1 \big| \mathcal{G}_t\big) = a_{i+}(t), \tag{11.40}$$

$$\lim_{h \downarrow 0} h^{-1} P\big(Q_i(t+h) - Q_i(t) \geq 2 \big| \mathcal{G}_t\big) = 0, \tag{11.41}$$

where $a_{i+}(t)$ is the right limit of $a_i(t)$ [1] [82, Theorem 4.2.1].

Result (11.39) extends (11.6) to the general intensity model. Note that (11.40) is equivalent to (11.39) if each individual can experience at most one event, as discussed in Section 11.2. From (11.41), given information up to time t, Q_i has at most one jump in the immediate future, or equivalently, there can be at most one event in the immediate future. Thus, it is impossible to have tied events.

From (11.39), $\lambda_{i+}[t; \boldsymbol{W}_i(t)]$ is the rate of change in the expectation of Q_i in the immediate future beyond time t, conditional on $\mathcal{G}_t$ which contains information on the history of Q_i up to t. Thus, it is likely that $\boldsymbol{W}_i(t)$ contains internal covariate components, such as the number and times of previous jumps. In these situations, similar to the discussion in Section 6.3, model (11.38) describes how the intensity process is influenced by $\boldsymbol{W}_i$. However, interpretation of treatment effect is challenging since the internal covariate may be responsive to the treatment. Further discussions on this topic can be found in Chapter Fifteen for analysis of recurrent event.

For the multiplicative intensity model (11.38), the partial likelihood inference theory still applies. Let

$$S^{(m)}(\boldsymbol{\beta}, t) = n^{-1} \sum_{i=1}^{n} \widetilde{Y}_i(t) \exp\left[\boldsymbol{\beta}^{\mathrm{T}} \boldsymbol{W}_i(t)\right] W_i(t)^{\otimes m},$$

for $m = 0, 1, 2$. The logarithm of the partial likelihood is

$$\ln L(\boldsymbol{\beta}) = \sum_{i=1}^{n} \int_0^{\infty} \boldsymbol{\beta}^{\mathrm{T}} \boldsymbol{W}_i(t) dQ_i(t) - \int_0^{\infty} \ln\left\{\sum_{i=1}^{n} \widetilde{Y}_i(t) \exp\left[\boldsymbol{\beta}^{\mathrm{T}} \boldsymbol{W}_i(t)\right]\right\} dQ.(t), \quad (11.42)$$

where $Q.(t) = \sum_{i=1}^{n} Q_i(t)$. Note that if the jump points of $Q_i(t)$ are $X_{i1} < \cdots < X_{iJ_i}$, $J_i \geq 1$, then

$$\int_0^{\infty} f(t) dQ_i(t) = \sum_{j=1}^{J_i} f(X_{ij}) \quad (11.43)$$

for any function f. Suppose $\boldsymbol{W}_i(t)$ is a $p \times 1$ vector process. Then the $p \times 1$ score vector $\boldsymbol{U}(\boldsymbol{\beta})$, with the ℓth component

$$\frac{\partial}{\partial \beta_\ell} \ln L(\boldsymbol{\beta}),$$

is

$$\boldsymbol{U}(\boldsymbol{\beta}) = \sum_{i=1}^{n} \int_0^{\infty} [\boldsymbol{W}_i(t) - E(\boldsymbol{\beta}, t)] dQ_i(t) \quad (11.44)$$

with $E(\boldsymbol{\beta}, t) = S^{(1)}(\boldsymbol{\beta}, t)/S^{(0)}(\boldsymbol{\beta}, t)$. The partial likelihood estimator $\widehat{\boldsymbol{\beta}}$ is the zero of $\boldsymbol{U}(\boldsymbol{\beta})$.

The information matrix is

$$\mathscr{I}(\boldsymbol{\beta}) = -\left(E \frac{\partial^2 \ln L}{\partial \beta_j \partial \beta_\ell}\right)_{p \times p} \quad (11.45)$$

and the observed information matrix is

$$\mathbb{I}(\boldsymbol{\beta}) = -\left(\frac{\partial^2 \ln L}{\partial \beta_j \partial \beta_\ell}\right)_{p \times p},$$

We have

$$\mathbb{I}(\boldsymbol{\beta}) = \sum_{i=1}^{n} \int_0^{\infty} \mathbf{V}(\boldsymbol{\beta}, t) dQ_i(t), \quad (11.46)$$

where as in (6.24),

$$\mathbf{V}(\boldsymbol{\beta}, t) = S^{(2)}(\boldsymbol{\beta}, t)/S^{(0)}(\boldsymbol{\beta}, t) - E(\boldsymbol{\beta}, t)^{\otimes 2}.$$

Under certain regularity conditions, it can be shown [8, 7] that, at the true value $\boldsymbol{\beta}_0$ of the parameter,

$$U(\boldsymbol{\beta}_0) \sim N\big(0, \mathscr{I}(\boldsymbol{\beta}_0)\big), \tag{11.47}$$

and

$$\widehat{\boldsymbol{\beta}} \sim N\big(\boldsymbol{\beta}_0, \mathscr{I}^{-1}(\boldsymbol{\beta}_0)\big). \tag{11.48}$$

Again, $\mathscr{I}(\boldsymbol{\beta}_0)$ in (11.47) and (11.48) can be replaced by $\mathbb{I}(\widehat{\boldsymbol{\beta}})$. These asymptotic results can be established using the martingale large sample theory in Section B.10 of Appendix B.

For the baseline cumulative hazard function $\int_0^t \lambda_0(s)ds$, the Breslow estimator is

$$\sum_{i=1}^{n} \int_0^t \frac{dQ_i(s)}{nS^{(0)}(\widehat{\boldsymbol{\beta}}, s)} = \sum_{i=1}^{n} \sum_{j=1}^{J_i} \frac{I(X_{ij} \le t)}{\sum_{m=1}^{n} \widetilde{Y}_m(X_{ij}) \exp\left[\widehat{\boldsymbol{\beta}}^{\mathrm{T}} \boldsymbol{W}_m(X_{ij})\right]}. \tag{11.49}$$

It is worth noting that, although the partial likelihood approach with multiplicative intensity models is most widely used, other models are possible, such as the accelerated failure time models [179] and transformation models [180].

12

Correlated Survival Data

12.1 Introduction

In the previous chapters, typically each participant in a trial contributes one time-to-event outcome, with data from different participants assumed to be independent. However, in certain clinical trials, such data structure is no longer present. This chapter focuses on the scenario when there are possibly correlated or clustered time-to-event outcomes subject to independent censoring. Other patterns of correlated outcomes will be discussed in Chapters Thirteen through Fifteen.

The types of data addressed in this chapter usually arise in two ways. First, participants in a trial can be assumed to act independently, but each individual contributes multiple correlated outcomes to be studied. Examples include conditions of the left and right eyes in an eye disease trial, or the occurrence of breast cancer, colorectal cancer, and heart disease in the WHI E+P trial. Second, a study may include clusters of participants sharing certain common genetic or environmental factors, resulting in correlated outcomes within a cluster. For instance, family members may be recruited into a genetic study, or students in the same school or community may participate in a group randomized trial.

12.2 Marginal Analysis

For correlated multivariate time-to-event outcomes, analysis must account for correlation among the outcomes. When the primary interest lies in comparing control and treatment groups for each component, and associations among outcomes are considered nuisance features to be accommodated, the marginal analysis approach is widely used due to its simplicity and often reasonable performance.

Testing the equality of two univariate survival distributions using weighted log-rank tests and their combinations has been discussed in Chapters Two and Nine. For comparing treatment and control groups with respect to K time-to-event variables subject to independent censoring, weighted log-rank tests can be

DOI: 10.1201/9780429324437-12

applied to each variable. The joint distribution of these test statistics can be established, properly accounting for correlations among variables in the analysis. Wei and Lachin [319] established the asymptotic normality of this joint distribution based on martingale convergence results by Gill [95].

For covariate-adjusted analysis, a marginal regression model is used to analyze the relationship between events and covariates for each outcome, leaving the correlation among events unspecified. Examples of works along this line include Wei, Lin and Weissfeld [320], Lee, Wei and Amato [159], and Spiekerman and Lin [286], among others.

12.2.1 Marginal Regression of K Different Types of Events

Let T_{ki} be time to the kth event of the ith unit, $k = 1,\ldots,K$, $i = 1,\ldots,n$. The corresponding time to censoring is C_{ki} and the associated covariate vector process is $\boldsymbol{W}_{ki}(t)$ which is $p \times 1$ and assumed to be external. The time to event vector $\boldsymbol{T}_i = (T_{1i},\ldots,T_{Ki})$ and the time to censoring vector $\boldsymbol{C}_i = (C_{1i},\ldots,C_{Ki})$ are assumed to be independent given all covariate paths $\mathbb{W}_i = (\boldsymbol{W}^*_{1i},\ldots,\boldsymbol{W}^*_{Ki})$. Let $X_{ki} = T_{ki} \wedge C_{ki}$, $\delta_{ki} = I(T_{ki} \le C_{ki})$. It is further assumed that $(\boldsymbol{T}_i, \mathbb{W}_i, \boldsymbol{C}_i)$, $1 \le i \le n$ are i.i.d. The observed data are $(\boldsymbol{X}_i, \delta_i, \mathbb{W}_i)$, $1 \le i \le n$, where $\boldsymbol{X}_i = (X_{1i},\ldots,X_{Ki})$, $\delta_i = (\delta_{1i},\ldots,\delta_{Ki})$, for $X_{ki} = T_{ki} \wedge C_{ki}$, $\delta_{ki} = I(T_{ki} \le C_{ki})$.

For the data structure given above, the marginal regression approach proposed by Wei, Lin and Weissfeld [320] postulates that given the entire covariate path $\boldsymbol{W}^*_{ki}$, the hazard function of the kth event for the ith individual is

$$\lambda_k[t; \boldsymbol{W}_{ki}] = \lambda_{0k}(t) \exp[\boldsymbol{\beta}_k^{\mathrm{T}} \boldsymbol{W}_{ki}(t)], \tag{12.1}$$

where $\lambda_{0k}(t)$, $k = 1,\ldots,K$, are unknown baseline hazard functions and $\boldsymbol{\beta}_k$, $k = 1,\ldots,K$, are $p \times 1$ vectors of unknown regression parameters.

In model (12.1), both $\boldsymbol{\beta}_k$ and $\lambda_{0k}(t)$ depend on k. A special case is when $\boldsymbol{\beta}_1 = \cdots = \boldsymbol{\beta}_K$. As illustrated in the review paper of Lin [170], by properly defining the covariate vector, it can always be achieved that $\boldsymbol{\beta}_1 = \cdots = \boldsymbol{\beta}_K$. This is because we can consider the $(Kp) \times 1$ covariate vector

$$\widetilde{\boldsymbol{W}}_{ki} = (\boldsymbol{0},\ldots,\boldsymbol{W}_{ki},\ldots,\boldsymbol{0}),$$

which consists of K blocks of p dimensional vectors with $\boldsymbol{W}_{Ki}$ being the kth block and all other blocks the zero vector. Similarly, define $\widetilde{\boldsymbol{\beta}}$ to be the $(Kp) \times 1$ parameter vector which consists of K blocks of p dimensional vectors, with $\boldsymbol{\beta}_k$ being the kth block. Then

$$\boldsymbol{\beta}_k^{\mathrm{T}} \boldsymbol{W}_{ki}(t) = \widetilde{\boldsymbol{\beta}}^{\mathrm{T}} \widetilde{\boldsymbol{W}}_{ki}(t)$$

and model (12.1) can be re-written as

$$\lambda_k[t; \widetilde{\boldsymbol{W}}_{ki}] = \lambda_{0k}(t) \exp[\widetilde{\boldsymbol{\beta}}^{\mathrm{T}} \widetilde{\boldsymbol{W}}_{ki}(t)],$$

a model in which all K events have a common regression parameter vector. Therefore it suffices to consider the model

$$\lambda_k[t; \boldsymbol{W}_{ki}] = \lambda_{0k}(t) \exp[\boldsymbol{\beta}^{\mathrm{T}} \boldsymbol{W}_{ki}(t)]. \tag{12.2}$$

Note that from (12.2), with attention only on the kth event for $i \geq 1$, a Cox multiplicative hazard model obtains. Let

$$S_k^{(m)}(\boldsymbol{\beta}, t) = n^{-1} \sum_{i=1}^{n} I(X_{ki} \geq t) \exp[\boldsymbol{\beta}^{\mathrm{T}} \boldsymbol{W}_{ki}(t)] \boldsymbol{W}_{ki}(t)^{\otimes m},$$

for $m = 0, 1, 2$ and $k = 1, \ldots, K$, where $\mathbf{V}^{\otimes m}$ for a vector $\mathbf{V}$ is as defined in (5.13). From the results in Section 6.3, with (6.18) adapted to the current situation, for the kth event the score function is

$$\boldsymbol{U}_k(\boldsymbol{\beta}) = \sum_{i=1}^{n} \delta_{ki} \left[\boldsymbol{W}_{ki}(X_{ki}) - \frac{S_k^{(1)}(\boldsymbol{\beta}, X_{ki})}{S_k^{(0)}(\boldsymbol{\beta}, X_{ki})} \right], \quad k = 1, \ldots, K. \tag{12.3}$$

Pulling the K score functions together, one obtains the estimating function

$$\boldsymbol{U}(\boldsymbol{\beta}) = \sum_{k=1}^{K} \boldsymbol{U}_k(\boldsymbol{\beta}) = \sum_{i=1}^{n} \sum_{k=1}^{K} \delta_{ki} \left[\boldsymbol{W}_{ki}(X_{ki}) - \frac{S_k^{(1)}(\boldsymbol{\beta}, X_{ki})}{S_k^{(0)}(\boldsymbol{\beta}, X_{ki})} \right]. \tag{12.4}$$

From Section 6.3, at the true parameter $\boldsymbol{\beta}_0$, each $\boldsymbol{U}_k(\boldsymbol{\beta}_0)$ is asymptotically normal with mean zero. It can be shown [320] that, under certain regularity conditions, $\boldsymbol{U}(\boldsymbol{\beta}_0)$ is also asymptotically normal with mean zero and the limiting covariance matrix of $n^{-1/2}\boldsymbol{U}(\boldsymbol{\beta}_0)$ is

$$\boldsymbol{A}(\boldsymbol{\beta}_0) = n^{-1} \sum_{i=1}^{n} \sum_{k=1}^{K} \sum_{\ell=1}^{K} \mathbf{V}_{ki}(\boldsymbol{\beta}_0) \mathbf{V}_{\ell i}(\boldsymbol{\beta}_0)^{\mathrm{T}},$$

where

$$\begin{aligned} \mathbf{V}_{ki}(\boldsymbol{\beta}) \quad = \quad & \delta_{ki} \left[\boldsymbol{W}_{ki}(X_{ki}) - \frac{S_k^{(1)}(\boldsymbol{\beta}, X_{ki})}{S_k^{(0)}(\boldsymbol{\beta}, X_{ki})} \right] \\ & - \sum_{j=1}^{n} \frac{\delta_{\ell j} I(X_{ki} \geq X_{kj}) \exp[\boldsymbol{\beta}^{\mathrm{T}} \boldsymbol{W}_{ki}(X_{kj})]}{n S_k^{(0)}(\boldsymbol{\beta}, X_{kj})} \left[\boldsymbol{W}_{ki}(X_{kj}) - \frac{S_k^{(1)}(\boldsymbol{\beta}, X_{kj})}{S_k^{(0)}(\boldsymbol{\beta}, X_{kj})} \right]. \end{aligned}$$

For the zero $\widehat{\boldsymbol{\beta}}$ of $\boldsymbol{U}(\boldsymbol{\beta})$, it can be shown that $\sqrt{n}(\widehat{\boldsymbol{\beta}} - \boldsymbol{\beta}_0)$ converges in distribution to a normal distribution with mean zero and covariance matrix which can be estimated by $\boldsymbol{B}(\widehat{\boldsymbol{\beta}})^{-1}\boldsymbol{A}(\widehat{\boldsymbol{\beta}})\boldsymbol{B}(\widehat{\boldsymbol{\beta}})^{-1}$, where

$$\boldsymbol{B}(\boldsymbol{\beta}) = \frac{1}{n}\sum_{i=1}^{n}\sum_{k=1}^{K}\delta_{ki}\left[\frac{S_k^{(2)}(\boldsymbol{\beta}, X_{ki})}{S_k^{(0)}(\boldsymbol{\beta}, X_{ki})} - \frac{S_k^{(1)}(\boldsymbol{\beta}, X_{ki})S_k^{(1)}(\boldsymbol{\beta}, X_{ki})^{\mathrm{T}}}{S_k^{(0)}(\boldsymbol{\beta}, X_{ki})^2}\right].$$

Note that $\boldsymbol{U}(\boldsymbol{\beta})$ would be exactly the score function in the partial likelihood approach if the K different events for each individual are independent. For this reason, the approach described above is often referred to as the independence working model approach.

12.2.2 Marginal Analysis for Clustered Observations

Next, consider the case when there are clustered observations that may be correlated. Suppose there are n clusters and the ith cluster has size $K_i, i = 1,\ldots,n$, with K_i's bounded by a constant. For $k = 1,\ldots,K_i$, $i = 1,\ldots,n$, let T_{ki} be time to event of the kth individual in the ith cluster, C_{ki} the corresponding time to censoring, and $\boldsymbol{W}_{ki}(t)$ the associated covariate vector process which is $p \times 1$ and external. The time to event vector $\boldsymbol{T}_i = (T_{1i},\ldots,T_{K_i i})$ and the time to censoring vector $\boldsymbol{C}_i = (C_{1i},\ldots,C_{K_i i})$ are assumed to be independent given all covariate paths $\mathbb{W}_i = (\boldsymbol{W}_{1i}^*,\ldots,\boldsymbol{W}_{K_i i}^*)$. Let $X_{ki} = T_{ki} \wedge C_{ki}$, $\delta_{ki} = I(T_{ki} \le C_{ki})$ and $\boldsymbol{X}_i = (X_{1i},\ldots,X_{K_i i})$. It is assumed that $(\boldsymbol{X}_i, \boldsymbol{C}_i, \mathbb{W}_i)$, $1 \le i \le n$ are independent, and that for all clusters of the same size $K_i = \ell$ with a fixed ℓ, the vectors $(\boldsymbol{T}_i, \boldsymbol{C}_i, \mathbb{W}_i)$ have a common joint distribution. Furthermore, the marginal distributions of $(T_{ki}, \boldsymbol{C}_{ki}, \boldsymbol{W}_{ki})$, $k = 1,\ldots,K_i, i = 1,\ldots,n$, are the same.

Lee, Wei and Amato [159] proposed the marginal analysis in which, conditional on $\boldsymbol{W}_{ki}^*$, the hazard function of the kth individual in the ith cluster is assumed to be

$$\lambda_k[t; \boldsymbol{W}_{ki}] = \lambda_0(t)\exp[\boldsymbol{\beta}^{\mathrm{T}}\boldsymbol{W}_{ki}(t)], \tag{12.5}$$

where $\lambda_0(t)$ is an unknown baseline hazard functions and $\boldsymbol{\beta}$ a $p \times 1$ vector of unknown regression parameters.

Let

$$S^{(m)}(\boldsymbol{\beta}, t) = n^{-1}\sum_{i=1}^{n}\sum_{k=1}^{K_i} I(X_{ki} \ge t)\exp[\boldsymbol{\beta}^{\mathrm{T}}\boldsymbol{W}_{ki}(t)]\boldsymbol{W}_{ki}(t)^{\otimes m},$$

for $m = 0, 1, 2$. The estimating function is now

$$\widetilde{\boldsymbol{U}}(\boldsymbol{\beta}) = \sum_{i=1}^{n}\sum_{k=1}^{K_i}\delta_{ki}\left[\boldsymbol{W}_{ki}(X_{ki}) - \frac{S^{(1)}(\boldsymbol{\beta}, X_{ki})}{S^{(0)}(\boldsymbol{\beta}, X_{ki})}\right]. \tag{12.6}$$

It can be shown that, under certain regularity conditions, at the true parameter $\boldsymbol{\beta}_0$, $\widetilde{\boldsymbol{U}}(\boldsymbol{\beta}_0)$ is asymptotically normal with mean zero and the limiting covariance matrix of $n^{-1/2}\widetilde{\boldsymbol{U}}(\boldsymbol{\beta}_0)$ is

$$\widetilde{\boldsymbol{A}}(\boldsymbol{\beta}_0) = n^{-1}\sum_{i=1}^{n}\sum_{k=1}^{K_i}\sum_{\ell=1}^{K_i}\widetilde{\mathbf{V}}_{ki}(\boldsymbol{\beta}_0)\widetilde{\mathbf{V}}_{\ell i}(\boldsymbol{\beta}_0)^{\mathrm{T}},$$

where

$$\begin{aligned}\widetilde{\mathbf{V}}_{ki}(\boldsymbol{\beta}) &= \delta_{ki}\left[\boldsymbol{W}_{ki}(X_{ki}) - \frac{S^{(1)}(\boldsymbol{\beta}, X_{ki})}{S^{(0)}(\boldsymbol{\beta}, X_{ki})}\right] \\ &\quad - \sum_{j=1}^{n}\sum_{\ell=1}^{K}\frac{\delta_{\ell j} I(X_{ki} \geq X_{\ell j})\exp\left[\boldsymbol{\beta}^{\mathrm{T}}\boldsymbol{W}_{ki}(X_{\ell j})\right]}{nS^{(0)}(\boldsymbol{\beta}, X_{\ell j})}\left[\boldsymbol{W}_{ki}(X_{\ell j}) - \frac{S^{(1)}(\boldsymbol{\beta}, X_{\ell j})}{S^{(0)}(\boldsymbol{\beta}, X_{\ell j})}\right].\end{aligned}$$

For the zero $\widehat{\boldsymbol{\beta}}$ of $\widetilde{\boldsymbol{U}}(\boldsymbol{\beta})$, it can be shown that $\sqrt{n}(\widehat{\boldsymbol{\beta}} - \boldsymbol{\beta}_0)$ converges in distribution to a normal distribution with mean zero and covariance matrix which can be estimated by $\widetilde{\boldsymbol{B}}(\widehat{\boldsymbol{\beta}})^{-1}\widetilde{\boldsymbol{A}}(\widehat{\boldsymbol{\beta}})\widetilde{\boldsymbol{B}}(\widehat{\boldsymbol{\beta}})^{-1}$, where

$$\widetilde{\boldsymbol{B}}(\boldsymbol{\beta}) = \frac{1}{n}\sum_{i=1}^{n}\sum_{k=1}^{K_i}\delta_{ki}\left[\frac{S^{(2)}(\boldsymbol{\beta}, X_{ki})}{S^{(0)}(\boldsymbol{\beta}, X_{ki})} - \frac{S^{(1)}(\boldsymbol{\beta}, X_{ki})S^{(1)}(\boldsymbol{\beta}, X_{ki})^{\mathrm{T}}}{S^{(0)}(\boldsymbol{\beta}, X_{ki})^2}\right].$$

Note that the formulas in Sections 12.2.1 and 12.2.2 are very similar. The model (12.5) can also be extended to allow different baseline hazard functions for the kth individual in the ith cluster. Spiekerman and Lin [286] proposed a general Cox-type marginal regression model that includes (12.1) and (12.5) as special cases. Models other than the Cox model have also been used to specify the marginal distributions. For example, Lee, Wei and Ying [160] considered the accelerated failure time model, and Cai, Wei and Wilcox [35] used linear transformation models. Additional models from Chapters Seven and Eight could also be applied to specify marginal distributions. Efficiency gains over independence working model approaches may be achieved by utilizing association structures among events, as demonstrated by Cai and Prentice [32, 33], Clegg, Cai and Sen [46], and Chen, Chen and Ying [39], among others.

12.3 Frailty Modeling for Association

When associations among events are of interest, frailty models provide a convenient approach to modeling these associations. Frailty models are similar to random effects models in that they incorporate additional unobserved variables, which introduce heterogeneity and association into the model. The difference is that in a frailty model, the unobserved variable is a multiplicative factor on the hazard function, whereas in a random effects model, it is an additive component in the outcome. Frailty models were first proposed for characterizing subject-specific heterogeneity in demographic models [311]. Oakes [213] provided an early work in the literature that explored a few attractive features of the frailty approach for the study of association between two survival times.

Suppose T is a time-to-event variable for a population such that given an unobserved positive variable γ, the conditional hazard function of T is

$$\lambda(t|\gamma) = \gamma\lambda_0(t), \tag{12.7}$$

where $\lambda_0(t)$ is a baseline hazard function. It follows that the conditional survival function of T is

$$S(t|\gamma) = \exp\left[-\gamma\Lambda_0(t)\right], \tag{12.8}$$

where $\Lambda_0(t)$ is the cumulative hazard function corresponding to $\lambda_0(t)$. γ is called a *frailty*, and an individual with a higher frailty is expected to have a higher risk of event and therefore is thought of as being more frail. In this context, γ represents the unobservable heterogeneity in the population. The frailty model (12.7) can also be viewed as a Cox proportional hazards model with an unobserved covariate. For identifiability of parameters, the frailty is usually scaled to have mean $E\gamma = 1$. By the law of iterated expectations (B.6) in Appendix B, the survival function of this heterogeneous population of individuals with different frailty values, is

$$P(T > t) = EP(T > t|\gamma) = E\exp\left[-\gamma\Lambda(t)\right] = \mathfrak{L}\big(\Lambda_0(t)\big), \tag{12.9}$$

where $\mathfrak{L}(x)$ is the Laplace transform of γ.

Now consider a bivariate vector (T_1, T_2) of two time-to-event variables. Suppose that correlation between the two event times is due to common genetic and/or environmental factors represented by a shared frailty γ, and that given γ, T_1, T_2 are conditionally independent. Furthermore, assume that, similar to (12.8), the conditional survival function of T_j given γ is

$$S_j(t|\gamma) = \exp\left[-\gamma\Lambda_{0j}(t)\right], \quad j = 1,2, \tag{12.10}$$

where $\Lambda_{0j}(t)$ are two baseline cumulative hazard functions. Then, by the conditional independence and (12.10), the conditional bivariate survival function given γ is

$$P(T_1 > t_1, T_2 > t_2|\gamma) = \exp\left\{-\gamma\left[\Lambda_{01}(t_1) + \Lambda_{02}(t_2)\right]\right\}.$$

Similarly to (12.9), it follows that the bivariate survival function is

$$S(t_1, t_2) = P(T_1 > t_1, T_2 > t_2) = \mathfrak{L}\big(\Lambda_{01}(t_1) + \Lambda_{02}(t_2)\big). \tag{12.11}$$

From this, the marginal survival functions of T_j are

$$\begin{aligned} S_1(t_1) &= S(t_1, 0) = \mathfrak{L}\big(\Lambda_{01}(t_1)\big), \\ S_2(t_2) &= S(0, t_2) = \mathfrak{L}\big(\Lambda_{02}(t_2)\big). \end{aligned}$$

Many frailty distribution have been studied in the literature, as shown in the review article by Hougaard [116], the tutorial by Balan and Putter [13], and books by Hougaard [117], Duchateau and Janssen [66], and Wienke [323]. The gamma distribution is often used for the frailty modeling. From Chapter Three, the gamma distribution with shape parameter α and rate parameter β has mean α/β and variance α/β^2 (Exercise 12.3). The restriction of $E\gamma = 1$ forces $\alpha = \beta$ and the variance becomes $1/\beta$. Let $\theta = 1/\beta$ denote the variance of this frailty distribution, It is left to Exercise 12.4 to verify that the joint and marginal survival functions of T_1, T_2 are given by

$$S(t_1, t_2) = \{1+\theta[\Lambda_{01}(t_1)+\Lambda_{02}(t_2)]\}^{-1/\theta}, \tag{12.12}$$

$$S_j(t_j) = [1+\theta\Lambda_{0j}(t_j)]^{-1/\theta}, \quad j=1,2. \tag{12.13}$$

From (12.13), the marginal hazard function $\lambda_j(t_j)$ of T_j is

$$\lambda_j(t_j) = -\frac{d\ln S_j(t_j)}{dt_j} = \frac{\lambda_{0j}(t_j)}{1+\theta\Lambda_{0j}(t_j)}, \tag{12.14}$$

where λ_{0j} is the hazard function corresponding to Λ_{0j}.

Next, suppose it is of interest to study relationships between the survival time T_j and the associated and observed $p \times 1$ covariate vector $\boldsymbol{W}_j, j = 1,2$. Assume that given $\boldsymbol{W}_1, \boldsymbol{W}_2$ and the shared frailty γ, T_1 and T_2 are independent, with the conditional hazard functions

$$\lambda_j(t_j|\boldsymbol{W}_1,\boldsymbol{W}_2,\gamma) = \lambda_j(t_j|\boldsymbol{W}_j,\gamma) = \gamma\exp(\boldsymbol{\beta}^{\mathrm{T}}\boldsymbol{W}_j)\lambda_{0j}(t_j), \quad j=1,2, \tag{12.15}$$

respectively. Note that the conditional hazard function of T_j does not depend on the covariate $\boldsymbol{W}_{3-j}$ of the other survival time. Let $S_j(t_j|\boldsymbol{W}_1,\boldsymbol{W}_2,\gamma)$ be the conditional survival function of T_j given $\boldsymbol{W}_1,\boldsymbol{W}_2,\gamma$. Since

$$\lambda_j(t_j|\boldsymbol{W}_1,\boldsymbol{W}_2,\gamma) = -\frac{d\ln S_j(t_j|\boldsymbol{W}_1,\boldsymbol{W}_2,\gamma)}{dt_j},$$

it follows from (12.15) that

$$S_j(t_j|\boldsymbol{W}_1,\boldsymbol{W}_2,\gamma) = S_j(t_j|\boldsymbol{W}_j,\gamma) = \exp[-\gamma\exp(\boldsymbol{\beta}^{\mathrm{T}}\boldsymbol{W}_j)\Lambda_{0j}(t_j)], \quad j=1,2. \tag{12.16}$$

Again, by the law of iterated expectations (B.6) in Appendix B, averaging over γ we obtain

$$\begin{aligned}
& P(T_1 > t_1, T_2 > t_2|\boldsymbol{W}_1,\boldsymbol{W}_2) \\
= \; & EP(T_1 > t_1, T_2 > t_2|\boldsymbol{W}_1,\boldsymbol{W}_2,\gamma) \\
= \; & E\Big[P(T_1 > t_1|\boldsymbol{W}_1,\boldsymbol{W}_2,\gamma)P(T_2 > t_2|\boldsymbol{W}_1,\boldsymbol{W}_2,\gamma)\Big] \\
= \; & \mathfrak{L}\Big(\exp(\boldsymbol{\beta}^{\mathrm{T}}\boldsymbol{W}_1)\Lambda_{01}(t_1)+\exp(\boldsymbol{\beta}^{\mathrm{T}}\boldsymbol{W}_2)\Lambda_{02}(t_2)\Big).
\end{aligned} \tag{12.17}$$

When the frailty γ has the gamma distribution with mean 1 and variance θ, similarly to (12.12) through (12.14),

$$\begin{aligned} & S(t_1, t_2 | \boldsymbol{W}_1, \boldsymbol{W}_2) \\ = & \left\{1+\theta\left[\exp(\boldsymbol{\beta}^{\mathrm{T}}\boldsymbol{W}_1)\Lambda_{01}(t_1)+\exp(\boldsymbol{\beta}^{\mathrm{T}}\boldsymbol{W}_2)\Lambda_{02}(t_2)\right]\right\}^{-1/\theta}, \end{aligned} \tag{12.18}$$

$$\begin{aligned} & S_j(t_j | \boldsymbol{W}_j) \\ = & \left[1+\theta\exp(\boldsymbol{\beta}^{\mathrm{T}}\boldsymbol{W}_j)\Lambda_{0j}(t_j)\right]^{-1/\theta}, \quad j=1,2, \end{aligned} \tag{12.19}$$

$$\begin{aligned} & \lambda_j(t_j | \boldsymbol{W}_j) \\ = & \frac{\exp(\boldsymbol{\beta}^{\mathrm{T}}\boldsymbol{W}_j)\lambda_{0j}(t_j)}{1+\theta\exp(\boldsymbol{\beta}^{\mathrm{T}}\boldsymbol{W}_j)\Lambda_{0j}(t_j)}, \quad j=1,2. \end{aligned} \tag{12.20}$$

If the above model is used for an unadjusted analysis in a two arm trial with $\boldsymbol{W}_j = Z_j, \boldsymbol{\beta}^{\mathrm{T}}\boldsymbol{W}_j = \beta Z_j$, where Z_j is the treatment group assignment indicator associated with T_j, then, similarly to (5.4) in Chapter Five,

$$\frac{\lambda_j(t_j | Z_j = 1, \gamma)}{\lambda_j(t_j | Z_j = 0, \gamma)} = \exp(\beta). \tag{12.21}$$

That is, the conditional hazard ratio (treatment over control) for those individuals with the same frailty γ is the constant $\exp(\beta)$. This might seem similar to (5.5) for a covariate-adjusted Cox model analysis. However, the difference here is that the frailty is unobservable.

If we drop conditioning on γ in the comparison, then from (12.20), the hazard ratio is

$$\frac{\lambda_j(t_j | Z_j = 1)}{\lambda_j(t_j | Z_j = 0)} = \frac{\exp(\beta)\left[1+\theta\Lambda_{0j}(t_j)\right]}{1+\theta\exp(\beta)\Lambda_{0j}(t_j)}. \tag{12.22}$$

This is referred to as the marginal hazard ratio. Note that it is only marginal with respect to γ as it depends on the conditional hazard function given Z_j. Compared with the conditional hazard ratio in (12.21), the marginal hazard ratio in (12.22) is a time-dependent function depending on all the model parameters β, θ and $\Lambda_{0j}(t)$.

When the treatment is beneficial ($\exp(\beta) < 1$), the marginal hazard ratio is an increasing function in t_j, starting at $\exp(\beta)$ when $t_j = 0$ and approaches 1 as $\Lambda_{0j}(t_j) \to \infty$. Therefore, the treatment effect indicated by the marginal hazard ratio is smaller than what the conditional hazard ratio suggests.

Similarly, when the treatment is harmful ($\exp(\beta) > 1$), the marginal hazard ratio is a decreasing function in t_j, starting at $\exp(\beta)$ when $t_j = 0$ and approaches 1 as $\Lambda_{0j}(t_j) \to \infty$. Thus the harmful effect is also smaller than what the conditional hazard ratio indicates. In either case, the hazard ratio is a time-dependent monotone function that is closer to 1 than the conditional hazard ratio $\exp(\beta)$.

It converges to 1 as $\Lambda_{0j}(t) \to \infty$, indicating that the treatment effect vanishes over time. Similar observations can be made for a covariate-adjusted analysis when $\boldsymbol{W}_j$ contains both Z_j and other explanatory variables.

Note that (12.21) remains valid for any frailty distribution. With frailty distributions other than the gamma distribution, the marginal hazard ratio typically is also time-dependent, except for the case when the frailty has the positive stable distribution, which preserves the proportional hazards assumption for the marginal hazards, but with different constants of proportionality [115].

The above discussion focuses on the frailty model with gamma frailty and Cox proportional hazards model conditional on the covariates and frailty. Other models and frailty distributions can also be considered. Depending on how the baseline hazard is modeled, appropriate parametric, semiparametric and nonparametric procedures can be obtained. More discussions and details can be found in the previous mentioned works [116, 13, 117, 66, 323] and references contained in them.

For gamma frailty, from (12.18) and (12.19) we have

$$S(t_1, t_2|\boldsymbol{W}_1, \boldsymbol{W}_2) = \left[S_1(t_1|\boldsymbol{W}_1)^{-\theta} + S_2(t_2|\boldsymbol{W}_2)^{-\theta} - 1\right]^{-1/\theta}. \tag{12.23}$$

Note that as $\theta \downarrow 0$,

$$S(t_1, t_2|\boldsymbol{W}_1, \boldsymbol{W}_2) \to S_1(t_1|\boldsymbol{W}_1)S_2(t_2|\boldsymbol{W}_2), \tag{12.24}$$

The significance of these results is that it looks possible to model the joint distribution by specifying the marginals together with an additional parameter that shapes the association between the two survival times, without the need for the conditional modeling approach via frailty. This will be discussed in the next section.

12.4 Copula Models

The frailty model has a natural appeal in certain situations, such as familial studies, where it can model the dependence of event times among family members due to shared genetic and environmental factors. However, this approach gives rise to model parameters that only have simple and clear interpretations conditionally, whereas the interest is usually in the unconditional description of relationships between observed covariates and survival times.

To circumvent the less straightforward interpretation of frailty models in terms of marginal survival and hazard functions, copula models provide an appealing alternative. Copula models specify the joint model using marginals plus an association parameter. The parameter interpretation is not conditional on an unobserved variable, making it more straightforward.

A K-dimensional *copula function* is a continuous joint cumulative distribution or survival function on the unit cube $[0,1]^K$ with uniform marginals. Earlier works on properties and applications of copula functions include Sklar [280], Marshall and Olkin [200], and Nelsen [211], among others. In the copula modeling approach, the joint survival function of K survival times is expressed in terms of the marginal survival functions and a copula function.

Suppose K events are of interest. Let T_k be time to the kth event and define the marginal survival functions

$$S_k(t) = P(T_k > t), \quad t \geq 0, \quad k = 1, \ldots, K,$$

and the joint survival function

$$S(t_1, \ldots, t_K) = P(T_1 > t_1, \ldots, T_K > t_K).$$

To motivate the copula representation, first assume that S_k's are continuous and strictly increasing. Then $T_k > t_k$ if and only if $S_k(T_k) > S_k(t_k)$. Thus

$$S(t_1, \ldots, t_K) = P\big(S_1(T_1) > S_1(t_1), \ldots, S_K(T_K) > S_K(t_K)\big). \tag{12.25}$$

Moreover, $S_k(T_k)$ can be shown to have the uniform distribution on $[0,1]$ (Exercise 12.8). Let $U_k = S_k(T_k)$ and C be the joint survival function of $U_1, \ldots, U_K$. Then (12.25) can be re-written as

$$S(t_1, \ldots, t_K) = C\big(S_1(t_1), \ldots, S_K(t_K)\big). \tag{12.26}$$

More generally, it can be shown [280] that any joint survival function S can be expressed in terms of its marginal survival functions and a copula function as in (12.26). Furthermore, when S is continuous, the copula C is unique and is given by

$$C(u1, \ldots, u_K) = S\big(S_1^{-1}(u_1), \ldots, S_K^{-1}(u_K)\big). \quad (u_1, \ldots, u_K) \in (0,1)^K,$$

where the inverse functions $S_1^{-1}, \ldots, S_K^{-1}$ are defined by

$$S_k^{-1}(x) = \inf\{t : S_k(t) \leq x\}, \quad x \in [0,1], \quad k = 1, \ldots, K.$$

The copula representation offers a way to model the joint distribution by separately modeling the marginals and the dependency structure, so that the marginal distributions do not depend on the dependency structure. This is similar to the case for the multivariate normal distribution, where the mean vector and the covariance matrix jointly determine the joint distribution and can be modeled separately.

An important sub-class of copula functions is the class of Archimedean copulas in which the copula is given by

$$C(u1,\ldots,u_K) = \phi\big(\phi^{-1}(u_1) + \cdots + \phi^{-1}(u_K)\big), \tag{12.27}$$

where ϕ is called an Archimedean generator. To ensure that the function C in (12.27) is a K-dimensional copula, ϕ needs to satisfy certain technical monotonicity conditions [201]. One such generator is the Laplace transform of a positive random variable. In particular, if $T_1,\ldots,T_K$ are conditionally independent given a positive variable A whose Laplace transform is ϕ, and

$$P(T_k > t \mid A) = \exp\left[-AH_k(t)\right]$$

for an increasing function H_k with $H_k(0) = 0$, then S can be obtained from taking expectation with respect to A and it will have the associated copula function of the form in (12.27). Thus the class of Archimedean copulas provides a connection between copula models and frailty models.

Example 12.1 The Clayton family of multivariate survival functions has the form

$$S(t_1,\ldots,t_K) = \left[\sum_{k=1}^{K} S_k(t_k)^{-\theta} - K + 1\right]^{-1/\theta}, \quad t_k > 0,\ k = 1,\ldots,K,\ \theta > 0. \tag{12.28}$$

The associated copula is an Archimedean copula with the generator $\phi(x) = (1 + x)^{-1/\theta}$, which is the Laplace transform of a gamma distribution.

12.5 Bivariate Dependence Measures

When it is of interest to study associations among multiple outcomes from the same individual or outcomes within a cluster, summary measures of dependence among outcomes are often useful. Consider the case for a bivariate random vector (T_1, T_2). In introductory statistics books, the Pearson correlation coefficient is typically the default measure of dependence or association between T_1 and T_2. While it provides a simple and convenient measure for approximately normally distributed data, it has limitations for survival analysis. Survival data are often skewed, deviating from the normal distribution assumption. Furthermore, in the presence of censoring, it can be challenging or even impossible to estimate the correlation coefficient reliably. To address these limitations, alternative measures have been proposed which are often better suited for describing dependence or correlation in survival data.

Let (T_{1i}, T_{2i}) and (T_{1j}, T_{2j}) be two independent copies of (T_1, T_2). The two pairs are *concordant* if $(T_{1i} - T_{1j})(T_{2i} - T_{2j}) \geq 0$, and *discordant* otherwise. Kendall's coefficient of concordance, τ, is defined by

$$\tau = P\big[(T_{1i} - T_{1j})(T_{2i} - T_{2j}) \geq 0\big] - P\big[(T_{1i} - T_{1j})(T_{2i} - T_{2j}) < 0\big]. \quad (12.29)$$

From the definition, τ depends only on ranks, not the exact values of the variables. Similar to the Pearson correlation coefficient, τ is bounded between -1 and 1, positive/negative if T_1 and T_2 are positively/negatively associated, and 0 if T_1 and T_2 are independent.

Another dependence measure is Spearman's correlation coefficient, defined by

$$\rho = 12E\big\{[S_1(T_1) - 1/2][S_2(T_2) - 1/2]\big\}, \quad (12.30)$$

where S_j is the survival function of T_j $j = 1,2$. That is, ρ is the correlation coefficient between the two uniform variables $S_1(T_1)$ and $S_2(T_2)$. If C is the copula associated with the joint survival function $S(t_1, t_2)$ of T_1 and T_2, then

$$\rho = 12\int_0^1\int_0^1 C(x, y)dxdy - 3. \quad (12.31)$$

Given a random uncensored sample $(T_{1i}, T_{2i}), i = 1,\ldots,n$, from (T_1, T_2), ρ is estimated by the sample (Pearson) correlation coefficient between the ranks of T_{1i}'s and T_{2i}'s. This is because $S_j(t)$ can be estimated by one minus the empirical CDF $F_{nj}(t)$ of T_j and $F_{nj}(T_{ji})$ is the rank of T_{ji} over n, $i = 1,\ldots,n$, $j = 1,2$.

When there is censoring, it may be impossible to nonparametrically identify the complete bivariate survival distribution, in which case none of Pearson correlation coefficient, Kendall's τ and Spearman's correlation coefficient can be nonparametrically estimated. On the other hand, if the bivariate survival function is assumed to be generated from an Archimedean copula, Genest and MacKay [90] showed that Kendall's τ is given by

$$\tau = 4\int_0^1 \kappa(t)dt + 1, \quad \kappa(t) = \frac{\psi(t)}{\psi'(t)}, \quad (12.32)$$

where $\psi'(t)$ is the derivative of $\psi(t)$ and $\psi(t) = \phi^{-1}(t)$, the inverse of the Archimedean generator in (12.27). Spearman's correlation coefficient can be obtained using (12.31). Note that Pearson correlation coefficient depends on the marginal distributions as well as the copula function, therefore its estimation is more involved even under the Archimedean copula model.

The above three measures each gives one numerical value to quantify the dependence between T_1 and T_2. Sometimes, it is of interest to assess how the dependence changes over time. Clayton [44] defined the cross-ratio function

$$\theta(t_1,t_2)=\frac{\lambda(t_1\big|T_2=t_2)}{\lambda(t_1\big|T_2>t_2)},\tag{12.33}$$

where $\lambda(t_1|T_2=t_2)$ and $\lambda(t_1|T_2>t_2)$ are the conditional hazard functions of T_1 given $T_2=t_2$ and $T_2>t_2$, respectively. The cross-ratio is a useful measure for the local dependence between T_1 and T_2 as it is the factor by which the risk of event T_1 at t_1 is increased if the associated T_2 occurs at time t_2 versus the alternate situation when $T_2>t_2$. From the hazard function definition and some algebra, we have

$$\theta(t_1,t_2)=\frac{S(t_1,t_2)\frac{\partial^2 S(t_1,t_2)}{\partial t_1\partial t2}}{\frac{\partial S(t_1,t_2)}{\partial t_1}\frac{\partial S(t_1,t_2)}{\partial t_2}}.\tag{12.34}$$

Also, the cross-ratio can be interpreted as the instantaneous odds ratio at (t_1,t_2) [5]. It equals 1 if and only if T_1 and T_2 are independent.

When the bivariate survival function $S(t_1,t_2)$ is generated by an Archimedean copula with generator ϕ, Oakes [213] showed that

$$\theta(t_1,t_2)=\eta\big[S(t_1,t_2)\big],\tag{12.35}$$

where

$$\eta(x)=-\frac{x\psi''(x)}{\psi'(x)},$$

where ψ'' is the second derivative of ψ, the inverse of ϕ.

Example 12.2 From (12.32), for the Clayton family of multivariate survival functions, Kendall's τ is given by

$$\tau=\frac{\theta}{\theta+2}.\tag{12.36}$$

Spearman's correlation coefficient can be obtained by numerical integration using (12.27) and (12.31). The inverse of the Archimedean copula generator is $\psi(x)=x^{-\theta}-1$. It follows from (12.35) that the cross ratio $\theta(t_1\,t_2)=1+\theta$, a constant function.

Note that from (12.36), the Clayton model only yields positive τ between the two variables. Genest and MacKay [90] extended the Clayton model to allow for negative dependency by using the generator $\phi(t)=(1-t)^{-1/\theta},\theta<0$ with the inverse function $\psi(t)=1-t^{-\theta}$. This function ϕ is no longer a Laplace transform, and in the bivariate case there is a restriction $\theta\geq-1$ [201]. In addition, to avoid negative probability in certain regions, the bivariate survival function is defined as

$$S(t_1,t_2) = \left[\max\{S_1(t_1)^{-\theta} + S_2(t_2)^{-\theta} - 1, 0\}\right]^{-1/\theta}, \quad t_1 > 0, t_2 > 0, -1 \le \theta \le 0. \quad (12.37)$$

More examples and discussions can be found in Genest and MacKay [90] and Genest and Rivest [91].

Let $\Lambda_j(t)$ be the cumulative hazard function of T_j for $j = 1,2$. Assume that the bivariate survival function of (T_1, T_2) is absolutely continuous. Let

$$M_j(t) = I(T_j \le t) - \Lambda_j(t \wedge T_j).$$

Prentice and Cai [246] introduced a covariance function

$$C(t_1,t_2) = Cov[M_1(t_1), M_2(t_2)] = E[M_1(t_1)M_2(t_2)]. \quad (12.38)$$

They showed that the bivariate survival function can be represented in terms of the marginal survivor functions and this covariance function. They also obtained a closely related representation expressing the bivariate survivor function in terms of marginal survivor functions and a conditional covariance function, which leads to a new nonparametric survivor function estimator.

Hsu and Prentice [118] proposed a global dependence measure defined by

$$\rho_\Lambda = Corr[\Lambda_1(T_1), \Lambda_2(T_2)]. \quad (12.39)$$

This measure can be easily estimated when there is no censoring. In the presence of independent right censorship, modeling assumptions are required for its estimation. They proposed a semiparametric class of bivariate failure time models in which a dependence parameter has a one-to-one relationship with ρ_Λ. An estimating function was obtained as a weighted sum over the grid formed by the observed failure times of differences between nonparametric and model-restricted estimates of covariance rates. For a more robustness inference, additional dependency measures were discussed and corresponding nonparametric estimators were proposed.

Using the cross-ratio function $\theta(t_1,t_2)$, Fan, Prentice and Hsu [74] proposed a class of weighted dependence measures

$$D(t_1,t_2) = \frac{\int_0^{t_1}\int_0^{t_2} \phi[\theta(s_1,s_2)]\, w(ds_1,ds_2)}{\int_0^{t_1}\int_0^{t_2} w(ds_1,ds_2)}, \quad (12.40)$$

where ϕ is a fixed function and w is a weight function. This class of measures includes the cross-ratio measure as a special case. Additionally, new cases are identified that avoid the need to estimate the bivariate survival function and permit explicit variance estimators. Nonparametric estimators of these measures were proposed, and consistency and asymptotic normality were established, with variances that can be consistently estimated.

12.6 Parameter Estimation

In copula models for bivariate survival data, the bivariate survival function is determined by the marginal survival functions and a copula function, which is often characterized with a single parameter. This parameter determines Kendall's τ and Spearman's ρ for the bivariate distribution. This simplifying feature suggests that parameters in the marginals and association parameter can be estimated separately by a two-stage procedure as follows:

1. Model and analyze the marginal distributions, for example by the methods in Section 12.1 when the relationships between marginal outcomes and covariates are of interest.

2. Model the dependence between marginal outcomes by an appropriate copula, and then estimate the association parameter using the pseudo-maximum likelihood approach by Gong and Samaniego [103], with estimators from stage one above replacing the parameters in the score function.

Genest, Ghoudi, and Rivest [89] proposed the procedure for uncensored data without covariates. Shih and Louis [278] extended the method to censored data, also without covariates. Glidden [101] further developed the approach by incorporating covariates in the marginal distributions with the proportional hazards model and using the Clayton copula for association.

For the two-stage procedure, estimators for marginal distribution parameters are consistent under the correctly specified marginal distributions, even when the copula model is misspecified. In addition, compared with the alternative approach of nonparametric maximum likelihood estimation, the two stage procedure is computationally stable and much more easily implemented. Details of the proposed estimation methods can be found in the references [278, 89, 101].

For multivariate survival data, in the absence of censoring, Prentice and Hsu [247] used the mean and covariance structure of the cumulative baseline hazard variates and standard baseline hazard function estimators to develop joint estimating equations for parameters in marginal hazard ratios and pairwise correlation models. Under quite general conditions, the resulting estimators are asymptotically normal, and the estimators for parameters in the mean structure are consistent and asymptotically normal, even if the covariance structure is misspecified. See Exercise 12.11 for some related details.

When there is independent right censoring, semiparametric models for pairwise survivor functions are required to generalize these equations. For the Clayton family of bivariate distributions, the resulting equations lead to joint estimators of hazard ratio and cross ratio parameters. Prentice and Hsu showed that the estimators derived from the estimating equations are consistent and asymptotically normal.

Li, Prentice and Lin [168] introduced a class of semiparametric normal transformation models for right censored bivariate failure times. Nonparametric hazard rate models are transformed to a standard normal model and a joint normal distribution is assumed for the bivariate vector of transformed variates. Parameters in the marginal survival distribution and the pairwise correlation were the estimated by maximizing a semiparametric likelihood. The estimators are consistent, asymptotically normal, and semiparametric efficient. See Exercise 12.12 for some related details.

12.7 Exercises and Complements

12.1 Show that the Jacobian matrix of $\boldsymbol{U}(\boldsymbol{\beta})$ in (12.4) is

$$\boldsymbol{B}(\boldsymbol{\beta}) = \frac{1}{n}\sum_{i=1}^{n}\sum_{k=1}^{K}\delta_{ki}\left[\frac{S_k^{(2)}(\boldsymbol{\beta}, X_{ki})}{S_k^{(0)}(\boldsymbol{\beta}, X_{ki})} - \frac{S_k^{(1)}(\boldsymbol{\beta}, X_{ki})S_k^{(1)}(\boldsymbol{\beta}, X_{ki})^{\mathrm{T}}}{S_k^{(0)}(\boldsymbol{\beta}, X_{ki})^2}\right].$$

12.2 Show that the Jacobian matrix of $\widetilde{\boldsymbol{U}}(\boldsymbol{\beta})$ in (12.6) is

$$\widetilde{\boldsymbol{B}}(\boldsymbol{\beta}) = \frac{1}{n}\sum_{i=1}^{n}\sum_{k=1}^{K_i}\delta_{ki}\left[\frac{S^{(2)}(\boldsymbol{\beta}, X_{ki})}{S^{(0)}(\boldsymbol{\beta}, X_{ki})} - \frac{S^{(1)}(\boldsymbol{\beta}, X_{ki})S^{(1)}(\boldsymbol{\beta}, X_{ki})^{\mathrm{T}}}{S^{(0)}(\boldsymbol{\beta}, X_{ki})^2}\right].$$

12.3 Show that the gamma distribution with shape parameter α and rate parameter β has mean α/β and variance α/β^2.

12.4 (a) Prove (12.12) and (12.13).

(b) Obtain the marginal PDFs $f_j(t_j),\ j = 1,2$.

(c) Suppose that the frailty γ has a positive stable distribution instead of a gamma distribution, with the Laplace transform

$$\mathfrak{L}(s) = \exp(-s^{\alpha}),$$

$0 < \alpha < 1$. Use (12.11) to obtain the bivariate survival function and the marginal survival functions.

12.5 For the marginal hazard ratio in (12.22), verify the monotonicity and boundedness properties mentioned in Section 12.3.

12.6 Verify (12.24).

12.7 For a CDF F, define

$$F^{-1}(x) = \inf\{t : F(t) \geq x\},\ x \in [0,1].$$

When the set is empty (as in the case of $x = 1$ with $F(t) < 1$ at any t), $F^{-1}(x)$ is defined to be ∞.

(a) Let F be discrete having mass 1/2 at 1 and 2. Plot F.

(b) Find F^{-1} and plot it. Show that the plot can be obtained from that of F by reflecting it over the diagonal line.

(b) Let y=$F^{-1}(x)$. Show that for $0 < x < 1$,

$$F_{-}(y) \leq x \leq F(y).$$

Hint: By the definition, there are $\xi_n \geq y$ and $\xi_n \downarrow y$ such that $F(\xi_n) \geq x$ for each n. Also recall that F is right continuous. Similarly, there are $\eta_n < y$ and $\eta_n \uparrow y$ such that $F(\eta_n) < x$ for each n.

12.8 By the change of variable formula (A.11) in Appendix A,

$$\int_0^t h'(G(x))dG(x) = h(G(t)) - h(G(0)) \tag{12.41}$$

for continuous G and differentiable h. Assume that $F(t)$ is continuous.

(a) Show that $F(T)$ has the uniform distribution on $[0,1]$.

Hint: Apply (12.41) to

$$P(F(T) \leq t) = EI(F(T) \leq t) = \int_0^\infty I(F(s) \leq t)dF(s).$$

(b) Show that $\Lambda(T)$ has the standard exponential distribution.

12.9 Verify the results in Example 12.2 for the Clayton bivariate survival function. That is,

$$\psi(x) = x^{-\theta} - 1,$$

and

$$\tau = \frac{\theta}{\theta+2}, \quad \theta(t_1, t_2) = 1 + \theta.$$

12.10 In the shared frailty setting described in Section 12.3 without covariates, use equation (12.34) to derive the cross-ratio function for the gamma frailty and the positive stable frailty.

12.11 Suppose that (T_1, T_2) has the Clayton bivariate survival function

$$S(t_1, t_2) = \left[S_1(t_1)^{-\theta} + S_2(t_1)^{-\theta} - 1\right]^{-1/\theta},$$

where S_j is the survival function of T_j for $j = 1,2$. Let Λ_j be the cumulative hazard function of T_j.

(a) Show that the survival function of $(\Lambda_1(T_1), \Lambda_2(T_2))$ is

$$S_\theta(t_1, t_2) = \left[e^{\theta t_1} + e^{\theta t_2} - 1\right]^{-1/\theta},$$

(b) Let $A(y_1, y_2)$ be the bivariate survival function of the nonnegative random variables Y_1 and Y_2. Show that

$$EY_1Y_2 = \int_0^\infty \int_0^\infty A(y_1, y_2)dy_1dy_2.$$

This result is the two-dimensional analog of the univariate result (2.61).

Hint: Use

$$A(y_1, y_2) = EI(Y_1 > y_1, Y_2 > y_2).$$

(c) Let

$$\rho = E\left[\Lambda_1(T_1)\Lambda_2(T_2))\right] - E\Lambda_1(T_1)E\Lambda_2(T_2),$$

the covariance between $\Lambda_1(T_1)$ and $\Lambda_2(T_2)$. Note that ρ is also the correlation between $\Lambda_1(T_1)$ and $\Lambda_2(T_2)$. Show that

$$\rho = \int_0^\infty \int_0^\infty S_\theta(y_1, y_2)dy_1dy_2 - 1.$$

Prentice and Hsu [247] used this result to connect the correlation parameter to the association parameter in the bivariate model.

12.12 Let (T_1, T_2) be a bivariate vector of event times. Assume that T_j has a continuous CDF $F_j(t)$, $j = 1,2$.

(a) Define $\tilde{T}_j = \Phi^{-1}\left[F_j(T_j)\right]$, where Φ^{-1} is the inverse of the standard normal CDF Φ. Show that $\tilde{T}_j$ has the standard normal distribution.

(b) Assume that $(\tilde{T}_1, \tilde{T}_2)$ is bivariate normal with standard normal marginals and correlation ρ. Let

$$\Psi(z_1, z_2) = P(\tilde{T}_1 > z_1, \tilde{T}_2 > z_2).$$

Show that the joint survival function $S(t_1, t_2)$ of (T_1, T_2) is

$$S(t_1, t_2) = \Psi\{\Phi^{-1}\left[F_1(t_1)\right], \Phi^{-1}\left[F_2(t_2)\right]\}.$$

Li, Prentice and Lin [168] used this type of normal transformations to introduced a class of semiparametric bivariate transformation models for right censored data.

12.13 Suppose two sequential events $Y_1 < Y_2$ are subject to independent censoring by C. The events Y_1 and Y_2 can be, for example, times to the first and second emergency room visits for treating a particular condition. Let (Y_{1i}, Y_{2i}, C_i) be i.i.d. copies of (Y_1, Y_2, C). The observable data are $(\widetilde{Y}_{1i}, \widetilde{Y}_{2i}, \delta_{1i}, \delta_{2i})$, where

$$\widetilde{Y}_{ji} = Y_{ji} \wedge C_i, \quad \delta_{ji} = I(Y_{ji} \le C_i), \quad j = 1,2, \ 1 \le i \le n.$$

Suppose the gap times $T_1 = Y_1$, $T_2 = Y_2 - Y_1$ are of interest. Note that T_2 is censored by $C - Y_1$ which is correlated to T_2. Thus methods assuming independent censoring are no longer valid for estimating the marginal distributions of T_2 and the joint distribution of (T_1, T_2). The nonparametric estimation method of Lin, Sun and Ying [175] is outlined below.

Assume that the joint distribution function F of (T_1, T_2) is continuous. Let

$$H(t_1, t_2) = P(T_1 \le t_1, T_2 > t_2).$$

Then $F(t_1, t_2) = H(t_1, 0) - H(t_1, t_2)$.

(a) Let (T_{1i}, T_{2i}), $1 \le i \le n$ be i.i.d. copies of (T_1, T_2). Note that $\widetilde{Y}_{2i} > \widetilde{Y}_{1i}$ implies that $\widetilde{Y}_{1i} = T_{1i}$. Use this fact to show that

$$I(\widetilde{Y}_{1i} \le t_1, \widetilde{Y}_{2i} - \widetilde{Y}_{1i} > t_2) = I(T_{1i} \le t_1, T_{2i} > t_2, C_i > T_{1i} + t_2).$$

(b) Show that

$$E\big[I(\widetilde{Y}_{1i} \le t_1, \widetilde{Y}_{2i} - \widetilde{Y}_{1i} > t_2) \big| T_{1i}, T_{2i}\big] = I(T_{1i} \le t_1, T_{2i} > t_2) G(T_{1i} + t_2),$$

where G is the survival function of C. Thus

$$E\left[\frac{I(\widetilde{Y}_{1i} \le t_1, \widetilde{Y}_{2i} - \widetilde{Y}_{1i} > t_2)}{G(T_{1i} + t_2)} \Big| T_{1i}, T_{2i}\right] = I(T_{1i} \le t_1, T_{2i} > t_2).$$

Note that this result requires that $G(T_{1i} + t_2) > 0$. It follows that

$$\widetilde{H}(t_1, t_2) = n^{-1} \sum_{i=1}^{n} \frac{I(\widetilde{Y}_{1i} \le t_1, \widetilde{Y}_{2i} - \widetilde{Y}_{1i} > t_2)}{G(\widetilde{Y}_{1i} + t_2)}$$

would be an unbiased estimator of $H(t_1, t_2)$ if G were known. Lin, Sun and Ying used the Kaplan-Meier estimator $\widehat{G}$ of G to obtain the estimator

$$\widehat{H}(t_1, t_2) = n^{-1} \sum_{i=1}^{n} \frac{I(\widetilde{Y}_{1i} \le t_1, \widetilde{Y}_{2i} - \widetilde{Y}_{1i} > t_2)}{\widehat{G}(\widetilde{Y}_{1i} + t_2)}.$$

Then $F(t_1, t_2)$ can be estimated by

$$\widehat{F}(t_1, t_2) = \widehat{H}(t_1, 0) - \widehat{H}(t_1, t_2).$$

13

Competing Risks Analysis

13.1 Introduction

Before Chapter Twelve, the focus was primarily on univariate analysis, where each individual contributes only one time-to-event outcome of a single type. In clinical trials, however, the benefit of a treatment is often reflected in multiple outcomes of interest. A common practice is to combine these outcomes and define a single time-to-event variable as the time to the first among outcomes considered, then apply the models and analysis techniques discussed in the previous chapters. This approach is sometimes referred to as the time-to-first-event analysis or a composite outcome analysis. Additionally, earlier discussions often assumed that the time-to-event and censoring variables were independent.

In Chapter Twelve, an individual contributes multiple time-to-event outcomes that are of interest and subject to independent censoring. The outcomes may be dependent, but they do not censor each other.

This chapter discusses an extension of univariate analysis to *competing risks*, where an individual is at risk of experiencing one of several event types. Crucially, once one event occurs, it prevents the observation of any other potential event types for that individual; i.e., it censors other event types. Since different events from the same individual are very likely dependent, this situation differs from what was considered in Chapter Twelve, where the censoring was assumed to be independent of the time-to-event variables. Another distinction is that in competing risks analysis, an individual contributes only one event, whereas in Chapter Twelve, an individual could potentially experience all the events of interest.

It will be shown, among other things, that the log-rank test and the Cox proportional hazards model remain applicable, but the results should be interpreted somewhat differently. Additionally, it will also be shown that the Kaplan-Meier estimator of event probability may lack validity or interpretability without additional assumptions.

In the competing risks framework, each individual still contributes only one event; however, there is now an additional variable that indicates the event type. This differs from semi-competing risks analysis, which will be discussed in the next chapter. This chapter focuses on major topics related to clinical trial applications. For more discussions and examples, readers can refer to textbooks and

DOI: 10.1201/9780429324437-13

tutorials by authors such as Kalbfleisch and Prentice [131], Crowder [56], Pintilie [233], and Putter [255].

13.2 Competing Risks Data and Related Functions

A typical example of competing risks is when death of a specific type is considered. In cardiovascular trials, the interest may be in cardiovascular death. Then, death due to other causes represents a competing risk. It is also possible to have several competing risks, by breaking non-cardiovascular death into different categories.

Note that censoring by death due to other causes is likely dependent on the event under study. This differs from censoring due to random loss to follow-up or the conclusion of a trial. In the latter two scenarios, censoring can reasonably be assumed to be independent of the event under study, given the treatment assignment.

The often adopted practice of using composite outcomes gives rise to a couple of competing risks scenarios. Suppose the primary endpoint of a trial is the composite of cardiovascular death and heart failure hospitalization. First, in the primary analysis, death due to other causes is the competing risk that censors the outcome of interest. Second, typically among secondary analyses of a trial, assessment of treatment effect on components of the composite primary endpoint is included. For the secondary analysis of treatment effect on heart failure hospitalization, all cause mortality is the competing risk that censors the event of interest.

In the above example, if the first event an individual experiences is heart failure hospitalization, typically the follow-up continues until death or censoring. But as far as the time-to-first-event analysis is concerned, the individual still contributes only one outcome, and the first-event-only restriction gives rise to a competing risks scenario. The next chapter will discuss analysis approaches that incorporate both heart failure hospitalization and cardiovascular death outcomes, when such data are available.

Suppose that the event an individual may experience is of K distinct types. In applications, it is possible to observe an event caused by more than one factor. In such cases, additional event types can be defined to account for these scenarios, ensuring that the assumption of K distinct event types still holds. Let T be the time until an event occurs and D the event type indicator, respectively, with D taking values $1,\ldots,K$. Assume that the distribution of T is absolutely continuous. From (2.4), the instantaneous rate of occurrence of event, without considering event types, is

$$\lambda(t) = \lim_{h\downarrow 0} P\left[t \le T < t+h \middle| T \ge t\right]/h, \text{ for } t \text{ with } P(T \ge t) > 0.$$

Now for event of type $D = k$, it is natural to extend the above definition to the *cause-specific hazard function*

$$\lambda_k(t) = \lim_{h\downarrow 0} P\left[t \le T < t+h, D = k \middle| T \ge t\right]/h, \text{ for } t \text{ with } P(T \ge t) > 0, \qquad (13.1)$$

$k = 1,\ldots,K$, where absolute continuity of the distribution of T with $D = k$ is assumed to ensure that the limits exist.

The cause-specific hazard function is the instantaneous rate of occurrence of a type k event given that no event of any type has occurred. In other words, it represents the instantaneous rate of a type k event in the presence of all other competing event types. From the definitions, it follows that

$$\lambda(t) = \sum_{k=1}^{K} \lambda_k(t). \qquad (13.2)$$

Similar to the cumulative hazard function of event $\Lambda(t) = \int_0^t \lambda(s)ds$, define the cumulative hazard function of type k event

$$\Lambda_k(t) = \int_0^t \lambda_k(s)ds. \qquad (13.3)$$

Then

$$\Lambda(t) = \sum_{k=1}^{K} \Lambda_k(t). \qquad (13.4)$$

Let $S(t) = P(T > t)$ be the overall survival function. From (2.8) and (13.2),

$$S(t) = \exp\{-\Lambda(t)\} = \exp\{-\sum_{k=1}^{K}\int_0^t \lambda_k(s)ds\}, \qquad (13.5)$$

For event of type k, define the (sub-) PDF

$$f_k(t) = \lim_{h\downarrow 0} P(t \le T < t+h, D = k)/h. \qquad (13.6)$$

From (13.1) and (13.5),

$$f_k(t) = \lambda_k(t)S_{-}(t) = \lambda_k(t)\exp\{-\sum_{\ell=1}^{K}\int_0^t \lambda_\ell(s)ds\}. \qquad (13.7)$$

Note that the PDF $f(t)$ of T is given by

$$f(t) = \sum_{k=1}^{K} f_k(t).$$

The *cumulative incidence function* (CIF) for event of type k is

$$F_k(t) = P(T \le t, D = k) = \int_0^t f_k(s)ds, \ t \ge 0, \tag{13.8}$$

$k = 1, \ldots, K$. $F_k(t)$ is the probability that an event occurs within time interval $[0, t]$ and the event type is k, or equivalently, the probability that type k event is observed within $[0, t]$, in the presence of other competing event types. It represents the expected proportion of individuals with event of type k over $[0, t]$. Note that $F_k(t)$ is a sub-distribution function and

$$\lim_{t\to\infty} F_k(t) = P(D = k), k = 1, \ldots, K, \tag{13.9}$$

with $\sum_{k=1}^{K} P(D = k) = 1$. From (13.7) and (13.8),

$$F_k(t) = \int_0^t f_k(s)ds = \int_0^t S_-(s)d\Lambda_k(s). \tag{13.10}$$

In the above setup, the functions are defined based on observable quantities. No assumptions are made about whether the underlying processes leading to events of different types are independent or not, nor about the nature of dependence structure if they are dependent. More discussions on this will be given in Section 13.6. Quantities discussed here have "crude" rather than "net" interpretation as discussed in Tsiatis [300].

To derive estimators of $\Lambda_k(t)$ and $F_k(t)$, consider the *random censorship model for competing risks data* specified as follows for ease of presentation: $(T_1, D_1), \ldots, (T_n, D_n)$ are *i.i.d.* copies of (T, D). The censoring variables $C_1, \ldots, C_n$ are independent which are also independent of $(T_1, D_1), \ldots, (T_n, D_n)$. The observed data are $(X_i, \delta_i), 1 \le i \le n$, where $X_i = T_i \wedge C_i$ and $\delta_i = D_i I(X_i = T_i)$. With these notations, δ_i indicates the event type when the event is observed, and $\delta_i = 0$ if the event is censored.

For $k \in \{1, \ldots, K\}$, define the counting process for the ith individual and event of type k

$$N_{ik}(t) = I(X_i \le t, \delta_i = k), \tag{13.11}$$

and let

$$H_k(t) = \sum_{i=1}^{n} N_{ik}(t). \tag{13.12}$$

Then $H_k(t)$ parallels $H(t)$ in (2.43). The Nelson-Aalen estimator of $\Lambda_k(t)$ is

$$\widehat{\Lambda}_k(t) = \int_0^t \frac{dH_k(s)}{K(s)}. \tag{13.13}$$

for $K(t)$ in (2.43), the number of individuals at risk of event at time t. Let

$$\widehat{F}_k(t) = \int_0^t \widehat{S}_-(s) d\widehat{\Lambda}_k(s), \tag{13.14}$$

where $\widehat{S}(t)$ is the Ka[plan-Meier estimator of $P(T > t)$. An argument similar to that in Section 2.4 can show that under the random censorship model, $\widehat{\Lambda}_k(t)$ and $\widehat{F}_k(t)$ are the nonparametric maximum likelihood estimators of $\Lambda_k(t)$ and $F_k(t)$, respectively.

Note that $H_k(t)$ counts the number of type k events in $[0, t]$. It is exactly $H(t)$ in (2.43) if events of other types are treated as part of censoring along with the C_i's. In other words, if the Nelson-Aalen estimator in (2.44) is naively applied to a scenario where censoring is due to both competing events and independent censoring, then it estimates $\Lambda_k(t)$. It can also be shown that the variance estimator in (2.46) remains valid. Thus, when the Nelson-Aalen estimator and its variance estimator are used in a competing risks setting— by treating it as a simple univariate problem—the function being estimated is $\Lambda_k(t)$, and the point and interval estimates remain unchanged,

The situation with Kaplan-Meier estimator is more complex. Caution is required when interpreting the Kaplan-Meier estimator $F_k^*(t) = 1 - \mathcal{P}_{(0,t]}(1 - d\widehat{\Lambda}_k)$ in the presence of competing events. Note that $F_k^*(t)$ estimates $\widetilde{F}_k(t) = 1 - \exp[-\Lambda_k(t)]$. In a hypothetical scenario where competing risks are removed, $F_k^*(t)$ would estimate the probability of type k event by time t. However, this hypothetical population, where competing risks are removed, may not be the most relevant for clinical or policy decision-making. This is because the instantaneous rate for a type k event in the presence of competing risks may differ from the rate in an environment where the competing risks are removed [131, 226].

For the Kaplan-Meier estimator to have a meaningful probability interpretation, two conditions have to be met:

1. Competing risks can be removed;

2. Such removal does not alter the risk for the event of interest.

These two assumptions may be reasonable in certain specific cases of industrial reliability studies. However, in clinical trials, they are often too stringent and rarely hold true, as discussed and demonstrated in Kalbfleisch and Prentice [131]. Without additional assumptions, the only estimable probability function related to event of type k is the CIF $F_k(t)$.

Note also that

$$\begin{aligned} F_k(t) &= \int_0^t \exp[-\Lambda(s)]d\Lambda_k(s) \\ &\le \int_0^t \exp[-\Lambda_k(s)]d\Lambda_k(s) \\ &= 1-\exp[-\Lambda_k(t)] = \widetilde{F}_k(t), \end{aligned} \qquad (13.15)$$

with strict inequality if $\Lambda_\ell(t_0) > 0$ for some $\ell \neq k$ and $t_0 > 0$. Thus in general, the Kaplan-Meier estimator $F_k^*(t)$ is greater than $\widehat{F}_k(t)$. In particular, if $F_k^*(t)$ is used to estimate the event probability for each type, then sum of all the estimates may exceed $\widehat{F}(t) = 1-\widehat{S}(t)$, the estimated probability of an event by time t regardless of the event type. Consequently, the sum may exceed 1.

13.3 Cause-Specific Hazards vs. Cumulative Incidence Functions

From (13.5), (13.10) and the definitions, we have

$$\begin{aligned} \lambda_k(t) &= \frac{f_k(t)}{S(t)} = \frac{f_k(t)}{1-\sum_{\ell=1}^K F_\ell(t)}, \\ F_k(t) &= \int_0^t f_k(s)ds = \int_0^t \lambda_k(s)\exp\left\{-\sum_{\ell=1}^K \int_0^s \lambda_\ell(x)dx\right\}ds. \end{aligned} \qquad (13.16)$$

Therefore, either $(\lambda_1,\ldots,\lambda_K)$ or $(F_1,\ldots,F_K)$ completely describes the distribution of (T,D). However, note that from (13.16), F_k depends not only on λ_k, but also on λ_ℓ, $\ell \neq k$, the cause-specific hazards of competing risks.

Typically, a trial focuses on a specific event type. While competing risks from other event types need to be properly accounted for in the analysis, the impact of the treatment on these other event types may not be of primary concern. This could explain, though not justify, the common misuse of the Kaplan-Meier estimator $1-\mathcal{P}_{(0,t]}(1-d\widehat{\Lambda}_k)$ when there are competing risks.

In such situations, instead of using the Kaplan-Meier estimator (which requires strong assumptions to be meaningful) or the CIF estimator (which depends on the treatment effects on competing risks), the Nelson-Aalen estimator, $\widehat{\Lambda}_k(t)$, can be used to indicate group differences in the risks for the event of interest, without distortion from other event types.

Dependence of F_k on competing event types may sometimes yield quite misleading results, as the following example illustrates.

Example 13.1. Suppose that in a two-arm trial, there are two competing event types and type 1 is of interest. Suppose further that events of both types are adverse. Assume that

$$\Lambda_{1C}(t) = t, \qquad \Lambda_{2C}(t) = 0.7t,$$

where Λ_{1C} and Λ_{2C} are the cumulative cause-specific hazard functions for type 1 and type 2 events in the control group, respectively. Assume also that the follow-up stops at $t = 1$.

Consider two treatment effect scenarios:

A.

$$\Lambda_{1T}(t) = 0.6\Lambda_{1C}(t), \qquad \Lambda_{2T}(t) = 0.6\Lambda_{2C}(t),$$

B.

$$\Lambda_{1T}(t) = \Lambda_{1C}(t), \qquad \Lambda_{2T}(t) = 2.2\Lambda_{2C}(t),$$

where Λ_{1T} and Λ_{2T} are the cumulative cause-specific hazard functions for type 1 and type 2 events in the treatment group, respectively. Note that both scenarios assume proportional treatment effects on the cause-specific hazards for both event types.

Scenario A depicts an ideal situation where the treatment reduces the hazards of both event types by 40%, despite the primary focus of the trial being on the type 1 event. On the other hand, in Scenario B, there is no treatment effect on the event type of interest, and, to complicate matters further, the treatment more than doubles the risk for type 2 event. While this scenario is extreme, it serves as a valuable example to illustrate some important points.

The cumulative hazard functions $\Lambda_{1C}(t)$ and $\Lambda_{1T}(t)$ clearly show the treatment's beneficial effect on type 1 event in Scenario A, and its null effect in Scenario B. The plots, which have been omitted as they are plots of simple linear functions with zero intercept, would show that, for type 1 event, the treatment reduces the cumulative hazard function in Scenario A, but yields no change in Scenario B.

However, Figure 13.1 shows that the treatment results in a reduced CIF in both scenarios. This may seem surprising at first, but there is a logical explanation: In Scenario B, the treatment increases the risk of type 2 event, leading to a higher number of type 2 events and consequently fewer type 1 events, as the occurrence of a type 2 event prevents a type 1 event from happening.

To distinguish between Scenario A and Scenario B using CIFs, one could supplement Figure 13.1 with CIF curves for the type 2 event. However, this approach would be more cumbersome and still would not directly address the question of whether the risk of type 1 event is reduced by the treatment—a question that can be simply answered using the cumulative hazard functions, Λ_{1C} and Λ_{1T}, for the type 1 event.

Scenario B represents an extreme case, as treatment effects typically trend in the same direction for different event types. However, even in such cases, the

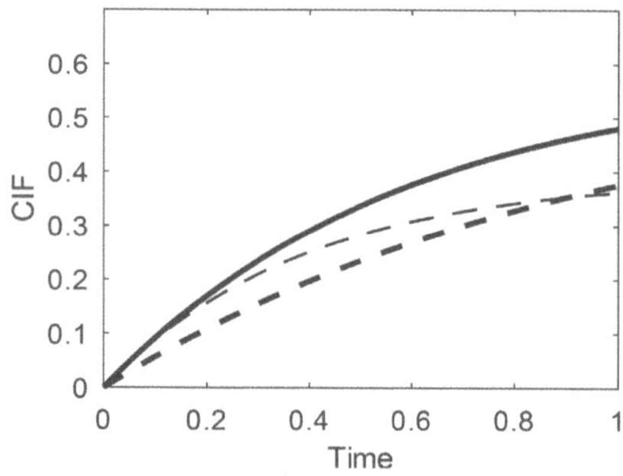

FIGURE 13.1
Cumulative incidence functions for type 1 event in Scenarios A and B. Solid—control group; thick dashed—treatment group in Scenario A; thin dashed—treatment group in Scenario B.

distortion caused by type 2 events remains present. Consider two more treatment effect scenarios:

C.
$$\Lambda_{1T}(t) = 0.6\Lambda_{1C}(t), \quad \Lambda_{2T}(t) = 0.4\Lambda_{2C}(t),$$

D.
$$\Lambda_{1T}(t) = 0.6\Lambda_{1C}(t), \quad \Lambda_{2T}(t) = 0.9\Lambda_{2C}(t),$$

Two conclusions can be drawn based on the assumed parameters:

1. If the attention is focused solely on type 1 event, the treatment is equally effective in both Scenarios C and D, demonstrating a 40% reduction in the hazard rate.

2. Overall, the treatment has a stronger beneficial effect in Scenario C than in Scenario D. Specifically, the hazard ratios for an event, regardless of type, are 0.52 and 0.72 in Scenarios C and D, respectively.

Figures 13.2. and 13.3 show the ratios

$$\frac{F_{1T}(t)}{F_{1C}(t)}, \quad \frac{-\log[1 - F_{1T}(t)]}{-\log[1 - F_{1C}(t)]}$$

for type 1 event in Scenario C and Scenario D, respectively. The second ratio is the ratio of cumulative sub-distribution hazards [104, 76]. These two ratios will be

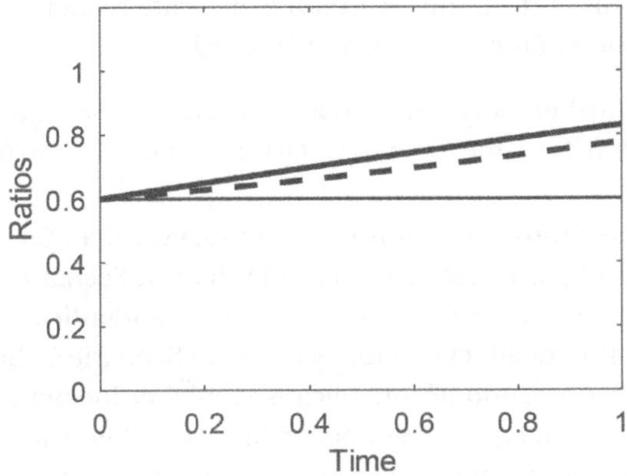

FIGURE 13.2
Cumulative hazard functions for type 1 event in Scenario C. Solid— $F_{1T}(t)/F_{1C}(t)$; dashed—$\log[1-F_{1T}(t)]/\log[1-F_{1C}(t)]$.

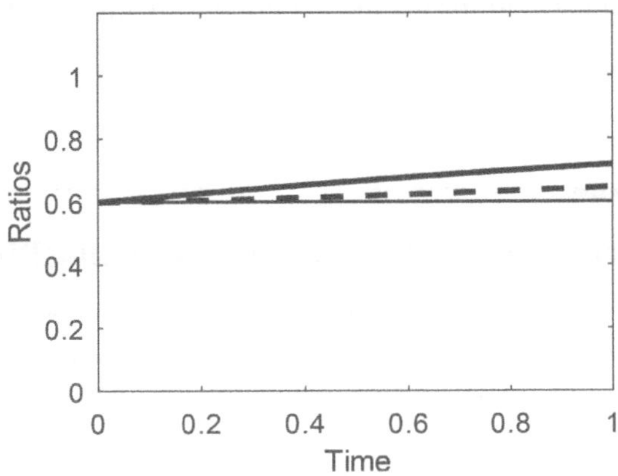

FIGURE 13.3
Cumulative hazard functions for type 1 event in Scenario D. Solid— $F_{1T}(t)/F_{1C}(t)$; dashed—$\log[1-F_{1T}(t)]/\log[1-F_{1C}(t)]$.

referred to as the CIF ratio and the CSDH ratio, respectively. Note that a beneficial treatment effect corresponds to a value < 1 for either ratio.

The plots show that:

1. In both Scenarios C and D, the treatment has a beneficial effect on type 1 event, with a CIF ratio or CSDH ratio between .6 and 1. However, either ratio increases over time, moving closer to 1 and further away from 0.6. In particular, for Scenario C, at $t = 1$, the CIF and CSDH ratios are 0.83 and 0.78,

respectively. This corresponds to about a 20% rate reduction, which is half of the rate reduction in the cause-specific hazard.

2. The ratios are further away from 1 in Scenario D than Scenario C. In particular, for Scenario D, at $t = 1$, the CIF and CSDH ratios are 0.72 and 0.65, respectively,

Therefore, these ratios might misleadingly suggest that, for type 1 event, the treatment has a stronger effect in Scenario D than in Scenario C. However, this impression is incorrect, as the effect on type 1 event is identical in both scenarios, and the overall treatment effect is actually better in Scenario C than in Scenario D. The misleading phenomenon occurs because a higher incidence of type 2 event reduces the likelihood of type 1 event occurring. Also, this example demonstrates that these ratios will usually be closer to 1 than the ratio of cause-specific hazards.

The CIF $F_k(t)$ is influenced by competing event types. However, clinical trials usually focus on one specific event type. Consequently, for etiological/causal inference of treatment effects, typically cause-specific hazard functions are used. CIFs are valuable tools for assessing and predicting absolute risks, and for informing decision-making regarding the net benefit of a treatment on a specific disease type [154, 137].

13.4 Comparison of Two Samples of Competing Risks Data

Similar to how the Nelson-Aalen estimator can be extended to competing risks data, weighted log-rank tests can be adapted to compare two cumulative hazard functions for event of type k. Denote the cumulative hazard functions for event of type k in the two groups by Λ_{kC}, Λ_{kT}, respectively. Assume that the quadruplets (T_i, D_i, Z_i, C_i), $i = 1, \ldots, n$, are independent, where T_i, D_i are time to event and event type indicator, respectively, Z_i is the indicator function of the treatment group, and $C_1, \ldots, C_n$ are the censoring variables. Assume also that given Z_i, (T_i, D_i) and C_i are independent and that the conditional cumulative hazard function for event of type k is $Z_i\Lambda_{kT} + (1 - Z_i)\Lambda_{kC}$, $k = 1, \ldots, K$. Furthermore, assume that for all event types the cumulative hazard functions are absolutely continuous. The available data are $(X_i, \delta_i, Z_i), 1 \le i \le n$, where

$$X_i = T_i \wedge C_i, \; \delta_i = D_i I(X_i = T_i), \; 1 \le i \le n.$$

For testing

$$H_0 : \Lambda_{kT} = \Lambda_{kC} \quad \text{vs.} \quad H_a : \Lambda_{kT} \ne \Lambda_{kC}, \tag{13.17}$$

the weighted log-rank test statistic with weight Φ is

$$\sum_{i=1}^{n} \int_0^\infty \Phi(t)\Big(Z_i - \frac{K_T(t)}{K(t)}\Big) dN_{ik}(t), \tag{13.18}$$

where Φ satisfies certain regularity conditions and K_C, K_T are as in (2.48). Similarly to (2.55), the statistic can be re-written as

$$\int_0^\infty \frac{K_C(t)K_T(t)}{K_C(t)+K_T(t)} d\big(\widehat{\Lambda}_{kT}(t) - \widehat{\Lambda}_{kC}(t)\big), \tag{13.19}$$

where

$$\widehat{\Lambda}_{kC}(t) = \int_0^t \frac{d\sum_{i=1}^n (1-Z_i)N_{ik}(t)}{K_C(t)}, \quad \widehat{\Lambda}_{kT}(t) = \int_0^t \frac{d\sum_{i=1}^n Z_i N_{ik}(t)}{K_T(t)}, \tag{13.20}$$

the Nelson-Aalen estimators of the cumulative hazard functions $\Lambda_{kC}(t)$, $\Lambda_{kT}(t)$, respectively.

Let

$$M_{ik}(t) = N_{ik}(t) - \int_0^t Y_i(s) d[Z_i\Lambda_{kT}(s) + (1-Z_i)\Lambda_{kC}(s)], \tag{13.21}$$

for $1 \le i \le n$, $1 \le k \le K$. Then, similar to the derivation in Section 11.2, it can be shown that $M_{ik}(t)$'s are martingales with predictable variation processes

$$\langle M_{ik}, M_{ik}\rangle(t) = \int_0^t Y_i(s) d[Z_i\Lambda_{kT}(s) + (1-Z_i)\Lambda_{kC}(s)], \quad 1 \le i \le n, \ 1 \le k \le K. \tag{13.22}$$

Furthermore, it can be shown [104, 95] that the martingales are orthogonal to each other:

$$\langle M_{ik}, M_{j\ell}\rangle(t) = 0 \quad \text{when } (i,k) \ne (j,\ell). \tag{13.23}$$

Thus when Φ is predictable, similarly to (2.53), it can be shown that the variance of the weighted log-rank statistic in (13.18) is

$$\int_0^\infty \frac{\Phi^2(t)K_C(t)K_T(t)}{K(t)} d\widehat{\Lambda}_k(t), \tag{13.24}$$

where $\widehat{\Lambda}_k(t)$ is as defined in (13.13) and, in this context, it is the pooled Nelson-Aalen estimator for the common cumulative hazard function for type k event under the null hypothesis H_0. Analogous to the discussions in Sections 6.6.2 and 9.2, for Φ that is not predictable, the variance formula (13.24) is also asymptotically valid under appropriate conditions.

The preceding discussion demonstrates that the weighted log-rank test and its variance formula are identical to those obtained from a univariate survival analysis when events of other types are treated as censoring. However, the relevant null hypothesis is the equality of the cumulative cause-specific hazard functions for type k event between the two groups, rather than the equality of two cumulative distribution functions.

Sometimes it may be of interest to test the hypothesis of equality between $F_{kT}(t)$ and $F_{kC}(t)$, the CIFs in the treatment and control groups for type k event, respectively. Gray [104] proposed the class of test statistics

$$\int_0^\infty \Phi(t)\Big[\frac{d\widehat{F}_{kT}(t)}{1-\widehat{F}_{kT-}(t)} - \frac{d\widehat{F}_{kC}(t)}{1-\widehat{F}_{kC-}(t)}\Big], \tag{13.25}$$

where $\Phi(t)$ is a weight function, $\widehat{F}_{kC}(t)$ is the estimated CIF for the control group, obtained similarly to (13.14) but using only the control group data, and $\widehat{F}_{kT}(t)$ is the corresponding estimated CIF for the treatment group. When $K=1$, this class of test statistics reduces to the class of weighted log-rank tests. In general, this statistic essentially compares weighted averages of $\lambda_k^* = f_k/(1-F_k)$ between the control and treatment groups. The function λ_k^* will be discussed further in Section 13.7. Under certain regularity conditions, Gray [104] established the asymptotic normality of these test statistics under both the null and local alternative hypotheses.

Pepe and Mori[226] proposed the class of test statistics

$$\int_0^\infty \Phi(t)\big[\widehat{F}_{kT}(t) - \widehat{F}_{kC}(t)\big]dt. \tag{13.26}$$

where $\Phi(t)$ is a weight function. This statistic is a weighted sum of differences in the values of the two estimated CIFs directly. Under appropriate regularity conditions, Pepe and Mori [226] established the asymptotic normality of these test statistics under the null hypothesis.

Lin [171] considered the Kolmogorov-Smirnov type statistic

$$\sup_t \Phi(t)\big|\widehat{F}_{kT}(t) - \widehat{F}_{kC}(t)\big|. \tag{13.27}$$

To obtain critical values of this test statistic, a Monte Carlo method similar to that in Section 6.5 was used. This Kolmogorov-Smirnov type test is consistent against any alternatives under which $F_{kT}(t) \neq F_{kC}(t)$ for some t in the data range. In contrast, the tests of Gray and Pepe and Mori can be more sensitive to certain specific departures from the null hypothesis of equal CIFs.

13.5 Regression

Suppose that in addition to (T, D), time-dependent covariate vector $\boldsymbol{W}(t)$ is also available. By (6.11), the conditional instantaneous rate of event given the covariate history, without considering event types, is

$$\lambda[t;\boldsymbol{W}(t)] = \lim_{h\downarrow 0} P\big[t \le T < t+h \big| T \ge t, \boldsymbol{W}^h(t)\big]/h.$$

Now for event of type $D = k$, given the covariate $\boldsymbol{W}(t)$, define the conditional cause-specific hazard function

$$\lambda_k[t;\boldsymbol{W}(t)] = \lim_{h\downarrow 0} P\big[t \le T < t+h, D=k \big| T \ge t, \boldsymbol{W}^h(t)\big]/h, \tag{13.28}$$

for $k = 1,\ldots,K$, where absolute continuity of relevant functions are assumed to ensure that the limits exist.

While more general results can be obtained for time-dependent covariates, both internal and external, under an appropriately formed independent censoring condition for modeling and analysis using cause-specific hazard functions [131, 7], it is important to note that, analogous to univariate analysis in Chapter Six, including internal covariates renders the estimation of the CIF or the covariate effects on CIF meaningless. To maintain the connection between the cause-specific hazard functions and the CIFs, we consider the random censorship model for competing risks data with time-dependent external covariates.

First, the definition of external covariates in Section 6.2 need to be extended to competing risks data. This extension is achieved by requiring conditions analogous to (6.12) for each cause-specific hazard function. For external covariate $\boldsymbol{W}(t)$, define the conditional (sub-) PDF by

$$f_k[t;\boldsymbol{W}(t)] = \lim_{h\downarrow 0} P\big[t \le T < t+h, D=k \big| \boldsymbol{W}^h(t)\big]/h, \tag{13.29}$$

assuming that the limits exist.

Similarly define the conditional survival function of T by

$$S[t;\boldsymbol{W}(t)] = P\big(T > t \big| \boldsymbol{W}^h(t)\big), \tag{13.30}$$

and the conditional cumulative incidence function

$$F_k(t;\boldsymbol{W}(t)] = P\big(T \le t, D=k \big| \boldsymbol{W}^h(t)\big). \tag{13.31}$$

To simplify notations, it is easier to work with the entire covariate path $\boldsymbol{W}_i^* = \{\boldsymbol{W}_i(t) : t \ge 0\}$. Similar to the discussion in Section 6.2, we have

$$\begin{aligned}
\lambda_k[t;\boldsymbol{W}(t)] &= \lambda_k[t;\boldsymbol{W}^*], \\
F_k[t;\boldsymbol{W}(t)] &= F_k[t;\boldsymbol{W}^*], \\
S[t;\boldsymbol{W}(t)] &= S[t;\boldsymbol{W}^*], \\
f_k[t;\boldsymbol{W}(t)] &= f_k[t;\boldsymbol{W}^*].
\end{aligned}$$

The random censorship model for competing risks data with time-dependent external covariates is specified as follows. The observations from n individuals are $(X_i, \delta_i, \boldsymbol{W}_i)$, where $X_i = T_i \wedge C_i$, $\delta_i = D_i I(T_i \leq C_i)$, with T_i, D_i, C_i, $\boldsymbol{W}_i(t)$ being, respectively, time to event, event type indicator, time to censoring and $p \times 1$ time-dependent external covariate vector process for the ith participant, $p \geq 1$, $i = 1, \cdots, n$. The quadruplets $\big(T_i,\ D_i,\ C_i,\ \{\boldsymbol{W}_i(t) : t \geq 0\}\big)$, $i = 1, \ldots, n$ are i.i.d. copies of $\big(T,\ D,\ C,\ \{\boldsymbol{W}(t) : t \geq 0\}\big)$ defined for the population from which the sample is drawn. Within each quadruplet, (T_i, D_i) and C_i are conditionally independent given the entire covariate path $\boldsymbol{W}_i^*$.

Similar to the argument leading to (2.25) in Chapter Two, for the observation X_i, when $\delta_i = k, 1 \leq k \leq K$, the contribution to the likelihood is $f_k(X_i; \boldsymbol{W}^*)$; when $\delta_i = 0$, the contribution is $S(X_i; \boldsymbol{W}^*)$. Let

$$\delta_{ik} = I(\delta_i = k), \quad 0 \leq k \leq K.$$

Note that δ_{ik} is the censoring indicator for type k event when competing types are treated as part of the censoring. Also, $\delta_{i0} = 1 - \sum_{k=1}^{K} \delta_{ik}$. Thus the contribution to the likelihood by the ith individual can be written as

$$\begin{aligned}
L_i &= \Big[\prod_{k=1}^{K} f_k(X_i; \boldsymbol{W}^*)^{\delta_{ik}}\Big] S(X_i; \boldsymbol{W}^*)^{\delta_{i0}} \\
&= \Big\{\prod_{k=1}^{K} \Big[\frac{f_k(X_i; \boldsymbol{W}^*)}{S(X_i; \boldsymbol{W}^*)}\Big]^{\delta_{ik}}\Big\} S(X_i; \boldsymbol{W}^*) \\
&= \Big\{\prod_{k=1}^{K} \lambda_k(X_i; \boldsymbol{W}^*)^{\delta_{ik}}\Big\} S(X_i; \boldsymbol{W}^*) \\
&= \prod_{k=1}^{K} \Big\{\lambda_k(X_i; \boldsymbol{W}^*)^{\delta_{ik}} \exp\Big[-\int_0^{X_i} \lambda_k(s; \boldsymbol{W}^*) ds\Big]\Big\}, \qquad (13.32)
\end{aligned}$$

where the identity $S(t; \boldsymbol{W}^*) = \exp\big[-\sum_{k=1}^{K} \int_0^t \lambda_k(s; \boldsymbol{W}^*) ds\big]$ has been used in obtaining the last equality. Therefore the likelihood is

$$\begin{aligned}
L &= \prod_{i=1}^{n} L_i \\
&= \prod_{k=1}^{K} \Big(\prod_{i=1}^{n} \Big\{\lambda_k(X_i; \boldsymbol{W}^*)^{\delta_{ik}} \exp\Big[-\int_0^{X_i} \lambda_k(s; \boldsymbol{W}^*) ds\Big]\Big\}\Big). \qquad (13.33)
\end{aligned}$$

This important result on likelihood factorization was given by Prentice et al. [248]. From (13.33), several important observations can be made:

1. The likelihood is completely determined by the cause-specific functions $\lambda_k(t; \boldsymbol{W}^*)$, $1 \le k \le K$, without any assumptions on the dependence structure among the processes generating the K event types.

2. The likelihood is a product of K factors, where the kth one depends solely on $\lambda_k(t; \boldsymbol{W}^*)$. Consequently, if there are no shared parameters across event types, inference for parameters in $\lambda_k(t; \boldsymbol{W}^*)$ can be made by maximizing the corresponding likelihood factor alone.

3. The likelihood factor for type k event is exactly the likelihood that would be obtained in Chapter Four by treating other event types as independent censoring. Therefore, hazard-based modeling and inference procedures discussed in previous chapters can be used for competing risks data with minimal adjustment, as illustrated by discussions on weighted log-rank test in the previous section.

These results significantly simplify the analysis of competing risks. They also help explain why survival analysis literature often overlooks the competing risks issue, frequently treating all censoring as independent.

However, it is crucial to recognize that this simplification is valid only when the focus is on a single event type, and the modeling and analysis are based on the hazard function. If one attempts to extend a survival probability-based analysis, such as the restricted mean survival time, or to jointly analyze multiple event types, a deeper and more extensive analysis is required. Ignoring the competing risks issues in these situations could yield invalid and misleading results, as discussed in Section 13.3. Chapter Fourteen provides related discussions on analysis of terminal and non-terminal events.

Suppose it is of interest to fit a Cox multiplicative hazards model to the cause-specific hazard for the type k event. The model is

$$\lambda_k\left[t; \boldsymbol{W}(t)\right] = \lambda_{k0}(t) \exp\left[\boldsymbol{\beta}^{\mathrm{T}} \boldsymbol{W}(t)\right], \tag{13.34}$$

where $\boldsymbol{W}(t)$ is a $p \times 1$ time-dependent external covariate vector, $\boldsymbol{\beta}$ the $p \times 1$ parameter, and λ_{k0} an unknown baseline hazard function. Treating events of other types as censoring and proceeding as in Chapter Six, inference on $\boldsymbol{\beta}$ and $\Lambda_{k0}(t) = \int_0^t \lambda_{k0}(t)$ can be made. With $\boldsymbol{W}$ containing either the treatment group indicator Z only, or Z together with other baseline covariates, the coefficient of Z in model (13.34) is the logarithm of the ratio (treatment over control) of the cause-specific hazard functions for event of type k, without covariate adjustment, or with covariates fixed at the same level in both groups, respectively.

Since a trial typically focuses on an event of a particular type, model (13.34) is often used once, for the event type of interest. The model can also be applied separately to several event types when necessary. If there is interest in studying all event types, and there is reason to believe that event of different types share some common parameters, then K models similar to (13.34) can be considered with proper modifications. Three examples are

1. $\lambda_{10} = \cdots = \lambda_{K0}$;

2. $\lambda_{10} = \cdots = \lambda_{K0}$, with $\boldsymbol{W}(t)$ containing an additional $(K-1) \times 1$ vector $\big(I(k = 2), \ldots, I(k = K)\big)^{\mathrm{T}}$;

3. common coefficient(s) for one or more components of the covariate vector.

Note that case (2) assumes that the baseline cause-specific hazard functions for all event types are proportional. In these cases, the analysis is more complicated and is postponed to Section 14.4 which deals with the more general multi-state setup.

In addition to (13.34), other models and inference procedures are possible, For example, the models of short-term and long-term hazard ratios (7.6), (7.46), (7.56) and (7.57), and the pseudo-likelihood methods, can be considered. Similar to the case for Cox regression, the variance estimators are also valid with proper modifications, provided that everything is expressed in terms of the cause-specific hazards rather than the survival functions. Again, these models can be applied to the event type of interest, without requiring the modeling or analysis of other competing event types. When several event types are of interest, the models can be applied separately to each. Extensions are also possible for cases when different event types share certain common parameters.

Nonparametric MLE provides another analytic option, as illustrated by Diao et al. [61] for a variation of model (7.57). Note that their work requires modeling all cause-specific hazard functions, and each function depends on the cause-specific hazards of competing risks through the overall event distribution. Consequently, while it may offer efficiency gains due to the comprehensive modeling and analysis, it does not isolate a specific event type. If the focus is on a specific event type or a subset of all cause-specific hazards, the pseudo-likelihood methods discussed in Chapter Seven should be used.

Let

$$M_{ik}(t) = N_{ik}(t) - \int_0^t Y_i(s)\lambda_k\big[s; \boldsymbol{W}(s)\big]ds, \quad 1 \le i \le n, \ 1 \le k \le K. \tag{13.35}$$

Similar to the derivation in Section 11.5.2, it can be shown that $M_{ik}(t)$'s are martingales with predictable variation processes

$$\langle M_{ik}, M_{ik}\rangle(t) = \int_0^t Y_i(s)\lambda_k\big[s; \boldsymbol{W}(s)\big]ds, \quad 1 \le i \le n, \ 1 \le k \le K. \tag{13.36}$$

Also, similar to the case without covariate, the martingales can be shown to be orthogonal to each other:

$$\langle M_{ik}, M_{j\ell}\rangle(t) = 0 \quad \text{when } (i,k) \ne (j,\ell). \tag{13.37}$$

These properties and the counting process and martingale techniques help simplify variance and covariance estimation, as well as the asymptotic analysis.

Example 13.1. In Example 2.2, various weighted log-rank tests were applied to the TOPCAT primary endpoint, which was the composite of death from cardiovascular causes, aborted cardiac arrest, or hospitalization for the management of heart failure. Justification of the asymptotic validity requires the independent censoring assumption, which is questionable as there was a substantial number of non-cardiovascular deaths that dependently censored the primary endpoint. To properly account for such competing risks, the hypothesis of no treatment effect must be modified to the hypothesis of equality between the two groups in terms of the cause-specific hazards for the primary endpoint.

With this modification, the weighted log-rank tests and their variance estimators remain valid and yield exactly the same numerical values as before. In particular, the P-value of the log-rank test remains 0.14.

Similarly, in Example 5.1, an unadjusted analysis using the Cox model (5.4) was performed for the TOPCAT primary endpoint, assuming independent censoring. To account for the competing risks from non-cardiovascular deaths, model (5.4) should be applied to the cause-specific hazard. The point estimator and its variance estimator remain valid under this modification, yielding the same numerical results as before. In particular, the ratio of cause-specific hazards is 0.89, with a 95% confidence interval 0.77–1.04.

Example 13.2. In Example 7.2, the short-term and long-tern hazard ratio model (7.6) was applied to the WHI E+P trial primary endpoint, which was the composite of non-fatal myocardial infarction and CHD death. Again, justification of the asymptotic validity requires the independent censoring assumption, which is questionable, as there were 165 and 166 deaths due to other causes in the two groups, compared with 164 and 122 CHD deaths [324].

To account for competing risks, the cause-specific hazard for the primary endpoint should be the target of modeling and analysis. Applying model (7.6) to this cause-specific hazard, the point and interval estimators of the parameters, and confidence bands for the ratio of cause-specific hazards between the two groups, are valid asymptotically and yield the same numerical values as before. In particular, Figure 7.4 should now be interpreted as showing point estimates and confidence intervals for the ratio of cause-specific hazards between the two groups.

Similarly, for secondary analyses on components in the TOPCAT primary endpoint, hazard-focused models and analyses in previous chapters can be applied to each component individually. However, for overall treatment effect assessment, a joint analysis of components—such as time to CVD death and time to heart failure hospitalization—is needed. This introduces additional complexity, which is addressed in Chapter Fourteen.

13.6 Latent Variables and Multiple Decrement Models

One approach to competing risks analysis utilizes latent variables or potential outcomes corresponding to different event types. This is known as *multiple decrement models* in actuarial statistics. Let $\widetilde{T}_1,\ldots,\widetilde{T}_K$ be the K different latent variables. The variable $\widetilde{T}_k$ represents time to event of type k in a hypothetical situation where there is no risk for other event types. The observed time to event is defined as

$$T = \min(\widetilde{T}_1,\ldots,\widetilde{T}_K),$$

and the event type D is k when $T = \widetilde{T}_k$, $1 \le k \le K$. Often there is an important assumption:

$$\text{The variables } \widetilde{T}_1,\ldots,\widetilde{T}_K \text{ are independent.} \tag{13.38}$$

Suppose an external covariate $\boldsymbol{W}(t)$ is available. define the joint survival function of $(\widetilde{T}_1,\ldots,\widetilde{T}_K)$ given the entire covariate path $\boldsymbol{W}^*$

$$\widetilde{S}(t_1,\ldots,t_K;\boldsymbol{W}^*) = P\big(\widetilde{T}_1 > t_1,\ldots,\widetilde{T}_K > t_K\big|\boldsymbol{W}^*\big). \tag{13.39}$$

By the definition of T, the survival function of T given $\boldsymbol{W}^*$ is

$$S(t;\boldsymbol{W}^*) = \widetilde{S}(t,\ldots,t;\boldsymbol{W}^*), \tag{13.40}$$

It is left to Exercise 13.10 to verify that the cause-specific hazard functions are given by

$$\lambda_k(t;\boldsymbol{W}^*) = -\frac{\partial \log \widetilde{S}(t_1,\ldots,t_K;\boldsymbol{W}^*)}{\partial t_k}\bigg|_{t_1=\cdots=t_K=t}, \quad 1\le k\le K. \tag{13.41}$$

The conditional CIF $F_k(t;\boldsymbol{W}^*)$ can also be defined and, analogous to (13.39), (13.40) and (13.10), it can be expressed in terms of $\widetilde{S}(t_1,\ldots,t_K;\boldsymbol{W}^*)$.

However, the joint survival function $\widetilde{S}(t_1,\ldots,t_K;\boldsymbol{W}^*)$ cannot be expressed in terms of $\lambda_k(t;\boldsymbol{W}^*), 1\le k\le K$. Intuitively, this is because, from (13.41), $\lambda_k(t)$ is only determined by the local behavior of $\widetilde{S}(t_1,\ldots,t_K;\boldsymbol{W}^*)$ on the diagonal line $t_1=\cdots=t_K=t$. Therefore, the joint survival function itself, the marginal survival functions

$$P(\widetilde{T}_k > t;\boldsymbol{W}^*) = \widetilde{S}(t_1,\ldots,t_K;\boldsymbol{W}^*)\big|_{t_k=t,t_\ell=0,\ell\neq k}, \quad 1\le k\le K, \tag{13.42}$$

and many other functions cannot be determined by $\lambda_k(t;\boldsymbol{W}^*), 1\le k\le K$. Since the likelihood is a function of the $\lambda_k(t;\boldsymbol{W}^*)$'s, it seems plausible that a non-identifiability issue exists.

Tsiatis [300] showed that, given the joint survival function $\widetilde{S}$ of any K latent variables $\widetilde{T}_1,\ldots,\widetilde{T}_K$ which are not independent and have an arbitrary dependence structure among them, there exists a joint survival function $\widetilde{S}^*$ for K independent latent variables $\widetilde{T}_1^*, \ldots, \widetilde{T}_K^*$, such that both joint survival functions $\widetilde{S}$, $\widetilde{S}^*$ yield the same set of cumulative incidence functions $F_1(t), \ldots, F_K(t)$. Consequently, the joint survival function $\widetilde{S}$ is unidentifiable from observed competing risks data (T, D), Therefore, the independent assumption (12.38) is crucial for identifiability. This assumption is often unrealistic. Furthermore, it cannot be tested using competing risks data alone.

The non-identifiability problem above pertains to nonparametric estimation in a homogeneous population. When covariates are available, if the joint survival function has a certain form, then with either the Cox proportional hazards model or the accelerated failure time model for the marginal distribution of each latent variable, the joint survival function is identifiable. Technical details can be found in Heckman and Honore [111].

It is crucial to note, however, that although there is no identifiability issue under these assumed models, checking the validity of the assumed models is inherently difficult because the true joint distribution remains inestimable nonparametrically from the observed data. Standard goodness-of-fit tests are often not directly applicable. Typically, researchers rely on indirect methods to assess model plausibility, such as evaluating result robustness under different model specifications, examining how well the model fits marginal distributions, etc. [10].

Even when there is no identifiability issue in the joint distribution due to an assumed model form, interpreting a marginal distribution and related parameters using the multiple decrement approach refers to a hypothetical population where competing risks are removed. Therefore, such interpretation requires the strong assumption of no impact removal of competing risks, similarly to the discussion on the Kaplan-Meier estimator in Section 13.2.

13.7 Sub-Distribution Hazard Regression with the Fine-Gray Model

Using the regression approach in Section 13.5, cause-specific hazard functions for a particular event type k can be modeled and compared, parametrically or semiparametrically, corresponding to covariate levels. This approach avoids modeling the distributions of cause-specific hazard functions for competing events.

To compare CIFs corresponding to specific covariate levels, one option is to model each cause-specific hazard and then use equations (13.10) and (13.5) to derive the associated CIFs. For instance, a proportional hazards model can be applied to all cause-specific hazards. In this approach, all scalar parameters and baseline functions in the cause-specific hazard functions must be estimated to describe the difference between two CIFs for a single event type.

Fine and Gray [76] proposed a model based on the function

$$\lambda_k^*(t) = \lim_{h\downarrow 0} P\left[t \le T < t+h, D=k \middle| \{T \ge t\} \cup \{T < t, D \ne k\}\right] / h, \tag{13.43}$$

for t with $P(\{T \ge t\} \cup \{T < t, D \ne k\}) > 0$, $k = 1, \ldots, K$, where absolute continuity of relevant functions are assumed to ensure that the limits exist. $\lambda_k^*(t)$ is called the *sub-distribution hazard function* and was introduced in Gray [104]. It satisfies

$$\begin{aligned} \lambda_k^*(t) &= \frac{f_k(t)}{1 - F_k(t)} \\ &= -\frac{d}{dt}\log\left[1 - F_k(t)\right]. \end{aligned} \tag{13.44}$$

Thus, the relationship between λ_k^* and F_k parallels that between the hazard function and CDF in univariate survival analysis.

To analyze the association between covariates and the CIF, Fine and Gray [76] considered the conditional sub-distribution hazard function

$$\lambda_k^*[t; \boldsymbol{W}(t)] = \lim_{h\downarrow 0} P\left[t \le T < t+h, D=k \middle| \{T \ge t\} \cup \{T < t, D \ne k\}, \boldsymbol{W}^h(t)\right] / h, \tag{13.45}$$

where $\boldsymbol{W}(t)$ is a $p \times 1$ external covariate vector process. They studied the model

$$\lambda_k^*[t; \boldsymbol{W}(t)] = \lambda_{k0}^*(t) \exp\left[\boldsymbol{\beta}^{\mathrm{T}} \boldsymbol{W}(t)\right], \tag{13.46}$$

where $\boldsymbol{\beta}$ is the $p \times 1$ parameter and $\lambda_{k0}(t)$ an unknown baseline function.

Similar to (13.44),

$$\lambda_k^*[t; \boldsymbol{W}(t)] = -\frac{d}{dt}\log\left\{1 - F_k\left[t; \boldsymbol{W}(t)\right]\right\}, \tag{13.47}$$

where $F_k\left[t; \boldsymbol{W}(t)\right] = P\left(T \le t, D = k \middle| \boldsymbol{W}^h(t)\right)$. Thus the relationship between $\lambda_k^*[t; \boldsymbol{W}(t)]$ and $F_k\left[t; \boldsymbol{W}(t)\right]$ parallels (2.7) between hazard and survival functions in the univariate case.

Note that $\lambda_k^*(t)$ is the instantaneous rate of occurrence of type k event, given that no event has occurred or a competing event has occurred before time t. This complicates the conceptualization of a risk set, as some individuals will not experience type k event. However, for time-independent covariates, the model and parameter $\boldsymbol{\beta}$ can be interpreted based on the expression

$$\log\frac{1}{1 - F_k(t; \boldsymbol{W})} = \exp(\boldsymbol{\beta}^{\mathrm{T}} \boldsymbol{W}) \int_0^t \lambda_{k0}^*(s) ds. \tag{13.48}$$

In this formulation, the covariate effect is a multiplicative factor $\exp(\boldsymbol{\beta}^{\mathrm{T}}\boldsymbol{W})$ on $-\log[1-F_k(t;\boldsymbol{W})]$.

To make inference on $\boldsymbol{\beta}$ and λ_{k0} in (13.46), Fine and Gray used an inverse probability of censoring weighting method to obtain an estimating function similar to (6.18), and established the asymptotic normality of the resulting estimator $\widehat{\boldsymbol{\beta}}$. Confidence intervals and bands were also derived for predicted cumulative incidence given specified covariates. Some probabilistic results related to the inverse probability weighting method are explored in Exercise 13.12.

Often, clinical trials are designed to have a primary analysis focusing on the cause-specific hazard function for the event type of interest, with Fine-Gray model-based analysis as a sensitivity analysis for CIF assessment.

13.8 Exercises and Complements

13.1 The CIF F_k is the sub-distribution of T with $D = k$. Thus,

$$EA(T)I(D=k) = \int_0^\infty A(x)dF_k(x),$$

for any function A such that the expectation exists. Assume that data are obtained from the random censorship model for competing risks data described in Section 13.2.

(a) Show that

$$P(T_i \le t, D_i = k, T_i \le C_i) = \int_0^t S_i^C(x)dF_k(x),$$

where $S_i^C(t) = P(C_i \ge t)$. This result is valid in general by (B.7) in Appendix B. However, you can assume that the distributions are continuous.

(b) Verify that the random censorship model for competing risks data satisfies the condition

$$\frac{dP(T_i \le t, D_i = k, T_i \le C_i)}{P(T_i \wedge C_i \ge t)} = d\Lambda_k(t), \quad k = 1,\ldots,K,$$

for t with $P(T_i \wedge C_i \ge t) > 0$. This condition is the *independent censoring condition for competing risks data.*

13.2 Suppose there are two competing causes, with $\lambda_k(t) = \theta_k$, $k = 1,2$. Obtain $S(t), f_k(t)$ and $F_k(t)$ in (13.5), (13.7) and (13.8).

13.3 Suppose there are two competing causes, with $\Lambda_k(t) = \alpha_k t^\beta$, $k = 1,2$. Obtain $S(t), f_k(t)$ and $F_k(t)$ in (13.5), (13.7) and (13.8).

13.4 Suppose there are two competing causes, with

$$\Lambda_k(t) = \frac{\eta_k}{\nu}\{\exp[\nu t)] - 1\},\ k = 1,2.$$

Obtain $S(t), f_k(t)$ and $F_k(t)$ in (13.5), (13.7) and (13.8).

13.5 Derive the CIFs for the control and treatment groups in Scenarios A through D in Example 13.1.

13.6 Use statistical software to reproduce Figures 13.2 and 13.3.

13.7 Suppose T_1 and T_2 are independent given gamma frailty γ with mean 1 and variance θ. Furthermore, assume that the conditional survival functions given frailty are as in (12.10). From (12.12),

$$P(T_1 \geq t, T_2 \geq t) = \{1 + \theta[\Lambda_{01}(t) + \Lambda_{02}(t)]\}^{-1/\theta}.$$

(a) Use the conditional independence to show that

$$\begin{aligned} & P(T_1 \in [t, t+\varepsilon), T_2 \geq t) \\ = \quad & E\{[\exp[-\gamma\Lambda_{01}(t)] - \exp[-\gamma\Lambda_{01}(t+\varepsilon)]]\exp(-\gamma\Lambda_{02}(t)\}. \end{aligned}$$

(b) Assume that the order of expectation and limit can be interchanged. Show that

$$\begin{aligned} & \lim_{\varepsilon \downarrow 0} P(T_1 \in [t, t+\varepsilon), T_2 \geq t)/\varepsilon \\ = \quad & \lambda_{01}(t)\{1 + \theta[\Lambda_{01}(t) + \Lambda_{02}(t)]\}^{-(1+1/\theta)}, \end{aligned}$$

where $\lambda_{01} = d\Lambda_{01}(t)/dt$.

(c) Show that the cause-specific hazard $\lambda_1^{cs}(t)$ of T_1 is

$$\frac{\lambda_{01}(t)}{1 + \theta[\Lambda_{01}(t) + \Lambda_{02}(t)]}. \tag{13.49}$$

Note that this differs from the marginal hazard function of T_1, which is

$$\lambda_1(t) = \frac{\lambda_{01}(t)}{1 + \theta\Lambda_{01}(t)}.$$

Hint:

$$\begin{aligned}\lambda_1(t) &= \lim_{\varepsilon\downarrow 0}\frac{P(T_1\in[t,t+\varepsilon),T_2>T_1)/\varepsilon}{P(T_1\ge t,T_2\ge t)}\\ &= \lim_{\varepsilon\downarrow 0}\frac{P(T_1\in[t,t+\varepsilon),T_2\ge t)/\varepsilon}{P(T_1\ge t,T_2\ge t)}.\end{aligned}$$

(d) Suppose $\Lambda_{02}(t)=c\Lambda_{01}(t)$ for a constant $c>0$. Then $\lambda_1^{cs}(t)$ is

$$\frac{\lambda_{01}(t)}{1+\theta(1+c)\Lambda_{01}(t)}.$$

When $\lambda_{01}(t)$ is a constant, $\lambda_1^{cs}(t)$ is not a constant since $\Lambda_{01}(t)$ is a linear function. For $\lambda_1^{cs}(t)$ to be a constant A, we can solve the first order differential equation

$$\frac{d\Lambda_{01}(t)}{dt}=A[1+\theta(1+c)\Lambda_{01}(t)].$$

More generally, for $\lambda_1^{cs}(t)$ to be Weibull, or $\lambda_1^{cs}(t)=At^{\alpha},\ A>0,\ \alpha>-1.$ $\Lambda_{01}(t)$ must satisfy the differential equation

$$\frac{d\Lambda_{01}(t)}{dt}=At^{\alpha}[1+\theta(1+c)\Lambda_{01}(t)].$$

The solution is

$$\Lambda_{01}(t)=\int_0^t \exp\left\{A\theta(1+c)\left[t^{1+\alpha}-x^{1+\alpha}\right]/(1+\alpha)\right\}Ax^{\alpha}dx. \tag{13.50}$$

In particular, for the exponential case $\alpha=0$, verify that (13.50) reduces to

$$\Lambda_{01}(t)=\left\{\exp[A\theta(1+c)t]-1\right\}/[\theta(1+c)],$$

or the Gompertz distribution with $\eta=A,\ \nu=A\theta(1+c)$. Correspondingly,

$$\Lambda_{02}(t)=c\left\{\exp[A\theta(1+c)t]-1\right\}/[\theta(1+c)],$$

This provides a way to generate Weibull cause-specific hazards for dependent competing causes.

13.8 (a) Verify that contribution from X_i to the likelihood for the competing risks problem is given in (13.32).

(b) Verify that the likelihood for the competing risks problem is given in (13.33).

13.9 Verify that when applying the two sample model of short-term and long-term hazard ratios (7.6) to the cause-specific hazard function for event of type k, the baseline function $R(t)$ is

$$\exp\left[\Lambda_{kC}(t)\right] - 1,$$

where $\Lambda_{kC}(t)$ is the cumulative hazard function for event of type k in the control group.

13.10 Verify (13.40) through (13.42).

13.11 Verify (13.44), (13. 47) and (13.48).

13.12 Assume that T and C are independent given $\boldsymbol{W}$. Let $X = T \wedge C$ and

$$G_{\boldsymbol{W}}(t) = P(C \geq t \big| \boldsymbol{W}).$$

(a) Show that

$$\frac{I(C \geq T \wedge x)}{G_{\boldsymbol{W}}(X \wedge x)} = \frac{I(C \geq T \wedge x)}{G_{\boldsymbol{W}}(T \wedge x)}.$$

Note that this result implicitly assumes that $G_{\boldsymbol{W}}(X \wedge x) > 0$.

Hint: Both sides are 0 if $C < T \wedge x$. When $C \geq T \wedge x$, simplify $X \wedge x = T \wedge C \wedge x$.

(b) Let

$$A(C, T, \boldsymbol{W}) = \frac{I(C \geq T \wedge x)}{G_{\boldsymbol{W}}(T \wedge x)}.$$

Then $E\big[A(C, T, \boldsymbol{W})\big| T, \boldsymbol{W}\big] = \phi(T, \boldsymbol{W})$, where

$$\begin{aligned}
\phi(t, \boldsymbol{w}) &= E\big[A(C, T, \boldsymbol{W})\big| T = t, \boldsymbol{W} = \boldsymbol{w}\big] \\
&= E\big[A(C, t, \boldsymbol{w})\big| T = t, \boldsymbol{W} = \boldsymbol{w}\big] \\
&= E\big[A(C, t, \boldsymbol{w})\big| \boldsymbol{W} = \boldsymbol{w}\big], \qquad (13.51)
\end{aligned}$$

where the last equality follows from property #13 in Section B.2 0f Appendix B. Show that the last quantity in (13.51) is identically 1.

(c) Combining results from (a) and (b), show that

$$E\Big[\frac{I(C \geq T \wedge x)}{G_{\boldsymbol{W}}(X \wedge x)} \big| T, \boldsymbol{W}\Big] = 1. \qquad (13.52)$$

Fine and Gray [76] established (13.52) and used it to develop an estimating function for $\boldsymbol{\beta}$ in (13.46). Note that from (13.52) and (B.4) in Appendix B,

$$E\Big[\frac{I(C \geq T \wedge x)}{G_{\boldsymbol{W}}(X \wedge x)} \big| \boldsymbol{W}\Big] = E\Big\{E\Big[\frac{I(C \geq T \wedge x)}{G_{\boldsymbol{W}}(X \wedge x)} \big| T, \boldsymbol{W}\Big] \big| \boldsymbol{W}\Big\} = 1. \qquad (13.53)$$

14

Analysis of Terminal and Non-Terminal Events

14.1 Introduction

In Chapter Twelve, the focus was on multiple potentially correlated events. These events are subject to independent censoring but do not censor one another. In Chapter Thirteen, competing risks data were examined. In this type of data, in addition to the usual independent censoring, the occurrence of one event censors the other events. This has two consequences: each individual contributes only one outcome to the analysis, and there is dependent censoring.

In clinical trials, it is almost always the case that multiple potentially correlated events are of interest. These events often comprise certain terminal and non-terminal events, where the terminal event may censor the non-terminal events, but not vice versa. To simplify the presentation, we focus on the case involving one non-terminal event (A) and one terminal event (B). Extensions to accommodate additional events are relatively straightforward.

As an example, let A be the time to heart failure hospitalization, and B be the time to cardiovascular death. Then there are four possible scenarios: 1. both A and B are observed, in that order; 2. only A is observed (when censoring occurs before B but after A); 3. only B is observed (when B occurs without A); 4. neither A or B is observed (when censoring occurs before either event). Thus, up to two events of interest may be observed from the same individual. This situation differs from that described in Chapter Twelve due to dependent censoring of A by B. It also differs from competing risks analysis, where only up to one event is observed for each individual, resulting in independent observations in the analysis.

When multiple events are of interest, traditionally it is common to use a composite outcome and adopt the time-to-first-event analysis. This reduces a multivariate analysis problem to a univariate analysis problem. Consequently, hypothesis testing and effect estimation can be conducted using methods such as the log-rank test, the Cox model, or other techniques discussed in Chapters Five through Nine. Combining multiple events into a composite outcome could potentially enhance statistical power. Furthermore, in scenarios involving both terminal and

DOI: 10.1201/9780429324437-14

non-terminal events, the composite outcome approach resolves the issue of censoring among the components within the composite.

Although the composite outcome analysis is appealing, there are several limitations. For the case with A and B in the example above, it treats all first events equally, regardless of their type. This can potentially mask treatment effects when they vary between A and B. Furthermore, in the case when both A and B are observed, it ignores event B, which is clinically more important.

This chapter focuses on the analysis of terminal and non-terminal events beyond the traditional composite outcome approach, utilizing fuller data to gain efficiency. This research area has received considerable attention recently. Depending on research objectives and the assumed absence or presence of competing risks, different methodological approaches have been proposed. Yang [340] provides a brief summary of some works with more established properties and asymptotic theory. This chapter expands on that work, providing a more in-depth analysis, a broader range of examples, and a more complete discussion of these methodological approaches.

Many of the existing methods focus on the simpler scenario where no additional competing risks exist for the terminal and non-terminal events. However, this is often unrealistic in clinical trials. For instance, in the example above with time to heart failure hospitalization (A) and time to cardiovascular death (B), an individual is subject to the competing risk of non-cardiovascular death. In many cardiology trials, the presence of competing risks can be substantial, as illustrated in two recent large trials that will be discussed in Section 14.9.

We will start with by examining the simpler case of no additional competing risks. Then, the more general case in the presence of competing risks will be discussed. Various recently developed methods are explored and compared, emphasizing necessary conditions, parameter interpretations, and their strengths and limitations. Crucially, with applications to recent large clinical trials, the chapter provides practical guidance to help researchers choose methods best suited to their specific study goals.

14.2 Copula Models

Let T_1^*, T_2^* be the non-terminal and terminal events, respectively, and assume that they are subject to censoring by an independent variable C. Fine et al. [77] considered such data and referred to this setting as "semi-competing risks," a term that has since been widely adopted. The term stems from the fact that T_2^* may censor T_1^* but not vice versa. In this setting, T_2^* is only subject to censoring by C. However, T_1^* is subject to censoring by both C and T_2^*. The work of Fine et al. was motivated by a situation where the terminal event can be prevented with no side-effect altering the non-terminal event.

Suppose that the observed data are i.i.d. copies $(X_i, \delta_i^x, Y_i, \delta_i^y)$, $i = 1, \ldots, n$, of $(X, \delta^x, Y, \delta^y)$, where

$$X = \min(T_1^*, T_2^*, C),\ \delta^x = I(X = T_1^*),\ Y = \min(T_2^*, C),\ \delta^y = I(Y = T_2^*).$$

Assume that $P(X > \tau) > 0$ for a fixed τ. Fine et al. extended an argument in Lin and Ying [182] to show that the joint distribution of (T_1^*, T_2^*) can be identified and estimated nonparametrically in the upper wedge where $T_1^* < T_2^*$. By the independence between C and (T_1^*, T_2^*), we have, for $0 \le t_1 \le t_2$,

$$\begin{aligned} P(X > t_1, Y > t_2) &= P(T_1^* > t_1, T_2^* > t_2, C > t_2) \\ &= P(T_1^* > t_1, T_2^* > t_2)P(C > t_2). \end{aligned}$$

Thus

$$P(T_1^* > t_1, T_2^* > t_2) = \frac{P(X > t_1, Y > t_2)}{P(C > t_2)}, \tag{14.1}$$

for $0 \le t_1 \le t_2 \le \tau$. Since the numerator and denominator in the ratio on the right-hand side of (14.1) can be estimated by $(1/n)\sum_{i=1}^n I(X_i > t_1, Y_i > t_2)$ and the Kaplan-Meier estimator of $P(C > t_2)$, respectively, it follows that, nonparametrically, the joint distribution of (T_1^*, T_2^*) can be identified and estimated in the upper wedge $T_1^* < T_2^*$.

The marginal survivor function of T_1^* is nonparametrically non-identifiable. However, under certain assumed models for the joint distribution, Fine et al. showed that the marginal distribution of T_1^* can be identified and consistently estimated. Let $S(t_1, t_2)$ be the joint survival function of (T_1^*, T_2^*). Fine et al. considered the Clayton bivariate survival function

$$S(t_1, t_2) = \left\{S_1(t_1)^{-\theta} + S_2(t_2)^{-\theta} - 1\right\}^{-1/\theta}, \ 0 \le t_1 \le t_2, \tag{14.2}$$

where S_1, S_2 meet the definition for survival function. The joint density on the lower wedge, $f_{t_2 < t_1}(t_1, t_2)$, is unspecified but satisfies

$$\left\{S_1(t_1)^{-\theta} + S_2(t_2)^{-\theta} - 1\right\}^{-1/\theta} = \int_{t_2}^{\infty}\int_{t_1}^{y} f_{t_1 \le t_2}(x, y)dxdy + \int_{t_2}^{\infty}\int_{y}^{\infty} f_{t_2 < t_1}(x, y)dxdy \tag{14.3}$$

for $t_1 \le t_2$, where $f_{t_1 \le t_2}(t_1, t_2)$ is the joint density on the upper wedge. Note that there are many solutions to (14.3) and the model on the lower wedge is unverifiable.

Fine et al. assumed that

$$S(t_1, t_2) = A\big(S_1(t_1), S_2(t_2)\big), \; t_2 < t_1, \tag{14.4}$$

where A is a copula function on the unit square. It is further assumed that $A\big(S_1(t), S_2(t)\big) = S(t,t)$ for $S(t_1, t_2)$ given by (14.2). Note that $S(t,t)$ and $S_2(t)$ are the survival functions of $T_1^* \wedge T_2^*$ and T_2^*, respectively, thus can be estimated by Kaplan-Meir estimators based on observed data. From (14.2),

$$S_1(t) = \left\{S(t,t)^{-\theta} + 1 - S_2(t)^{-\theta}\right\}^{-1/\theta}, \; t \geq 0. \tag{14.5}$$

Using (14.6), and an estimator for θ, Fine et al. obtained a plug-in estimator for the marginal distribution of T_1^*. The plug-in estimator was shown to be uniformly consistent and to converge weakly to a Gaussian process.

Later, Peng and Fine [223] extended the model and analysis to incorporate covariates and study their effects on the distributions of T_1^* and T_2^*, using a time-dependent copula model in the observable region of the data. Nonparametric estimators for the marginal and dependence models were derived under the model and shown to be uniformly consistent and to converge weakly to Gaussian processes.

For semi-competing risks data, the non-identifiability issue is less severe than in the competing risks setting, although it is not entirely absent. The model assumption (14.5) cannot be verified using only the observed data. Similar to the multiple decrement model for competing risks, interpretation of the marginal distribution of T_1^* is hypothetical.

Often, the interest is usually on the covariate effect. Association between the terminal and non-terminal events needs to be accounted for in the analysis, but may not be of primary interest. The works on semi-competing risks data along the lines of Fine et al. and Peng and Fine are useful in situations where the terminal event can be prevented with no side effect altering the non-terminal event distribution, and where the association parameter and the marginal distribution of the non-terminal event are important.

14.3 The Win Ratio

Consider again the semi-competing risks setting described in Section 14.2. The win ratio [79, 238] has gained much attention for its simplicity and prioritized nature of comparison. Additional references on win ratio and related prioritized comparison include works by Buyse [30], Luo et al. [191], Bebu and Lachin [17], and Mao [196], among others.

To obtain the win ratio, pairwise comparisons are made between the control and treatment groups. For each pair, comparisons are made hierarchically. The treatment is declared a winner if the individual in the treatment group has a better outcome on T_2^*, and a loser if the individual in the control group does better. If comparison on T_2^* is inconclusive due to censoring, then the comparison moves to T_1^*, and the treatment is declared a winner or loser in a similar fashion. If comparison on T_1^* is also inconclusive, no winner or loser is declared.

The total win score W^* for the treatment is the number of pairs in which the treatment is declared a winner. The loss score L^* is obtained similarly. The win ratio is then defined as L^*/W^*, consistent with the hazard ratio convention, with a value < 1 indicating beneficial treatment effect. If $W^* = 0$, the ratio can be redefined to be a large value and the large sample properties will not be affected. For cases with more than two events in an hierarchical order, the win ratio can be extended in an obvious way.

Suppose there are n individuals in the trial. For the ith individual, denote the collection of times to non-terminal and terminal events and to censoring, in that order, by $(T_{1i}^*, T_{2i}^*, C_i)$, $i = 1, \ldots, n$. Arrange the labels such that the first n_1 observations, $n_1 < n$, constitute the control group. Assume that $\lim_n n_1/n = \zeta \in (0,1)$. Furthermore, assume that the first n_1 quadruplets $(T_{1i}^*, T_{2i}^*, C_i)$, $i \le n_1$ are i.i.d., as are the remaining $n - n_1$ quadruplets. The two collections of quadruplets are also assumed to be independent of each other. The observed data are $(Y_{1i}^*, Y_{2i}^*, \delta_{1i}^*, \delta_{2i}^*)$, $i = 1, \ldots, n$ where

$$Y_{1i}^* = T_{1i}^* \wedge T_{2i}^* \wedge C_i,\ \delta_{1i}^* = I(Y_{1i}^* = T_{1i}^*),$$

$$Y_{2i}^* = T_{2i}^* \wedge C_i,\ \delta_{2i}^* = I(Y_{2i}^* = T_{2i}^*).$$

Due to right censoring, the comparison on either T_2^* or T_1^* is conclusive only if the smaller value in a pair is uncensored. Thus for individual i in the treatment group and j in the control group, the win indicators for the terminal and non-terminal events are $W_{2ij}^* = \delta_{2j}^* I(Y_{2i}^* \ge Y_{2j}^*)$ and $W_{1ij}^* = \delta_{1j}^* I(Y_{1i}^* \ge Y_{1j}^*)$, respectively. Similarly the loss indicators for the terminal and non-terminal events are $L_{2ij}^* = \delta_{2i}^* I(Y_{2i} \le Y_{2j}^*)$ and $L_{1ij}^* = \delta_{1i}^* I(Y_{1i}^* \le Y_{1j}^*)$, respectively. Therefore, in the i, j comparison, the treatment is a winner if

$$W_{2ij}^* + (1 - W_{2ij}^*)(1 - L_{2ij}^*) W_{1ij}^* = 1,$$

and a loser if

$$L_{2ij}^* + (1 - W_{2ij}^*)(1 - L_{2ij}^*) L_{1ij}^* = 1.$$

Consequently,

$$W^* = \sum_{i > n_1} \sum_{j \le n_1} \left[W_{2ij}^* + (1 - W_{2ij}^*)(1 - L_{2ij}^*) W_{1ij}^* \right],$$

$$L^* = \sum_{i > n_1} \sum_{j \le n_1} \left[L_{2ij}^* + (1 - W_{2ij}^*)(1 - L_{2ij}^*) L_{1ij}^* \right].$$

For (T_1^*, T_2^*), define the conditional hazard function for the non-terminal event

$$\lambda^*(s|t) = \lim_{h\downarrow 0} P[s \leq T_1^* < s+h | T_1^* \geq s, T_2^* \geq t]/h, \ 0 < s \leq t. \tag{14.6}$$

Let $\lambda_{1C}^*(s|t)$, $\lambda_{1T}^*(s|t)$ be the conditional hazard functions of the non-terminal event in the control and treatment groups, respectively. Denote by λ_{2C}^* and λ_{2T}^* the hazard functions of the terminal event in the control and treatment groups, respectively. Luo et al. [191] showed that the win ratio can be used to test the global null hypothesis $H_{01}^* \cap H_{02}^*$, where

$$\begin{aligned} H_{01}^* : \lambda_{1T}^*(s|t) &= \lambda_{1C}^*(s|t), \ 0 < s \leq t. \\ H_{02}^* : \lambda_{2T}^*(t) &= \lambda_{2C}^*(t), \ t > 0. \end{aligned}$$

The win ratio test is nonparametric, and the global null hypothesis $H_{01}^* \cap H_{02}^*$ pertains to functions that can be estimated using observed data. Luo et al. proposed the weighted win loss statistics, derived closed-form variance estimators and established the asymptotic normality of related tests under the null hypothesis $H_{01}^* \cap H_{02}^*$.

Note that $\lambda^*(s|t)$ is a bivariate function of s and t, where $0 < s \leq t$. It represents the instantaneous rate of the non-terminal event occurring in the immediate future, given that it has not yet happened, and that the terminal event will occur beyond a specific future time t. At $t = s$, $\lambda^*(s|t)$ reduces to the cause-specific hazard $\lambda^*(s)$ of the non-terminal event under the competing risk from T_2^*. Therefore, H_{01}^* is stronger than the condition of the equality of $\lambda^*(s)$ in the two groups.

In applications, beyond hypothesis testing, the win ratio is often used as an effect measure. For general priority comparison procedures including the win ratio, Bebu and Lachin [17] established the asymptotic normality of significance tests and confidence intervals for effect measures. Their work is based on the large sample theory of the multivariate multi-sample U-statistics by Lehmann [165].

It is important to note that as the sample size increases, the limit of the win ratio generally has a complicated expression. This expression depends not only on the distributions of (T_1^*, T_2^*), but also on the censoring distributions. Therefore, the validity of win ratio as an effect measure is questionable. However, in certain specific scenarios, the win ratio can be a valid effect measure. Oakes [214] showed that if

$$S_T(t_1, t_2) = S_C(t_1, t_2)^\theta, \tag{14.7}$$

for some $\theta > 0$, where S_T, S_C are the bivariate survival functions of the two groups, then the limit of the win ratio is censoring-free and equals θ. Some probabilistic results related to the work of Oakes are explored in Exercise 14.6.

The win ratio can be calculated easily and the comparison prioritizes the more important event, thus is quite appealing. It can be used to test the global null hypothesis $H_{01}^* \cap H_{02}^*$ which is formulated in terms of estimable functions based on observed data. Unlike the methods discussed in Section 14.2, the win ratio test does not require assumptions on the joint distribution of (T_1^*, T_2^*).

However, the power of the win ratio test might be low if the treatment effect is primarily on T_1^*. In the extreme case when all terminal events are observed (e.g., with long follow-up and no censoring), non-terminal events have no impact at all on the win ratio. Conversely, when censoring on the terminal event is substantial and the number of terminal events is small relative to the non-terminal events, the win ratio is primarily driven by the non-terminal events—somewhat undermining its intended emphasis on the terminal event. Such sensitivity of the win ratio to censoring or follow-up duration and its implications for comparing trial results was discussed in Shaw [277]. Exercise 4.19 provides a simple hypothetical example to illustrate this issue.

Condition (14.7) ensures that the win ratio has a valid censoring-free estimand. It relates to the joint survival distribution of (T_1^*, T_2^*). This condition implies that the marginals of both T_1^* and T_2^* obey a proportional hazards model, and the constants of proportionality in both marginal models are the same. Similar to the discussions in the previous section, condition (14.7) is unverifiable on the lower wedge. Moreover, treatment often has differential effects on the terminal and non-terminal events. In such situations, the win ratio converges to a complicated mixture of these effects that depends on the censoring distributions. Another important point is that θ in (14.7) is not based on the cause-specific hazard functions of T_1^*, thus the influence on T_1^* of the competing risk from T_2^* may not be properly accounted for. Due to these issues, using the win ratio as a measure of effect size is questionable. Furthermore, the win ratio might have more fluctuations than alternative summary measures of the overall treatment effect, as will be illustrated in Section 14.9.

The win ratio approach was initially developed for semi-competing risks data without additional competing risks. When there are additional competing risks, as will be discussed in later sections, it may be complicated, if possible, to obtain conditions similar to (14.7) that ensures a valid estimand for the win ratio in the presence of competing risks. Furthermore, such extensions would quite possibly involve the cumulative incidence functions rather than the cause-specific hazard functions. In these scenarios, under appropriate conditions, the win ratio might be used to make inference on the cumulative incidence functions, or for prediction of event probabilities over time, rather than for causal inference on treatment effects, as previously noted in Section 13.3.

14.4 Multi-State Models

Multi-state models provide an alternative framework to the analysis of survival data, in which an event occurrence is viewed as a transition from one state to another in a finite state space. Traditional univariate survival analysis, competing risks and semi-competing risks analyses, and many more problems, can be recast under the multi-state model framework. Discussions of multi-state models are included in this chapter because this is where the framework offers modeling and analytic approaches different from many other methods.

A *multi-state model* is a process $X(t),\ t \in \mathscr{T}$, where $\mathscr{T}$ is a finite or infinite interval starting from $t = 0$, and $X(t)$ is the state in a finite state space S that an individual occupies at time t. The process $X(t)$ is assumed to have right-continuous sample paths. A state is absorbing if transitions out of that state is impossible, and transient otherwise.

The process $X(t)$ generates a history $\mathfrak{X}(t)$ consisting of information on X over time interval $[0, t]$. Let $\mathfrak{X}(t_-) = \lim_{\Delta\downarrow 0} \mathfrak{X}(t - \Delta)$. The transition probabilities are

$$P_{jk}(s,t) = P\big[X(t) = k\big|X(s) = j, \mathfrak{X}(s_-)\big] \tag{14.8}$$

for $s \le t,\ j,k \in \mathrm{S}$. $P_{jk}(s,t)$ is the conditional probability of being in state k at a future time t, given the state at the current time s and the history prior to s. The process is a *Markov process* if

$$P_{jk}(s,t) = P\big[X(t) = k\big|X(s) = j\big] \tag{14.9}$$

for $s \le t,\ j,k \in \mathrm{S}$. That is, the probability of transitioning to any future state depends only on the current state and not the prior history.

The transition intensities are

$$\lambda_{jk}(t) = \lim_{\Delta\downarrow 0} \frac{P\big[X((t+\Delta)_-) = k\big|X(t_-) = j, \mathfrak{X}(t_-)\big]}{\Delta}, \tag{14.10}$$

for $s \le t \le \tau, j \ne k, j,\ k \in \mathrm{S}$, assuming that the limits exist. Note that, by definition, the transition intensity functions typically depend on the history $\mathfrak{X}(t_-)$, except in the case of a Markov process. Multi-state model analysis usually deals with inference on transition intensities. Some or all of the transition intensities may be of interest, depending on the research objectives. A multi-state model can be graphically illustrated by a diagram, with boxes and arrows representing the states and possible transitions, respectively.

Example 14.1. (competing risks analysis) For simplicity assume there are only 2 competing risks, yielding a 3 state multi-state model. An individual starts from state 1 (event-free) at time 0, then moves to either state 2 (type 1 event) or state 3 (type 2 event) after some time. It can be shown that the transition intensities are the cause-specific hazards $\lambda_1(t)$, $\lambda_2(t)$, respectively. The model is Markovian since the history prior to time t does not contribute any additional information.

Example 14.2. (illness-death model) Let T_1^* and T_2^* represent times to illness and death, respectively. An individual begins in state 1 (healthy) at time 0, then transitions to either state 2 (ill) or state 3 (dead). If the transition is to illness,

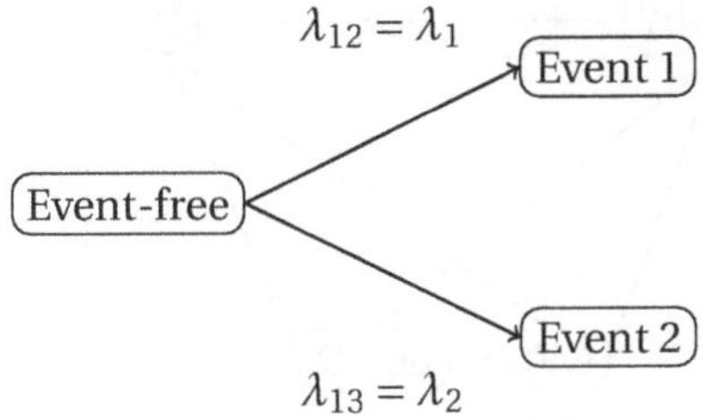

FIGURE 14.1
Competing risks model with two types of events.

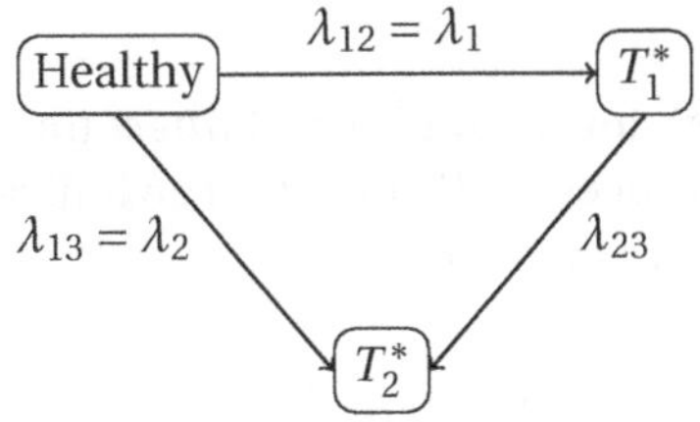

FIGURE 14.2
Illness-death model.

a subsequent transition to death follows. The transition intensities λ_{12} and λ_{13} correspond to the cause-specific hazards λ_1 and λ_2 for T_1^* and T_2^*, respectively, in the competing risks analysis of the first event $T_1^* \wedge T_2^*$. λ_{23} is more complicated. Similar to Example 14.1, The transition probabilities P_{12} and P_{13} satisfy the Markovian condition (14.9). However, P_{23} may depend on the history.

The illness-death model above is an example of a *progressive* multi-state model, in which only forward transitions, or transitions to a worse condition, are possible. A *non-progressive* multi-state model is one which allows backwards transitions to model reversible diseases or conditions. Note also that the data structure in Example 14.2 is the same as that in the semi-competing risks setting.

The next example shows that competing risks can be easily handled in the multi-state model framework, by adding states representing the competing risks.

Example 14.3. Suppose that time to heart failure hospitalization (H) and time to cardiovascular death (CVD) are of interest, and that both are subject to the competing risk of non-cardiovascular death (nCVD). Then the data can be modeled by a multi-state model described in the diagram below.

For a Markov process, the usual counting process and martingale techniques, which readers may be familiar with in the context of univariate survival analysis, remain applicable. Specifically, let

$$\begin{aligned} N_{jk}^*(t) &= \#\{s \le t : X(s_-) = j, X(s) = k\}, \ k \ne j, \\ K_j^*(t) &= I\big(X(t_-) = j\big). \end{aligned}$$

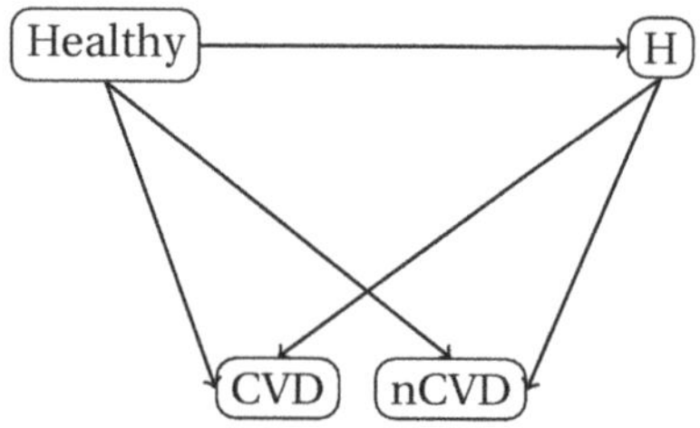

FIGURE 14.3
A multi-state model for the heart failure hospitalization (H) and cardiovascular death (CVD), when both are subject to the competing risk of non-cardiovascular death (nCVD).

$N^*_{jk}(t)$ is the counting process for the number of *direct* transitions from j to k in $[0, t]$, and $K^*_j(t)$ is the at-risk process indicating that an individual is in state j prior to time t. Define the cumulative intensity functions

$$\Lambda_{jk}(t) = \int_0^t \lambda_{jk}(s)ds, \; j \neq k, \tag{14.11}$$

and let

$$M^*_{jk}(t) = N^*_{jk}(t) - \int_0^t K^*_j(s)d\Lambda_{jk}(s), \; j \neq k, \; j,k \in \mathrm{S}.$$

Then the $M^*_{jk}(t)$'s are martingales [122] [7, Theorem II.6.8].

Due to censoring by C, the observed counting and at-risk processes are

$$N_{jk}(t) = N^*_{jk}(t \wedge C), \; K_j(t) = I(C \geq t)K^*_j(t),$$

respectively. Suppose there are i.i.d. copies $X_i(t), i = 1,\ldots,n$, of $X(t)$, and i.i.d. censoring variables $C_1,\ldots,C_n$ that are independent of $X_i(t)$'s. For $1 \leq i \leq n$, let N_{jki}, K_{ji} be the observed counting and at-risk processes for individual i:

$$\begin{aligned} N_{jki}(t) &= \#\{s \leq t \wedge C_i : X_i(s_-) = j, X_i(s) = k\}, \\ K_{ji}(t) &= I(C_i \geq t)I\big(X_i(t_-) = j\big), \; j \neq k \in \{1,\ldots,K\}. \end{aligned} \tag{14.12}$$

These processes completely describe the data, analogously to the univariate case.

Let

$$N_{jk\cdot}(t) = \sum_{i=1}^n N_{jki}(t), \; K_{j\cdot}(t) = \sum_{i=1}^n K_{ji}(t)$$

and define

$$M_{jk}(t) = N_{jk\cdot}(t) - \int_0^t K_{j\cdot}(x)d\Lambda_{jk}(x) = N_{jk\cdot}(t) - \int_0^t K_{j\cdot}(x)\lambda_{jk}(x)dx.$$

Then M_{jk} are martingales and

$$Var\left(\int_0^t h(x)dM_{jk}(x)\right) = E\int_0^t h^2(x)K_{j\cdot}(x)d\Lambda_{jk}(x)$$

for predictable h. Note that censoring by the independent variables $C_1, \ldots, C_n$ does not alter the intensity functions. A censoring scheme with this property is referred to as independent censoring in the literature. Under this scheme, censoring variables are not necessarily independent of the processes $X_i(t)$'s. This is analogous to the discussion in Section 2.7 for the univariate analysis case. For simplicity, we will focus on the case with independent censoring variables C_i's.

Similar to the univariate case, Λ_{jk} can be estimated by the Nelson-Aalen estimator

$$\widehat{\Lambda}_{jk}(t) = \int_0^t \frac{dN_{jk\cdot}(x)}{K_{j\cdot}(x)}, \ k \neq j, \tag{14.13}$$

and the variance estimator is

$$\int_0^t \frac{dN_{jk\cdot}(x)}{K_{j\cdot}^2(x)}, \ k \neq j. \tag{14.14}$$

Due to similarities between univariate survival analysis and Markov multi-state models, many familiar procedures, such as weighted log-rank tests, Cox model and GREs, can be extended to the study of Markov multi-state models. The martingale structure and properties provide an asymptotic analysis analogous to that in the univariate case [7]. For example, consider the null hypothesis

$$H_{0jk} : \lambda_{jkT}(t) = \lambda_{jkC}(t), \ t > 0, \tag{14.15}$$

where $\lambda_{jkC}(t)$, $\lambda_{jkT}(t)$ are the (j,k) transition intensity functions for the control and treatment groups, respectively. The log-rank test statistic for H_{0jk} is

$$U_{jk} = \int_0^\infty \frac{K_{jC}(t)K_{jT}(t)}{K_{jC}(t)+K_{jT}(t)} d\left[\widehat{\Lambda}_{jkT}(t) - \widehat{\Lambda}_{jkC}(t)\right], \tag{14.16}$$

where $\widehat{\Lambda}_{jkC}(t)$, $\widehat{\Lambda}_{jkT}(t)$ are the Nelson-Aalen estimators for the cumulative (j,k) transition intensity functions in the control and treatment groups, respectively, and $K_{jC}(t)$, $K_{jT}(t)$ are the at-risk processes for the (j,k) transition in the control and treatment groups, respectively. The variance of U_{jk} is estimated by

$$V_{jk} = V_\Phi = \sum_{i=1}^n \int_0^\infty \frac{K_{jC}(t)K_{jT}(t)}{\left[K_{jC}(t)+K_{jT}(t)\right]^2} dN_{jki}(t). \tag{14.17}$$

Similarly, under the two-sample Cox model that for some $\theta > 0$,

$$\lambda_{jkT}(t) = \theta\lambda_{jkC}(t), \ t > 0, \tag{14.18}$$

the log-rank GTE is

$$\widehat{\theta}_{jk} = \frac{\int_0^\infty \Phi_j(t)d\widehat{\Lambda}_{jkT}(t)}{\int_0^\infty \Phi_j(t)d\widehat{\Lambda}_{jkC}(t)}, \tag{14.19}$$

with

$$\Phi_j(t) = \frac{K_{jC}(t)K_{jT}(t)}{K_{jC}(t)+K_{jT}(t)}.$$

For covariate adjusted analysis in a general multi-state process that may not be Markovian, intensity models discussed in Chapter Eleven can be used. Suppose $\mathfrak{C}$ is the collection of (j,k) transitions of interest, and the collection of counting processes $N_{jki}(t)$ for $(j,k) \in \mathfrak{C}, 1 \le i \le n$ do not jump at the same time. Let $\boldsymbol{W}_i(t)$ be a time-dependent covariate vector for the ith individual. Suppose that, with respect to an increasing family of σ-algebras $\{\mathscr{F}_t\}$ where $\mathscr{F}_t$ contains information on the counting processes and covariate vectors over $[0,t)$, $\boldsymbol{W}_i(t)$ is predictable and the intensity process $\lambda_{jki}[t;\boldsymbol{W}_i(t)]$ of $N_{jki}(t)$ has the form

$$\lambda_{jki}[t;\boldsymbol{W}_i(t)] = K_{ji}(t)\lambda_{0jk}(t)\exp[\boldsymbol{\beta}^{\mathrm{T}}\boldsymbol{W}_i(t)], \quad t>0, \tag{14.20}$$

for some parameter vector $\boldsymbol{\beta}$ and baseline function λ_{0jk}. Note that $\boldsymbol{\beta}$ and $\boldsymbol{W}$ do not depend on the transition type (j,k). This allows certain transitions to share some common parameters, in situations such as those discussed in Section 13.5 for competing risks analysis.

For partial likelihood inference, the score function is

$$\boldsymbol{U}^{ms}(\boldsymbol{\beta}) = \sum_{(j,k)\in\mathfrak{C}} \left\{ \sum_{i=1}^{n} \int_0^\infty \left[\boldsymbol{W}_i(t) - E_j(\boldsymbol{\beta},t)\right] dN_{jki}(t) \right\}, \tag{14.21}$$

where

$$E_j(\boldsymbol{\beta},t) = \frac{\sum_{i=1}^n K_{ji}(t)\exp[\boldsymbol{\beta}^{\mathrm{T}}\boldsymbol{W}_i(t)]\boldsymbol{W}_i(t)}{\sum_{i=1}^n K_{ji}(t)\exp[\boldsymbol{\beta}^{\mathrm{T}}\boldsymbol{W}_i(t)]}.$$

This is analogous to the discussions in Section 6.3, except for the modifications that the score now is the sum of several score functions, one for each (j,k) in $\mathfrak{C}$, and that the individual at-risk process is $K_{ji}(t)$ for a (j,k) transition. Derivation of the observed information matrix is left to Exercise 14.9.

Next, for analysis on transition probabilities, let $\boldsymbol{P}(s,t) = \left(P_{j\ell}(s,t)\right)_{K\times K}$. Define

$$\lambda_{jj}(t) = -\sum_{\ell\neq j}\lambda_{j\ell}(t), \quad \Lambda_{jj}(t) = -\sum_{\ell\neq j}\Lambda_{j\ell}(t). \quad j=1,\ldots,K, \tag{14.22}$$

and let $\boldsymbol{\Lambda} = \left(\Lambda_{j\ell}\right)_{K\times K}$, Note that $\boldsymbol{\Lambda}(t)$ is a $K\times K$ matrix of cadlag functions. Let $\boldsymbol{I}$ be the $K\times K$ identity matrix. Define

$$\mathscr{P}_{(s,t]}\left[\boldsymbol{I}+d\boldsymbol{\Lambda}(u)\right] = \lim \prod_{k=1}^{L}\left[\boldsymbol{I}+\boldsymbol{\Lambda}(u_k)-\boldsymbol{\Lambda}(u_{k-1})\right], \tag{14.23}$$

where $\prod$ is the matrix product in its natural order from left to right, and the limit is taken as $\max_i(u_i - u_{i-1}) \to 0$ for a partition $s = u_0 < u_1 < \cdots < u_L = t$ of $(s,t]$. This extends the univariate product-integration in (2.18) and (2.19) to the matrix case.

For a Markov process, an important relationship between $\boldsymbol{P}(s,t)$ and $\boldsymbol{\Lambda}(t)$ is given by

$$\boldsymbol{P}(s,t) = \mathscr{P}_{(s,t]}\left[\boldsymbol{I} + d\boldsymbol{\Lambda}(u)\right]. \tag{14.24}$$

More details regarding this connection can be found in Theorem II.6.7 in Andersen et al. [7]. From this and continuity of the product-integration, $\boldsymbol{P}$ can be consistently estimated by

$$\widehat{\boldsymbol{P}}(s,t) = \mathscr{P}_{(s,t]}\left[\boldsymbol{I} + d\widehat{\boldsymbol{\Lambda}}(u)\right],$$

where $\widehat{\boldsymbol{\Lambda}}(t) = \left(\widehat{\Lambda}_{j\ell}(t)\right)_{K\times K}$, with $\widehat{\Lambda}_{jj}(t) = -\sum_{\ell\neq j}\widehat{\Lambda}_{j\ell}(t)$. $\widehat{\boldsymbol{P}}(t)$ is called the Aalen-Johansen estimator. Furthermore, the matrix product-integration can be shown to be differentiable, from which the asymptotic normality of $\widehat{\boldsymbol{P}}(s,t)$ can be established. More details regarding continuity and differentiability of the product-integration can be found in Gill and Johansen [99].

The matrix product-integration in (14.24) offers a succinct expression connecting $\boldsymbol{P}(s,t)$ and $\boldsymbol{\Lambda}(t)$. However, in a concrete model, it may be easier to obtain a specific transition probability using the Kolmogorov forward equations [75]:

$$\frac{\partial P_{jk}(s,t)}{\partial t} = \sum_{\ell} P_{j\ell}(s,t)\lambda_{\ell k}(t). \tag{14.25}$$

These equations can be obtained from the Markov and conditional probability properties as follows. For $\Delta > 0$, we have

$$\begin{aligned}
& P\left[X(t+\Delta) = k \middle| X(s) = j\right] \\
= \; & \sum_{\ell} P\left[X(t+\Delta) = k, X(t) = \ell \middle| X(s) = j\right] \\
= \; & \sum_{\ell} P\left[X(t) = \ell \middle| X(s) = j\right] P\left[X(t+\Delta) = k \middle| X(t) = \ell, X(s) = j\right] \\
= \; & \sum_{\ell} P_{j\ell}(s,t) P\left[X(t+\Delta) = k \middle| X(t) = \ell\right] \\
= \; & \sum_{\ell\neq k} P_{j\ell}(s,t) P\left[X(t+\Delta) = k \middle| X(t) = \ell\right] \\
& + P_{jk}(s,t) P\left[X(t+\Delta) = k \middle| X(t) = k\right].
\end{aligned} \tag{14.26}$$

Thus

$$
\begin{aligned}
& P_{jk}(s,t+\Delta)-P_{jk}(s,t) \\
= & \sum_{\ell\neq k} P_{j\ell}(s,t)P\big[X(t+\Delta)=k\big|X(t)=\ell\big]-P_{jk}(s,t)\{1-P\big[X(t+\Delta)=k\big|X(t)=k\big]\} \\
= & \sum_{\ell\neq k} P_{j\ell}(s,t)P\big[X(t+\Delta)=k\big|X(t)=\ell\big]-P_{jk}(s,t)\sum_{\ell\neq k} P\big[X(t+\Delta)=\ell\big|X(t)=k\big].
\end{aligned}
$$

If follows from the definitions of $\lambda_{jk}(t)$'s that

$$
\begin{aligned}
& \frac{\partial P_{jk}(s,t)}{\partial t} \\
= & \sum_{\ell\neq k} P_{j\ell}(s,t)\lambda_{\ell k}(t)-P_{jk}(s,t)\sum_{\ell\neq k}\lambda_{k\ell}(t) \\
= & \sum_{\ell} P_{j\ell}(s,t)\lambda_{\ell k}(t). \qquad (14.27)
\end{aligned}
$$

It is left to Exercise 14.10 to verify some of the details in obtaining of (14.26) and (14.27).

Example 14.4. Consider the illness-death model in Example 14.2 with a Markov process. Then $P_{11}(s,t)$ is the conditional probability that the individual remains healthy at time t, given that the individual is healthy at s. We have

$$\frac{\partial P_{11}(s,t)}{\partial t}=\sum_{\ell} P_{1\ell}(s,t)\lambda_{\ell 1}(t). \qquad (14.28)$$

It is left to Exercise 14.11 to show that the intensity matrix is

$$\begin{bmatrix} -\lambda_{12}-\lambda_{13} & \lambda_{12} & \lambda_{13} \\ 0 & -\lambda_{23} & \lambda_{23} \\ 0 & 0 & 0 \end{bmatrix}. \qquad (14.29)$$

Thus equation (14.28) is simplified to

$$\frac{\partial P_{11}(s,t)}{\partial t}=-P_{11}(s,t)\big[\lambda_{12}(t)+\lambda_{12}(t)\big].$$

Solving this differential equation in $t\geq s$ for fixed s (Exercise 14.13), and using $P_{11}(s,s)=1$, we get

$$P_{11}(s,t)=\exp\Big\{-\big[\Lambda_{12}+\Lambda_{13}\big]\big|_s^t\Big\}=\exp\big[-\Lambda_m\big|_s^t\big], \qquad (14.30)$$

where $\xi\big|_s^t = \xi(t) - \xi(s)$ for a function ξ, and Λ_m is the cumulative hazard function of $T_1 \wedge T_2$.

Under the Markov condition, counting process and martingale techniques can be used to simply the analysis. However, the Markov condition may not hold for a particular model or data set. For the illness-death model in Example 14.2, it is Markov if the intensity function $\lambda_{23}(t)$ does not depend on the history. For this model, a simple ad hoc test of the Markov condition can be obtained by fitting the intensity model

$$\lambda_{23i}(t\big|T_{1i}^*) = \lambda_{023}(t)\exp(\beta T_{1i}^*) \tag{14.31}$$

to the counting process N_{23i}, and testing the hypothesis

$$H_{0m} : \beta = 0 \tag{14.32}$$

[134]. A statistically significant result for testing H_{0m} is an indication that the Markov condition is questionable. This test is simple but circumstantial. It relies on the proportionality assumption and the particular functional form of the covariate built into model (14.31). Consequently, the test may fail to detect violations of the Markov Condition [284]. Other tests and related discussions can be found in Titman and Putter [299] and Soutinho and Meira-Machado [284].

To analyze a non-Markovian process $X(t)$, an often used and convenient approach is to consider a covariate-adjusted analysis using an intensity model, by including the entry time into the current state as a covariate. This is exemplified in model (14.31). However, it is important to note that T_1^* is a post-randomization covariate and may be responsive to the treatment. Consequently, there are complications as discussed in Section 6.2, and caution should be exercised when the objective is causal inference on the treatment effect.

A broad category of non-Markovian processes is the class of *semi-Markov processes,* in which $\lambda_{jk}(t)$ only depends on (j,k) and the time spent in the state j for each (j,k) transition. Such processes are also called *Markov-renewal processes.* The special case in the illness-death model of Example 14.2 is discussed below.

In the illness-death model, the transition intensity $\lambda_{23}(t)$ is in general a function of both t and the duration $d = t - T_1^*$ since entering the current state (state 2). A Markov process obtains if $\lambda_{23}(t,d)$ depends only on t. On the other hand, if $\lambda_{23}(t,d)$ depends only on the duration d, then the process is a semi-Markov process. This is because t and duration in the current state are the same for the $(1,2)$ and $(1,3)$ transitions.

For a semi-Markov process, instead of the time scale t that starts from the time since the initial state, duration or time since entering the current state can also be used as the time scale. The approach of working with the duration time scale is sometimes referred to as the "clock- reset" approach. In this method, the focus is on the time spent in the current state. In contrast, the usual approach with the total time scale is sometimes referred to as the "clock- forward" approach.

In the case of illness-death model for a semi-Markov process, a multiplicative intensity model obtains, and tools such as log-rank-test, GRE, and Cox model partial likelihood inference remain applicable. However, for a non-progressive semi-Markov process that allows transitions back and forth, alternative techniques to the martingale asymptotic theory are needed. More detailed discussions on the duration time scale can be found in Andersen et al. [7, Ch. X].

In the illness-death model for a semi-Markov process, for the (2,3) transition, the counting and at-risk processes are now

$$N_{23\cdot}^{r}(d) = \sum_{i=1}^{n} N_{23i}(d + T_{1i}^{*}), \ K_{2\cdot}^{r}(d) = \sum_{i=1}^{n} K_{2i}(d + T_{1i}^{*}),$$

where T_{1i}^{*}'s are the times to the non-terminal event. Note that $N_{23i} = K_{2i} = 0$ if T_{1i}^{*} is censored. Results parallel to those in (14.13) through (14.21) can then be obtained with obvious modifications.

Similar to the case for Markov processes, it is also important to check the semi-Markov condition that $\lambda_{23}(t,d)$ depends only on the duration d and not on t. From $d = t - T_1^*$, we get $t = d + T_1^*$. Let $K_{23}(t)\lambda(t|T_1^*)$ be the conditional intensity process given T_1^* for the (2,3) transition. A simple informal way to check the semi- Markov condition is to test the hypothesis

$$H_{0sm} : \beta = 0, \tag{14.33}$$

where β is the regression parameter in the model

$$\lambda(t|T_1^*) = \lambda_0(d)\exp(\beta T_1^*).$$

The test can be done with the partial likelihood framework applied to the variable $T_2^* - T_1^*$ in the subset for which T_1^* has occurred. That is, the time scale is the duration time scale. A statistically significant result is an indication that the semi-Markov condition is questionable. Limitations of this test and the related covariate-adjusted analysis are similar to those for testing (14.32) and using model (14.31). A non-significant test result does not directly establish that $\lambda_{23}(t,d)$ is only a function of the duration d. Therefore, more formal procedures are needed.

Results on more elaborate multi-state models and examples can be found in various sources, including Andersen et al. [7], Putter et al. [256], Meira-Machado et al. [204], Xu et al. [326], and Cook and Lawless [49].

Example 14.5. For the primary outcome data from the TOPCAT trial, let the terminal event be CVD, and the non-terminal event the composite of aborted cardiac arrest and hospitalization for the management of heart failure. Assume that the data follow the Markov illness-death model and that

$$\lambda_{jk}(t|Z) = \lambda_{0jk}(t)\exp(\beta_{jk}Z), \ t \geq 0, \ j,k \in \{(1,2),(1,3),(2,3)\},$$

TABLE 14.1
Log-rank test P-values and related GREs for the TOPCAT data.

	$\exp(\beta_{12})$	$\exp(\beta_{13})$	$\exp(\beta_{23})$
Log-rank GRE	0.82	1.07	0.83
Log-rank P-value	0.03	0.61	0.32

for some $\beta_{jk} > 0$, where Z is the treatment group indicator. The P-values for the log-rank tests of $H_{0jk} : \beta_{jk} = 0$, and the related log-rank GREs for $\exp(\beta_{jk})$ are summarized in Table 14. 1.

The above results assume that the Markov condition holds. Unfortunately, the score test for H_{0m} in (14.32) shows a P-value of 0.01. Thus the Markov assumption is questionable. Now assume that the semi-Markov condition holds. Then, under the proportional intensity model

$$\lambda_{23}(t|Z) = \lambda_{023}(d)\exp(\beta_{23}^* Z),$$

the log-rank GRE for $\exp(\beta_{23}^*)$ is 0.79, and the P-value for equality of the transition intensity functions in the control and treatment groups is 0.22. The score test for H_{0sm} in (14.33) has a non-significant P-value of 0.19. Note that under either the Markov or semi-Markov assumption, there is a noticeable difference between $\exp(\beta_{23})$ (or $\exp(\beta_{23}^*)$) and $\exp(\beta_{13})$, for T_2^* after T_1^* and T_2^* without T_1^*, respectively.

Multi-state models provide a framework for a refined analysis of complex disease progression processes. Often, intermediate events may change the natural history of disease progression, leading to different rates of terminal events in different transient states. Multi-state models allow separate modeling of terminal events with or without intermediate events, and account for how intermediate events may alter disease progression rates. Unlike the multiple increment models for competing risks or copula models for semi-competing risks, multi-state models work with transition intensity functions which are estimable using observed data. Additional competing risks to the terminal and non-terminal events can also be easily incorporated.

However, in the multi-state model framework, for the semi-competing risks setting which can be described by two hazard functions, three transition intensity functions are needed to specify the model. Assessing the overall risk of T_2^* is complex, as the relevant hazard function is a complicated functional of these three transition intensity functions. Moreover, the Markov or even semi-Markov assumption may be strong in some cases. Extensions to non-Markovian processes can further complicate the analysis and the results may be less straightforward to interpret.

A more significant consideration for causal inference in multi-state analysis arises because the definitions of states depend on the post-randomization covariate T_1^*. Consequently, even if all transitions are Markovian and treatment effect is proportional for all transition intensities, the intensity ratios still may not fully capture the treatment effect on the disease process. This is because individuals who have experienced T_1^* and are at risk for T_2^* may not be a representative subset of the sample at randomization. A significant ratio for (2,3) transition intensities may be due to the difference in T_1^* for the subsets of individuals who transit from state 2 to state 3, and it is difficult, if not impossible, to formulate or correct for such difference. This complication makes the assessment of treatment effects challenging.

The multi-state model approach is highly valuable for estimating and predicting actual risks across various outcome scenarios. This capability is particularly beneficial for prognosis and informed decision-making in clinical settings. The detailed scenario analysis provided by multi-state models can effectively complement a primary analysis for the etiologic summary assessment of treatment effects.

14.5 Restricted Mean Time Related Approaches

For univariate T, the restricted mean survival time (RMST), as discussed in Section 7.6.3, provides an intuitive and model-free summary of survival experience within the interval $[0,\tau]$. It is defined as

$$RMST = ET \wedge \tau = \int_0^\tau S(t)dt,$$

where $S = 1 - F$ is the survival function of T. A related measure is the restricted mean time lost (RMTL)

$$RMTL = \int_0^\tau F(t)dt.$$

For competing risks data, Zhao et al. [364] proposed using

$$RMTL_k = \int_0^\tau F_k(t)dt, \tag{14.34}$$

where F_k is the CIF of type k event. The RMTL_k is a model-free measure and represents the mean time lost due to cause k during $[0,\tau]$. Differences or ratios of RMTL_k can quantify treatment group disparities. Note that RMTL_k depends on competing risks through F_k. As previously discussed, treatment effect assessment typically is based on cause-specific hazards. However, Similar to the discussion in Section 13.3 on the CIF, RMTL_k-based measures can be valuable in epidemiological profiling of a population and risk prediction.

For multi-state processes, Mao [198] proposed the restricted mean time in favor (RMT-IF) of treatment. This nonparametric effect size quantifies the net average time individuals in the treatment group spend in a more favorable state than those in the control group, within a pre-specified time window.

To apply this method to the semi-competing risks data, as in the Section 14.3 setup, we define states $0, 1, 2$ to represent being event free, having had the non-terminal event but not yet the terminal event, and having had the terminal event, respectively. Denote by $Y(t)$ the state of a individual at time t, and let $Y^C(t)$, $Y^T(t)$ be the $Y(t)$ process for the control and treatment groups, respectively. The RMT-IF of treatment is

$$a_{TC} = E\int_0^{\tau} I\left(Y^T(t) < Y^C(t)\right) dt.$$

Note that the labels $0, 1, 2$ for the states are treated as ordinal for the purpose of computing a_{TC}. The net win time over $[0, \tau]$ is

$$\mu(\tau) = a_{TC} - a_{CT} = \int_0^{\tau} \{S_2^T(t)[1 - S_1^C(t)] - S_2^C(t)[1 - S_1^T(t)]\} dt, \tag{14.35}$$

where S_1 and S_2 denote the survival functions of $T_1^* \wedge T_2^*$ and T_2^*, respectively, with the superscript indicating control (C) or treatment (T) group.

The RMT-IF approach is intuitively simple and appealing. It is a generalization of the RMST to semi-competing risks data, since $\mu(\tau)$ reduces to the restricted mean survival difference in univariate survival analysis when there is only one event. Note that the net win time is a difference, not a ratio that some other methods employ. The approach does not accommodate additional competing risks to T_1^* and T_2^*, although it is possible to extend the method to accommodate competing risks using the cumulative incidence functions [198].

14.6 Data Structure and Global Testing

14.6.1 Terminal and Non-Terminal Events Subject to Competing Risks

Among the methods discussed so far in this chapter, only multi-state models and RMTL_k-based procedures can accommodate additional competing risks to both terminal and non-terminal events. However, these methods have their own limitations, as discussed in the previous sections. For a primary analysis assessing the overall treatment effect in the presence of competing risks, it is preferable to focus on risks for the events of interest while accounting for competing risks, and to formulate the problem with minimal model assumptions and parameters to be estimated.

To this end, an approach proposed by Yang [340] formulates the problem as one of two correlated competing risks. This formulation is slightly more general than related works proposed earlier [348, 349].

To help understand the data structure to be described, it is illustrative to think of an example where heart failure hospitalization and cardiovascular death are of interest. In this case, heart failure hospitalization is subject to the competing risk of all-cause mortality, while cardiovascular death is subject to the competing risk of non-cardiovascular death.

Let T_2 be the time to a terminal event which is either the terminal event of interest or a competing terminal event that stops further follow-up, and T_1 be the time to the first among events of interest or competing risks. Let D_1 and D_2 be the event type indicators corresponding to T_1 and T_2, taking values in $\{1,\ldots,K_1\}$, $\{1,\ldots,K_2\}$, respectively. Let $D_1 = 1$, $D_2 = 1$ indicate the non-terminal and terminal event of interest, respectively. In the example above, T_1 is the time to either heart failure hospitalization or all-cause mortality, and T_2 is the time to death. Additionally, $D_1 = 1$ and $D_2 = 1$ indicate heart failure hospitalization and cardiovascular death, respectively. When necessary, additional event types can be specified by additional values of D_1 and D_2. For example, if it is also of interest to study death from cancer, then $D_2 = 2$ can be defined to indicate cancer death.

Note that the formulation involves no latent variables, and the distributions of (T_j, D_j), $j = 1,2$, can be estimated nonparametrically without additional assumptions on the joint and marginal distributions. Let C be the censoring time independent of (T_j, D_j), $j = 1,2$. It is assumed that the distribution of T_j with $D_j = k_j$ is absolutely continuous, $k_j \leq K_j$, $j = 1,2$, while the censoring distribution may have discrete components.

Suppose there are n individuals in the trial, with those in the control group labeled $1,\ldots,n_1$, where $n_1 < n$. The quintuplets of time to the first event, time to a terminal event, event type indicators, and censoring time are denoted by

$$(T_{1i}, D_{1i}, T_{2i}, D_{2i}, C_i), \; i = 1,\ldots,n.$$

In the remainder of this chapter, the vectors $(T_{1i}, D_{1i}, T_{2i}, D_{2i}, C_i)$, $i \leq n_1$, are assumed to be i.i.d., as are the vectors $(T_{1i}, D_{1i}, T_{2i}, D_{2i}, C_i)$, $i > n_1$. These two collections of vectors are also assumed to be independent of each other. Due to censoring, the observed data are $(Y_{1i}, Y_{2i}, \delta_{1i}, \delta_{2i})$, $i = 1,\ldots,n$ where $Y_{1i} = T_{1i} \wedge C_i$, $Y_{2i} = T_{2i} \wedge C_i$, $\delta_{1i} = D_{1i} I(Y_{1i} = T_{1i})$ and $\delta_{2i} = D_{2i} I(Y_{2i} = T_{2i})$.

14.6.2 Global Null Hypothesis of No Treatment Effect

Let $\lambda_{jC}(t)$ and $\lambda_{jT}(t)$, for $j = 1,2$, be the cause-specific hazard functions of the non-terminal ($j = 1$) and terminal ($j = 2$) events of interest in the control (C) and treatment (T) groups, respectively:

$$\begin{aligned}\lambda_{jC}(t) &= \lim_{\Delta\downarrow 0}\frac{P\left[t \le T_{j1} < t+\Delta, D_{j1}=1 \middle| T_{j1} \ge t\right]}{\Delta}, \\ \lambda_{jT}(t) &= \lim_{\Delta\downarrow 0}\frac{P\left[t \le T_{jn} < t+\Delta, D_{jn}=1 \middle| T_{jn} \ge t\right]}{\Delta}, \ j=1,2. \qquad (14.36)\end{aligned}$$

For a primary analysis assessing the overall treatment effect, consider the null hypotheses

$$\begin{aligned} H_{01}: &\quad \lambda_{1T}(t) = \lambda_{1C}(t), \\ H_{02}: &\quad \lambda_{2T}(t) = \lambda_{2C}(t). \qquad (14.37)\end{aligned}$$

The global null hypothesis is defined as $H_{01} \cap H_{02}$.

The two component null hypotheses H_{01} and H_{02} focus on the treatment effects in terms of the cause-specific hazards for the events of interest, in the presence of competing risks. These hypotheses involve quantities that can be estimated from observable data without additional model assumptions. Formulating the global null hypothesis in this way leaves the joint distribution of the terminal and non-terminal events unspecified. This approach offers greater flexibility and allows for a more robust primary analysis. Furthermore, it avoids modeling assumptions involving unobservable data and unverifiable conditions.

It is important to note that the global hypothesis comprises only two component hypotheses. This contrasts with a multi-state model approach, which involves three: one for the non-terminal event, one for the terminal event occurring without non-terminal event, and one for the terminal event occurring after the non-terminal event. While the difference between two and three may seem minor, it can have a noticeable impact on the power for testing the global null hypothesis. For example, if the Bonferroni method is used, the P-value significance thresholds would be $0.05/2 = 0.025$ and $0.05/3 \approx 0.0167$, respectively.

Note that formulation of this global null hypothesis of no treatment effect accommodates competing risks to both the terminal and non-terminal events. When the only competing risk is the terminal event to the non-terminal event—for example, when the terminal and non-terminal events of interest are death and hospitalization, respectively, and death is the only terminating event—the win ratio tests the global null $H_{01}^* \cap H_{02}^*$ in Section 14.3, which involves the more complicated hazard function $\lambda^*(s|t)$. In comparison, the global null in (14.37) involves the much simpler cause-specific hazards whose integrals can be easily estimated by the Nelson-Aalen estimators.

14.7 Event-Specific Win Ratios

The event-specific win ratios (ESWR) were proposed by Yang and Troendle [348], who used them to form various tests of the overall treatment effect. The ESWRs are obtained through pairwise comparisons, similar to the win ratio. However, while the win ratio combines different events in a prioritized manner during these comparisons, ESWRs are calculated separately for each event. Under proportional hazards models for the cause-specific hazard functions of the non-terminal and terminal events, Yang et al. [349] showed that the ESWRs converge to the cause-specific hazard ratios. Asymptotic distributions of the ESWRs were also established and used to construct confidence intervals and test the global hypothesis that, for both the non-terminal and terminal events, the cause-specific hazard functions are the same in the control and treatment groups.

In the rest of this section, the ESWRs and related inference procedures will be introduced using the notations from Section 14.6, which provides a slightly more general framework than the original setup. Testing and estimation procedures developed in Yang and Troendle [348] and Yang et al. [349] remain valid under this framework.

For individual i in the treatment group and j in the control group, or $i > n_1, j \leq n_1$, the win indicators for the terminal and non-terminal events are $W_{2ij} = I(\delta_{2j} = 1, Y_{2i} \geq Y_{2j})$ and $W_{1ij} = I(\delta_{1j} = 1, Y_{1i} \geq Y_{1j})$ respectively. Similarly, the loss indicators for the terminal and non-terminal events are $L_{2ij} = \delta_{2i} I(Y_{2i} \leq Y_{2j})$ and $L_{1ij} = \delta_{1i} I(Y_{1i} \leq Y_{1j})$ respectively. This is analogous to the discussion on the win ratio in Section 14.3. Yang and Troendle [348] considered event-specific scores for terminal and non-terminal events separately. Let

$$
\begin{aligned}
W_\ell &= \sum_{i>n_1} \sum_{j \leq n_1} W_{\ell ij}, \\
L_\ell &= \sum_{i>n_1} \sum_{j \leq n_1} L_{\ell ij}, \quad \ell = 1, 2,
\end{aligned}
$$

The event-specific win ratios are

$$
R_\ell = \frac{L_\ell}{W_\ell}, \quad \ell = 1, 2.
$$

Consistent with the convention for hazard ratio and win ratio, the ESWRs are defined such that a ratio < 1 indicates beneficial effect.

14.7.1 Asymptotic Distributions of the ESWRs

Let

$$\mathbf{R} = (R_1, R_2)^{\mathrm{T}}, \quad \mathbf{1} = (1,1)^{\mathrm{T}}.$$

Using the multivariate U-statistics theory by Lehmann [165], Yang and Troendle [348] showed that, under the null hypothesis $H_{10} \cap H_{20}$, $\sqrt{n}(\mathbf{R} - \mathbf{1})$ has a limiting bivariate normal distribution with mean zero and covariance matrix $\boldsymbol{\Omega}$ which can be consistently estimated. Based on this asymptotic result, Yang and Troendle combined the ESWRs to form χ^2, linear combination, and maximum tests of $H_{01} \cap H_{02}$.

In a subsequent work, Yang et al. [349] constructed analogous tests using a different estimator of $\boldsymbol{\Omega}$, which remains consistent under certain alternative hypotheses as well as under the null hypothesis $H_{10} \cap H_{20}$. Since tests from Yang et al. typically have similar or slightly improved power, we will focus on their work In the presentation here.

Recall the win indicator $W_{\ell ij} = I(\delta_{\ell j} = 1, Y_{\ell i} \geq Y_{\ell j})$ for the (i, j) comparison and $\ell = 1, 2$. By the definition of Lebesgue-Stieltjes integral, we have

$$W_{\ell ij} = \int_0^\infty I(Y_{\ell i} \geq t) dI(\delta_{\ell j} = 1, Y_{\ell j} \leq t).$$

For $\ell = 1, 2$, let

$$K_{\ell C}(t) = \sum_{i \leq n_1} I(Y_{\ell i} \geq t)/n, \; N_{\ell C}(t) = \sum_{i \leq n_1} I(\delta_{\ell i} = 1, Y_{\ell i} \leq t)/n,$$

$$K_{\ell T}(t) = \sum_{i > n_1} I(Y_{\ell i} \geq t)/n, \; N_{\ell T}(t) = \sum_{i > n_1} I(\delta_{\ell i} = 1, Y_{\ell i} \leq t)/n.$$

Then

$$\begin{aligned} W_\ell &= \sum_{i > n_1} \sum_{j \leq n_1} W_{\ell ij} \\ &= \sum_{i > n_1} \int_0^\infty I(Y_{\ell i} \geq t) d\left[\sum_{j \leq n_1} I(\delta_{\ell j} = 1, Y_{\ell j} \leq t)\right] \\ &= n^2 \int_0^\infty K_{\ell C}(t) dN_{\ell T}(t). \end{aligned}$$

Similarly,

$$L_\ell = n^2 \int_0^\infty K_{\ell T}(t) dN_{\ell C}(t).$$

Let $\Lambda_{\ell C}(t), \Lambda_{\ell T}(t)$, $\ell = 1, 2$, be the cumulative cause-specific hazard functions corresponding to $\lambda_{\ell C}(t), \lambda_{\ell T}(t)$, $\ell = 1, 2$, respectively. From (13.13) and with the notations here, the Nelson-Aalen estimators of $\Lambda_{\ell C}(t)$ and $\Lambda_{\ell T}(t)$ are

$$\widehat{\Lambda}_{\ell C}(t) = \int_0^t \frac{dN_{\ell C}(s)}{K_{\ell C}(s)}, \quad \widehat{\Lambda}_{\ell T}(t) = \int_0^t \frac{dN_{\ell T}(s)}{K_{\ell T}(s)}, \ \ell = 1,2. \tag{14.38}$$

Thus

$$\begin{aligned} R_\ell &= \frac{\int_0^\infty K_{\ell C}(t) dN_{\ell T}(t)}{\int_0^\infty K_{\ell T}(t) dN_{\ell C}(t)} \\ &= \frac{\int_0^\infty K_{\ell C}(t) K_{\ell T}(t) d\widehat{\Lambda}_{\ell T}(t)}{\int_0^\infty K_{\ell C}(t) K_{\ell T}(t) d\widehat{\Lambda}_{\ell C}(t)}, \ \ell = 1,2. \end{aligned} \tag{14.39}$$

It follows that, under certain regularity conditions, R_ℓ converges to the limit

$$r_\ell = \frac{\int_0^\infty S_{CC}(t) S_{CT}(t) S_{\ell C}(t) S_{\ell T}(t) d\Lambda_{\ell T}(t)}{\int_0^\infty S_{CC}(t) S_{CT}(t) S_{\ell C}(t) S_{\ell T}(t) d\Lambda_{\ell C}(t)}, \quad \ell = 1,2, \tag{14.40}$$

where

$$S_{CC}(t) = P[C_1 \geq t], \ S_{jC}(t) = P[T_{j1} \geq t],$$

$$S_{CT}(t) = P[C_n \geq t], \ S_{jT}(t) = P[T_{jn} \geq t].$$

Therefore, under $H_{01} \cap H_{02}$, R_ℓ converges to 1, $\ell = 1,2$.

In general, the limit in (14.40) depend on the censoring distributions. Now consider the proportional hazards hypotheses for the non-terminal and terminal events, respectively:

$$H_{1PH}: \quad \lambda_{1T}(t) = \theta_1 \lambda_{1C}(t), \ \text{for some } \theta_1 > 0, \tag{14.41}$$

$$H_{2PH}: \quad \lambda_{2T}(t) = \theta_2 \lambda_{2C}(t), \ \text{for some } \theta_2 > 0. \tag{14.42}$$

It can be seen that, under the hypothesis $H_{\ell PH}$, $r_\ell = \theta_\ell$, $\ell = 1,2$, free of the censoring distributions. From (14.39), it can also be recognized that R_1, R_2 are of the forms similar to the GREs for univariate survival analysis in Section 5.7.

By the martingale theory, $\sqrt{n}(R_1 - \theta_1)$ and $\sqrt{n}(R_2 - \theta_2)$ each have a limiting normal distribution. However, the martingale structure no longer holds for the joint analysis of non-terminal and terminal events, and additional analytical steps are required.

Using the theory of empirical processes, it can be shown that, under $H_{1PH} \cap H_{2PH}$, $\sqrt{n}(\widehat{\mathbf{R}} - \boldsymbol{\theta})$ has a limiting bivariate normal distribution with mean vector zero and covariance matrix $\boldsymbol{\Omega}(\boldsymbol{\theta})$ which has a consistent estimator $\widehat{\boldsymbol{\Omega}}$.

14.7.2 Tests of the Global Null Hypothesis

Since the global null hypothesis $H_{01} \cap H_{02}$ implies $H_{1PH} \cap H_{2PH}$, the asymptotic results in the previous subsection can be used to establish asymptotically valid tests for $H_{01} \cap H_{02}$.

The χ^2 test is a traditional approach for combining multiple tests and has often been used in many statistical problems. In this setting, the test statistic is

$$\chi^2 = n(\mathbf{R}-\mathbf{1})\widehat{\boldsymbol{\Omega}}^{-1}(\mathbf{R}-\mathbf{1})^T.$$

The null hypothesis $H_{01} \cap H_{02}$ is rejected at a significance level α if $\chi^2 > \chi_2^2(\alpha)$.

However, the χ^2 test does not correspond to an effect measure for the overall treatment effect. An alternative to the χ^2 test is the linear combination test. Let

$$\widehat{T}_1 = \sqrt{n}(R_1 - 1),\ \widehat{T}_2 = \sqrt{n}(R_2 - 1).$$

The test statistic is

$$\eta\widehat{T}_1 + (1-\eta)\widehat{T}_2 = \sqrt{n}\big[\eta R_1 + (1-\eta)R_2 - 1\big], \tag{14.43}$$

for a pre-determined and fixed $\eta \in (0,1)$, The simple average corresponds to $\eta = 1/2$. The linear combination test is often used when the treatment effects are expected to be in the same direction for both terminal and non-terminal events. This test statistic also provides $\eta R_1 + (1-\eta)R_2$ as an overall treatment effect measure.

Let σ_1^2, σ_2^2, and ρ be the marginal variances and correlation coefficient of the covariance matrix $\boldsymbol{\Omega}(\boldsymbol{\theta})$. Under the null $H_{10} \cap H_{20}$, the statistic in (14.43) is asymptotically normal with mean zero and variance

$$\sigma^2(\eta) = \eta^2\sigma_1^2 + (1-\eta)^2\sigma_2^2 + 2\eta(1-\eta)\sigma_1\sigma_2\rho. \tag{14.44}$$

Thus an asymptotic level α test rejects $H_{10} \cap H_{20}$ if

$$\left|\ell^{\mathrm{T}}\mathbf{R} - 1\right|\left(\frac{\ell^{\mathrm{T}}\widehat{\boldsymbol{\Omega}}\ell}{n}\right)^{-1/2} > z(\alpha/2), \tag{14.45}$$

where $\ell = (\eta, 1-\eta)^{\mathrm{T}}$.

The linear combination test with a fixed η allows for a simper analysis and a clearer demonstration of the contribution from each event type. Additionally, a data-dependent value of η can be used to satisfy a particular optimality criterion. For example, the asymptotic variance is minimized at

$$\eta_0 = \frac{\sigma_2^2 - \sigma_1\sigma_2\rho}{\sigma_1^2 + \sigma_2^2 - 2\sigma_1\sigma_2\rho},$$

which can be estimated by

$$\widehat{\eta} = \frac{\widehat{\sigma}_2^2 - \widehat{\sigma}_1\widehat{\sigma}_2\widehat{\rho}}{\widehat{\sigma}_1^2 + \widehat{\sigma}_2^2 - 2\widehat{\sigma}_1\widehat{\sigma}_2\widehat{\rho}}, \tag{14.46}$$

where $\widehat{\sigma}_1^2, \widehat{\sigma}_2^2$, and $\widehat{\rho}$ are the marginal variances and correlation coefficient of the covariance matrix estimator $\widehat{\boldsymbol{\Omega}}$. Now let

$$L(\mathbf{R}) = \widehat{\eta}\widehat{R}_1 + (1-\widehat{\eta})\widehat{R}_2, \tag{14.47}$$

$$\widehat{T}_{LD} = \widehat{\eta}\widehat{T}_1 + (1-\widehat{\eta})\widehat{T}_2 = \sqrt{n}(L(\mathbf{R}) - 1). \tag{14.48}$$

Under $H_{10} \cap H_{20}$, $L(\mathbf{R})$ approaches 1 as n increases. It can be shown that $\widehat{T}_L$ has a limiting normal distribution with mean zero and variance $\sigma^2(\eta)$ in (14.44), with $\eta = \eta_0$. A consistent estimator $\widehat{\sigma}_{LD}^2$ of $\sigma^2(\eta_0)$ can be obtained by replacing η_0, ρ and σ_ℓ in (14.44) with $\widehat{\eta}$, $\widehat{\rho}$ and $\widehat{\sigma}_\ell$, respectively, for $\ell = 1, 2$. Consequently, a test for the global null $H_{10} \cap H_{20}$ at significance level α rejects it when

$$\frac{|\widehat{T}_{LD}|}{\widehat{\sigma}_{LD}} > z(\alpha/2).$$

To better control the type one error rate in finite samples for the linear combination test with data-driven coefficients, Yang et al. [349] considered a transformed version of the test. In addition, Yang [340] introduced a correction factor to further improve size control for small samples. Let $\widehat{\ell} = (\widehat{\eta}, 1-\widehat{\eta})^{\mathrm{T}}$ for $\widehat{\eta}$ in (14.46). Using transformation Q and correction factor c_n, the corresponding test rejects $H_{01} \cap H_{02}$ if

$$\sqrt{n}\left|Q(\widehat{\ell}^{\mathrm{T}}\mathbf{R}) - Q(1)\right| \Big/ \left[c_n q(\widehat{\ell}^{\mathrm{T}}\mathbf{R})\sqrt{\widehat{\ell}^{\mathrm{T}}\widehat{\boldsymbol{\Omega}}\widehat{\ell}}\right] > z_{\alpha/2}. \tag{14.49}$$

By the delta method, under the null $H_{01} \cap H_{02}$, the statistic on the left-hand side of (14.49) has the same limiting distribution as $|\widehat{T}_L|/\widehat{\sigma}_L$. Thus the test in (14.49) is asymptotically valid.

The maximum test offers another option to form a global test based on the ESWRs. Let

$$\widehat{T}_M = \max(|\widehat{T}_1/\widehat{\sigma}_1|, |\widehat{T}_2/\widehat{\sigma}_2|).$$

The maximum test at level α rejects $H_{10} \cap H_{20}$ when $\widehat{T}_M > t_\alpha(\widehat{\rho})$, where $t_\alpha(\rho)$ satisfies:

$$1 - \alpha = \int_{-t_\alpha(\rho)}^{t_\alpha(\rho)} \left\{ \Gamma\left(\frac{t_\alpha(\rho) - \rho w}{\sqrt{1-\rho^2}}\right) - \Gamma\left(\frac{-t_\alpha(\rho) - \rho w}{\sqrt{1-\rho^2}}\right) \right\} \gamma(w) dw, \tag{14.50}$$

with γ and Γ being the $p.d.f.$ and $c.d.f.$ of the standard normal distribution respectively. In the literature, the χ^2 test can often be improved by the linear combination and the maximum tests [342].

Again, better control of the type one error rate can be achieved with an appropriate transformation and correction factor. Define

$$\widehat{T}_{MQ}(\boldsymbol{\theta}) = \sqrt{n}\max\left(\frac{|Q(R_1)-Q(\theta_1)|}{c_n q(R_1)\widehat{\sigma}_1}, \frac{|Q(R_2)-Q(\theta_2)|}{c_n q(R_2)\widehat{\sigma}_2}\right). \tag{14.51}$$

By the delta method, under the null $H_{01} \cap H_{02}$, $\widehat{T}_{MQ}(\mathbf{1})$ has the same limiting distribution as $\widehat{T}_M$. This yields a test that rejects $H_{10} \cap H_{20}$ if

$$\widehat{T}_{MQ}(\mathbf{1}) > t_\alpha(\widehat{\rho}). \tag{14.52}$$

The χ^2 test can be similarly modified. For the linear combination test with fixed η, it is unnecessary to use a transformation or correction factor.

The procedure for using any one of the global tests is as follows:

1. Determine if the particular global test is significant at the α level.
2. If the global test is significant, determine if

$$\frac{Q(R_j)-Q(1)}{c_n q(R_j)\widehat{\sigma}_j} < -z_{\alpha/2} \text{ or } > z_{\alpha/2},\ j = 1,2,$$

and declare beneficial or harmful effect on the components accordingly.

Note that all the global tests are two sided. A test being significant means that the observed data provides strong evidence to reject the null hypothesis $H_{10} \cap H_{20}$. More comments and discussions regarding global testing can be found in Yang and Troendle [348]. Note that these global tests utilize the available data more fully than the win ratio test, which does not use the non-terminal events if the pairwise comparison is conclusive with the terminal events.

14.7.3 Test of the Proportional Hazards Assumptions

As discussed in Section 14.7.1, the ESWRs converge to limits that in general depend on censoring distributions, unless the proportional hazards assumptions H_{1PH} and H_{2PH} hold. Thus, it is important to test those assumptions. The simple test of Gill and Schumacher [100] in Section 6.6.1 can be extended to the current setting.

For the non-terminal event, consider the weighted event-specific win ratio

$$R_{1\Phi} = \frac{\int_0^\infty \Phi K_{1C}(t)K_{1T}(t)d\widehat{\lambda}_{1T}(t)}{\int_0^\infty \Phi K_{1C}(t)K_{1T}(t)d\widehat{\lambda}_{1C}(t)}.$$

Under H_{1PH}, for two weights Φ_1, Φ_2, it can be shown that $\sqrt{n}(R_{1\Phi_2} - R_{1\Phi_1})$ is asymptotically normal with mean 0. Similarly, for the terminal event, consider the weighted event-specific win ratio

$$R_{2\Psi} = \frac{\int \Psi K_{2C}(t) K_{2T}(t) d\widehat{\lambda}_{2T}(t)}{\int \Psi K_{2C}(t) K_{2T}(t) d\widehat{\lambda}_{2C}(t)}.$$

Under H_{2PH}, for two weights Ψ_1, Ψ_2, $\sqrt{n}(R_{1\Psi_2} - R_{1\Psi_1})$ is also asymptotically normal with mean 0.

Let $\mathbf{RD} = (R_{1\Phi_2} - R_{1\Phi_1}, R_{2\Psi_2} - R_{2\Psi_1})^{\mathrm{T}}$. Under $H_{1PH} \cap H_{2PH}$, it can be shown that $\sqrt{n}\mathbf{RD}$ has a limiting normal distribution with mean vector zero and a covariance matrix $\mathbf{V}$ which has a consistent estimator $\widehat{\mathbf{V}}$. Technical details can be found in Yang et al. [349]. Let $\widehat{v}_k$, $k = 1,2$ and $\widehat{\mu}$ be the marginal standard deviations and correlation coefficient from $\widehat{\mathbf{V}}$. Then a maximum test for $H_{1PH} \cap H_{2PH}$ rejects it at significance level α if

$$\sqrt{n}\max\left(|R_{1\Phi_2} - R_{1\Phi_1}|/\widehat{v}_1, |R_{2\Psi_2} - R_{2\Psi_1}|/\widehat{v}_2\right) > t_\alpha(\widehat{\mu}) \tag{14.53}$$

for t_α in (14.50). Yang et al. showed that, if Φ_2/Φ_1 and Ψ_2/Ψ_1 are both monotone non-constant functions, then the test is consistent against the alternative that either $\lambda_{1T}(t)/\lambda_{1C}(t)$ or $\lambda_{2T}(t)/\lambda_{2C}(t)$ is a monotone non-constant function of t.

On recommendations from Gill and Schumacher, the pairs of Φ functions and Ψ functions are chosen to correspond to, respectively, the log-rank test statistics and test statistics similar to the Peto-Prentice weighted log-rank test statistics, for both the non-terminal and terminal events. Specifically,

$$\begin{aligned} \Phi_{LR} &= \frac{1}{K_{1C} + K_{1T}}, \quad \Phi_{PP} = \frac{\exp(-\widehat{\Lambda}_{1P})}{K_{1C} + K_{1T}}, \\ \Psi_{LR} &= \frac{1}{K_{2C} + K_{2T}}, \quad \Psi_{PP} = \frac{\exp(-\widehat{\Lambda}_{2P})}{K_{2C} + K_{2T}}, \end{aligned} \tag{14.54}$$

where $\widehat{\Lambda}_{kP}$, $k = 1,2$ are the Nelson-Aalen estimators from the pooled sample for the non-terminal and terminal events respectively. Other choices for the weights are possible. For example, $\exp(-\widehat{\Lambda}_{kP})$, $k = 1,2$ can be replaced by the estimated cumulative incidence functions which usually yield similar results. Note that $R_{1\Phi}$ and $R_{2\Psi}$ with weights Φ_{LR} and Ψ_{LR} are the log-rank GREs for the non-terminal and terminal events, respectively.

14.7.4 Effect Measures

The PH assumptions (14.41) and (14.42) are on the cause-specific hazards which are estimable using observed data. In addition, they do not restrict the proportionality constants to be the same. Therefore, the ESWRS have more interpretable estimands, under conditions more flexible than condition (14.7) for the win ratio.

Based on the results of Section 14.8.1, confidence intervals for various effect measures can be derived. Using a transformation Q and correction factor c_n, a $100(1-\alpha)\%$ confidence interval for θ_k is

$$\left[Q^{-1}\left(Q(R_k) - z_{\alpha/2}\frac{c_n q(R_k)\widehat{\sigma}_k}{\sqrt{n}}\right), Q^{-1}\left(Q(R_k) + z_{\alpha/2}\frac{c_n q(R_k)\widehat{\sigma}_k}{\sqrt{n}}\right)\right], \quad k = 1,2, \quad (14.55)$$

where Q^{-1} is the inverse of Q.

As mentioned before, when the treatment effects are expected to be in the same direction for both terminal and non-terminal events, a weighted average $\ell'\boldsymbol{\theta}$ is often used as a measure for an overall effect, where $\ell = (\eta, 1-\eta)^{\mathrm{T}}$ for a fixed $\eta \in (0,1)$. A $100(1-\alpha)\%$ confidence interval for $\ell'\boldsymbol{\theta}$ is

$$\left[\left(\ell'\mathbf{R} - z_{\alpha/2}\sqrt{\frac{\ell'\widehat{\boldsymbol{\Omega}}\ell}{n}}\right)_+, \ell'\mathbf{R} + z_{\alpha/2}\sqrt{\frac{\ell'\widehat{\boldsymbol{\Omega}}\ell}{n}}\right], \quad (14.56)$$

where $(a)_+ = \max(a, 0)$.

The confidence intervals in (14.55) provide separate probability statements. In some cases, simultaneous confidence intervals may be desirable. From

$$P[\widehat{T}_{MQ}(\boldsymbol{\theta}) > t_\alpha(\widehat{\rho})] \to 1-\alpha, \quad (14.57)$$

$100(1-\alpha)\%$ simultaneous confidence intervals for θ_1, θ_2 can be obtained as

$$\left[Q^{-1}\left(Q(R_k) - t_\alpha(\widehat{\rho})\frac{c_n q(R_k)\widehat{\sigma}_k}{\sqrt{n}}\right), Q^{-1}\left(Q(R_k) + t_\alpha(\widehat{\rho})\frac{c_n q(R_k)\widehat{\sigma}_k}{\sqrt{n}}\right)\right], \quad k = 1,2, \quad (14.58)$$

For tests and interval estimation, certain test-estimation coherency results can be established. The linear combination test in (14.45) rejects $H_{01} \cap H_{02}$ if and only if the confidence interval in (14.56) excludes 1. Furthermore, the maximum test in (14.52) rejects $H_{01} \cap H_{02}$ if and only if at least one of the simultaneous confidence intervals in (14.58) excludes 1.

However, for the linear combination test with data-driven coefficients, under $H_{1PH} \cap H_{2PH}$, the test statistic $L(\mathbf{R})$ converges to a limit that, in general, depends on the censoring distributions. Let

$$H_{EPH}: \lambda_{jT}(t) = \theta\lambda_{jC}(t), \ j = 1,2, \ \text{for some } \theta > 0. \quad (14.59)$$

Suppose that H_{EPH} holds. It can be shown that the limit of $L(\mathbf{R})$ depends only on the cause-specific hazard functions of interest. Therefore, $L(\mathbf{R})$ has a valid estimand. The test in (14.50) rejects $H_{01} \cap H_{02}$ if and only if 1 is excluded from the confidence interval $[\widehat{l}, \widehat{u}]$, where

$$\begin{aligned}\widehat{l} &= Q^{-1}\Big(Q(\widehat{\ell}^{\mathrm{T}}\mathbf{R}) - z(\alpha/2)c_n q(\widehat{\ell}^{\mathrm{T}}\mathbf{R})\sqrt{\widehat{\ell}^{\mathrm{T}}\widehat{\boldsymbol{\Omega}}\widehat{\ell}/n}\Big),\\ \widehat{u} &= Q^{-1}\Big(Q(\widehat{\ell}^{\mathrm{T}}\mathbf{R}) + z(\alpha/2)c_n q(\widehat{\ell}^{\mathrm{T}}\mathbf{R})\sqrt{\widehat{\ell}^{\mathrm{T}}\widehat{\boldsymbol{\Omega}}\widehat{\ell}/n}\Big).\end{aligned} \tag{14.60}$$

Based on various numerical studies and applications to clinical trial data, for ESWR-based χ^2 and maximum tests of $H_{01} \cap H_{02}$, as well as for the global testing procedures and the confidence intervals in (14.55), It is recommended [349, 340] that the transformation and correction factor be used:

$$Q(x) = -\ln\big(-\ln\frac{\exp(x)-1}{\exp(x)+1}\big),\ c_n = 1 + 15/\max(n, 100). \tag{14.61}$$

For the linear combination test with data-driven coefficients, the log transformation and $c_n = 1 + 10/\max(n, 100)$ are recommended. No transformation is needed for the linear combination test with fixed coefficients.

To help implement the ESWR-based procedures, the R package EventWinRatios is available at the Comprehensive R Archive Network [218]. Given input data, the package generates global testing and confidence interval results, as well as the results of testing for $H_{1PH} \cap H_{2PH}$ and H_{EPH}.

14.8 Nonparametric Testing and Estimation Procedures

As discussed in Sections 14.3 and 14.7, both the win ratio and linear combinations of the ESWRs can be used to measure the overall treatment effect. However, the win ratio requires condition (14.7), while the ESWRs rely on the proportional hazards conditions (14.41) and (14.42). Those conditions are semiparametric, with unspecified baseline functions. Yang [340] proposed new testing and estimation procedures that are entirely nonparametric.

Recall the restricted mean time lost due to cause k in Section 14.5. To avoid dependence on competing risks, Yang proposed using the integrated cumulative hazard (ICH) $\int_0^\tau \Lambda_k(t)dt$ as a measure for the total risk of type k event over $[0, \tau]$, where Λ_k is the cumulative cause-specific hazard function for type k event. This measure retains the intuitive area-under-the-curve interpretation, but depends solely on the cause-specific hazard of type k event. The ratios of those measures can then be used to describe the treatment effect on the non-terminal ($j = 1$) and terminal ($j = 2$) events:

$$r_j = \frac{\int_0^\tau \Lambda_{jT}(s)ds}{\int_0^\tau \Lambda_{jC}(s)ds},\ j = 1, 2. \tag{14.62}$$

For $j = 1,2$, under H_{jPH} in (14.41) and (14.42), $r_j = \theta_j$. Thus r_j is a nonparametric extension of the hazard ratio. r_1, r_2 can be nonparametrically estimated by $\widehat{r}_1$, $\widehat{r}_2$, respectively, which are obtained by plugging in the Nelson-Aalen estimators.

More generally, for a monotone smooth transformation Φ, Yang considered the integrated transformed cumulative hazard (ITCH) $\int_0^\tau \Phi(\Lambda_k(t))dt$, and defined

$$r_{j\Phi} = \frac{\int_0^\tau \Phi(\Lambda_{jT}(t))dt}{\int_0^\tau \Phi(\Lambda_{jC}(t))dt}, \quad j = 1,2. \tag{14.63}$$

The corresponding estimators are

$$\widehat{r}_{j\Phi} = \frac{\int_0^\tau \Phi(\widehat{\Lambda}_{jT}(t))dt}{\int_0^\tau \Phi(\widehat{\Lambda}_{jC}(t))dt}, \quad j = 1,2. \tag{14.64}$$

When there are no competing risks, the quantity $r_{j\Phi_0}$ with $\Phi_0(t) = 1 - \exp(-t)$ reproduces the ratio of restricted mean times lost in the univariate case. In general, however, as discussed in Chapter Thirteen, the interpretation as the restricted mean time lost is not applicable unless the strong assumption of no-impact removal of competing risks holds. When Λ_{jC}, Λ_{jT} are small over $[0,\tau]$, as in the case of heavy censoring,

$$1 - \exp(-\Lambda_{jC}) \simeq \Lambda_{jC}, \quad 1 - \exp(-\Lambda_{jT}) \simeq \Lambda_{jT}.$$

Thus $r_{j\Phi_0} \simeq r_j$, $j = 1,2$.

Regarding the choice of τ, it is ideal to include most or all data when assessing the overall treatment effect in a clinical trial. However, the Nelson-Aalen estimator is often unstable near the upper end of the data range. To balance representativeness and robustness, Yang recommended setting τ as 90% of the total trial duration, or even 80% for longer trials. Regardless of the specific value for τ, it is important that the choice be pre-specified before data unblinding.

Let

$$\widehat{\boldsymbol{\Upsilon}} = (\widehat{r}_{1\Phi}, \widehat{r}_{2\Phi})^{\mathrm{T}}, \quad \boldsymbol{\Upsilon} = (r_{1\Phi}, r_{2\Phi})^{\mathrm{T}}.$$

Under regularity conditions, Yang showed that $\widehat{r}_{j\Phi}$ consistently estimates $r_{j\Phi}$ for $j = 1,2$, and that $\sqrt{n}(\widehat{\boldsymbol{\Upsilon}} - \boldsymbol{\Upsilon})$ converges in distribution to a bivariate normal with mean zero and covariance matrix which has a consistent estimator $\widehat{\mathbf{A}}_N$. Based on these asymptotic results, Yang [340] studied the maximum and linear combination tests using ICH or ITCH with $\Phi_0 = 1 - \exp(-t)$. Confidence intervals were also established. These results parallel those for ESWR-based inference, with $\widehat{\boldsymbol{\Upsilon}}$ and $\boldsymbol{\Upsilon}$ replacing $\mathbf{R}$ and $\boldsymbol{\theta}$, respectively. Yang [340] also recommended using the same transformation and correction factor in (14.61) for the maximum tests of $H_{01} \cap H_{02}$ and the global testing procedures. No transformation is needed for the linear combination test with fixed coefficients.

TABLE 14.2
Observed events by treatment group in the TOPCAT trial.

Observed Events	Treatment	Control	All
H only	160	175	335
H & CVD	48	74	122
CVD only	112	102	214
NCVD	97	97	194
Censored	1306	1274	2580

14.9 Illustrations with the TOPCAT and SPRINT Data

To illustrate the tests and confidence intervals from various methods, we apply them to the primary outcome data from the TOPCAT and SPRINT trials in this section. First, consider the TOPCAT trial. The primary endpoint of the trial was the composite of cardiovascular death (CVD), aborted cardiac arrest, and heart failure hospitalization. It was shown in Example 5.1 that, under the proportional hazards model (5.4), the estimated hazard ratio for the primary composite is 0.89, with a 95% confidence interval 0.77–1.04. For the null hypothesis of no treatment effect, the Wald test has a P-value of 0.14. It was also shown in Example 6.3 that model (5.4) is reasonable. These results were derived assuming independent censoring.

To illustrate some of the methods discussed in this chapter, the terminal event of interest is CVD, and the non-terminal event of interest is the composite of aborted cardiac arrest and heart failure hospitalization (H). The breakdown of observed events is provided in Table 14.2.

From Table 14.2, 122 trial participants experienced both H and CVD. Thus 122 CVD events were excluded from the primary analysis of TOPCAT. There were $122+214=336$ CVD events, and 194 NCVD events, indicating that the presence of competing risks was substantial.

Table 14.3 provides the results of tests and confidence intervals (when applicable) from various methods. Results for the log-rank test, the two-sample Cox models on the primary and component endpoints, the win ratio test, and the test based on the restricted mean time in favor of treatment, are in the rows denoted by LR and COX, WR, and RMT-IF, respectively, Results for LR, WR, and RMT-IF, are from Yang [340].

The results based on ESWR, the weighted ESWR with the log-rank weights in (14.54), ICH, and ITCH with Φ_0 are denoted by ESWR, LRGRE, ICH, and ITCH, respectively. The linear and maximum tests are indicated by the subscripts L and M, respectively. The linear combination test using ESWR with data-driven coefficients is denoted by ESWR_{LD}. The column "P-value" gives results for testing

TABLE 14.3
Testing and confidence interval results for the TOPCAT data. Results for LR, WR, and RMT-IF, are from Table 5 in Yang [340].

Method	P-value	Effect_1 (CI)	Effect_2 (CI)	Overall Effect (CI)
LR	0.142			
Cox	0.142	0.82 (0.68,0 .98)	0.90 (0.73, 1.12)	0.89 (0.77, 1.04)
WR	0.089			0.87 (0.75, 1.02)
RMT-IF	0.115			0.10 (-0.12, 0.23)
ESWR_L	0.014	0.79 (0.64, 0.94)	0.88 (0.68, 1.08)	0.83 (0.70, 0.97)
ESWR_{MX}	0.015	0.79 (0.64, 0.94)	0.88 (0.68, 1.08)	
ESWR_{LD}	0.012	0.79 (0.64, 0.94)	0.88 (0.68, 1.08)	0.82 (0.70, 0.96)
LRGRE_L	0.040	0.82 (0.67, 0.97)	0.90 (0.71, 1.10)	0.86 (0.73, 0.99)
LRGRE_{MX}	0.044	0.82 (0.67, 0.97)	0.90 (0.71, 1.10)	
ICH_L	0.033	0.82 (0.67, 0.97)	0.89 (0.71, 1.09)	0.86 (0.72, 0.99)
ICH_{MX}	0.040	0.82 (0.67, 0.97)	0.89 (0.71, 1.09)	
ITCH_L	0.032	0.83 (0.69, 0.97)	0.90 (0.72, 1.09)	0.86 (0.74, 0.99)
ITCH_{MX}	0.038	0.83 (0.69, 0.97)	0.90 (0.72, 1.09)	

the null of no treatment effect. The columns Effect_1, Effect_2, and Overall Effect provide point and interval estimates for the effects on H, CVD, and the overall effect, respectively.

For the ICH- and ITCH- based methods, Yang recommended setting τ to 90% of the trial duration, which is 6.15. The results using $\tau = 6.15$ can be founded in Yang [340]. To illustrate the influence of τ on the results, the current illustration uses $\tau = 5.81$, or 85% of the trial duration. Note that for ESWR, LRGRE, there is no need to restrict the integration range and all data can be used, as shown in (14.39). However, for a direct comparison with results for ICH and ITCH, the integration range $[0, 5.81]$ is also applied to the point estimates and variance estimates for ESWR, LRGRE.

Table 14.3 shows that tests in rows five through thirteen are significant at the 0.05 level. Following rejection of the global null, each of these methods shows a significant reduction in the cause-specific hazard of H. However, none of the methods show a significant effect on CVD.

Note that for the asymptotic validity of the WR or RMT-IF methods, it is assumed that no competing risks are present. This effectively assumes that the NCVD events are independent of CVD and H events. For effect estimation using the WR or ESWR-based methods, condition (14.7) and the assumption $H_{1PH} \cap H_{2PH}$ are required, respectively. In addition, for estimating the overall effect using ESWR-based linear combination with data-driven coefficients, condition H_{EPH} is assumed. From Yang et al. [348], the P-values for testing $H_{1PH} \cap H_{2PH}$ and H_{EPH}

are 0.32 and 0.44, respectively. However, for condition (14.7) related to the WR method, no formal testing procedures are currently available in the literature.

From Table 14.3, the ESWR-, LRGRE-, ICH- and ITCH-based methods demonstrate greater sensitivity to group differences in TOPCAT compared to other methods. Two contributing factors are that these methods make fuller use of the available data and that they rely on cause-specific hazards, which isolate the risk of interest from competing events.

Under the proportional hazards model, the minimal variance for generalized rank estimators is achieved with the weight corresponding to LRGRE [95]. However, although the proportional hazards models are reasonable for CVD and H, Table 14.3 shows that the ESWR-based tests are more sensitive than those based on LRGRE. This is because the cause-specific hazard ratio for H increases slightly over time, similar to the case for the composite outcome shown in Figure 7.11. The ESWRs, which use Gehan weights, emphasize early event times more than LRGREs which use the log-rank weights. As a result, ESWRs are better at detecting group differences in the TOPCAT data. This example demonstrates that, even when the proportional hazards assumption holds, the log-rank test may be less sensitive than the Gehan-weighted log-rank test if the treatment effect is more pronounced at early event times.

To assess the sensitivity of WR to follow-up duration, Figure 14.4 plots WR, ICH_L, and ratios of the estimated integrated cumulative cause-specific hazards $\widehat{r}_{CVD}$ and $\widehat{r}_H$, for CVD and H, respectively, using TOPCAT data artificially censored by t across various values of t. Such comparison is particularly informative because the nonparametric $\widehat{r}_{CVD}$ and $\widehat{r}_H$ converge to limits determined solely by the respective cause-specific hazard functions—free of censoring and without relying on any model assumptions. ICH_L also maintains these properties as the average of $\widehat{r}_{CVD}$ and $\widehat{r}_H$.

The figure reveals that for small t, WR fluctuates more than the other curves. As expected, WR tends to be closer to $\widehat{r}_{CVD}$ most of the time. However, for $t \in [2.5, 4.5]$, WR occasionally falls outside the range between $\widehat{r}_{CVD}$ and $\widehat{r}_H$. From year 4.5 onward, WR gradually approaches ICH_L, the average of $\widehat{r}_{CVD}$ and $\widehat{r}_H$.

These patterns suggest that WR for a specific follow-up interval $[0, t]$ is a complex mixture of the effects on CVD and H, influenced by the number of CVD and H events, as well as censored data within that interval. This can vary unpredictably as t changes.

Next, for the SPRINT trial, the primary endpoint was the composite of myocardial infarction, other acute coronary syndromes, stroke, heart failure, or death from cardiovascular causes. For the illustration here, the terminal event of interest is CVD, and the non-terminal event of interest is the composite of non-fatal events, namely, time to the first event among myocardial infarction, other acute coronary syndromes, stroke, and heart failure (NF). In this setup, more data are utilized compared to the SPRINT primary endpoint, but non-fatal events after the first one are not considered. This is to keep the problem's dimension low. For the

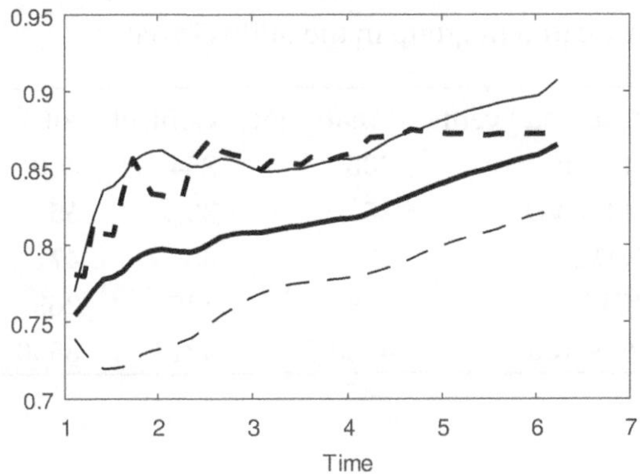

FIGURE 14.4
WR, ICH_L, and ratios of the estimated integrated cumulative cause-specific hazards $\hat{r}_{CVD}$ and $\hat{r}_H$, for CVD and H, respectively, for TOPCAT data artificially censored by t for various values of t in the data range. Thick solid: ICH_L; Thick dashed: WR; thin solid: ratio of the estimated integrated cumulative cause-specific hazards for CVD; thin dashed: ratio of the estimated integrated cumulative cause-specific hazards for H.

maximum tests based on ESWR, LRGRE, ICH, and ITCH, the power may decrease as the number of component tests increase. However, linear combination tests are generally less affected by the number of components. The breakdown of observed events is provided in Table 14.4.

From Table 14.4, 55 trial participants experienced both NF and CVD. There were 102 CVD events, and 263 NCVD events. Thus NCVD events represent a much larger proportion of total deaths in SPRINT compared to TOPCAT, indicating that competing risks are more severe in the SPRINT trial.

Table 14.5 presents the results of tests and confidence intervals for methods in Table 14.3 that accommodate competing risks. The row and column titles are consistent with those in Table 14.3, with NF replacing H. For the ICH-, ITCH- ESWR-, and LRGRE- based methods, $\tau = 4.31$, which represents 90% of the trial duration of 4.79.

Table 14.5 shows all tests considered are significant at the 0.05 level for their corresponding null hypotheses. Following rejection of the global null, each of the ESWR-, LRGRE-, ICH-, and ITCH-based methods shows a significant reduction in the cause-specific hazard of CVD. For NF, all methods except $ITCH_L$ and $ITCH_{MX}$ show a significant effect, although the P-values of the latter two tests are very close to 0.05.

Comparing Tables 14.3 and 14.5, the results of the ESWR-, LRGRE-, ICH-, and ITCH-based methods are much closer to those of LR and Cox in Table 14.5. One contributing factor for this similarity in SPRINT may be that the number of CVD

TABLE 14.4
Observed events by treatment group in the SPRINT trial.

Observed Events	Treatment	Control	All
NF only	206	254	460
NF& CVD	25	30	55
CVD only	12	35	47
NCVD	118	145	263
Censored	4322	4214	8536

TABLE 14.5
Testing and confidence interval results for methods accommodating competing risks, using the SPRINT data.

Method	P-value	Effect_1 (CI)	Effect_2 (CI)	Overall Effect (CI)
LR	0.0009			
Cox	0.0010	0.81 (0.68,0.96)	0.57 (0.38, 0.85)	0.75 (0.64, 0.89)
ESWR_L	0.00001	0.82 (0.68, 0.97)	0.55 (0.34, 0.80)	0.68 (0.54, 0.83)
ESWR_{MX}	0.001	0.82 (0.68, 0.97)	0.55 (0.34, 0.80)	
ESWR_{LD}	0.0009	0.82 (0.68, 0.97)	0.55 (0.34, 0.80)	0.75 (0.64, 0.89)
LRGRE_L	< 0.00001	0.81 (0.67, 0.95)	0.57 (0.36, 0.81)	0.69 (0.55, 0.82)
LRGRE_{MX}	0.002	0.81 (0.67, 0.95)	0.57 (0.36, 0.81)	
ICH_L	0.0002	0.84 (0.70, 0.999)	0.59 (0.36, 0.85)	0.72 (0.57, 0.86)
ICII_{MX}	0.005	0.84 (0.70, 0.999)	0.59 (0.36, 0.85)	
ITCH_L	0.0002	0.85 (0.70, 1.001)	0.59 (0.36, 0.85)	0.72 (0.57, 0.87)
ITCH_{MX}	0.005	0.85 (0.70, 1.001)	0.59 (0.36, 0.85)	

events after NF events represents a much smaller percentage of the total number of observed events. Consequently, the benefit of utilizing the additional events is reduced compared to the case in TOPCAT.

Note that in Table 14.5, LRGRE_{LD} is less sensitive to the group differences compared to ESWR_L. This is opposite of the phenomenon observed for TOPCAT (Table 14.3). This discrepancy arises because in both trials, as in many others, the number of non-terminal events is much larger than the number of terminal events, Consequently, the data-driven weight favors the test statistic for the non-terminal events. In SPRINT, the hazard reduction in NF is smaller than in CVD. Therefore, the data-driven weight yields a smaller hazard reduction than that in the simple average used in ESWR_L. In contrast, for TOPCAT, the hazard reduction in H is larger than in CVD, meaning the data-driven weight yields a larger hazard reduction than the simple average used in ESWR_L. This explains the discrepancy between Tables 14.3 and 14.5.

For ESWR- and LRGRE-based methods, again the assumption $H_{1PH} \cap H_{2PH}$ is required. In addition, for the average effect estimate by ESWR_{LD} to have a valid estimand, the assumption H_{EPH} must hold. For the SPRINT data, the P-values for testing these two hypotheses are 0.13 and 0.04, respectively. This provides strong evidence against the assumption of H_{EPH}. Consequently, while the ESWR_{LD}-based test of the global null $H_{01} \cap H_{01}$ is valid, the use of ESWR_{LD} as an average effect measure is questionable.

Since the analysis plan must be pre-specified before data unblinding, ESWR_L with a pre-determined and fixed η is recommended. ESWR_{LD} can be used if the goal is solely to test the global null, rather than to test and estimate the overall treatment effect.

The significant P-value for testing H_{EPH} further suggests that use of the win ratio as an overall effect measure in SPRINT may also be questionable. While condition (14.7) for the win ratio differs from H_{EPH}—with the two focusing on the joint distribution of NF and CVD, and the cause-specific hazards, respectively—the results in Table 14.5 suggest that condition (14.7) is highly unlikely to hold. This is in addition to the identifiability and estimability issues related to terminal and non-terminal events, as discussed in Section 14.3.

To assess change over time of WR with respect to the follow-up duration, Figure 14.5 plots WR, ICH_L, and ratios of the estimated integrated cumulative cause-specific hazards $\hat{r}_{CVD}$ and $\hat{r}_{NF}$, for CVD and NF, respectively, using SPRINT data artificially censored by t for various values of t. The figure shows that during most of the time interval $[0,2]$, WR is closer to $\hat{r}_{CVD}$ than ICH_L is, as expected. From year 2 to 3, however, WR is almost identical to ICH_L. Then, from year 3 onward, WR moves slightly away from ICH_L and closer to $\hat{r}_{NF}$, which corresponds to the less important endpoint.

Thus, in many respects, the behavior of WR in SPRINT differs from that in TOPCAT, as displayed in Figure 14.4. These phenomena again highlight the complexity of WR, which reflects a mixture of effects on both terminal and non-terminal events and is further influenced by censoring.

Analysis of terminal and non-terminal events under competing risks is an evolving area of research, with many new methods emerging recently. As such, it is impossible to cover all or even most of the results in this field. This chapter focuses on methods with more established properties and asymptotic theory. The choice of analysis method for a particular trial or study depends on the research objectives. Based on various simulation studies and trial data applications, recommendations have been made in Yang [340].

When the focus is on disease prognosis and event prediction, multi-state models provide a natural framework. However, when the interest lies in assessing and summarizing treatment effects, methods based on ESWR, LRGRE, ICH, and ITCH are more appropriate. If competing risks are minimal, or can reasonably be assumed to be independent of the events under study, the win ratio and RMT-IF may also be considered.

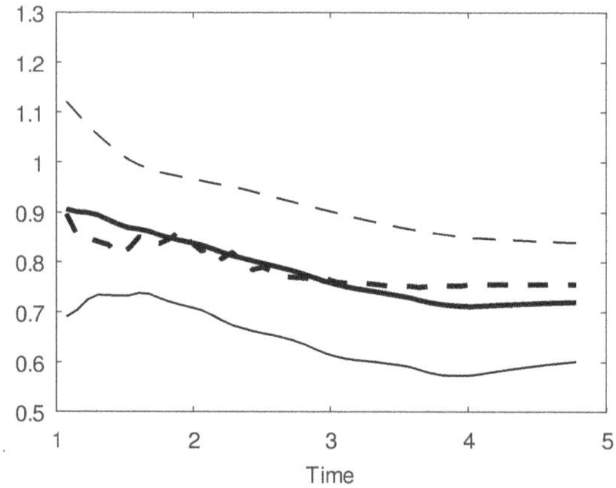

FIGURE 14.5
WR, ICH_L, and ratios of the estimated integrated cumulative cause-specific hazards $\hat{r}_{CVD}$ and $\hat{r}_{NF}$, for CVD and NF, respectively, for SPRINT data artificially censored by t for various values of t in the data range. Thick solid: ICH_L; Thick dashed: WR; thin solid: ratio of the estimated integrated cumulative cause-specific hazards for CVD; thin dashed: ratio of the estimated integrated cumulative cause-specific hazards for H.

The composite endpoint approach using time to the first event, may be appealing when there is only a small chance of observing both terminal and non-terminal events, or when the treatment effect is similar for both. In such cases, this approach offers relatively high efficiency with a simplified analysis.

If the primary interest is to test the treatment effect on the terminal event, the win ratio test is a good choice. However, interpreting the value of the win ratio itself as an effect measure relies on strong assumptions and should be done with caution, and the resulting estimate may not be generalizable to other settings or populations where censoring patterns differ. When the goal is to assess the treatment effect without distinguishing whether it shows up more prominently in the terminal event or non-terminal events—especially when differential effects are expected—then ESWR-, ICH-, or ITCH-based methods are preferred.

If the condition $H_{1PH} \cap H_{2PH}$ is expected to hold, ESWR-based methods are preferred. However, if there are concerns about the validity of $H_{1PH} \cap H_{2PH}$, , ICH or ITCH-based methods provide robustness and high efficiency. For any of these methods—ESWR, ICH, or ITCH—the maximum test should be used when treatment effects are expected to influence terminal and non-terminal events in opposite directions.

In some scenarios, more than one test may be reasonable. Since the significance of secondary analyses can only be claimed if the primary analysis yields a significant result, it is important to choose a primary analysis test with high statistical power to reject the global null hypothesis of no treatment effect.

To implement the procedures in Sections 14.7 and 14.8, the R package TxEffectsSurvival is available from the Comprehensive R Archive Network (CRAN). Given input data, it produces global tests and confidence intervals based on ESWR, LRGRE, ICH, and ITCH, as well as tests for the proportional hazards assumptions and for equality of hazard ratios. For comparison, it also reports results using the win ratio described in Section 14.3. Although the package is designed for analyses of terminal and non-terminal events in the presence of competing risks, univariate survival data can also be handled by assigning the same univariate outcomes to both the terminal and non-terminal event inputs.

14.10 Exercises and Complements

14.1 Provide details for the derivation of (14.1).

14.2 Derive (14.6) from (14.3).

14.3 Consider the semi-competing risks setting as described in Section 14.2 and the conditional hazard function of T_1^*:

$$\lambda^*(s|t) = \lim_{h \downarrow 0} P\left[s \le T_1^* < s+h \middle| T_1^* \ge s, T_2^* \ge t\right]/h,\ 0 < s \le t.$$

For the conditional distribution of T_1^* given T_2^*, we have

$$P(T_1^* > t_1 | T_2^* > t_2) = P(T_1^* > t_1 | T_2^* \ge t_2) = \exp\left[-\int_0^{t_1} \lambda^*(x|t_2)dx\right],\ t_1 \le t_2.$$

Use this result to show that

$$P(T_1^* > t_1, T_2^* > t_2) = \exp\left[-\int_0^{t_2} \lambda_2(x)dx - \int_0^{t_1} \lambda^*(x|t_2)dx\right],$$

on $t_1 \le t_2$, where λ_2 is the hazard function of T_2^*.

14.4 For the Clayton bivariate survival function $S(s,t)$, obtain the joint PDF $f(s,t)$. Then express $\lambda^*(s|t)$ in (14.6) in terms of $S(s,t)$ and $f(s,t)$.

14.5 Show that

$$\lambda^*(s|t) = \frac{\partial \log S(s,t)}{\partial s}.$$

14.6 Consider the semi-competing risks setting. Let T_{1C}^* and T_{2C}^* denoted the times to the non-terminal event and the terminal event in the control group, respectively. Define T_{1T}^* and T_{2T}^* similarly for the treatment group. Furthermore, the censoring variables are denoted by C_C and C_T for the two groups, respectively.

Then, the event in the probability space that the treatment group wins on the terminal event comparison is

$$\{T_{2C}^* \le C_C\} \cap \{T_{2C}^* \le T_{2T}^* \wedge C_T\} = \{T_{2C}^* \le \min(C_C, C_T, T_{2T}^*)\}.$$

Similarly, the event in the probability space that the treatment group loses on the terminal event comparison is

$$\{T_{2T}^* \le C_T\} \cap \{T_{2T}^* \le T_{2C}^* \wedge C_C\} = \{T_{2T}^* \le \min(C_C, C_T, T_{2C}^*)\}.$$

The event that comparison on the terminal event is indeterminable is

$$\begin{aligned}
&\{T_{2C}^* \le \min(C_C, C_T, T_{2T}^*)\}^c \cap \{T_{2T}^* \le \min(C_C, C_T, T_{2C}^*)\}^c \\
= \; &\{T_{2C}^* > \min(C_C, C_T, T_{2T}^*),\ T_{2T}^* > \min(C_C, C_T, T_{2C}^*\} \\
= \; &\{T_{2C}^* > \min(C_m, T_{2T}^*),\ T_{2T}^* > \min(C_m, T_{2C}^*\}, \qquad (14.65)
\end{aligned}$$

where A^c denotes the complement of an event A and $C_m = \min(C_C, C_T)$.

(a) Show that the last expression in (14.65) can be simplified to

$$\{T_{2C}^* > C_m,\ T_{2T}^* > C_m\}.$$

(b) Show that for the prioritized comparison used in win ratio, the probability of a treatment group win is

$$P\big(T_{2C}^* \le \min(C_m, T_{2T}^*)\big) + P\big(T_{2C}^* > C_m,\ T_{2T}^* > C_m, T_{1C}^* \le \min(C_m, T_{1T}^*)\big).$$

(c) Use the law of iterated expectations (B.6) in Appendix B to show that the probability of a treatment group win is $\int_0^\infty \phi(x) dF_{cm}(x)$, where F_{cm} is the CDF of C_m and

$$\phi(x) = P\big(T_{2C}^* \le \min(x, T_{2T}^*)\big) + P\big(T_{2C}^* > x,\ T_{2T}^* > x, T_{1C}^* \le \min(x, T_{1T}^*)\big).$$

(d) Define

$$F_{1C}(w|x) = P\big(T_{1C}^* \le w \big| T_{2C}^* > x, T_{2T}^* > x\big) = P\big(T_{1C}^* \le w \big| T_{2C}^* > x\big),$$

$$F_{1T}(w|x) = P\big(T_{1T}^* \le w \big| T_{2C}^* > x, T_{2T}^* > x\big) = P\big(T_{1T}^* \le w \big| T_{2T}^* > x\big),$$

and $S_{1C}(w) = 1 - F_{1C}(w)$, $S_{1T}(w) = 1 - F_{1T}(w)$. Also, let

$$S_{2C}(x) = P\big(T_{2C}^* > x\big),\ S_{2T}(x) = P\big(T_{2T}^* > x\big).$$

Note that

$$\begin{aligned} & P\big(T_{2C}^* > x,\ T_{2T}^* > x, T_{1C}^* \leq \min(x, T_{1T}^*)\big) \\ = \quad & S_{2C}(x)S_{2T}(x)P\big(T_{1C}^* \leq \min(x, T_{1T}^*)\big| T_{2C}^* > x, T_{2T}^* > x\big). \end{aligned}$$

Apply the law of iterated expectation a few more times to show that

$$\begin{aligned} & \phi(x) \\ = \quad & \int_0^x S_{2T}(w)dF_{2C}(w) + S_{2C}(x)S_{2T}(x)\int_0^x S_{1T}(w|x)dF_{1C}(w|x), \end{aligned}$$

Oakes [214] derived this type of results to establish condition (14.7) for the win ratio to be a valid effect measure.

14.7 For the illness-death model, express $\lambda_{jk}(t)$ in (14.10) in terms of T_1^* and T_2^*.

14.8 For the model in Example 14.3, express $\lambda_{jk}(t)$ in (14.10) in terms of the events involved.

14.9 Show, by taking derivative in $\boldsymbol{\beta}$ in (14.21), that the observed information matrix corresponding to $\boldsymbol{U}^{ms}(\boldsymbol{\beta})$ is

$$\mathbb{I}^{ms}(\boldsymbol{\beta}) = \sum_{(j,k)\in\mathfrak{C}} \sum_{i=1}^{n} \int_0^\infty \mathbf{V}_{jk}(\boldsymbol{\beta}, t)dN_{jki}(t), \tag{14.66}$$

where $\mathbf{V}_{jk}(\boldsymbol{\beta}, t)$ is the matrix

$$\mathbf{V}_{jk}(\boldsymbol{\beta}, t) = \frac{\sum_{i=1}^n K_{ji}(t)\exp[\boldsymbol{\beta}^{\mathrm{T}} \boldsymbol{W}_i(t)]\boldsymbol{W}_i(t)\boldsymbol{W}_i(t)^{\mathrm{T}}}{\sum_{i=1}^n K_{ji}(t)\exp[\boldsymbol{\beta}^{\mathrm{T}}\boldsymbol{W}_i(t)]} - E_{jk}(\boldsymbol{\beta}, t)^{\otimes 2}, \tag{14.67}$$

where $\mathbf{V}^{\otimes 2} = \mathbf{V}\mathbf{V}^{\mathrm{T}}$ for a vector $\mathbf{V}$.

14.10 Fill in the details of (14.26) and (14.27) to establish the Kolmogorov forward equations.

14.11 Show that the intensity matrix for the illness-death model is given by (14.29).

14.12 Prove the Kolmogorov backward equations:

$$\frac{\partial P_{jk}(s,t)}{\partial s} = -\sum_{\ell} P_{\ell k}(s,t)\lambda_{j\ell}(s).$$

14.13 (a) Suppose that A, B, f are functions on an interval $[a, b]$ and $f > 0$. Verify that the solution of the differential equation

$$\frac{df(x)}{dx} = A(x)f(x) + B(x), \quad f(a) = f_0$$

is

$$f(x) = \exp\left[\int_a^x A(w)dw\right]\left\{\int_a^x B(w)\exp\left[-\int_a^w A(y)dy\right]dw + f_0\right\}.$$

(b) For the model in Example 14.2, use the result in (a) to obtain the transition probabilities $P_{22}(s,t)$, $P_{23}(s,t)$, $P_{12}(s,t)$ and $P_{13}(s,t)$, in that order, so that a quantity can be expressed in terms of quantities obtained previously, including $P_{11}(s,t)$ in (14.30).

14.14 Consider the multi-state model for a single event H. Let the states 0 and 1 represent being event free and having had the event. Obtain the RMT-IF and show that the net win time over $[0, \tau]$ is

$$\mu(\tau) = \int_0^t [F_C(x) - F_T(x)]dx = \int_0^t [S_T(x) - S_C(x)]dx,$$

where F and S are the CDF and survival function, respectively, with subscript indicating treatment group.

14.15 Suppose there are two cumulative hazard functions $\Lambda_j(t)$, $j = 1, 2$, with corresponding survival functions $S_j(t)$, $j = 1, 2$. Let $\Lambda(t) = \Lambda_1(t) + \Lambda_2(t)$ and denote the survival function associated with $\Lambda(t)$ by $S(t)$. Show that

$$S(t) = S_1(t)S_2(t).$$

Hint: Recall Exercise 2.6.

14.16 Consider the random censorship model defined in Section 2.4, with the additional assumption that the censoring variables C_i's are i.i.d. with CDF $G(t)$. Suppose there are no common discontinuity points between $F(t)$ and $G(t)$. Then the mathematical structure in the censoring problem is symmetric in T and C. Let $\widehat{S}_C(t)$ and $\widehat{S}_T(t)$ be the Kaplan-Meier estimators for $1 - F(t)$ and $1 - G(t)$, respectively. Use Exercise 14.15 to show that

$$\frac{1}{n}K(t) = \widehat{S}_T(t)\widehat{S}_C(t), \tag{14.68}$$

where $K(t)$ is the at-risk process in (2.43).

14.17 To avoid dependence on censoring in the limit, the inverse probability weighting method can be used, which replaces R_ℓ in (14.39) by

$$\widetilde{R}_\ell = \frac{\int_0^\tau K_{\ell C}(t)K_{\ell T}(t)\left[\widehat{S}_{CC}(t)\widehat{S}_{CT}(t)\right]^{-1} d\widehat{\Lambda}_{\ell T}(t)}{\int_0^\tau K_{\ell C}(t)K_{\ell T}(t)\left[\widehat{S}_{CC}(t)\widehat{S}_{CT}(t)\right]^{-1} d\widehat{\Lambda}_{\ell C}(t)}, \quad \ell = 1,2,$$

for some $\tau > 0$, where $\widehat{S}_{CC}(t)$ and $\widehat{S}_{CT}(t)$ are the Kaplan-Meier estimators of the survival functions of the control and treatment group censoring distributions, respectively (be mindful of the requirement of positive denominator, which necessitates a restriction to a proper integration range $[0,\tau]$). Use (14.68) to show that

$$\widetilde{R}_\ell = \frac{\int_0^\tau \widehat{S}_{\ell C}(t)\widehat{S}_{\ell T}(t) d\widehat{\Lambda}_{\ell T}(t)}{\int_0^\tau \widehat{S}_{\ell C}(t)\widehat{S}_{\ell T}(t) d\widehat{\Lambda}_{\ell C}(t)}, \quad \ell = 1,2,$$

where $\widehat{S}_{\ell C}(t)$ and $\widehat{S}_{\ell T}(t)$ are the Kaplan-Meier estimators of $\boldsymbol{S}_{\ell C}(t)$ and $\boldsymbol{S}_{\ell T}(t)$ in (14.40), respectively.

14.18 Verify (14.44) and (14.46).

14.19 Suppose that the control and treatment groups each consist of five individuals, and the data for the terminal and non-terminal events are as follows:

	Control					Treatment				
Non-Terminal	1	2	3	4	5	1.2	2.4	3.6	4.8	6
Terminal	6	7	8	9	10	5.4	6.3	7.2	8.1	9

where the first individual in the control group has times to non-terminal and terminal events given by the first and second rows in the first column, and so on. It can be seen that the treatment decelerates (delays) the non-terminal event by 20%, which is a positive effect. However, it accelerates the terminal event by 10%, which is a negative effect. Use the R package TxEffectsSurvival to obtain the event-specific win ratios for the terminal and non-terminal events, the ratios based on LRGRE, ICH, and ITCH, and the overall win ratio, in the following three cases (setting $\text{tau}_r = 1$):

(a) when there is no censoring;

(b) when there is type I censoring at the constant $c = 8.5$; and

(c) when there is type I censoring at the constant $c = 6.5$.

Note: The results indicate that the overall win ratio may fluctuate between values less than 1 and greater than 1 depending on the censoring level, despite being designed to emphasize the terminal event, while the other measures and the average ratios based on them are more robust against changes in censoring levels.

15

Recurrent Event Analysis

In the previous chapters, typical scenarios are when an individual experiences either a single event or one of $K \geq 2$ types of events. However, there are situations where an individual can experience recurrent events, such as repeated infections or tumor recurrences. In this chapter, we discuss modeling and analysis of such data. The traditional Andersen-Gill model and the Prentice-Williams-Peterson models, and the more recent marginal mean/rate models, are explored. To help readers gain a deeper understanding of the marginal models and become more comfortable studying their properties, discussions are provided on formal model definitions. Modeling and analysis in the presence of death are also addressed.

15.1 Intensity Models

15.1.1 The Andersen-Gill Model

As discussed in Chapter Eleven, intensity models can be obtained for a counting process using the Doob-Meyer decomposition. Let $\widetilde{N}_i^*(t)$ be an underlying counting process that counts the number of recurrent events for the ith individual in interval $[0, t]$. Since time to event is positive, $\widetilde{N}_i^*(0) = 0$. In addition, $\widetilde{N}_i^*(t)$ is a cadlag increasing step function taking nonnegative integer values.

Suppose $\widetilde{N}_i^*(t)$ is under observation for $t \leq C_i$, where C_i is the censoring variable. In this section and the next, it is assumed that the counting process is only subject to independent censoring. The exact meanings of this assumption will be clarified later. It is also assumed that the censoring times $C_i, 1 \leq i \leq n$, are known, representing the end points of observation periods of the counting processes. In Section 15.3, the presence of death, which terminates the observation period and dependently censors the process, will be discussed.

Due to censoring, the observed counting process $\widetilde{N}_i(t)$ is

$$\widetilde{N}_i(t) = \widetilde{N}^*(t \wedge C_i) = \int_0^t C_i(s) d\widetilde{N}_i^*(s), \qquad (15.1)$$

DOI: 10.1201/9780429324437-15

where $C_i(t) = I(C_i \geq t)$ is the censoring process indicating whether the individual is under observation or censored at time t. $\widetilde{N}_i$ counts the number of observed events in $[0, t]$, and jumps at t if and only if $\widetilde{N}_i^*$ jumps at t and $C_i \geq t$.

Let $\boldsymbol{W}_i(t)$ be a time-dependent covariate process for the ith individual. Suppose it is of interest to study the behavior of $\widetilde{N}_i^*$ in association with $\boldsymbol{W}_i(t)$, Let $\{\mathscr{F}_t\}$ be a family of increasing σ-algebras such that $\widetilde{N}_i^*(t)$ is adapted to $\mathscr{F}_t$ and $\boldsymbol{W}_i(t)$ is $\mathscr{F}_t$-predictable for each i and t. For example, $\mathscr{F}_t$ can be the σ-algebra generated by information on $[0, t]$ from all n individuals on events and the covariate history $\boldsymbol{W}_i^h(t) = \{\boldsymbol{W}_i(s), 0 \leq s < t\}$. Since $\widetilde{N}_i^*$ is increasing, it satisfies (11.20). Assume that $E\widetilde{N}_i^*(t) < \infty$ for any t, then by the Doob-Meyer decomposition, $\widetilde{N}_i^*(t)$ has a predictable compensator. The Andersen-Gill (AG) model [8] assumes that for $i \in \{1, \ldots, n\}$, $\widetilde{N}_i^*(t)$ has the intensity process

$$a_i(t) = \lambda_0(t) \exp\left[\boldsymbol{\beta}^{\mathrm{T}} \boldsymbol{W}_i(t)\right]. \tag{15.2}$$

That is,

$$\int_0^t \lambda_0(x) \exp\left[\boldsymbol{\beta}^{\mathrm{T}} \boldsymbol{W}_i(x)\right] dx < \infty,$$

for any $t < \infty$, and $\widetilde{N}_i^*(t)$ satisfies the intensity model

$$E\left[d\widetilde{N}_i^*(t) \middle| \mathscr{F}_{t-}\right] = \lambda_0(t) \exp\left[\boldsymbol{\beta}^{\mathrm{T}} \boldsymbol{W}_i(t)\right] dt. \tag{15.3}$$

Note that $\mathscr{F}_t$ may not contain information on censoring. The censoring by C_i is *independent* for the counting process $\widetilde{N}_i^*(t)$ if there is a family of increasing σ-algebras $\{\mathscr{G}_t\}$ such that, for each t, $\mathscr{F}_t \subset \mathscr{G}_t$ and the censoring process $C_i(t)$ is $\mathscr{G}_t$-predictable for each i, and that $a_i(t)$ remains the intensity process of $\widetilde{N}_i^*(t)$ with respect to the enlarged family $\{\mathscr{G}_t\}$. It can be shown that if the censoring variables are independent of the underlying counting processes, then the independent censoring condition is satisfied. The condition is also satisfied for type II censoring. More discussions and examples of censoring and intensity process can be found in Section III.2 of Andersen et al. [7].

From (15.1), (15.3), under the independent censoring condition,

$$E\left[d\widetilde{N}_i(t) \middle| \mathscr{G}_{t-}\right] = C_i(t) \lambda_0(t) \exp\left[\boldsymbol{\beta}^{\mathrm{T}} \boldsymbol{W}_i(t)\right] dt. \tag{15.4}$$

That is, $\widetilde{N}_i(t)$ satisfies the intensity model (15.4), with intensity process $C_i(t)a_i(t)$.

Let

$$S^{(m)}(\boldsymbol{\beta}, t) = n^{-1} \sum_{i=1}^{n} C_i(t) \exp\left[\boldsymbol{\beta}^{\mathrm{T}} \boldsymbol{W}_i(t)\right] \boldsymbol{W}_i(t)^{\otimes m},$$

for $m = 0, 1, 2$. Under model (15.4), the partial likelihood inference is still valid [7]. The score function is

$$\boldsymbol{U}(\boldsymbol{\beta}) = \sum_{i=1}^{n} \int_0^{\infty} [\boldsymbol{W}_i(t) - E(\boldsymbol{\beta}, t)] d\widetilde{N}_i(t), \tag{15.5}$$

with

$$E(\boldsymbol{\beta}, t) = S^{(1)}(\boldsymbol{\beta}, t)/S^{(0)}(\boldsymbol{\beta}, t) = \frac{\sum_{i=1}^{n} C_i(t)\exp[\boldsymbol{\beta}^{\mathrm{T}}\boldsymbol{W}_i(t)]\boldsymbol{W}_i(t)}{\sum_{i=1}^{n} C_i(t)\exp[\boldsymbol{\beta}^{\mathrm{T}}\boldsymbol{W}_i(t)]}. \tag{15.6}$$

Let

$$M_i(t) = \widetilde{N}_i(t) - \int_0^t C_i(x)\exp\left[\boldsymbol{\beta}^{\mathrm{T}}\boldsymbol{W}_i(x)\right]\lambda_0(x)dx, \tag{15.7}$$

the martingale associated with the ith individual. It is left to Exercise 15.1 to show that

$$\boldsymbol{U}(\boldsymbol{\beta}) = \sum_{i=1}^{n}\int_0^{\infty}\left[\boldsymbol{W}_i(x) - E(\boldsymbol{\beta}, x)\right]dM_i(x). \tag{15.8}$$

The observed information matrix is

$$\mathbb{I}(\boldsymbol{\beta}) = \sum_{i=1}^{n}\int_0^{\infty}\mathbf{V}(\boldsymbol{\beta}, t)d\widetilde{N}_i(t), \tag{15.9}$$

where as in (6.24),

$$\mathbf{V}(\boldsymbol{\beta}, t) = S^{(2)}(\boldsymbol{\beta}, t)/S^{(0)}(\boldsymbol{\beta}, t) - E(\boldsymbol{\beta}, t)^{\otimes 2}.$$

Let $\widehat{\boldsymbol{\beta}}$ be partial likelihood estimator of the true parameter value $\boldsymbol{\beta}_0$. Analogous to the discussions in Chapter Eleven,

$$U(\boldsymbol{\beta}_0) \sim N\big(0, \mathbb{I}(\boldsymbol{\beta}_0)\big),$$

and

$$\widehat{\boldsymbol{\beta}} \sim N\big(\boldsymbol{\beta}_0, \mathbb{I}^{-1}(\boldsymbol{\beta}_0)\big).$$

Furthermore, $\boldsymbol{\beta}_0$ in the limiting distributions can be replaced by $\widehat{\boldsymbol{\beta}}$.

For the baseline cumulative hazard function

$$\Lambda_0(t) = \int_0^t \lambda_0(s)ds, \tag{15.10}$$

the Breslow estimator $\widehat{\Lambda}(t)$ is

$$\widehat{\Lambda}(t) = \sum_{i=1}^{n}\int_0^t \frac{d\widetilde{N}_i(s)}{nS^{(0)}(\widehat{\boldsymbol{\beta}}, s)} = \sum_{i=1}^{n}\sum_{j=1}^{J_i}\frac{I(X_{ij} \le t)}{\sum_{m=1}^{n} C_m(X_{ij})\exp\left[\widehat{\boldsymbol{\beta}}^{\mathrm{T}}\boldsymbol{W}_m(X_{ij})\right]}, \tag{15.11}$$

where $X_{i1}, \ldots, X_{iJ_i}$ are the observed events for the ith individual.

From the result (11.39) on intensity process, $a_{i+}(t)$ is the instantaneous rate of change in the expected number of events in the immediate future, given information on event, censoring and covariate history in $\mathscr{G}_t$. Thus, $\boldsymbol{W}_i(t)$ may contain internal covariates from event history such as the number and timing of previous events.

In the special case when $\boldsymbol{W}_i(t)$ consists of only fixed covariates, the model implies a memory-less property that future event occurrence does not depend on past events. This condition may be too restrictive, and the model may not adequately describe the instantaneous rate of change in the expected number of events given information on event history. On the other hand, a model in which $\boldsymbol{W}_i(t)$ contains covariates based on past events makes the interpretation of treatment effect difficult, since those covariates may be responsive to the treatment. Alternative modeling approaches will be discussed in Section 15.2.

When there are several types of recurrent events, the asymptotic theory discussed in this section can be applied to each of the event types. If the treatment effects on different events are expected to be in the same direction, and the interest is on how the treatment affects all events, the counting process can be defined as the total number of events in the time interval $[0, t]$, and the asymptotic theory remains valid. In this combined-events approach, $a_{i+}(t)$ is the sum of the instantaneous rates of change over all event types.

15.1.2 The Prentice-Williams-Peterson Models

Under the AG model, past events can influence the occurrence of a future one through components of $\boldsymbol{W}_i$ that depend on event history. However, the baseline function is $\lambda_0(t)$ regardless of how many events have occurred prior to time t. The Prentice-Williams-Peterson (PWP) models [252] consider time-dependent stratified analysis where the strata are determined by the number of events prior to t. All individuals are at risk for the first event, but only those with an event in the kth stratum are at risk for the $(k+1)$th event, $k \geq 1$. The baseline functions are different for different strata in the multiplicative models, as will be described below. Such models are important when the research interest is in analysis of a future event given prior events.

Since the multi-state models have been introduced and used in the previous chapter, it is convenient to describe the PWP models using multi-state processes. Suppose that the number of recurrent events is less than or equal to a fixed integer $J \geq 2$. A multi-state process $X(t)$ can be obtained by specifying that $X(t)$ starts from the state 1 at $t = 0$, and for $j > 1$, $X(t) = j$ as soon as $j - 1$ events are observed, $j = 2, \ldots, J$. For the counting process $N_{jki}(t)$ that counts the number of observed direct transitions from j to k in $[0, t]$ for the ith individual, defined in (14.12), a multiplicative intensity model can be obtained by specifying that the intensity process $\lambda_{jki}[t; \boldsymbol{W}_i(t)]$ of $N_{jki}(t)$ has the form

$$\lambda_{jki}[t; \boldsymbol{W}_i(t)] = K_{ji}(t)\lambda_{0jk}(t)\exp\left[\boldsymbol{\beta}^{\mathrm{T}}\boldsymbol{W}_i(t)\right], \quad t > 0, \tag{15.12}$$

for $k = j+1, j = 1, \ldots, J-1$, where $K_{ji}(t)$ is the at-risk process as given in (14.12). This recovers the PWP model with time scale since $t = 0$, or the total time scale.

Compared with (15.2), the functions $\lambda_{0jk}(t)$ in (15.12) are different for each (j,k) transition. As in Chapter Fourteen, the parameter $\boldsymbol{\beta}$ and the covariate $\boldsymbol{W}_i$ do not depend on the transition type (j,k) to allow shared parameters, or equivalently, to allow both overall and transition/event-specific effects for each covariate.

Since an individual can only experience the kth event if the first $k-1$ events have occurred, the risk sets for later transitions may be too small to yield reliable results. Thus typically, the model is only applied to the first few transitions. If $\mathfrak{C}$ is the collection of the first few transitions of interest, then partial likelihood analysis of $\boldsymbol{\beta}$ can be performed with score function in (14.21) and information matrix in (14.66).

In the context of semi-Markov process analysis in Chapter Fourteen, a different time scale, the time since entrance to the current state, provides an alternative to the total time scale. This time scale is useful when the research interest is on predicting the occurrence of the next event based on past history, rather than on analyzing the total number of events over a given time period. Instead of (15.12), the intensity model assumes that

$$\lambda_{jki}[t;\boldsymbol{W}_i(t)] = K_{ji}(t)\lambda_{0jk}(d)\exp[\boldsymbol{\beta}^{\mathrm{T}}\boldsymbol{W}_i(t)], \quad t > 0, \tag{15.13}$$

where d is the time since occurrence of the previous event. This recovers the PWP model with the gap time. Similarly to the discussion on semi-Markov models for the illness-death model in Chapter Fourteen, $\boldsymbol{\beta}$ can be estimated with appropriate modifications, working with the gap time scale instead of the total time scale.

In the PWP models, even if $\boldsymbol{W}_i(t)$ does not contain variables that depend on past history, the strata or states depend on the number of previous events which is a post-randomization variable. Thus caution is needed for treatment effect assessment as discussed in Section 14.4. It is important to note that while trial participants are randomized for the first event, there is no such randomization for subsequent events. The imbalance in confounders may progressively worsen with each additional event.

15.2 The Marginal Mean/Rate Models

15.2.1 The General Regression Model

The intensity models discussed in the preceding section are useful for analyzing how event history affect the chance of a new event. Often, the research focus is on the effect of covariates on the recurrent events, rather than the effect of past events on future ones. As mentioned before, there are challenges in treatment effect interpretation if $\boldsymbol{W}_i(t)$ contains variables defined on the previous history. Conversely, if $\boldsymbol{W}_i(t)$ contains only baseline covariates, the model might not adequately describe the expected instantaneous rate of events given event history. To circumvent this issue, the marginal mean/rate model [224, 155, 156, 177] provides an alternative.

In the AG model (15.3), the right-hand side depends only on $\boldsymbol{W}_i(t)$, whereas the left-hand side is an expectation conditional on the event and covariate history before t. By (B.4), equation (15.3) implies that the expectation conditional on $\boldsymbol{W}_i(t)$ is also given by the same expression:

$$E\left[d\widetilde{N}_i^*(t)\middle|\boldsymbol{W}_i(t)\right] = \lambda_0(t)\exp\left[\boldsymbol{\beta}^{\mathrm{T}}\boldsymbol{W}_i(t)\right]dt. \tag{15.14}$$

Instead of been viewed as a consequence of model (15.3), expression (15.14) can serve as the definition of a new model. It specifies a multiplicative form for the marginal rate of the counting process conditional on $\boldsymbol{W}_i(t)$. Lin et al. [177] referred to this model as the proportional rates model.

Model (15.14) is more flexible than model (15.3) since it is only conditional on the covariates of interest. $\boldsymbol{W}_i(t)$ may contain a specific part of the event history, but it may also not involve the event history at all.

15.2.2 Model Definitions and Implications*

Note that the model definition (15.14) stems from the informal, although illuminating, expression (15.3). For intensity models, the informal expression is backed by rigorous counting process and martingale theory. However, for the marginal model, since $\boldsymbol{W}_i(t)$ does not contain information on the entire history of $\widetilde{N}_i^*(t)$, $\widetilde{N}_i^*(t)$ is not adapted to $\sigma\{\boldsymbol{W}_i(t)\}$, the σ-algebra generated by $\boldsymbol{W}_i(t)$. The family $\left\{\sigma\{\boldsymbol{W}_i(t)\}, t \geq 0\right\}$ is not even nested. Consequently, the theory of martingales and intensity models is not applicable.

Therefore, the precise meaning of the marginal model critically requires clarification. A notable gap in the existing literature is that the model definition typically does not extend beyond the informal expression (15.14). This lack of formalization hinders rigorous analysis and application. In this section, we discuss options for formally defining marginal models. This section is marked with an asterisk (*). Master's students may choose to bypass it on a first reading or focus on the motivation for the discussion and the resulting Definition A and Definition A′, without going into the detailed derivations.

Suppose that $a_i(t)$ is the intensity process of $Q_i(t)$ with respect to an increasing family of σ-algebras $\{\mathscr{G}_t\}$. By the definition of a martingale, this assumption can be equivalently expressed as

$$E\left\{[Q_i(t) - Q_i(s)]\middle|\mathscr{G}_s\right\} = E\left[\int_s^t a_i(x)dx\middle|\mathscr{G}_s\right], \tag{15.15}$$

for any $0 \leq s \leq t$. Analogous to (15.15), one option to define model (15.14) is to specify that,

$$E\widetilde{N}^*(t) < \infty, \quad E\int_0^t \lambda_0(x)\exp\left[\boldsymbol{\beta}^{\mathrm{T}}\boldsymbol{W}_i(x)\right]dx < \infty, \quad \text{for any } t < \infty, \tag{15.16}$$

and that for any $0 \leq s \leq t$,

$$E\Big\{\big[\widetilde{N}_i^*(t) - \widetilde{N}_i^*(s)\big]\big|\boldsymbol{W}_i(s)\Big\} = E\Big[\int_s^t \lambda_0(x)\exp\left[\boldsymbol{\beta}^{\mathrm{T}}\boldsymbol{W}_i(x)\right]dx\big|\boldsymbol{W}_i(s)\Big]. \tag{15.17}$$

Let $\mathscr{F}_t^w = \sigma\{\boldsymbol{W}_i(t), i = 1,\cdots,n\}$, the σ-algebra generated by $\{\boldsymbol{W}_i(t), i = 1,\cdots,n\}$. Suppose data from the n individuals are independent. By (15.17) and property #12 of the conditional expectation in Section B.2 of Appendix B, for any $0 \leq s \leq t$,

$$E\Big\{\big[\widetilde{N}_i^*(t) - \widetilde{N}_i^*(s)\big]\big|\mathscr{F}_s^w\Big\} = E\Big[\int_s^t \lambda_0(x)\exp\left[\boldsymbol{\beta}^{\mathrm{T}}\boldsymbol{W}_i(x)\right]dx\big|\mathscr{F}_s^w\Big]. \tag{15.18}$$

Since the martingale theory is not applicable to the marginal rate model, we need to examine the implications of (15.18) in statistical applications, which often involve integrals of the type $\int_0^t A(x)d\widetilde{N}_i^*(x)$, where $A(x)$ is a data-dependent function with necessary measurability and integrability properties. To simplify the presentation, we introduce the following definition:

Definition. For counting processes $\widetilde{N}_i^*(\cdot)$, $i = 1,\ldots,n$, and a family of σ-algebras $\{\mathscr{G}_t,\ t \geq 0\}$, a process $\{A(x)\}$ is said to be $(\widetilde{N}^*,\mathscr{G})$-regular if its sample paths are bounded, with at most countably many points of discontinuity, and continuous at each jump point of $\widetilde{N}_1^*(\cdot),\ldots,\widetilde{N}_n^*(\cdot)$, and $A(x)$ is $\mathscr{G}_x$-measurable for each $x \geq 0$.

Suppose that $\{A(x)\}$ is $(\widetilde{N}^*,\mathscr{F}^w)$-regular. By (A.17) in Appendix A, the Lebesgue-Stieltjes integral is the same as the Riemann-Stieltjes integral:

$$\int_0^t A(x)d\widetilde{N}_i^*(x) = \int_0^t A(x)\mathfrak{D}\widetilde{N}_i^*(x). \tag{15.19}$$

Let $0 = x_0 < \cdots < x_k = t$ be a partition of $[0, t]$ into sub-intervals with equal length $\Delta = t/k$, and $I_j = [x_{j-1}, x_j]$, $1 \leq j \leq n$. Then

$$\int_0^t A(x)\mathfrak{D}N_i^*(x) = \lim_{k\to\infty}\sum_{j=1}^k A(x_{j-1})\left[N_i^*(x_j) - N_i^*(x_{j-1})\right]. \tag{15.20}$$

By the law of iterated expectations (B.5),

$$
\begin{aligned}
& E\left\{A(x_{j-1})[N_i^*(x_j) - N_i^*(x_{j-1})]\right\} \\
= \; & EE\left\{A(x_{j-1})[N_i^*(x_j) - N_i^*(x_{j-1})]|\mathscr{F}_{x_{j-1}}\right\} \\
= \; & E\left\{A(x_{j-1})E\{[N_i^*(x_j) - N_i^*(x_{j-1})]|\mathscr{F}_{x_{j-1}}\}\right\} \\
= \; & E\left\{A(x_{j-1})E\left\{\int_{I_j} \lambda_0(x)\exp\left[\boldsymbol{\beta}^{\mathrm{T}}\boldsymbol{W}_i(x)\right]dx|\mathscr{F}_{x_{j-1}}\right\}\right\} \\
= \; & E\left\{\int_{I_j} A(x_{j-1})\lambda_0(x)\exp\left[\boldsymbol{\beta}^{\mathrm{T}}\boldsymbol{W}_i(x)\right]dx\right\} \\
= \; & EA(x_{j-1})[G(x_j) - G(x_{j-1})],
\end{aligned}
\tag{15.21}
$$

where $G(s) = \int_0^s \lambda_0(x)\exp\left[\boldsymbol{\beta}^{\mathrm{T}}\boldsymbol{W}_i(x)\right]dx$. From (15.19)–(15.21), by linearity of the expectation and the dominated convergence theorem,

$$
\begin{aligned}
& E\int_0^t A(x)\mathfrak{D}\widetilde{N}_i^*(x) \\
= \; & E\lim_{k\to\infty}\sum_{j=1}^{k} A(x_{j-1})[N_i^*(x_j) - N_i^*(x_{j-1})] \\
= \; & \lim_{k\to\infty}\sum_{j=1}^{k} E\left\{A(x_{j-1})[N_i^*(x_j) - N_i^*(x_{j-1})]\right\} \\
= \; & \lim_{k\to\infty}\sum_{j=1}^{k} E\left\{A(x_{j-1})[G(x_j) - G(x_{j-1})]\right\} \\
= \; & E\left\{\lim_{k\to\infty}\sum_{j=1}^{k} A(x_{j-1})[G(x_j) - G(x_{j-1})]\right\} \\
= \; & E\int_0^t A(x)\lambda_0(x)\exp\left[\boldsymbol{\beta}^{\mathrm{T}}\boldsymbol{W}_i(x)\right]dx,
\end{aligned}
\tag{15.22}
$$

where, in obtaining the last equality, property #7 in Section A.5 of Appendix A has been used (see Exercise 15.2).

Putting these results together, we have

$$E\int_0^t A(x)d\widetilde{N}_i^*(x) = E\int_0^t A(x)\lambda_0(x)\exp\left[\boldsymbol{\beta}^{\mathrm{T}}\boldsymbol{W}_i(x)\right]dx. \qquad (15.23)$$

This important property is sufficient for many applications. Note that it is for the expectation of an integral, not for the conditional expectation of an integral.

If a stronger version of result (15.23), for conditional expectations, is desired, one option is to define the model in parallel to (15.16) and (15.17), but with the conditioning σ-algebra generated by $\{\boldsymbol{W}_i(s), s \le t\}$. That is, the conditioning σ-algebras are nested. Formally, by the model

$$E\left\{d\widetilde{N}_i^*(t)\middle|\boldsymbol{W}_i(s), s \le t\right\} = \lambda_0(t)\exp\left[\boldsymbol{\beta}^{\mathrm{T}}\boldsymbol{W}_i(t)\right]dt, \qquad (15.24)$$

it is meant that condition (15.16) holds and for any $0 \le s \le t$,

$$\begin{aligned} &E\left\{\left[\widetilde{N}_i^*(t) - \widetilde{N}_i^*(s)\right]\middle|\boldsymbol{W}_i(u), u \le s\right\} \\ = \;& E\left\{\int_s^t \lambda_0(x)\exp\left[\boldsymbol{\beta}^{\mathrm{T}}\boldsymbol{W}_i(x)\right]dx\middle|\boldsymbol{W}_i(u), u \le s\right\}. \end{aligned} \qquad (15.25)$$

Let $\widetilde{\mathscr{F}}_t^w = \sigma\{\boldsymbol{W}_i(s), s \le t, i = 1, \cdots, n\}$, the σ-algebra generated by $\{\boldsymbol{W}_i(s), s \le t, i = 1, \cdots, n\}$. Then

$$\widetilde{\mathscr{F}}_s^w \subset \widetilde{\mathscr{F}}_t^w, s \le t. \qquad (15.26)$$

In comparison, the σ-algebras $\mathscr{F}_s^w$ and $\mathscr{F}_t^w$ may not be nested for $s \le t$.

Suppose that data from the n individuals are independent. Then condition (15.25) implies that for any $0 \le s \le t$,

$$E\left[\left[\widetilde{N}_i^*(t) - \widetilde{N}_i^*(s)\right]\middle|\widetilde{\mathscr{F}}_s^w\right] = E\left\{\int_s^t \lambda_0(x)\exp\left[\boldsymbol{\beta}^{\mathrm{T}}\boldsymbol{W}_i(x)\right]dx\middle|\widetilde{\mathscr{F}}_s^w\right\}. \qquad (15.27)$$

By (15.27) and the dominated convergence theorem (f) in Section B.2 of Appendix B, an argument similar to that used for the derivations of (15.21) through (15.23), but using (B.4) instead of (B.5), shows that, for a $(\widetilde{N}^*, \widetilde{\mathscr{F}}^w)$-regular process $\{A(x)\}$, we have, for any $0 \le s \le t$,

$$E\left\{\int_s^t A(x)d\widetilde{N}_i^*(x)\middle|\widetilde{\mathscr{F}}_s^w\right\} = E\left\{\int_s^t A(x)\lambda_0(x)\exp\left[\boldsymbol{\beta}^{\mathrm{T}}\boldsymbol{W}_i(x)\right]dx\middle|\widetilde{\mathscr{F}}_s^w\right\}. \qquad (15.28)$$

Verification of the details is left to Exercise 15.3.

Note that (15.27) follows from (15.28) by taking $A(x) \equiv 1$. Thus (15.27) and (15.28) are equivalent.

The martingale definition with its related properties, the relationships between (15.18) and (15.23), and the equivalence between (15.27) and (15.28) can all be viewed as extensions and related properties of the conditional expectation concept reviewed in Appendix B. These extensions are crucial for situations in which the conditioning σ-algebra changes over time. The martingale theory provides an elegant framework for analyzing survival data with simple variance and covariance formulas. In contrast, conditions (15.17) and (15.25) for marginal models provide simpler and more flexible model formulations.

An important observation is that, in deriving results (15.21) through (15.28), we do not need the baseline function to be absolutely continuous with derivative $\lambda_0(t)$. We only need the equivalence condition (A.17) in Appendix A between the Riemann-Stieltjes integral and the Lebesgue-Stieltjes integral. This condition holds even when the integrator is discrete, or a mixture of an absolutely continuous function and a discrete function.

To provide flexibility for both the absolutely continuous and the discrete cases, the model definitions and related properties are rewritten in terms of $\Lambda_0(t)$ below.

Definition A (*Marginal models with unnested σ-algebras*): By the marginal rate model

$$E\left[d\widetilde{N}_i^*(t)\middle|\boldsymbol{W}_i(t)\right] = \exp\left[\boldsymbol{\beta}^{\mathrm{T}}\boldsymbol{W}_i(t)\right]d\Lambda_0(t),$$

it is meant that $\Lambda_0(t)$ is a deterministic increasing cadlag function that is either absolutely continuous, discrete, or a mixture of both,

$$E\widetilde{N}^*(t) < \infty, \quad E\int_0^t \exp\left[\boldsymbol{\beta}^{\mathrm{T}}\boldsymbol{W}_i(x)\right]d\Lambda_0(x) < \infty, \quad \text{for any} \quad t < \infty,$$

and for any $0 \le s \le t$,

$$E\left\{\left[\widetilde{N}_i^*(t) - \widetilde{N}_i^*(s)\right]\middle|\boldsymbol{W}_i(s)\right\} = E\left\{\int_s^t \exp\left[\boldsymbol{\beta}^{\mathrm{T}}\boldsymbol{W}_i(x)\right]d\Lambda_0(x)\middle|\boldsymbol{W}_i(s)\right\}.$$

Assume that data from the n individuals are independent. Then the model definition implies that

$$E\int_0^t A(x)d\widetilde{N}_i^*(x) = E\int_0^t A(x)\exp\left[\boldsymbol{\beta}^{\mathrm{T}}\boldsymbol{W}_i(x)\right]d\Lambda_0(x) \tag{15.29}$$

for any $(\widetilde{N}^*, \mathscr{F}^w)$-regular process $\{A(x)\}$.

Definition A' (*Marginal models with nested σ-algebras*): By the marginal rate model

$$E\left[d\widetilde{N}_i^*(t)\middle|\boldsymbol{W}_i(s), s \le t\right] = \exp\left[\boldsymbol{\beta}^{\mathrm{T}}\boldsymbol{W}_i(t)\right]d\Lambda_0(t),$$

it is meant that $\Lambda_0(t)$ is a deterministic increasing cadlag function that is either absolutely continuous, discrete, or a mixture of both,

$$E\widetilde{N}^*(t) < \infty, \quad E\int_0^t \exp\left[\boldsymbol{\beta}^{\mathrm{T}}\boldsymbol{W}_i(x)\right]d\Lambda_0(x) < \infty, \quad \text{for any} \quad t < \infty,$$

and for any $0 \le s \le t$,

$$\begin{aligned} & E\Big\{[\widetilde{N}_i^*(t) - \widetilde{N}_i^*(s)]\big|\boldsymbol{W}_i(u), u \le s\Big\} \\ = & E\Big\{\int_s^t \exp[\boldsymbol{\beta}^{\mathrm{T}}\boldsymbol{W}_i(x)]d\Lambda_0(x)\big|\boldsymbol{W}_i(u), u \le s\Big\}. \end{aligned} \tag{15.30}$$

Assume that data from the n individuals are independent. Then the model definition implies that

$$E\Big\{[\widetilde{N}_i^*(t) - \widetilde{N}_i^*(s)]\big|\widetilde{\mathscr{F}}_s^w\Big\} = E\Big\{\int_s^t \exp[\boldsymbol{\beta}^{\mathrm{T}}\boldsymbol{W}_i(x)]d\Lambda_0(x)\big|\widetilde{\mathscr{F}}_s^w\Big\}. \tag{15.31}$$

Condition (15.31) holds if and only if

$$E\Big\{\int_s^t A(x)d\widetilde{N}_i^*(x)\big|\widetilde{\mathscr{F}}_s^w\Big\} = E\Big\{\int_s^t A(x)\exp[\boldsymbol{\beta}^{\mathrm{T}}\boldsymbol{W}_i(x)]d\Lambda_0(x)\big|\widetilde{\mathscr{F}}_s^w\Big\} \tag{15.32}$$

for any $(\widetilde{N}^*, \widetilde{\mathscr{F}}^w)$-regular process $\{A(x)\}$.

In the literature, modeling and analysis typically focus on the absolutely continuous case. The above definitions and related properties make it possible to explore the less-developed theory for the discrete case, and to present a unified approach when $\Lambda_0(t)$ is a mixture of absolutely continuous and discrete functions. To streamline the presentation, though, subsequent discussions will generally focus on models such as (15.14), for the absolutely continuous case and with conditioning σ-algebras that may not be nested.

From (15.23),

$$E\widetilde{N}_i^*(t) = E\int_0^t d\widetilde{N}_i^*(x) = E\int_0^t \exp[\boldsymbol{\beta}^{\mathrm{T}}\boldsymbol{W}_i(x)]\lambda_0(x)dx. \tag{15.33}$$

When $\boldsymbol{W}_i(t)$ is a fixed covariate vector, Lin et al. [177] referred to model (15.14) as the proportional means model. Note that in this case, for any t, $\mathscr{F}_t^w = \sigma\{\boldsymbol{W}_1, \cdots, \boldsymbol{W}_n\}$. Therefore, $\widetilde{N}^*(t)$ also satisfies model (15.24). By (15.32),

$$\begin{aligned} E[\widetilde{N}_i^*(t)|\boldsymbol{W}_i] &= E\Big\{\int_0^t d\widetilde{N}_i(x)\big|\boldsymbol{W}_i\Big\} \\ &= E\Big\{\int_0^t \exp[\boldsymbol{\beta}^{\mathrm{T}}\boldsymbol{W}_i(x)]\lambda_0(x)dx\big|\boldsymbol{W}_i\Big\} \\ &= \exp[\boldsymbol{\beta}^{\mathrm{T}}\boldsymbol{W}_i]\Lambda_0(t), \end{aligned} \tag{15.34}$$

for $\Lambda_0(t)$ in (15.10). This justifies the model's name. For fixed covariates, $\Lambda_0(t)$ in model (15.14) is the baseline expected number of events by time t, and $\boldsymbol{W}_i$ modifies that expected number by a factor of $\exp\left[\boldsymbol{\beta}^{\mathrm{T}}\boldsymbol{W}_i\right]$.

Model (15.14) is imposed on the underlying counting process $\widetilde{N}_i^*(t)$. Due to censoring, only $\widetilde{N}_i(t)$ is observable. Suppose the censoring by C_i is such that

$$E\left[d\widetilde{N}_i^*(t)\middle|\mathscr{F}_t^{wc}\right] = E\left[d\widetilde{N}_i^*(t)\middle|\mathscr{F}_t^{w}\right], \tag{15.35}$$

where $\mathscr{F}_t^{wc}$ is the σ-algebra generated by $\mathscr{F}_t^{w}$ and $\{C_1(s),\ldots,C_n(s), s \le t\}$. Then the censoring by C_i is called independent censoring. If C_i's are independent of the processes $\{\widetilde{N}_\ell^*(\cdot), \boldsymbol{W}_i(\cdot), 1 \le \ell \le n\}$, then the independent censoring condition is satisfied. It is also satisfied If data from the n individuals are independent, $\boldsymbol{W}_i(t) = \boldsymbol{W}_i$ is a fixed covariate vector, and C_i is independent of $\widetilde{N}_\ell^*(\cdot)$ given $\boldsymbol{W}_i$.

Under model (15.14) with independent censoring,

$$E\left[d\widetilde{N}_i^*(t)\middle|\mathscr{F}_t^{wc}\right] = \lambda_0(t)\exp\left[\boldsymbol{\beta}^{\mathrm{T}}\boldsymbol{W}_i(t)\right]dt.$$

From $d\widetilde{N}(t) = C_i(t)d\widetilde{N}^*(t)$, the marginal rate model for the observed process $\widetilde{N}(t)$ is

$$E\left[d\widetilde{N}_i(t)\middle|\mathscr{F}_t^{wc}\right] = C_i(t)\lambda_0(t)\exp\left[\boldsymbol{\beta}^{\mathrm{T}}\boldsymbol{W}_i(t)\right]. \tag{15.36}$$

Analogous to the discussion on model (15.14), model (15.36) can be made precise by a condition parallel to (15.18), replacing $\mathscr{F}_t^{w}$ by $\mathscr{F}_t^{wc}$ (Exercise 15.4).

15.2.3 Inference

For estimating $\boldsymbol{\beta}$ under model (15.14), the score function $\boldsymbol{U}(\boldsymbol{\beta})$ in (15.5) for model (15.3) can be used, in which case the point estimates from model (15.14) and the AG model are the same. Although the martingale structure is lost, $\boldsymbol{U}(\boldsymbol{\beta})$ remains an unbiased estimating function under mild conditions. It is left to Exercise 15.4 (b) to verify this assertion.

Since the martingale structure is lost, derivation of large sample properties requires tools different from the martingale asymptotic theory. Assume that $\left(\widetilde{N}_i^*(t), \boldsymbol{W}_i(t), C_i(t)\right), 1 \le i \le n$, are i.i.d. processes. Using empirical process theory, Lin et al. [177] showed that, under certain regularity conditions, at the true value $\boldsymbol{\beta}_0$ of the parameter, $n^{-1/2}\boldsymbol{U}(\boldsymbol{\beta}_0)$ converges in distribution to a zero mean multivariate normal distribution with covariance matrix $\Sigma(\boldsymbol{\beta}_0)$, where

$$\Sigma(\boldsymbol{\beta}) = E\left\{\int_0^\infty \left[\boldsymbol{W}_i(x) - \overline{w}(\boldsymbol{\beta},x)\right]dM_i(x)\int_0^\infty \left[\boldsymbol{W}_i(x) - \overline{w}(\boldsymbol{\beta},x)\right]^{\mathrm{T}} dM_i(x)\right\},$$

with $\overline{w}(\boldsymbol{\beta},x)$ being the limit of $E(\boldsymbol{\beta},x)$ in (15.6). Furthermore, $n^{1/2}(\widehat{\boldsymbol{\beta}} - \boldsymbol{\beta}_0)$ converges in distribution to a zero mean multivariate normal distribution with covariance matrix $A^{-1}(\boldsymbol{\beta}_0)\Sigma(\boldsymbol{\beta}_0)A^{-1}(\boldsymbol{\beta}_0)$, where

$$A(\boldsymbol{\beta}) = E\int_0^\infty \left[\boldsymbol{W}_i(x) - \overline{w}(\boldsymbol{\beta}, x)\right]^{\otimes 2} C_i(t)\exp\left[\boldsymbol{\beta}^{\mathrm{T}}\boldsymbol{W}(t)\right]\lambda_0(t)dt.$$

Note that under the AG model (15.3), $\boldsymbol{A}(\boldsymbol{\beta}_0)$ is the covariance matrix in the limiting distribution of $n^{-1/2}\boldsymbol{U}(\boldsymbol{\beta}_0)$, and $\boldsymbol{A}^{-1}(\boldsymbol{\beta}_0)$ is the covariance matrix in the limiting distribution of $n^{1/2}(\widehat{\boldsymbol{\beta}} - \boldsymbol{\beta}_0)$. However, under model (15.14), In general, $\Sigma(\boldsymbol{\beta}_0) \neq A(\boldsymbol{\beta}_0)$ and $A^{-1}(\boldsymbol{\beta}_0)\Sigma(\boldsymbol{\beta}_0)A^{-1}(\boldsymbol{\beta}_0) \neq A^{-1}(\boldsymbol{\beta}_0)$.

Once the estimator $\widehat{\boldsymbol{\beta}}$ is obtained, the Breslow estimator $\widehat{\Lambda}(t)$ in (15.11) can also be used to estimate $\Lambda_0(t)$ under model (15.14). Using empirical process theory, it can be shown that at each t, $\widehat{\Lambda}(t)$ is asymptotically normal with mean $\Lambda(t)$ and a covariance matrix that can be consistently estimated [177].

15.2.4 The One-Sample Case

Suppose individuals are from a homogeneous population and there are no covariates. The model is

$$Ed\widetilde{N}_i^*(t) = d\Lambda_0(t). \tag{15.37}$$

By the discussions in Section 15.2.2, this means (Exercise 15.5) that $\Lambda_0(t)$ is a deterministic increasing cadlag function, which is either absolutely continuous, discrete, or a mixture of both, and for any t,

$$E\widetilde{N}_i^*(t) = \Lambda_0(t). \tag{15.38}$$

This implies that, for any continuous function $A(x)$,

$$E\int_0^t A(x)d\widetilde{N}_i^*(x) = E\int_0^t A(x)d\Lambda_0(x). \tag{15.39}$$

Let $\mathscr{F}_t^c$ be the σ-algebra generated by $C_1(t),\ldots,C_n(t)$. Independent censoring by C_i in this context means that

$$E\left[d\widetilde{N}_i^*(t)|\mathscr{F}_{t-}^c\right] = d\Lambda_0(t). \tag{15.40}$$

This is satisfied if data from the n individuals are independent and C_i is independent of $\widetilde{N}^*(\cdot)$.

Under independent censoring, from $d\widetilde{N}(t) = C_i(t)d\widetilde{N}^*(t)$, the observed process $\widetilde{N}(t)$ satisfies the model

$$Ed\widetilde{N}_i(t) = C_i(t)d\Lambda_0(t), \tag{15.41}$$

which means that for any $0 \le s \le t$,

$$E\Big\{[\tilde{N}_i(t) - \tilde{N}_i(s)]\big|\mathcal{F}_s^c\Big\} = E\Big\{\int_s^t C_i(x)d\Lambda_0(x)\big|\mathcal{F}_s^c\Big\}. \tag{15.42}$$

This implies that

$$E\int_0^t A(x)d\tilde{N}_i(x) = E\int_0^t C_i(x)A(x)d\Lambda_0(x) \tag{15.43}$$

for any $(\tilde{N},\mathcal{F}^c)$-regular process $\{A(x)\}$. That is, the sample paths of $\{A(x)\}$ are bounded, continuous at the event times of the n individuals, and have at most countably many points of discontinuity.

Let

$$K(t) = \sum_{i=1}^{n} I(C_i \ge t) = \sum_{i=1}^{n} C_i(t).$$

The Nelson-Aalen estimator for $\Lambda_0(t)$ is

$$\widehat{\Lambda}_0(t) = \int_0^t \frac{\sum_{i=1}^n d\tilde{N}_i(x)}{K(x)}. \tag{15.44}$$

Under mild regularity conditions, it can be shown that $\widehat{\Lambda}_0(t)$ is consistent for $\Lambda_0(t)$.

Let $J(t) = I(K(t) > 0) = I(\max_i C_i \ge t)$. With the convention $0/0 = 0$, from (15.43) and (15.44),

$$\begin{aligned} E\widehat{\Lambda}_0(t) &= E\int_0^t \frac{J(x)\sum_{i=1}^n d\tilde{N}_i(x)}{K(t)} \\ &= E\int_0^t \frac{J(x)\sum_{i=1}^n C_i(x)d\Lambda_0(x)}{K(x)} \\ &= E\int_0^t J(x)d\Lambda_0(x) \\ &= E\Lambda_0(t \wedge \max_i C_i) \\ &= \int_0^t P(\max_i C_i \ge x)d\Lambda_0(x). \end{aligned} \tag{15.45}$$

Therefore, $E\widehat{\Lambda}_0(t) \le \Lambda_0(t)$, or $\widehat{\Lambda}_0(t)$ is biased downward for $\Lambda_0(t)$.

If C_i's are i.i.d., then

$$\begin{aligned}
\left|E\widehat{\Lambda}_0(t)-\Lambda_0(t)\right| &= \left|E\int_0^t I(\max_i C_i \geq x)d\Lambda_0(x)-\Lambda_0(t)\right| \\
&= \left|\int_0^t \left[1-\prod_i P(C_i<x)\right]d\Lambda_0(x)-\Lambda_0(t)\right| \\
&= \left|-\int_0^t G_C^n(x-)d\Lambda_0(x)\right| \\
&\leq G_C^n(t-)\Lambda_0(t), \qquad (15.46)
\end{aligned}$$

where G_C is the common CDF of C_i. Verification of this result is left to Exercise 15.7.

Result (15.46) shows that, for t satisfying $G_C(t-)<1$, the bias of $\widehat{\Lambda}_0(t)$ converges to zero at an exponential rate.

15.2.5 The Two-Sample Case

For an unadjusted analysis, from Definition A in Section 15.2.2 with $\boldsymbol{\beta}^{\mathrm{T}}\boldsymbol{W}_i=\beta Z_i$, the model specifies that

$$E\left[d\widetilde{N}_i^*|Z_i\right]=\exp(\beta Z_i)d\Lambda_0(t), \qquad (15.47)$$

which means that $\Lambda_0(t)$ is a deterministic increasing cadlàg function that is either absolutely continuous, discrete, or a mixture of both, and for any $0\leq s\leq t$,

$$\begin{aligned}
&E\left\{\left[\widetilde{N}_i^*(t)-\widetilde{N}_i^*(s)\right]|Z_i\right\} \\
&= E\left\{\int_s^t \exp(\beta Z_i)d\Lambda_0(x)|Z_i\right\} \\
&= \exp(\beta Z_i)\left[\Lambda_0(t)-\Lambda_0(s)\right]. \qquad (15.48)
\end{aligned}$$

Condition (15.48) can be simplified to requiring that, for any t,

$$E\left[\widetilde{N}_i^*(t)|Z_i\right]=\exp(\beta Z_i)\Lambda_0(t). \qquad (15.49)$$

Let $\Lambda_C^r(t)$ and Λ_T^r be the expected number of events by time t in the control and treatment groups, respectively. The model then assumes that for any $t>0$,

$$\Lambda_T^r(t)=\exp(\beta)\Lambda_C^r(t). \qquad (15.50)$$

This is similar to the two-sample Cox model for a single time-to-event variable.

Model (15.50) assumes that the ratio of the expected numbers of events during $[0, t]$ in the two groups is identically $\exp(\beta)$ for any $t > 0$. Thus β is the logarithm of the ratio of the expected numbers of events.

Note that Λ^r_C and Λ^r_T can be nonparametrically estimated using only the control group data and the treatment group data, respectively, as described in Section 15.2.4. Specifically,

$$\widehat{\Lambda}^r_C(t) = \sum_{Z_i=0}\sum_{j=1}^{J_i} \frac{I(X_{ij} \le t)}{\sum_{Z_m=0} C_m(X_{ij})},$$

$$\widehat{\Lambda}^r_T(t) = \sum_{Z_i=1}\sum_{j=1}^{J_i} \frac{I(X_{ij} \le t)}{\sum_{Z_m=1} C_m(X_{ij})}. \tag{15.51}$$

Similar to the discussions in Sections 9.3.4 and 14.8, the area-under-the-curve-based ratio

$$REAN_\tau = \frac{\int_0^\tau \Lambda^r_T(t)dt}{\int_0^\tau \Lambda^r_C(t)dt}, \tag{15.52}$$

for a predefined τ, can be considered as an alternative to the model-based parameter $\exp(\beta)$. It serves as a nonparametric summary measure for the treatment effect in the time interval $[0, \tau]$, without requiring the proportional means assumption (15.50).

By dividing both the numerator and denominator by τ, $REAN_\tau$ can be interpreted as the ratio of the average expected numbers of events over the interval $[0, \tau]$. A beneficial treatment effect corresponds to a value less than 1. A nonparametric estimator of $REAN_\tau$ can be obtained using $\widehat{\Lambda}^r_C$ and $\widehat{\Lambda}^r_T$.

Similar to the discussion in Section 9.3.4, the difference between the two area-under-the-curve measures can also be considered.

15.3 The Presence of Death or Dependent Censoring

In the previous two sections, the independent censoring condition was assumed. However, clinical trials often encounter dependent censoring where a dependent event, such as death, can censor recurrent events and end the observation period, in addition to the usual independent censoring due to trial completion or random loss to follow-up.

When the dependent event is a terminal event such as death, there will be no further recurrent events afterwards. Models are available in the literature with either a latent recurrent event process, or with an observable process. An observable processes-based model offers easier interpretation, and usually requires fewer assumptions, and has a reduced model complexity and risk of model identifiability issues. For latent variable models, it is important to have transparent assumptions with justifications, and be interpretable in a clinically meaningful way. This is similar to the situations for analyses when competing risks are present, as discussed in Chapters Thirteen and Fourteen.

When the dependent censoring is due to informative dropout, recurrent events are still possible beyond the dropout, but the information is not available to the trial investigators. In this situation, the latent model approach is more meaningful than when the recurrent event process is terminated by an event such as death.

Dependent censoring significantly complicates the analysis and interpretation of results. The subsections below focus on recurrent event analysis in the presence of death, or an event that terminates the recurrent event process (as opposed to an event that stops the observation of the recurrent event process). This is a more recent research area compared to topics in previous chapters. Various methodologies have been proposed, each with its own advantages and limitations. Some of these approaches will be briefly discussed.

15.3.1 Recurrent Event Counting Process in the Presence of Death

For the underlying counting process $\widetilde{N}_i^*(t)$ that counts the number of recurrent events for the ith individual, naturally its value stops changing once death occurs. Let D_i be the time to death for the ith individual. To account for the presence of death, define $\widetilde{N}_i^*(t)$ to be the number of recurrent events in $[0,t]$ if $D_i \geq t$, and $\widetilde{N}_i^*(t) = \widetilde{N}_i^*(D_i)$ for $t > D_i$. Thus $\widetilde{N}_i^*(t) = \widetilde{N}_i^*(t \wedge D_i)$.

In the presence of death, for more straightforward interpretation, the covariate $\boldsymbol{W}_i(t)$ must be restricted to be external, in the sense that, for $0 \leq s \leq t$, the distribution of $\left(\widetilde{N}_i^*(t), D_i\right)$ given $\boldsymbol{W}_i(t)$ is the same as the distribution of $\left(\widetilde{N}_i^*(t), D_i\right)$ given $\left\{\boldsymbol{W}_i(x) \middle| x \geq t\right\}$.

The modified definition of $\widetilde{N}_i^*(t)$ is natural in the presence of death, and $\widetilde{N}_i^*(t)$ remains a counting process. When $\boldsymbol{W}_i(t)$ is a baseline covariate vector $\boldsymbol{W}_i$, from (15.34),

$$E\left[\widetilde{N}_i^*(t \wedge D_i) \middle| \boldsymbol{W}_i\right] = E\left[\widetilde{N}_i^*(t) \middle| \boldsymbol{W}_i\right] = \exp\left[\boldsymbol{\beta}^{\mathrm{T}} \boldsymbol{W}_i\right] \Lambda_0(t). \tag{15.53}$$

Thus, for the recurrent event process in the presence of death, $\Lambda_0(t)$ remains the baseline expected number of recurrent events by time t, and $\boldsymbol{W}_i$ is the multiplicative factor. For an unadjusted analysis with $\boldsymbol{\beta}^{\mathrm{T}} \boldsymbol{W}_i(t) = \beta Z_i$, $\exp(\beta)$ is the ratio of the expected numbers of events of the stopped process for the treatment group relative to the control group.

Similar to discussions in Sections 15.1 and 15.2, An AG model or a marginal rate model on $\widetilde{N}_i^*(t)$ implies a corresponding model for the observed process $\widetilde{N}_i(t) = \int_0^t C_i(x) d\widetilde{N}_i^*(x)$, where as before, C_i is the independent censoring variable and $C_i(t) = I(C_i \geq t)$. Under the AG model or a marginal rate model, the estimating function $\boldsymbol{U}(\boldsymbol{\beta})$ in (15.5) remains unbiased.

However, in the presence of death, the processes $C_1, \ldots, C_n$, may not be fully observable. Therefore, $\boldsymbol{U}(\boldsymbol{\beta})$ cannot be used. For a trial, C_i is the time elapsed from randomization to study completion or random loss to follow-up. When the individual dies during the trial, C_i is unknown because the potential loss to follow-up cannot be determined. A naive approach might be to define C_i as the time to trial completion when death occurs. However, this makes C_i dependent on D_i, thus no longer representing independent censoring.

To address the issue that $C_i(t)$ is not always observable, Ghosh and Lin [93] proposed using inverse probability weighting to replace it with a determinable quantity, $\widehat{C}_i(t)$. Two specific inverse probability weighting options were considered: the inverse probability of censoring weighting and the inverse probability of survival weighting (see Exercise 15.8). Use of $\widehat{C}_i(t)$ yields the estimating function

$$\widetilde{\boldsymbol{U}}(\boldsymbol{\beta}) = \sum_{i=1}^{n} \int_0^{\infty} \left\{ \boldsymbol{W}_i(t) - \frac{\sum_{i=1}^{n} \widehat{C}_i(t) \exp[\boldsymbol{\beta}^{\mathrm{T}} \boldsymbol{W}_i(t)] \boldsymbol{W}_i(t)}{\sum_{i=1}^{n} \widehat{C}_i(t) \exp[\boldsymbol{\beta}^{\mathrm{T}} \boldsymbol{W}_i(t)]} \right\} \widehat{C}_i(t) d\widetilde{N}_i(t). \qquad (15.54)$$

When C_i and D_i are conditionally independent given $\boldsymbol{W}_i^*$, calculation of $\widehat{C}_i(t)$ requires fitting a proportional hazards model on either C_i or D_i. Details can be found in their work. Under the assumptions that $\left(\widetilde{N}_i^*(\cdot), \boldsymbol{W}_i(\cdot), D_i, C_i\right), i = 1, \cdots, n$, are i.i.d., along with other boundedness and stability conditions, the asymptotic normality of the estimators can be established [93].

In the one sample case, assume that the C_i's are i.i.d. Then for $\widehat{\Lambda}_0(t)$ in (15.44), from (15.46), $E\widehat{\Lambda}_0(t)$ converges to $\Lambda_0(t) = E\widetilde{N}_i^*(t)$ at an exponential rate for t satisfying $P(C_1 < t) < 1$. To approximate $K(t) = \sum_{i=1}^{n} I(C_i \ge t)$ in $\widehat{\Lambda}_0(t)$ that is not always observable, the inverse probability of survival weighting can be used (see Exercise 15.8 (b)), which replaces $I(C_1 \ge t)$ by $I(B_i \ge t)/\widehat{S}_D(t)$, where $B_i = D_i \wedge C_i$ and $\widehat{S}_D(t)$ is the Kaplan-Meier estimator of $P(D_i \ge t)$. This results in an estimator $\widetilde{\Lambda}_0(t)$ of $E\widetilde{N}_i^*(t)$:

$$\begin{aligned} \widetilde{\Lambda}_0(t) &= \int_0^t \left[\frac{\sum_{i=1}^{n} I(B_i \ge x)}{\widehat{S}_D(x)} \right]^{-1} d\left[\sum_{i=1}^{n} \widetilde{N}_i(x) \right] \\ &= \int_0^t \frac{\widehat{S}_D(x) d\left[\sum_{i=1}^{n} \widetilde{N}_i(x)\right]}{\sum_{i=1}^{n} I(B_i \ge x)}. \qquad (15.55) \end{aligned}$$

15.3.2 Recurrent Events Conditional on Survival

For recurrent event analysis in the presence of death, another approach is to define a conditional marginal rate model given survival:

$$E\left[d\widetilde{N}_i^*(t) \middle| D_i \ge t, \boldsymbol{W}_i(t)\right] = \lambda_0^s(t) \exp\left[\boldsymbol{\beta}^{\mathrm{T}} \boldsymbol{W}_i(t)\right] dt, \qquad (15.56)$$

where the covariate $\boldsymbol{W}_i(t)$ is external, and the baseline function λ_0^s has a superscript to indicate the conditional on survival approach. Some discussions on conditional modeling were given in Cook and Lawless [48]. This model was briefly mentioned in Lin et al. [177], and related models have been used by other authors [189, 270, 271].

One option to formally define model (15.56) is, analogous to (15.17), to specify that, for any $0 \le s \le t$,

$$\begin{aligned} & E\Big\{[\widetilde{N}_i^*(t) - \widetilde{N}_i^*(s)]\big|D_i(s), \boldsymbol{W}_i(s)\Big\} \\ = \quad & E\Big[\int_s^t \lambda_0^s(x)\exp\big[\boldsymbol{\beta}^{\mathrm{T}}\boldsymbol{W}_i(x)\big]dx\big|D_i(s), \boldsymbol{W}_i(s)\Big], \end{aligned}$$

where $D_i(t) = I(D_i \ge t)$. However, there is little interest in $\widetilde{N}_i(t)$ when $D_i < t$. Therefore, it may make more sense to formally define model (15.56) by specifying that,

$$E\widetilde{N}^*(t) < \infty, \quad E\int_0^t \lambda_0^s(x)\exp\big[\boldsymbol{\beta}^{\mathrm{T}}\boldsymbol{W}_i(x)\big]dx < \infty, \quad \text{for any } t < \infty, \tag{15.57}$$

and that for any $0 \le s \le t$,

$$\begin{aligned} & E\Big\{[\widetilde{N}_i^*(t) - \widetilde{N}_i^*(s)]\big|D_i(t), \boldsymbol{W}_i(t)\Big\} \\ = \quad & E\Big\{\int_s^t \lambda_0^s(x)\exp\big[\boldsymbol{\beta}^{\mathrm{T}}\boldsymbol{W}_i(x)\big]dx\big|D_i(t), \boldsymbol{W}_i(t)\Big\}. \end{aligned} \tag{15.58}$$

Let $\mathscr{F}_t^{dw} = \sigma\{D_i(t), \boldsymbol{W}_i(t), i = 1, \cdots, n\}$, the σ-algebra generated by $\{D_i(t), \boldsymbol{W}_i(t), i = 1, \cdots, n\}$. Suppose that data from the n individuals are independent. Similar to (15.18), from (15.58) we obtain, for any $0 \le s \le t$,

$$E\Big\{[\widetilde{N}_i^*(t) - \widetilde{N}_i^*(s)]\big|\mathscr{F}_t^{dw}\Big\} = E\Big[\int_s^t \lambda_0^s(x)\exp\big[\boldsymbol{\beta}^{\mathrm{T}}\boldsymbol{W}_i(x)\big]dx\big|\mathscr{F}_t^{dw}\Big]. \tag{15.59}$$

To examine implications of (15.59) for an integral $\int_0^t A(x)d\widetilde{N}_i^*(x)$, assume that $\{A(x)\}$ is a $(\widetilde{N}^*, \mathscr{F}^{dw})$-regular process. Then (15.19) continues to hold. Consider again the partition of $[0, t]$ used in (15.20). Then

$$\int_0^t A(x)\mathfrak{D}N_i^*(x) = \lim_{k\to\infty}\sum_{j=1}^k A(x_j)\big[N_i^*(x_j) - N_i^*(x_{j-1})\big]. \tag{15.60}$$

Analogous to (15.21),

$$\begin{aligned} & E\Big\{A(x_j)\big[N_i^*(x_j) - N_i^*(x_{j-1})\big]\Big\} \\ = \quad & EE\Big\{A(x_j)\big[N_i^*(x_j) - N_i^*(x_{j-1})\big]\big|\mathscr{F}_{x_j}\Big\} \\ = \quad & EA(x_j)\big[G(x_j) - G(x_{j-1})\big], \end{aligned} \tag{15.61}$$

where $G(s) = \int_0^s \lambda_0^s(x)\exp\left[\boldsymbol{\beta}^{\mathrm{T}}\boldsymbol{W}_i(x)\right]dx$. Verification of the details is left to Exercise 15.9. Similar to (15.22), we once again have

$$\begin{aligned}
& E\int_0^t A(x)\mathfrak{D}\widetilde{N}_i^*(x) \\
= \; & \lim_{k\to\infty} E\left\{\sum_{j=1}^k A(x_j)\left[G(x_j)-G(x_{j-1})\right]\right\} \\
= \; & E\left\{\lim_{k\to\infty}\sum_{j=1}^k A(x_j)\left[G(x_j)-G(x_{j-1})\right]\right\} \\
= \; & E\int_0^t A(x)\lambda_0^s(x)\exp\left[\boldsymbol{\beta}^{\mathrm{T}}\boldsymbol{W}_i(x)\right]dx. \qquad (15.62)
\end{aligned}$$

Consequently,

$$E\int_0^t A(x)d\widetilde{N}_i^*(x) = E\int_0^t A(x)\lambda_0^s(x)\exp\left[\boldsymbol{\beta}^{\mathrm{T}}\boldsymbol{W}_i(x)\right]dx. \qquad (15.63)$$

From (15.58), $\lambda_0^s(t)$ and $\exp\left[\boldsymbol{\beta}^{\mathrm{T}}\boldsymbol{W}_i(t)\right]$ can be interpreted as, respectively, the baseline and multiplicative factor of the rate function of $\widetilde{N}_i^*(t)$, conditional on the covariate and on the individual being alive. For interpretation in terms of mean functions, consider the case when $\boldsymbol{W}_i(t)$ is a fixed covariate: $\boldsymbol{W}_i(t) = \boldsymbol{W}_i$. From (15.58), for $0 \le s \le t$,

$$E\left[\widetilde{N}_i^*(t) - \widetilde{N}_i^*(s)\middle|D_i \ge t, \boldsymbol{W}_i\right] = \exp\left[\boldsymbol{\beta}^{\mathrm{T}}\boldsymbol{W}_i\right]\left[\Lambda_0^s(t) - \Lambda_0^s(s)\right], \qquad (15.64)$$

where

$$\Lambda_0^s(t) = \int_0^t \lambda_0^s(x)dx.$$

In particular, setting $s = 0$, we obtain

$$E\left[\widetilde{N}_i^*(t)\middle|D_i \ge t, \boldsymbol{W}_i\right] = \exp\left[\boldsymbol{\beta}^{\mathrm{T}}\boldsymbol{W}_i\right]\Lambda_0^s(t), \qquad (15.65)$$

Thus $\exp\left[\boldsymbol{\beta}^{\mathrm{T}}\boldsymbol{W}_i\right]\Lambda_0^s(t)$ is the expected number of recurrent events in $[0,t]$ given the covariate and the condition that the individual is alive prior to t. In particular, for an unadjusted analysis with $\boldsymbol{\beta}^{\mathrm{T}}\boldsymbol{W}_i = \beta Z_i$, $\exp(\beta)$ is the ratio of conditional mean numbers of recurrent events in $[0,t]$ given survival prior to t.

Note that from (15.64) and (15.65),

$$\begin{aligned}
& E\left[\widetilde{N}_i^*(t) - \widetilde{N}_i^*(s)\middle|D_i \ge t, \boldsymbol{W}_i\right] \\
= \; & E\left[\widetilde{N}_i^*(t)\middle|D_i \ge t, \boldsymbol{W}_i\right] - E\left[\widetilde{N}_i^*(s)\middle|D_i \ge s, \boldsymbol{W}_i\right].
\end{aligned}$$

It follows that, for $0 \le s \le t$,

$$E\big[\widetilde{N}_i^*(s)\big|D_i \ge t, \boldsymbol{W}_i\big] = E\big[\widetilde{N}_i^*(s)\big|D_i \ge s, \boldsymbol{W}_i\big]. \tag{15.66}$$

That is, the expected number of recurrent events in $[0, s]$ given survival on $[0, s]$ is the same as the expected number in $[0, s]$ given that the individual is alive beyond a further point $t > s$. Therefore, the model implies a weak dependence of the expected number on survival. If the expected number of recurrent events depends strongly on how long the individual survives, then model (15.55) may not be applicable.

For the expected number of recurrent events in $[0, t]$ without conditioning on being alive prior to t, an argument similar to (15.60)–(15.62), with $A(x) = D_i(x)$ and with the expectation replaced by the conditional expectation given $\boldsymbol{W}_i$, shows that

$$\begin{aligned} E\big[\widetilde{N}_i^*(t)\big|\boldsymbol{W}_i\big] &= E\Big\{\int_0^t D_i(x)d\widetilde{N}_i^*(x)\big|\boldsymbol{W}_i\Big\} \\ &= E\Big\{\int_0^t D_i(x)\exp\big[\boldsymbol{\beta}^{\mathrm{T}}\boldsymbol{W}_i\big]\lambda_0^s(x)dx\big|\boldsymbol{W}_i\Big\} \\ &= \exp\big[\boldsymbol{\beta}^{\mathrm{T}}\boldsymbol{W}_i\big]\int_0^t P\big(D_i \ge x\big|\boldsymbol{W}_i\big)\lambda_0^s(x)dx, \end{aligned} \tag{15.67}$$

This important result extends the result in Ghosh and Lin [92] for the one sample case, which can be thought of as when $\boldsymbol{W}_i \equiv 0$.

Model (15.56) is imposed on the counting process $\widetilde{N}_i^*$. Due to censoring, only

$$\widetilde{N}_i(t) = \widetilde{N}_i^*(t \wedge C_i) = \widetilde{N}_i^*(t \wedge D_i \wedge C_i) = \int_0^t B_i(x)d\widetilde{N}_i^*(x) \tag{15.68}$$

is observed, where

$$B_i(t) = I(D_i \wedge C_i \ge t).$$

Suppose C_i satisfies

$$E\big[d\widetilde{N}_i^*(t)\big|\mathscr{F}_{t-}^{dwc}\big] = E\big[d\widetilde{N}_i^*(t)\big|\mathscr{F}_{t-}^{dw}\big], \tag{15.69}$$

where $\mathscr{F}_t^{dwc}$ is the σ-algebra generated by $\mathscr{F}_t^{dw}$ and $\{C_i(s)\big|\ 1 \le i \le n,\ 0 \le s \le t\}$. Then the censoring by C_i is called independent censoring. Under this condition, and assuming that data from the n individuals are independent, from (15.68) the marginal rate model for the observed process $\widetilde{N}(t)$ is

$$E\big[d\widetilde{N}_i(t)\big|\mathscr{F}_t^{dwc}\big] = B_i(t)\lambda_0^s(t)\exp\big[\boldsymbol{\beta}^{\mathrm{T}}\boldsymbol{W}_i(t)\big]. \tag{15.70}$$

By this model, it is meant that condition (15.57) holds and that for any $0 \le s \le t$,

$$E\{[\tilde{N}_i(t) - \tilde{N}_i(s)] | \mathscr{F}_t^{dwc}\}$$

$$= E\{\int_s^t \lambda_0^s(x) \exp[\boldsymbol{\beta}^{\mathrm{T}} \boldsymbol{W}_i(x)] dx | \mathscr{F}_t^{dwc}\}. \tag{15.71}$$

This implies that for an $(\tilde{N}, \mathscr{F}^{dwc})$-regular $\{A(x)\}$,

$$E\int_0^t A(x) d\tilde{N}_i(x) = E\int_0^t A(x)\lambda_0^s(x) \exp[\boldsymbol{\beta}^{\mathrm{T}} \boldsymbol{W}_i(x)] dx. \tag{15.72}$$

For the marginal rate model (15.70), the estimating function is

$$\boldsymbol{U}_s(\boldsymbol{\beta}) = \sum_{i=1}^n \int_0^\infty \left\{ \boldsymbol{W}_i(t) - \frac{\sum_{i=1}^n B_i(t) \exp[\boldsymbol{\beta}^{\mathrm{T}} \boldsymbol{W}_i(t)] \boldsymbol{W}_i(t)}{\sum_{i=1}^n B_i(t) \exp[\boldsymbol{\beta}^{\mathrm{T}} \boldsymbol{W}_i(t)]} \right\} d\tilde{N}_i(t). \tag{15.73}$$

Under mild conditions on $\boldsymbol{W}_i(t)$, the integrands in (15.73) are $(\tilde{N}, \mathscr{F}^{dwc})$-regular. Hence $\boldsymbol{U}_s(\boldsymbol{\beta})$ is an unbiased estimating function for the parameter $\boldsymbol{\beta}$ (Exercise 15.10).

Note that model (15.56) is conditional on a post-randomization covariate D_i. Therefore, although the model is useful in describing how $\boldsymbol{W}_i(t)$ influences the marginal rate among survivors, caution should be exercised in the interpretation of the treatment effect.

Under the model in Section 15.3.1, $E[\tilde{N}_i^*(t) | \boldsymbol{W}_i]$ has a simpler expression compared to (15.67) for model (15.56) conditional on survivors. However, in the former approach, the estimating function involves $\hat{C}_i(t)$ which requires fitting a Cox model for C_i or D_i given the covariates. Consequently, the estimator depends on the distribution of C_i or D_i in a complex and opaque manner.

The conditional model given survivor in this section yields expression (15.67) which clearly shows the explicit form of the dependence on $P(D_i \ge t | \boldsymbol{W}_i)$. On the other hand, as noted before, model (15.56) may not be applicable when the expected number of recurrent events depends strongly on how long the individual survives.

For the one sample case, from (15.65),

$$E[\tilde{N}_i^*(t) | D_i \ge t] = \Lambda_0^s(t). \tag{15.74}$$

Let

$$\hat{\Lambda}_0^{\#}(t) = \int_0^t \frac{\sum_{i=1}^n d\tilde{N}_i(x)}{\sum_{i=1}^n B_i(x)} = \int_0^t \frac{\sum_{i=1}^n d\tilde{N}_i(x)}{\sum_{i=1}^n I(D_i \wedge C_i \ge x)}.$$

Similar to (15.45) and (15.46), it can be shown (Exercise 15.11) that

$$E\widehat{\Lambda}_0^{\#}(t) = \int_0^t P(\max_i D_i \wedge C_i \geq x) d\Lambda_0^s(x), \tag{15.75}$$

and that, if C_i's are i.i.d.,

$$\left| E\widehat{\Lambda}_0^{\#}(t) - \Lambda_0^s(t) \right| \leq \left[P(D_i \wedge C_i < t) \right]^n \Lambda_0^s(t). \tag{15.76}$$

$\widehat{\Lambda}_0^{\#}(t)$ only estimates the conditional expected number of recurrent events given survival. To estimate the unconditional expected number of recurrent events, $E\widetilde{N}^*(t)$, from the one-sample case of (15.67), i.e., with $\boldsymbol{W}_i \equiv 0$, we have

$$E\widetilde{N}_i^*(t) = \int_0^t P(D_i \geq x) d\Lambda_0^s(x). \tag{15.77}$$

By replacing $\Lambda_0^s(t)$ with $\widehat{\Lambda}_0^{\#}(t)$, and $P(D_i \geq t)$ with the Kaplan-Meier estimator $\widehat{S}_D(t)$, we can obtain an estimator of $E\widetilde{N}_i^*(t)$ as

$$\int_0^t \widehat{S}_D(x) d\widehat{\Lambda}_0^{\#}(x) = \int_0^t \frac{\widehat{S}_D(x) d\left[\sum_{i=1}^n \widetilde{N}_i(x)\right]}{\sum_{i=1}^n B_i(x)}., \tag{15.78}$$

which is precisely the estimator $\widetilde{\Lambda}_0(t)$ defined in (15.55). However, it is important to note that derivation of the estimator in (15.78) relies on model (15.74). This model may not be appropriate when the expected number of recurrent events is highly dependent on an individual's survival time. In contrast, the estimator $\widetilde{\Lambda}_0(t)$ in (15.55) is derived without any such restrictive modeling assumptions.

15.3.3 Death Plus Recurrent Events

Suppose it is expected that the treatment has similar effects on recurrent events and death. When the goal is to assess the total treatment effect on all adverse events—death or recurrent events—the simple approach of combining all events may seem appealing. In this context, $\widetilde{N}_i^{*a}(t)$ can be defined to count both types of events, or more generally, to count the total number of adverse events, which may be of several types.

Assuming there are no tied events, $\widetilde{N}_i^{*a}(t)$ defined this way remains a counting process, jumping by 1 at each adverse event. Therefore, one may consider applying the AG intensity model (15.3). However, note that the AG model assumes that, given event history, an individual is at risk for a future event. This assumption is violated when death has occurred, as the individual is no longer at risk of any future event.

The marginal mean/rate model (15.14) provides a good alternative to avoid the issue mentioned above. However, the estimating function (15.5) uses the censoring variables in (15.6), which might not always be available. Additionally, using estimated quantities, as in (15.54), can introduce a dependence of the estimator on the assumed distribution of C_i or D_i in an opaque manner.

Furthermore, it's worth noting that treatment may affect death and recurrent events in different ways. Combining them could obscure these distinct effects, similar to what is observed in time-to-first-event analysis. One consequence of this obscured effect is that the power may be lower than alternative methods. For these reasons, approaches that acknowledge the different natures of death and recurrent events and present treatment effects in a more direct and clear manner, are generally favored.

Note that for a marginal model on death plus recurrent events, death is a jump point of $\tilde{N}_i^{*a}(t)$ and also likely a discontinuity point of the integrand in (15.54). Therefore, the estimating function would no longer have a regular process as its integrand, and discussions in Sections 15.2.2 and 15.3.2 using the Riemann-Stieltjes integral no longer apply. Further work is necessary to explore ways to formally define these models and establish relevant properties.

15.4 Other Models

Recurrent event analysis is an active research area with various modeling approaches beyond those discussed in the previous sections. In addition to the multiplicative intensity or rate models, other models can also be considered, such as transformation models [180], additive models [271], and the accelerated life model [94]. Methods for multiple types of events [34] or clustered data [270] are also available. When there are different event types, a linear combination of counting processes, one for each event type, with weights reflecting their degree of severity, was also proposed [199].

For analysis of recurrent events under informative censoring, Wang, Qin and Chiang [314] considered multiplicative intensity models conditional on a latent variable and developed methods for estimation of the cumulative rate functions and regression parameters. The distributions of both the censoring and latent variables are treated as nuisance parameters. Liu et al. [189], Huang and Wang [119], Ye et al. [353], and Zeng and Lin [362] studied frailty models where the intensity or rate function of the recurrent and terminal events share an unobserved frailty. For dependent censoring, Miloslavsky et al. [208] extended the AG model and showed that the regression parameter estimator remains consistent if the censoring mechanism is estimated consistently. In their work, dependent censoring is treated as a nuisance, and the focus is on the parameters in the model for the latent counting process of recurrent events. Comparisons of some of the models and related simulation studies were provided in Luo et al. [192] and Charles-Nelson et al. [37]. For recurrent event analysis in the presence of death, there have also been works on the "while-alive" strategy adjusting for the average restricted survival [316, 197].

In many recurrent event models, typically there is only one type of terminal event that dependently censors the recurrent events, and the treatment effect on this terminal event is also of interest. In some situations, there may be multiple types of terminal events, but only one of them is of interest. For example, in a cardiovascular trial, the recurrent events may be censored by death. However, the primary interest may be on the treatment effects for the recurrent events and cardiovascular death. In this case, non-cardiovascular death presents a competing risk to both outcomes. Further research and more sophisticated modeling approaches are needed for assessing treatment effect in the presence of such competing risks.

15.5 Recurrent Event Analysis Versus Single Event Analysis

When each individual experiences at most one event, similarities between the estimating function in (15.5) and the one for univariate analysis in Chapter Six might lead to the impression that they are the same. However, this is not the case. In the univariate case, the individual is no longer under observation once the event or censoring has occurred. Therefore, at each observed event time X_i with $\delta_i = 1$, the risk set in (6.17) comprises individuals with $X_\ell \wedge C_\ell \geq X_i$.

In contrast, under the recurrent event framework, from (15.6), at an event time X_{ij}, the risk set is the set of individuals with $C_\ell \geq X_{ij}$, which can be a much larger set. In the extreme scenario of fixed censoring with $C_i \equiv c$ for some $c > 0$, at all event times observed in $[0, c]$, everyone is in the risk set. Therefore, using the recurrent event analysis in such case can distort estimation of the treatment effect. Specifically, the estimating function in (15.5) might lead to an effect estimate that amplifies the effect at early event times, since those who experienced early events remain in the risk set at later event times. Furthermore, C_i may not be available when the event is observed, and use of estimated quantiles as in (15.54) introduces complications as discussed in Section 15.3.2. Therefore, when everyone experiences at most one event, univariate time-to-event analysis should be used.

The above point might seem moot since it is unlikely that recurrent event analysis will be performed if everyone experiences at most one event. However, a somewhat related scenario is that, in certain clinical trials, among participants who experience any events, most typically have only one, while a very small number of individuals experience multiple events. In such situations of highly skewed recurrent events distributions, a recurrent event analysis might offer little improvement in efficiency or statistical power compared to the analysis approaches discussed in Chapter Fourteen. Furthermore, concerns could arise about the robustness and generalizability of recurrent event analysis results, as they could be disproportionately influenced by the few individuals with numerous events. Additionally, the key quantity in a recurrent event analysis is the expected number of events, $E\widetilde{N}_i^*(t)$, within the time interval $[0, t]$. When competing risks, such as death, are present and most individuals experience at most one recurrent event, this quantity is very close to the cumulative incidence function (CIF) discussed in Chapter Thirteen. As noted in that chapter, the CIF is influenced by the cause-specific hazards of competing risks. It may give a misleading impression of the treatment effect. Thus, caution should be exercised in its interpretation.

When the recurrent events distribution is highly skewed, for the primary analysis of a trial on the causal inference of treatment effect, it is recommended to use models and analysis approaches discussed in Chapter Fourteen. These methods focus on the terminal event and the first of the recurrent events. They isolate risks of the outcomes of interest while accounting for competing risks, using quantities that are generally better understood. This leads to simpler analysis, more transparent results, and clearer interpretations. Furthermore, results are more robust to outliers who have a large number of recurrent events. This enhances generalizability and replicability.

Recurrent event models and analyses are highly valuable for prediction and subgroup analysis, particularly for patients with specific disease progression patterns. They can enhance understanding of treatment effects by providing a detailed treatment effect profile and offering insights for patients with different disease progression patterns, helping to refine care strategies.

15.6 Combined Events Process Analysis Versus Analysis of Multiple Endpoints

As mentioned in Chapter Fourteen, in clinical trials, multiple adverse events or endpoints are often of interest, usually comprising certain terminal and non-terminal events. If the treatment is expected to have similar effects on these events and one wishes to assess the total treatment effect on all events, it may be tempting to consider the AG intensity model or a marginal mean/rate model using the counting process $\widetilde{N}_i^{*a}$ of all events. This is similar in spirit to the discussion of death plus recurrent events in Section 15.3.3.

However, caution should be exercised in using this approach. Consider a simple case where time to heart failure hospitalization (H), time to stroke (S), and time to cardiovascular death (CVD) are of interest. In this scenario, the competing risk for H and S is time to death, and the competing risk for CVD is time to non-cardiovascular death. We have

$$E\widetilde{N}_i^{*a}(t) = CIF_H(t) + CIF_S(t) + CIF_{CVD}(t),$$

where $CIF_H(t)$, $CIF_S(t)$ and $CIF_{CVD}(t)$ are the cumulative incidence functions of H, S and CVD, respectively. It can be seen that $E\widetilde{N}_i^{*a}(t)$ depends on the cause-specific hazards of competing events through the cumulative incidence functions.

Even if the component CVD is replaced by all-cause mortality (D), so that there are no competing risks for D, there is still the competing risk from D for H and S. As discussed in Chapter Thirteen, the presence of competing risks in $E\widetilde{N}_i^{*a}(t)$ may lead to a distorted estimate of the treatment effect and reduced power in treatment effect testing. Two other limitations of this approach, which are shared by the recurrent events plus death analysis, are that combining the events can obscure or mask the distinct treatment effects on individual events, and that integrals with respect to $\widetilde{N}_i^{*a}(t)$ may have an integrand and integrator both sharing common discontinuity points. The latter scenario prevents a model formulation and interpretation using the Riemann-Stieltjes integral; thus more work is needed to rigorously define the marginal model and analyze its associated properties.

The methods based on cause-specific hazards in Chapter Fourteen isolate the risks of events of interest while appropriately accounting for competing risks. It is recommended that these methods be used for treatment effect assessment due to their clear interpretation, simple implementation, and good power performance.

On the other hand, analysis based on $E\widetilde{N}_i^{*a}(t)$ is very useful for predicting total adverse events and assessing absolute treatment effect on the observed events. These analyses can complement those based on the cause-specific hazards, helping to provide a more complete understanding of the treatment effects.

15.7 Exercises and Complements

15.1 Verify the expression of $\boldsymbol{U}(\boldsymbol{\beta})$ in (15.8).

15.2 Provide the details in justifying the last equality in (15.22) using (A.17).

15.3 Provide the details in deriving (15.28) for model (15.24).

Hint: Let $s = x_0 < \cdots < x_k = t$ be a partition of $[s,t]$ into sub-intervals with equal length $\Delta = (t-s)/k$, and $I_j = [x_{j-1}, x_j]$, $1 \le j \le n$. Then

$$E\Big(\int_s^t A(x)\mathfrak{D}N_i^*(x)|\widetilde{\mathscr{F}}_s^w\Big) = E\Big(\lim_{k\to\infty}\sum_{j=1}^k A(x_{j-1})[N_i^*(x_j) - N_i^*(x_{j-1})]|\widetilde{\mathscr{F}}_s^w\Big).$$

Furthermore, since $\widetilde{\mathscr{F}}_s^w \subset \widetilde{\mathscr{F}}_{x_{j-1}}^w$, it follows from (B.4) in Appendix B that

$$E\Big(A(x_{j-1})\big[N_i^*(x_j) - N_i^*(x_{j-1})\big]\big|\widetilde{\mathscr{F}}_s^w\Big)$$

$$= E\Big\{E\Big(A(x_{j-1})\big[N_i^*(x_j) - N_i^*(x_{j-1})\big]\big|\widetilde{\mathscr{F}}_{x_{j-1}}^w\Big)\big|\widetilde{\mathscr{F}}_s^w\Big\}.$$

Note that the above equality would not hold if $\widetilde{\mathscr{F}}_t^w$ is not nested.

15.4 (a) Based on discussions regarding (15.14), provide a formal definition of model (15.36).

(b) Find conditions to ensure that, for model (15.14), $\boldsymbol{U}(\boldsymbol{\beta})$ remains an unbiased estimating function.

Hint: Identify the $\{A(x)\}$ process in (15.19) for $\boldsymbol{U}(\boldsymbol{\beta})$ and then find the conditions on $\boldsymbol{W}_i(t)$, etc., to guarantee that this $\{A(x)\}$ process is $(\widetilde{N}, \mathscr{F}^{wc})$-regular.

(c) Consider the case for nested σ-algebras. Let $\widetilde{\mathscr{F}}_t^{wc}$ be the σ-algebra generated by $\widetilde{\mathscr{F}}_t^w$ and $\{C_i(s)\big|\ 1 \le i \le n,\ 0 \le s \le t\}$. The censoring by C_i's is independent for model (15.24) if

$$E\big[d\widetilde{N}_i^*(t)\big|\widetilde{\mathscr{F}}_t^{wc}\big] = E\big[d\widetilde{N}_i^*(t)\big|\widetilde{\mathscr{F}}_t^w\big].$$

Assume that data from the n individuals are independent. Under model (15.24) with independent censoring,

$$E\big[d\widetilde{N}_i(t)\big|\widetilde{\mathscr{F}}_t^{wc}\big] = C_i(t)\lambda_0(t)\exp\big[\boldsymbol{\beta}^{\mathrm{T}}\boldsymbol{W}_i(t)\big]. \qquad (15.79)$$

Analogous to Definition A', provide a formal definition of the marginal model (15.79).

15.5 Based on discussions regarding (15.14), provide formal definitions of models (15.37) and (15.41) in the one-sample case.

15.6 Verify (15.45).

15.7 Verify (15.46).

15.8 Consider model (15.14) for the recurrent event counting process stopped by death in Section 15.3.1. To approximate the unknown censoring process $I(C_i \ge t)$, Ghosh and Lin [93] proposed two options. One is based on an identity similar to (13.52) that Fine and Gray [76] used for their sub-distribution hazard regression model. Assume that time to death, D, and time to censoring, C, are independent given the covariate vector $\boldsymbol{W}$. Let $X = D \wedge C$ and

$$G(t; \boldsymbol{W}) = P\big(C \ge t\big|\boldsymbol{W}\big).$$

Then similar to (13.53),

$$E\left[\frac{I(C \geq D \wedge t)}{G(X \wedge t; \boldsymbol{W})} \Big| \boldsymbol{W}\right] = 1. \tag{15.80}$$

Note that this implicitly requires the assumption that the denominator inside the expectation is positive in the data range.

(a) Show that

$$E\left[\frac{G(t; \boldsymbol{W}) I(C \geq D \wedge t)}{G(X \wedge t; \boldsymbol{W})} \Big| \boldsymbol{W}\right] = E\big[I(C \geq t) \big| \boldsymbol{W}\big]. \tag{15.81}$$

Based on this identity, Ghosh and Lin proposed an estimating function that uses $\widehat{G}(t; \boldsymbol{W}_i) I(C_i \geq D_i \wedge t)[\widehat{G}(X_i \wedge t; \boldsymbol{W}_i)]^{-1}$ instead of $I(C_i \geq t)$, where $\widehat{G}(t; \boldsymbol{W}_i)$ is the estimator of $G(t; \boldsymbol{W}_i)$ under a multiplicative hazards model.

Note that, as a process in t, the indicator $C_i(t) = I(C_i \geq t)$ takes the value 1 up to C_i, and 0 afterwards. Thus, knowledge of C_i is required to determine $C_i(t)$. In comparison, the indicator $I_i(t) = I(C_i \geq D_i \wedge t)$ is always observable. When $C_i \leq D_i$, which implies that C_i is observable, $I_i(t)$ takes value 1 up to C_i and 0 afterwards. When $C_i > D_i$, which implies that D_i is observable, $I_i(t)$ is identically 1 for all t.

(b) Let

$$S_D(t; \boldsymbol{W}) = P\big(D \geq t \big| \boldsymbol{W}\big).$$

Show that

$$E\left[\frac{I(X \geq t)}{S_D(t; \boldsymbol{W})} \Big| \boldsymbol{W}\right] = E\big[I(C \geq t) \big| \boldsymbol{W}\big]. \tag{15.82}$$

Note that this implicitly requires the assumption that the denominator inside the expectation is positive in the data range.

Based on this identity, Ghosh and Lin proposed another estimating function that uses $I(X_i \geq t)[\widehat{S}_D(t; \boldsymbol{W}_i)]^{-1}$ instead of $I(C_i \geq t)$, where $\widehat{S}_D(t; \boldsymbol{W}_i)$ is the estimator of $S_D(t; \boldsymbol{W}_i)$ under a multiplicative hazards model.

15.9 Use an argument parallel to that for (15.21) to fill out the details in obtaining (15.61).

15.10 For marginal rate models (15.70), obtain conditions on $\boldsymbol{W}_i(t)$ to ensure that $\boldsymbol{U}_s(\boldsymbol{\beta})$ is an unbiased estimating function.

15.11 Use arguments analogous to those for (15.45) and (15.46) to prove (15.75) and (15.76).

A

Measure and Integration Theory Basics

A.1 Introduction

Integration theory is an important tool in statistics. In survival analysis, integration plays an even more prominent role as integrals of the form $\int f dG$ on an interval $[a, b]$ are frequently encountered. The Riemann-Stieltjes integral is defined using partitions of $[a, b]$, or $x-$axis, and is best understood and motivated when f is continuous and G differentiable. Although this is often adequate, there are some limitations such as difficulty in exchanging the order of integration and summation/differentiation, passing limit inside the integral, and possible non-existence when f, G have common discontinuity points.

This appendix first presents a brief summary of basic results from measure theory and Lebesgue-Stieltjes integration. Following this, Section A.5 discusses Riemann-Stieltjes integrals and related concepts.

Riemann-Stieltjes integrals are highly relevant in survival analysis, particularly for numerical approximations and intuitive derivations. However, it is often not well explored, partly overshadowed by the success of counting process and martingale theory, and the established Lebesgue-Stieltjes integration theory. Chapter Fifteen demonstrates the utility of Riemann-Stieltjes integration theory. Based on these considerations, Section A.5 contains a more in-depth discussion compared to Sections A.1 through A.4.

For a more comprehensive understanding of measure and Lebesgue-Stieltjes integration theory, readers are directed to standard texts on real analysis and probability theory [138, 9, 265, 268, 11]. For Riemann-Stieltjes and related integrals, more detailed results are available in Wheeden and Zygmund [322] and Rudin [268]. Riemann-Stieltjes integrals are used in establishing various properties of rigorously formulated marginal rate/mean models in Chapter Fifteen, and in certain intuitive derivations for martingales in Chapter Eleven.

Loosely speaking, Lebesgue integration more often works with partitioning of the range of f, or $y-$axis. Thus Riemann and Lebesgue integration are often referred to as the x-axis approach and y-axis approach, respectively.

DOI: 10.1201/9780429324437-A

A.2 Measures and Measurable Functions

Let X be a set. A collection $\mathscr{A}$ of subsets in X is a *σ−algebra*, or a *σ−field*, if:

1. The empty set $\emptyset \in \mathscr{A}$;
2. The complement $A^c = \mathsf{X} - A \in \mathscr{A}$ whenever $A \in \mathscr{A}$; and
3. $\bigcup A_i \in \mathscr{A}$ whenever $A_i \in \mathscr{A}$, $i = 1, 2, \cdots$.

Examples of X include the real line R, the closed interval $[a, b]$ for some $a < b$, and the Euclidean k-space R^k. The Borel algebra on R is the smallest σ-algebra that contains all open intervals $(a, b), a < b$. A set in the Borel algebra is called a Borel set.

A function μ from $\mathscr{A}$ to $[0, \infty]$ is a *measure* if

1. $\mu(A) \geq 0$ for any $A \in \mathscr{A}$;
2. $\mu(\emptyset) = 0$; and
3. for countably many A_i, $i = 1, 2, \cdots$, of pairwise disjoint sets in $\mathscr{A}$,

$$\mu\left(\bigcup A_i\right) = \sum_{i=1}^{n} \mu(A_i).$$

The triplet $(\mathsf{X}, \mathscr{A}, \mu)$ is called a measure space. A measure space is *complete*, or μ or $\mathscr{A}$ is *complete* for short, if every subset of a set of measure zero is in $\mathscr{A}$.

Although there are many Borel measures for the Borel algebra on R, the choice of Borel measure that assigns

$$\mu((a, b]) = b - a \quad \text{for every half-open interval} \quad (a, b], \tag{A.1}$$

is sometimes called "the" Borel measure.

The Lebesgue algebra on R is the smallest σ−algebra that contains all Borel sets, as well as any subset of a Borel set A with $\mu(A) = 0$ for μ in (A.1). The Lebesgue algebra is the completion of the Borel algebra, meaning

1. it is the smallest σ−algebra that contains all the Borel sets; and
2. it has a complete measure μ_L such that

$$\mu_L(A) = \mu(A) \text{ for } \mu \text{ in (A.1) and any Borel set } A.$$

A function $f : \mathsf{X} \mapsto \mathsf{R}$ is *measurable* if the pre-image $\{x : f(x) > c\} \in \mathscr{A}$ for any $c \in \mathsf{R}$. It can be shown that a function f is measurable if and only if the pre-image of any Borel set on R is in $\mathscr{A}$. A *simple function* $f : \mathsf{X} \mapsto \mathsf{R}$, defined as a function taking at most countably many distinct values $r_i, i = 1, \cdots$, is measurable if and only if $\{x : f(x) = r_i\} \in \mathscr{A}, i = 1, \cdots$. A function is measurable if and only if it is the limit of a uniformly convergent sequence of simple functions.

A property is said to hold *almost everywhere* (on a Borel set A) if it holds on a subset $B \subset A$ and $B^c \cap A$ has measure zero. Suppose f, g are measurable and f_n is a sequence of measurable functions. Below are some measurability properties:

1. cf is measurable for any real c;
2. $|f|$, $f+g$, fg, $\max\{f,g\}$, $\min\{f,g\}$ are measurable;
3. f/g is measurable if $g \neq 0$;
4. $\sup_n f_n(x)$, $\inf_n f_n(x)$, $\limsup_n f_n(x)$ and $\liminf_n f_n(x)$ are all measurable;
5. If $\lim_n f_n(x)$ exists for every x, then the limit is measurable;
6. If $h = f$ almost everywhere then h is measurable provided that μ is complete; and
7. If $\lim_n f_n(x)$ exists almost everywhere on $A \in \mathscr{A}$, then $\lim_n f_n(x)$ is measurable provided that μ is complete.

A.3 Lebesgue Integral

Construction of the Lebesgue integral starts with a measurable simple function f taking at most countably many distinct values $r_i, i = 1, \cdots$. Let A be a Borel set of X with finite measure. The Lebesgue integral of f over A is defined as

$$\int_A f(x)d\mu = \sum_i r_i \mu(A_i),$$

where $A_i = \{x : x \in A, f(x) = r_i\}, i = 1, \cdots$, provided that the series is absolutely convergent, in which case the simple function is said to be integrable. A measurable f is *integrable* over A if there exists a sequence of integrable simple functions f_n converging uniformly to f on A. The limit

$$\lim_n \int_A f_n(x)d\mu$$

is then called the Lebesgue integral of f over A, and is denoted by $\int_A f(x)d\mu$ or $\int_A f d\mu$.

Below are some important properties:

1. (*Linearity*) If f, g are integrable on A, then for real numbers a, b, $af+bg$ is integrable, and
$$\int_A (af(x)+bg(x))d\mu = a\int_A f(x)d\mu + b\int_A g(x)d\mu;$$
2. If f is integrable on A, $|f|$ is integrable;
3. (*Nonnegativity*) If f, is integrable on A, and $f \geq 0$ almost everywhere on A, then
$$\int_A f(x)d\mu \geq 0,$$
with equality if and only if $f=0$ almost everywhere on A;
4. (*Dominance*) If f is integrable on A, $|h(x)| \leq f(x)$ almost everywhere on A, then h is also integrable on A and
$$|\int_A h(x)d\mu| \leq \int_A |f(x)|d\mu;$$
5. ($\sigma-$*additivity*) If $A=\bigcup A_i$ for a countable union of pairwise disjoint measurable sets $A_i, i=1,\cdots$, and f is integrable on A, then f is integrable on each A_i and
$$\int_A f(x)d\mu = \sum_i \int_{A_i} f(x)d\mu,$$
where the series on the right is absolutely convergent.
6. If a sequence f_n of measurable functions converges uniformly on A to an integrable f, then
$$\lim_n \int_A f_n(x)d\mu = \int_A f(x)d\mu.$$
7. (*Dominated convergence theorem*) If a sequence f_n of integrable functions converges to f on A and $|f_n(x)| \leq \phi(x)$ where ϕ is integrable on A, then f is integrable on A and
$$\lim_n \int_A f_n(x)d\mu = \int_A f(x)d\mu.$$
The convergence of f_n can be relaxed to hold only almost everywhere. The statement remains the same if μ is complete. If μ is not complete, and a measurable function $\tilde{f}$ is such that $\tilde{f}(x) = \lim_n f_n(x)$ almost everywhere, then $\tilde{f}$ is integrable, and
$$\lim_n \int_A f_n(x)d\mu = \int_A \tilde{f}(x)d\mu.$$
8. (*Levi's Monotone convergence theorem*) Suppose $f_1(x) \leq f_2(x) \leq \cdots \leq f_n(x)$ on a set A, where the functions f_n are all integrable and $\int_A f_n(x)d\mu \leq M, n=1,\cdots$

for some $M < \infty$. Then the limit $f(x) = \lim_n f_n(x)$ exists almost everywhere on A, f is measurable and integrable, and

$$\lim_n \int_A f_n(x)d\mu = \int_A f(x)d\mu.$$

The monotonicity of f_n can be relaxed to hold only almost everywhere. The statement remains the same if μ is complete. If μ is not complete, the limit $f(x) = \lim_n f_n(x)$ still exists almost everywhere, and If a measurable function $\tilde{f}$ is such that $\tilde{f}(x) = \lim_n f_n(x)$ almost everywhere, then $\tilde{f}$ is integrable, and

$$\lim_n \int_A f_n(x)d\mu = \int_A \tilde{f}(x)d\mu.$$

9. (*Fatou's lemma*) Suppose a sequence f_n of nonnegative integrable functions on A converges almost everywhere to f and

$$\int_A f_n(x)d\mu \leq M, n = 1, \cdots,$$

for some $M < \infty$. If Then, f is measurable and integrable, and

$$\int_A f(x)d\mu \leq M.$$

The convergence of f_n can be relaxed to hold only almost everywhere if μ is complete. When the convergence of f_n holds only almost everywhere and μ is not complete, if a measurable function $\tilde{f}$ is such that $\tilde{f}(x) = \lim_n f_n(x)$ almost everywhere, then $\tilde{f}$ is integrable, and

$$\int_A \tilde{f}(x)d\mu \leq M.$$

10. (*Connection with the Riemann integral*) Suppose f is a bounded function on a compact interval $[a, b]$. Then

    (a) If the Riemann integral $\int_a^b f(x)dx$ exists, then f is Lebesgue integrable on $[a, b]$ and the two integrals are equal. Due to this and for brevity, the Lebesgue integral on $[a, b]$ will also be denoted by $\int_a^b f(x)dx$.

    (b) f is Riemann integrable if and only if it is continuous almost everywhere (in the sense of Lebesgue measure) in $[a, b]$.

The definitions and properties discussed above pertain to a set A of finite measure. However, in many practical applications, we encounter sets of infinite measure. A common example is when A is the real line equipped with the Borel measure. Assume that a set X can be represented as

$$X = \bigcup_n X_n,$$

where $\mu(X_n) < \infty$ and $X_1 \subset X_2 \subset \cdots$. A measurable function f on X is said to be integrable on X if it is integrable on any subset of X that has a finite measure, and the limit $\lim_n \int_{X_n} f(x)d\mu$ exists. The limit is denoted by $\int_X f(x)d\mu$ and is called the integral of f on X. It can be shown that the limit does not depend on the choice of the sequence X_n. For Lebesgue integrals on X, most of the commonly used properties listed above continue to hold, with the notable exception of the uniform convergence theorem in #6.

A.4 Lebesgue-Stieltjes Integral

A function $G: [a,b] \mapsto R$ has *bounded variation* if

$$\sup_{P \in \mathscr{P}} \sum_{i=0}^{n-1} |G(x_{i+1}) - G(x_i)| < \infty,$$

where $\mathscr{P}$ is the collection of all partitions P with $x_0 < x_1 < \cdots < x_n$ and $x_i \in [a,b], i = 0,1,\ldots,n$. The supremum is called the total variation of G on $[a,b]$ and is denoted by $\bigvee_a^b(G)$. We have

$$G = G_1 - G_2 \quad \text{where} \quad G_1(x) = \bigvee_a^x(G), \; G_2(x) = G_1(x) - G(x). \tag{A.2}$$

It can be shown that both G_1 and G_2 are increasing. That is, $G_j(s) \le G_j(t),\; j = 1,2$ for any $a \le s \le t \le b$.

The limit $\lim_{t \downarrow x} G(t)$, if it exists, is called the right limit of G at x and is denoted by $G_+(x)$. G is *right-continuous* at x if $G(x) = G_+(x)$. Similarly the left limit $G_-(x)$ and left continuity of G can be defined. If G is monotone on $[a,b]$, then $G_-(x)$ exists for all $x \in (a,b]$ and $G_+(x)$ exists for all $x \in [a,b)$. For brevity, a function G on $[a,b]$ is said to be right-continuous if it is right-continuous at every $x \in [a,b)$. Similarly, G has left limits if $G_-(x)$ exists for all $x \in (a,b]$.

G is said to be cadlag on $[a,b]$ if G is right-continuous and has left limits, and G is said to be caglad on $[a,b]$ if G is left-continuous and has left limits. This overview of the Lebesgue-Stieltjes Integral will focus on the case when the integration is with respect to a cadlag function. The case with a caglad function follows a parallel development and is therefore omitted for brevity.

The jump $\Delta G(x)$ at $x \in (a,b]$ of a cadlag function G is defined by

$$\Delta G(x) = G(x) - G_-(x).$$

If G is right-continuous with bounded variation, then both G_1, G_2 in the decomposition (A.2) are right-continuous and increasing.

A function $G : [a,b] \mapsto \mathrm{R}$ is *absolutely continuous* if, for any $\epsilon > 0$, there exists a $\delta > 0$ such that

$$\sum_{i=1}^{k} |G(b_i) - G(a_i)| < \epsilon$$

for every finite collection of pairwise disjoint sub-intervals

$$(a_i, b_i) \subset [a,b], \quad i = 1, \cdots, k$$

with total length $\sum_{i=1}^{k}(b_i - a_i) < \delta$. From the definitions, absolute continuity implies bounded variation. If G is absolutely continuous, then both G_1, G_2 in the decomposition (A.2) are absolutely continuous. An absolutely continuous G has derivative G' that exists almost everywhere, measurable and integrable on $[a,b]$ and

$$G(t) = G(a) + \int_a^t G'(x)dx. \tag{A.3}$$

A function of bounded variation on $[a,b]$ is *singular* if it is continuous and non-constant, and its derivative exists and equals zero almost everywhere. A singular function cannot be absolutely continuous, since by (A.3), an absolutely continuous function whose derivative is zero almost everywhere must be a constant function.

A right-continuous function G on $[a,b]$ with bounded variation can be written

$$G(x) = \Phi_1(x) + \Phi_2(x) + \Psi(x),$$

where Φ_1 is absolutely continuous, Φ_2 is singular, and Ψ is a right-continuous jump function. That is, Ψ can be written as

$$\Psi(x) = \sum_{a_i \le x} h_i,$$

where $\{a_1, \ldots\}$ is a set of countably many points in $[a,b]$, $\sum_i h_i$ is an absolutely convergent series. This follows from the Lebesgue decomposition. Note that $\Psi(x)$ can be written

$$\Psi(x) = \Psi(a) + \sum_{a<s\le x} \Delta G(s) = \Psi(a) + \sum_{a<a_i\le x} \Delta G(a_i),$$

where $\sum_i |\Delta G(a_i)| < \infty$ and summation over an empty set is 0. It is thus sometimes called the discrete part of $G(x)$. The continuous part of G, denoted by $G^c(x)$, is

$$\Phi_1(x) + \Phi_2(x) = G(x) - \Psi(s).$$

$\Phi_1(x)$ can be recovered from its derivative using (A.3) and $\Psi(x)$ can be determined by the jumps of $G(x)$. However, $\Phi_2(x)$ cannot be obtained from either the derivative or the jumps. Consequently, in statistics literature, CDFs and related distributional functions are often assumed to be a mixture of an absolutely continuous part and a discrete part, omitting the singularly continuous component.

For a right-continuous function G on $[0, b]$ with bounded variation, let G_1, G_2 be as in the decomposition (A.2) with $a = 0$. Let $\mathscr{F}$ be the collection of finite unions of sets of the form $\{0\}$ or $(c, d] \subset [0, b]$. A finitely additive set function μ_{01} can be defined on $\mathscr{F}$ by

$$\mu_{01}((c,d]) = G_1(d) - G_1(c), \quad (c,d] \subset [a,b], \quad \text{and} \quad \mu_{01}(\{0\}) = 0.$$

Let $\mathscr{B}([0, b])$ be the Borel algebra on $[0, b]$. It can be shown that $\mathscr{B}([0, b])$ is generated by $\mathscr{F}$. There is an extension theorem, due to Caratheodory, which states that a unique measure μ_1 exists on $\mathscr{B}([0, b])$ such that $\mu_1(A) = \mu_{01}(A)$ for all $A \in \mathscr{F}$. The measure μ_1 will be referred to as the measure generated by G_1. Similarly, a measure μ_2 on $\mathscr{B}([0, b])$ is generated by G_2.

For a $\mathscr{B}([0, b])$ measurable function h and $B \in \mathscr{B}([0, b])$, the Lebesgue-Stieltjes integral $\int_B h(x)dG(x)$ is defined by

$$\int_B h(x)dG(x) = \int_B h(x)d\mu_1 - \int_B h(x)d\mu_2, \tag{A.4}$$

provided both integrals on the right-hand side exist. The functions h, G are referred to as the integrand and integrator, respectively. For a simpler notation, sometimes the integral is denoted by

$$\int_B hdG.$$

If G can be written $G = G_1^* - G_2^*$ for a different pair of increasing right-continuous functions which generate measures μ_1^*, μ_2^*, respectively, it can be shown that

$$\int_B h(x)d\mu_1^* - \int_B h(x)d\mu_2^* = \int_B h(x)d\mu_1 - \int_B h(x)d\mu_2.$$

Therefore the integral $\int_B h(x)dG(x)$ is uniquely defined by (A.4).

A measure μ is a finite measure if it does not take the value ∞. A finite signed measure is defined similarly to a finite measure but with the non-negativity requirement removed. For μ_1, μ_2 in (A.4), $\mu_1 - \mu_2$ is a finite signed measure.

By the Caratheodory extension theorem, the finitely additive set function $\mu_{01} - \mu_{02}$ on $\mathscr{F}$ can also be uniquely extended to a finite signed measure on $\mathscr{B}([0,b])$. Thus $\mu_1 - \mu_2$ must be that extension. G uniquely determines $\mu_{01} - \mu_{02}$ and thus $\mu_1 - \mu_2$ as well. We will denote $\mu_1 - \mu_2$ by μ_G and refer to it as the signed measure generated by G. Uniqueness of μ_G ensures that $\int_s^t f(x)dG(x)$ in (A.4) depends only on G and not on how G is decomposed as the difference of two increasing functions.

For μ_G, there exist measurable disjoint sets A^+, A^- such that $A^+ \bigcup A^- = [0,b]$ and for any Borel measurable E, $E \cap A^+$, $E \cap A^-$ are Borel measurable and

$$\mu_G(E \cap A^+) \geq 0,\ \mu_G(E \cap A^-) \leq 0.$$

The decomposition is unique up to sets with μ_G measure zero. This is called the Hahn decomposition theorem.

Define a pair of finite measures λ_G, ν_G by

$$\lambda_G(E) = \mu_G(E \cap A^+),\ \nu_G(E) = -\mu_G(E \cap A^-).$$

Then $\mu_G = \lambda_G - \nu_G$. This is called the Jordan decomposition. Define a measure $|\mu_G| = \lambda_G + \nu_G$. This is called the total variation of μ_G. The relationship between the total variation of the function G and total variation of the signed measure μ_G is that if $G(0) = 0$, then the signed measure generated by the function $\bigvee_0^x(G)$ is $|\mu_G|$. This signed measure is a measure since $\bigvee_0^x(G)$ is increasing.

In applications, the set B in the Lebesgue-Stieltjes integral $\int_B h(x)dG(x)$ is usually an interval. The integral $\int_{(s,t]} h(x)d\mu$ will be denoted by $\int_s^t h(x)dG(x)$ for brevity, where $0 \leq s < t \leq b$. The half open interval $(s,t]$ is used to avoid ambiguity caused by possible discontinuity of G at s or t. Note that $\int_s^s h(x)dG(x)$ since $(s,s] = \emptyset$.

Below are some important properties of Lebesgue-Stieltjes integral:

1. (*Existence*) Suppose G is right-continuous with bounded variation on $[0,b]$. If h is either continuous or with bounded variation or bounded and Borel measurable on $[0,b]$, then $\int_0^b h(x)dG(x)$ exists and

$$\left|\int_0^b h(x)dG(x)\right| \leq \int_0^b |h(x)|d|\mu_G| < \infty. \tag{A.5}$$

2. (*Linearity*) Since Lebesgue-Stieltjes integral is a Lebesgue integral, it is linear in its integrand. Moreover, it is also linear in its integrator. If h is integrable with respect to both G and H, then

$$\int_0^b h(x)d\big(\alpha G(x) + \beta H(x)\big) = \alpha\int_0^b h(x)dG(x) + \beta\int_0^b h(x)dH(x) \tag{A.6}$$

for real α, β.

3. (*Absolutely continuous case*) If G is absolutely continuous and h bounded Borel measurable, both being functions on $[0,b]$, then the Lebesgue-Stieltjes integral exists and

$$\int_0^b h(x)dG(x) = \int_0^b h(x)G'(x)dx. \tag{A.7}$$

   This can be written more succinctly as

$$dG(x) = G'(x)dx.$$

4. (*Discrete case*) If G is a right-continuous step function of bounded variation that jumps at countably many points a_i, $i \geq 1$, and h is bounded and Borel measurable, then

$$\int_0^b h(x)dG(x) = \sum_{0<a_i\leq b} h(a_i)\Delta G(a_i). \tag{A.8}$$

   This can be written as

$$dG = \Delta G$$

5. (*Associativity*) If h is Borel measurable and $\int_0^b |h(x)|d|\mu_G| < \infty$. Then the function $H(t) = \int_0^t h(x)dG(x)$ is right-continuous with bounded variation on $[0,b]$, and

$$\int_0^b g(x)dH(x) = \int_0^b g(x)h(x)dG(x). \tag{A.9}$$

   This will be denoted by $dH = hdG$. Note that $H(0) = 0$ since $(0,0] = \emptyset$.

6. (*Integration by parts*) Let F, G be right-continuous functions with bounded variation on $[0,b]$. Then for $0 < t \leq b$,

$$F(t)G(t) = F(0)G(0) + \int_0^t F_-(t)dG(t) + \int_0^t G(t)dF(t), \tag{A.10}$$

   or

$$d(FG) = F_-G + GdF.$$

7. (*Change of variable*) Let G be a right-continuous function with bounded variation on $[0,b]$ and h continuously differentiable on a closed interval containing the range of G. Then $h(G)$ is right-continuous with bounded variation and

$$\begin{aligned} & h(G(t)) - h(G(0)) \\ = & \int_0^t h'(G(x))dG^c(x) + \sum_{0<s\leq t} \Delta h(G(s)), \end{aligned} \tag{A.11}$$

where $\Delta h(G(s)) = h(G(s)) - h(G_-(s))$ and $G^c(t)$ is the continuous part of G:

$$G^c(t) = G(t) - \sum_{0 \le s \le t} \Delta G(s)$$

Note that both sides are 0 at $t = 0$ as $(0, 0] = \emptyset$. This result can be written as

$$dh(G) = h'(G)dG^c + \Delta h(G).$$

8. If G is measurable, bounded and has left limits, and h is right-continuous with bounded variation, then $\int_0^b h(x)dG(x)$ can be defined using integration by parts formula:

$$\int_0^b h(x)dG(x) = h(b)G(b) - h(0)G(0) - \int_0^b G_-(x)dh(x). \tag{A.12}$$

In the above discussion, the Lebesgue-Stieltjes integral is defined on a bounded interval $[0, b]$. More generally, it can be defined on an interval $[a, b]$ or even on unbounded intervals such as $(0, \infty)$ or (∞, ∞), For unbounded intervals, the integrals are defined as limits:

$$\int_0^\infty h(x)dG(x) = \lim_{M\to\infty} \int_0^M h(x)dG(x)$$

and

$$\int_{-\infty}^\infty h(x)dG(x) = \lim_{M\to\infty, N\to-\infty} \int_N^M h(x)dG(x)$$

respectively, assuming that $G(x)$ is cadlag and of bounded variation on $(0, \infty)$ and (∞, ∞), respectively, and that the limits exist. Properties #1-#5 can be extended in an obvious manner for these integrals.

In probability and statistics, such integrals on an unbounded range are often encountered. For example, the expectation of a random variable X is defined as

$$EX = \int_{-\infty}^\infty x dF(x),$$

when the integral on the right-hand side exists, where $F(x)$ is the CDF of X. When $F(x)$ is absolutely continuous. its derivative $f(x)$ exists almost everywhere and the integral reduces to

$$\int_{-\infty}^\infty x f(x) dx.$$

When $F(x)$ is discrete with probability mass function

$$f(x_k) = P(X = x_k),\ k \ge 1,$$

for x_k's on the real line, the integral reduces to

$$\sum_k x_k f(x_k).$$

Under the random censorship model described in Section 2.4, let $\widehat{F}$ be the Kaplan-Meier estimator of the CDF F of the time-to-event variable. There is an important identity that links $\widehat{F} - F$ to a martingale integral which is stated in the following proposition. The result can be proved by decomposing the cumulative hazard function Λ corresponding to F as the sum of the continuous and discrete parts ([95, Lemma 3.2.1], [279, Theorem 7.2.1]). Here the proof uses properties of the Lebesgue-Stieltjes Integral. Let

$$\tau_F = \sup\{t : F(t) < 1\}, \quad L = \max_i X_i, \quad J(t) = I(K(t) > 0) = I(t \le L). \tag{A.13}$$

Proposition A.1. *Assume that data are from the random censorship model. Then, for any $t < \tau_F$,*

$$\frac{\widehat{F}(t) - F(t)}{1 - F(t)} = \int_0^t \frac{1 - \widehat{F}_-(x)}{1 - F(x)} d\big[\widehat{\Lambda}(x) - \Lambda(x)\big], \tag{A.14}$$

where $\widehat{\Lambda}$ is the Nelson-Aalen estimator of Λ in (2.44).

Proof. Let $\widehat{S}(t) = 1 - \widehat{F}(t)$ and $S(t) = 1 - F(t)$. From (2.20),

$$F(t) = \int_0^t S_-(x) d\Lambda(x). \quad \text{for } t < \tau_F,$$

and

$$\widehat{F}(t) = \int_0^t \widehat{S}_-(x) d\widehat{\Lambda}(x).$$

Thus when $t < \tau_F$, both equations hold. Succinctly, they can be written as

$$d\widehat{F} = \widehat{S}_- d\widehat{\Lambda}, \quad dF = S_- d\Lambda.$$

Let

$$A(t) = \widehat{F}(t) - F(t), \quad B(t) = \int_0^t \widehat{S}_-(x) d\big[\widehat{\Lambda}(x) - \Lambda(x)\big].$$

Then

$$\begin{aligned} dA &= \widehat{S}_- d\widehat{\Lambda} - S_- d\Lambda \\ &= \widehat{S}_- d\Lambda + \widehat{S}_- d(\widehat{\Lambda} - \Lambda) - S_- d\Lambda \\ &= -A_- d\Lambda + dB \\ &= -A_- \frac{dF}{S_-} + dB. \end{aligned}$$

On the other hand, from the integration by parts formula,

$$\begin{aligned} dA &= d[\frac{A}{S} S] \\ &= \frac{A_-}{S_-} dS + Sd[\frac{A}{S}]. \end{aligned}$$

It follows that $Sd[\frac{A}{S}] = dB$. or

$$\frac{A(t)}{S(t)} - \frac{A(0)}{S(0)} = \int_0^t \frac{dB(x)}{S(x)}.$$

This proves (A.14). □

A.5 Riemann-Stieltjes Integral and Darboux-Stieltjes Integral

The Lebesgue integral overcomes some difficulties associated with the Riemann integral studied in introductory calculus courses. However, the Riemann integral remains valuable for motivating various approximations, as it is defined as the limit of Riemann sums over an interval.

Similarly, although the Lebesgue-Stieltjes integral is used throughout most of this book and in most research articles, it is beneficial to introduce a Riemann-type Stieltjes integral. This Riemann-Stieltjes integral can help understand various properties of martingales in Chapter Eleven and the intensity models in Chapter Fifteen.

Despite its importance for providing insight and intuition, this topic is not explored as much as it should be in survival analysis. One reason might be its somewhat confusing nature, stemming from different definitions in the literature and the existence of pathological cases regardless of the definition used.

Let $I = [a, b]$ be a closed interval on the real line and P a partition of I with $a = x_0 < x_1 < \cdots < x_n = b$. Let G and h be functions on I, where G is increasing cadlag and f is bounded. For $k = 0, \ldots, n-1$, let

$$I_k = [x_k, x_{k+1}], \quad \Delta G_k = G(x_{k+1}) - G(x_k),$$

and

$$R_P = \sum_{k=0}^{n-1} h(\xi_k)\Delta G_k,$$

where $\xi_k \in I_k$, $0 \le k \le n-1$, are arbitrarily selected intermediate points. R_P is called a Riemann-Stieltjes sum.

Define the norm of the partition as $|P| = \sup_{0\le k\le n-1}(x_{k+1} - x_k)$. Suppose there is a real number A with the property that, for any $\epsilon > 0$, there exists a $\delta > 0$ such that,

$$\left|A - R_P\right| < \epsilon \tag{A.15}$$

whenever $|P| < \delta$, regardless of the selections of intermediate points $\xi_k \in I_k$, $0 \le k \le n-1$. That is,

$$\lim_{|P|\to 0} R_P$$

exists and is finite. Then h is said to be Riemann-Stieltjes integrable on I with respect to G, or Riemann-Stieltjes integrable for short if G and I are clear from the context. This property is denoted by

$$h \subset RS(G, I).$$

A is called the Riemann-Stieltjes integral of h on I with respect to G, and is denoted by

$$\int_a^b h\mathfrak{D}G \quad \text{or} \quad \int_a^b h(x)\mathfrak{D}G(x).$$

Note that the integral definition inherently includes a uniformity in the selections of ξ_k's. This turns out to be very important in applications such as formulations of marginal models for recurrent events in Chapter Fifteen.

The integrand G is required to be cadlag here. In real analysis books, the Stieltjes integral is often defined for an increasing function, which necessarily has right and left limits but may not be right-continuous. However, the cadlag requirement is not really a restriction in statistical applications, as it is often either guaranteed or needed due to other considerations in the analysis. Additionally, it avoids unnecessary complications due to ambiguity at discontinuity points of G.

As mentioned before, a confusing aspect of this topic is the existence of several definitions in the real analysis literature. often, these different integrals have the same name "Riemann-Stieltjes integral." One alternative definition is provided below. To differentiate from the definition in (A.15), we will refer to this alternately defined integral as Darboux-Stieltjes integral.

Let

$$m_k = \inf\{h(x) : x \in I_k\}, \quad M_k = \sup\{h(x) : x \in I_k\},$$

and define

$$l(h, G, P) = \sum_{k=0}^{n-1} m_k \Delta G_k, \quad u(h, G, P) = \sum_{k=0}^{n-1} M_k \Delta G_k.$$

Finally let

$$L(h, G, I) = \sup_P l(h, G, P), \quad U(h, G, I) = \inf_P u(h, G, P),$$

where the supremum and Infimum are taken over the collection $\mathscr{P}$ of all partitions P of I. It can be shown that $L(h, G, I)$ and $U(h, G, I)$ always exist due to the boundedness of h and G. The function h is *Darboux-Stieltjes integrable* on I with respect to G, or Darboux-Stieltjes integrable for short if G and I are clear from the context, if

$$L(h, G, I) = U(h, G, I). \tag{A.16}$$

This property is denoted by

$$h \in DS(G, I).$$

The common value is called the *Darboux-Stieltjes integral* of h on I with respect to G and is denoted by

$$\int_a^b h \mathbb{D} G \quad \text{or} \quad \int_a^b h(x) \mathbb{D} G(x).$$

When Stieltjes first introduced the integral, the definition in (A.15) was used. The Riemann and Stieltjes integrals are then defined as the limit of Riemann sums

$$\sum_{i=0}^{n-1} h(\xi_i)(x_{i+1} - x_i)$$

and Riemann-Stieltjes sums

$$\sum_{i=0}^{n-1} h(\xi_i)\left[G(x_{i+1}) - G(x_i)\right]$$

respectively, Darboux later showed that upper and lower sums could be used in defining the Riemann integral.

While using either Riemann sums or upper and lower sums will give the same result for the Riemann integral (i.e., $G(x) \equiv x$), for the Stieltjes integral, the two approaches generally result in different classes of integrable functions. Kolmogrov and Fomin [138], Royden and Fitzpatrick [265], and Wheeden and Zygmund [322] considered the Riemann-Stieltjes integral, and Rudin [268] considered the Darboux-Stieltjes integral. There are also definitions of the Stieltjes integral other than those in (A.15) and (A.16).

The real analysis literature often prefers the Darboux-Stieltjes integral definition because it exists more generally and offers a richer set of mathematical properties, making proofs and theoretical explorations more straightforward in some cases. However, the Darboux-Stieltjes integral definition loses the convenience of approximation by Riemann-Stieltjes sums. This limits its direct application in survival analysis. Riemann-Stieltjes sums are incredibly useful for numerical approximation and for intuitively understanding the integral's meaning in fields such as survival analysis, where discrete data points and cumulative changes are common. In contrast, the Darboux-Stieltjes integral involves suprema and infima, which are more cumbersome in applications.

Since the Lebesgue-Stieltjes integral is the most general and analytically powerful approach, and the main use of the Riemann-Stieltjes integral is to provide approximations and intuitive reasoning, we will focus on definition (A.15) using its link to (A.16).

In addition to the usual linearity properties for

$$\int_a^b [\alpha_1 h_1(x) + \alpha_2 h_2(x)]\mathfrak{D}G(x)$$

and

$$\int_a^b h(x)\mathfrak{D}[\beta_1 G_1(x) + \beta_2 G_2(x)]$$

which parallel those for the Lebesgue-Stieltjes integral, where $\beta_j > 0$, some important properties of the Riemann-Stieltjes integral are summarized below. More detailed discussions on the Riemann-Stieltjes integral and the Darboux-Stieltjes integral can be found in Wheeden and Zygmund [322] and Rudin [268], respectively.

1. Suppose that on I, h is bounded and G is increasing and cadlag. Then

   (a) h is Riemann-Stieltjes integrable if and only if for any $\varepsilon > 0$, there exists a $\delta > 0$ such that

   $$\left|R_P - R_{P^*}\right| < \varepsilon$$

   for any two partitions P and P^* of I satisfying $|R_P| < \delta$ and $|R_{P^*}| < \delta$, regardless of the selection of the intermediate points.

   (b) h is Darboux-Stieltjes integrable if and only if for any $\varepsilon > 0$, there exists a partition P of I such that

   $$U(h, G, I) - L(h, G, I) < \varepsilon.$$

   (c) Riemann-Stieltjes integrability of h implies Darboux-Stieltjes integrability, and

$$\int_a^b h\mathfrak{D}G = \int_a^b h\mathbb{D}G.$$

(d) If, in addition, G is continuous, then Darboux-Stieltjes integrability of h implies Riemann-Stieltjes integrability,

2. Suppose that on I, h is continuous and G is increasing and cadlag. Then h is Riemann-Stieltjes integrable and its Riemann-Stieltjes integral is the same as its Lebesgue-Stieltjes integral:

$$\int_a^b h\mathfrak{D}G = \int_a^b h dG.$$

3. If, on I, h is bounded and has at most finitely many discontinuity points, and G is increasing and cadlag, and is continuous at each of the discontinuity point of f, then h is Riemann-Stieltjes integrable and

$$\int_a^b h\mathfrak{D}G = \int_a^b h dG.$$

4. Suppose that on I, h is bounded and monotone, and G is increasing and continuous. Then h is Riemann-Stieltjes integrable.

5. Suppose that on I, h is bounded and G is increasing and cadlag. Let $c \in (a,b)$. If h is Riemann-Stieltjes integrable on $[a,b]$, then it is Riemann-Stieltjes integrable on both $[a,c]$ and $[c,b]$, and

$$\int_a^b h\mathfrak{D}G = \int_a^c h\mathfrak{D}G + \int_c^b h\mathfrak{D}G.$$

However, Riemann-Stieltjes integrability on $[a,c]$ and $[c,b]$ does not guarantee Riemann-Stieltjes integrability on $[a,b] = [a,c] \cup [c,b]$, as the example after the list of properties shows.

6. Suppose that on I, h is bounded and G is increasing and cadlag. If h is Riemann-Stieltjes integrable, then h and G have no common points of discontinuity.

7. (*Absolutely continuous case*) Suppose that on I, G is increasing and absolutely continuous, h is bounded and has at most countably many points of discontinuity. Then h is Riemann-Stieltjes integrable, and

$$\int_a^b h\mathfrak{D}G = \int_a^b h dG = \int_a^b h(x)G'(x)dx.$$

This can be written as

$$h(x)\mathfrak{D}G(x) = h(x)dG(x) = h(x)G'(x)dx.$$

8. (*Discrete case*) Suppose G is a right-continuous increasing jump function:

$$G(x) = \sum_{a_i \le x} h_i,$$

where $\{a_1, \ldots, \} \subset (a, b]$ and $\sum_i g_i$ is an absolutely convergent series with $g_i \ge 0, i \ge 1$. Suppose furthermore that h is bounded and has at most countably many points of discontinuity, and that h and G have no common points of discontinuity. Then h is Riemann-Stieltjes integrable, and

$$\int_a^b h(x)\mathfrak{D}G(x) = \sum_{a_i} h(a_i)\Delta G(a_i) = \int_a^b h(x)dG(x).$$

This can be written as

$$h(x)\mathfrak{D}G(x) = h(x)\Delta G(x) = h(x)dG(x).$$

9. If h is Riemann-Stieltjes integrable, then $|h|$ is Riemann-Stieltjes integrable and
$$\left|\int_a^b h(x)\mathfrak{D}G(x)\right| \le \int_a^b |h(x)|\mathfrak{D}G(x).$$

10. If h_1, h_2 are Riemann-Stieltjes integrable and $h_1 \le h_2$, then

$$\int_a^b h_1(x)\mathfrak{D}G(x) \le \int_a^b h_2(x)\mathfrak{D}G(x).$$

11. A constant c is Riemann-Stieltjes integrable on I with respect to any increasing cadlag G and
$$\int_a^b c\mathfrak{D}G(x) = c\left[G(b) - G(a)\right].$$

From properties #7 and #8, if G is an increasing cadlag function on I, and is either absolutely continuous or a jump function, then for a bounded integrand h that has at most countably many points of discontinuity and is continuous at each discontinuity point of G, the Riemann-Stieltjes integral exists and

$$\int_a^b h(x)\mathfrak{D}G(x) = \int_a^b h(x)dG(x). \tag{A.17}$$

By the linearity of the Riemann-Stieltjes and Lebesgue-Stieltjes integrals with respect to the integrator, and by the Lebesgue decomposition discussed in Section A.4, result (A.17) is valid when G is an increasing cadlag function with no singular component, while h satisfies the same conditions as before.

Define a function

$$H(x) = I(x \geq 1), \qquad x \in [0,2].$$

Using property #1(a), it can be shown that $H_-(x) = I(x > 1)$ is not Riemann-Stieltjes integrable with respect to H on $[0,2]$.

However, note that H_- is continuous on $[0,1]$ and H is continuous on $[1,2]$. Therefore, by properties #2 and #3, respectively, H_- is Riemann-Stieltjes integral integrable with respect to H on both $[0,1]$ and$[1,2]$, and

$$\int_0^1 H_-(x)\mathfrak{D}DH(x) = \int_0^1 H_-(x)dH(x) = 0,$$

$$\int_1^2 H_-(x)\mathfrak{D}DH(x) = \int_1^2 H_-(x)dH(x) = 0,$$

Moreover, using property #1(b), it can be verified that H_- is Darboux-Stieltjes integrable with respect to H on $[0,2]$, and

$$\int_0^2 H_-(x)\mathbb{D}H(x) = 0.$$

As a simple example of the non-existence of either the Riemann-Stieltjes integral or the Darboux-Stieltjes integral, note that H is not integrable with respect to H on $[0,2]$ under either definition (A.15) or (A.16). This simple example illustrates the complications and subtleties inherent in Riemann-Stieltjes and Darboux-Stieltjes integrals.

For applications to marginal models in Chapter Fifteen, the integrand and integrator typically satisfy the conditions for properties #7 and #8, so that (A.17) holds. On the other hand, for univariate survival analysis, the simple Nelson-Aalen estimator would not exist as a Riemann-Stieltjes integral, although the Darboux-Stieltjes integral does exist. The latter claim is based on the following property:

12. Suppose G is a right-continuous increasing jump function:

$$G(x) = \sum_{a_i \leq x} g_i,$$

where $\{a_1, \ldots,\} \subset (a,b]$ and $\sum_i g_i$ is an absolutely convergent series. Suppose furthermore that h is bounded and left continuous. Then h is Darboux-Stieltjes integrable, and

$$\int_a^b h(x)\mathbb{D}G(x) = \sum_{a_i} h(a_i)\Delta G(a_i) = \int_a^b h(x)dG(x).$$

This property can be proved adapting the arguments in the proofs of Theorems 6.15 and 6.16 in Rudin [268], relaxing the continuity requirement to left-continuity.

For martingales discussed in Chapter Eleven, result (11.9) there gives a hint at a property for the martingale integrals as suggested by the informal notation in (11.10). A rigorous statement and its proof are, it turns out, unnecessary at that point, since the martingale property can be verified directly, as shown in Sections11.2 and 11.4. For marginal models, rigorous statements and proofs can be established using Riemann-Stieltjes integral properties, as illustrated in Chapter Fifteen.

B

Counting Process and Martingale Theory Basics

B.1 Introduction

Counting process and martingale theory provides an elegant framework for analyzing survival data. While its theoretical appeal is noteworthy, for applications, perhaps a more practical significance is the straightforward variance and covariance formulas, for scenarios where alternative methods, such as the commonly used i.i.d. representations found in many statistics textbooks and journal articles, often require complex algebraic manipulations and result in cumbersome expressions. This simplification not only streamlines calculations, but also enhances the interpretability of results in survival analysis.

This appendix provides an overview of the counting process and martingale approach. This methodology was first introduced in Aalen's 1975 Berkeley Ph.D. thesis [1] and made its initial journal appearance in Aalen's subsequent publication [2]. Books offering a more comprehensive treatment include Gill [95], Fleming and Harrington [82], and Andersen et al. [7]. Among the three books, the first is among the earliest applications of this probabilistic theory to one- and two-sample problems with rigorous justification. The second gives a thorough treatment of survival analysis and counting processes. The third has the most comprehensive coverage of asymptotic analysis, Markov models, and multivariate counting processes, with many illustrative examples.

The overview starts with probability space and conditional expectation,, topics thoroughly explored in texts such as Billingsley [23]. For counting process and martingale theory, to streamline the presentation, the focus is on basic concepts and commonly used properties rather than exhaustive coverage or the most general results. For a more comprehensive treatment, readers can refer to the three books mentioned above, among others.

This appendix provides more than just an overview of basic results from counting process and martingale theory. It also includes several propositions and theorems on the convergence of various processes. While not all are new, nor are they always the most general or based on the weakest conditions, the emphasis here is on rigor at an accessible level. They are presented with elementary proofs and

DOI: 10.1201/9780429324437-B

under easily verifiable conditions that commonly hold in practice. Some gaps in the existing literature are also found and filled. Together, these convergence results demonstrate to students and beginning researchers how the theory can justify the asymptotics for the Kaplan-Meier estimator and weighted log-rank tests. Propositions B.1 and B.2 are also general enough for the readers to apply them in a wide range of other survival analysis contexts.

It is worth noting that although empirical process theory with convergence in abstract spaces, to be discussed in Appendix C, is in general a more powerful tool for asymptotic analysis, counting process and martingale theory offers a more intuitive and simpler approach for traditional topics in survival analysis, particularly for type II censoring and more complicated censoring patterns. Aalen [3] discussed several notable properties of the martingale approach and made a strong argument for its inclusion as an important part of the graduate-level curriculum.

B.2 Probability Space and Conditional Expectation

A *probability space* is a measure space triplet $(\Omega, \mathscr{F}, P)$ where Ω is the space of outcomes of a random experiment, $\mathscr{F}$ a σ-algebra on Ω, and P a measure such that $P(\Omega) = 1$. Since a probability space is a measure space, results for a general measure space presented in Appendix A apply here.

A *random variable* is a function $X: \Omega \mapsto \mathrm{R}$ that is measurable with respect to $\mathscr{F}$. That is, the pre-image of any Borel set on R is in $\mathscr{F}$. X is integrable if the integral of X, as a function of $\omega \in \Omega$, exists with respect to the measure P. This integral is called the *expectation* of X and is denoted by EX. For brevity, the argument ω of a random variable is usually suppressed. Two random variables X and Y are *equivalent* if $P(X \neq Y) = 0$.

Let F be the CDF of X. Suppose that the expectation of $g(X)$ exists, where g is a measurable function. Then

$$Eg(X) = \int_{-\infty}^{\infty} g(x) dF(x).$$

In probability theory, the phrase “almost everywhere" from measure theory has synonyms “almost all," “almost surely ($a.s.$)," and “with probability one." These phrases are used interchangeably. Two random variables X and Y are *equivalent* if $X = Y$ $a.s.$

In introductory statistics books, conditional expectation is usually defined separately for absolutely continuous and discrete cases. It represents the expected value of a random variable given additional information. This concept will now be defined more generally.

A *sub-σ-algebra* $\mathscr{G}$ of $\mathscr{F}$ is a σ-algebra such that $\mathscr{G} \subset \mathscr{F}$. For a random variable X and a sub-σ-algebra $\mathscr{G}$, let Y be a random variable such that

1. Y is $\mathscr{G}$-measurable; and

2. $\int_A Y dP = \int_A X dP$ for all $A \in \mathscr{G}$.

Then Y is called the *conditional expectation* of X given $\mathscr{G}$, and is denoted by $E(X|\mathscr{G})$. If Y and W both satisfy the conditions, they are called *versions* of the conditional expectation, and it can be shown that Y and W are equivalent.

If $E|X| < \infty$, then $E(X|\mathscr{G})$ exists. For an event $A \in \mathscr{F}$, the conditional probability $P(A|\mathscr{G})$ is defined as $E[I(A)|\mathscr{G}]$.

Since there are different versions of a conditional expectation and they are all equivalent, unless otherwise specified, statements regarding conditional expectations such as $E(X|\mathscr{G}) = E(Y|\mathscr{G})$ are understood to be true *a.s.*

As $\mathscr{G}$ increases, more information is provided. If $\mathscr{G} = \{\emptyset, \Omega\}$, the smallest σ-algebra, then $E(X|\mathscr{G}) = EX$, because this $\mathscr{G}$ does not contain any additional information. At the other extreme, $E(X|\mathscr{F}) = X$ with probability one. The random variable $E(X|\mathscr{G})$ at ω is interpreted as the expectation of X when it is known for each $G \in \mathscr{G}$ whether or not it contains ω.

For a collection $\mathscr{E}$ of sets or random variables or both in a measure space, the σ-algebra generated by $\mathscr{E}$ is denoted by $\sigma\{\mathscr{E}\}$ and it is given by $\bigcap \mathscr{G}$, where the intersection is taken over all σ-algebras with respect to which elements in $\mathscr{E}$ are measurable. The set of σ-algebras in the intersection is non-empty since it contains $\mathscr{F}$. Thus $\sigma\{\mathscr{E}\}$ exists for any $\mathscr{E}$.

Assume that X, Y, X_n have expectations (i.e., are integrable). The following are some frequently used properties.

1. If $X = a$ a.s. for a constant a, then $E(X|\mathscr{G}) = a$.

2. (*Discrete case*) If $\mathscr{G}$ is generated by a countable partition $A_1, \ldots$ of Ω, that is, events $A_i, i = 1, \ldots$, are pairwise disjoint and $\bigcup A_i = \Omega$, then

$$E(X|\mathscr{G})(\omega) = \frac{1}{P(A_i)} \int_{A_i} X dP, \quad \text{for } \omega \in A_i \text{ with } P(A_i) > 0.$$

   If $P(A_i) = 0$, then the value of $E(X|\mathscr{G})$ over A_i is defined arbitrarily.

   This result shows that the more general conditional expectation here coincides with the calculus level definition of conditional expectation for the discrete case.

3. (*Linearity*) For real numbers a, b, $E(aX + bY|\mathscr{G})$ exists and

$$E(aX + bY|\mathscr{G}) = aE(X|\mathscr{G}) + bE(Y|\mathscr{G}).$$

4. (*Dominance*) If $X \le Y$ *a.s.*, then

$$E(X|\mathscr{G}) \le E(Y|\mathscr{G}).$$

5. ($\sigma-$*additivity*) If $A = \bigcup A_i$ for a countable union of pairwise disjoint events $A_i, i = 1, \cdots$, then

$$E(I(A)X|\mathscr{G}) = \sum_i E(I(A_i)X|\mathscr{G}).$$

6. (*Dominated convergence theorem*) If, with probability one, $\lim_n X_n = X$ and $|X_n| \le Y$, then

$$\lim_n E(X_n|\mathscr{G}) = E(X|\mathscr{G}). \tag{B.1}$$

7. If $\mathscr{H}$ is generated by a countable partition $\{A_i \mid i \ge 1\}$ of Ω, and $\mathscr{H} \vee \mathscr{G}$ denotes the σ-algebra generated by $\mathscr{H} \cup \mathscr{G}$, then

$$P(B|\mathscr{H} \vee \mathscr{G}) = \sum_i I(A_i) \frac{P(B \cap A_i|\mathscr{G})}{P(A_i|\mathscr{G})},$$

   where, if $P(A_i|\mathscr{G}) = 0$, then the value of $P(B|\mathscr{H} \vee \mathscr{G})$ over A_i is defined arbitrarily.

8. (*Convergence under increasing σ-algebras*) If σ-algebras $\mathscr{G}_n$ are nested: $\mathscr{G}_1 \subset \mathscr{G}_2 \subset \cdots$, and $\mathscr{G}_\infty$ is the σ-algebra generated by $\bigcup \mathscr{G}_n$, then

$$\lim_n E(X|\mathscr{G}_n) = E(X|\mathscr{G}_\infty). \tag{B.2}$$

9. (*Product rule of conditional expectation*) If Y, XY are integrable and X is $\mathscr{G}$-measurable, then

$$E(XY|\mathscr{G}) = XE(Y|\mathscr{G}) \tag{B.3}$$

   That is, given $\mathscr{G}$, a $\mathscr{G}$-measurable variable is determined, or effectively a constant.

10. If $\mathscr{G}_1 \subset \mathscr{G}_2$, then

$$E\big[\big(E(X|\mathscr{G}_2)\big)|\mathscr{G}_1\big] = E(X|\mathscr{G}_1) \tag{B.4}$$

   In particular, with $\mathscr{G}_1 = \{\emptyset, \Omega\}$,

$$E\big[E(X|\mathscr{G})\big] = EX, \tag{B.5}$$

   for any σ-algebra $\mathscr{G} \subset \mathscr{F}$.

   When $\mathscr{G}$ is generated by a random vector $\mathbf{V}$, meaning it is a σ-algebra and is contained in any σ-algebra with respect to which $\mathbf{V}$ is measurable, the conditional expectation is often written as $E(X|\mathbf{V})$ and (B.5) becomes

$$E\left[E(X|\mathbf{V})\right] = EX. \tag{B.6}$$

Formula (B.6) is sometimes called the *law of iterated expectations* when **V** is a random variable. For brevity, (B.4) and (B.5) will also be referred to by the same name.

11. If X and Y are independent and $E|A(X,Y)| < \infty$, then

$$E\left[A(X,Y)|X\right] = \phi(X), \tag{B.7}$$

where

$$\phi(x) = EA(x,Y).$$

From (B.6) and (B.7), it follows that

$$EA(X,Y) = E\phi(X).$$

12. If a random vector $\boldsymbol{W}$ is independent of (X,Y), and $E|A(X)| < \infty$, then

$$E\left[A(X)|Y,\boldsymbol{W}\right] = E\left[A(X)|Y\right].$$

13. If X and Y are independent given $\boldsymbol{W}$, and $E|A(X)| < \infty$, then

$$E\left[A(X)|Y,\boldsymbol{W}\right] = E\left[A(X)|\boldsymbol{W}\right].$$

Properties #1–#6 above show that conditional expectations behave very much like the usual expectations. Property #7 is perhaps the most routinely used in survival analysis, in justifying the formula for conditional hazard function given covariates. Property #8 justifies the intuitive approach of discretizing a random variable when $\mathcal{G}_\infty = \sigma(Y)$ and the $\mathcal{G}_n$'s are a nested sequence of σ-algebras generated by discretized versions of Y, using a sequence of nested partitions of the interval over which Y is defined.

There is no need to memorize the iteration order on the left-hand side of (B.4), since the other way is trivially true:

$$E\left[\left(E(X|\mathcal{G}_1)\right)|\mathcal{G}_2\right] = E(X|\mathcal{G}_1).$$

With either iteration order, the right-hand side (the simper expression) always involves the smaller σ-algebra.

B.3 Stochastic Processes

A *stochastic process* is a family of random variables $\mathscr{X} = \{X(t) : t \in \mathsf{A}\}$ indexed by a set A, where all variables are defined on a common probability space $(\Omega, \mathscr{F}, P)$. Often, the stochastic process is referred to as "the process $X(t)$." Since for each t, $X(t)$ is a random variable or a mapping $\Omega \mapsto \mathsf{R}$, the stochastic process is actually a mapping $X(t,\omega)$ from $\mathsf{A} \times \Omega$ to R, although the dependence on ω is often suppressed.

The counting process and martingale theory applies generally to an index set A that is a finite or infinite interval on the real line. However, for simpler presentation, in the rest of this appendix, the set A is taken to be a sub-interval of $[0, \infty)$ containing 0.

The process $X(t)$ is *measurable* if the mapping $X(\cdot,\cdot) : \mathsf{A} \times \Omega \mapsto \mathsf{R}$ is measurable, where A is equipped with the Borel σ-algebra. For $\omega \in \Omega$, the function $X(\cdot, \omega) : \mathsf{A} \mapsto \mathsf{R}$ is called a *sample path* of the process $X(t)$. A process is measurable if all of its sample paths are right-continuous or if all of its sample paths are left-continuous. It follows that a process is also measurable if it is obtained through finitely many steps of addition and multiplication from processes whose sample paths are either all right-continuous or all left-continuous. For a measurable process, its sample paths are measurable functions from A to R.

The left limit version $\{X_-(t)\}$ of $X(t)$ is a process which at $\omega \in \Omega$ takes the value $X_-(t)$ for all t, for almost all $\omega \in \Omega$. In subsequent development, unless explicitly stated otherwise, a process is said to have certain property, such as being right-continuous with left limit, or cadlag, if that property holds for ω in a probability one set in Ω. A process $\mathscr{X}$ is a modification of $\mathscr{Y} = \{Y(t) : t \in \mathsf{A}\}$ if $X(t)$ and $Y(t)$ are equivalent for any $t \in \mathsf{A}$.

If, from two processes $X(t)$ and $Y(t)$, the Lebesgue-Stieltjes integral

$$X^*(t) = \int_0^t X dY$$

can be defined for almost all sample paths, then this defines a new process $X^*(t)$, which in general may not be measurable even if $X(t)$ and $Y(t)$ are. However, suppose that for any $t > 0$, the sample paths of $Y(t)$ are right-continuous with bounded variation on $[0, t]$, and the sample paths of $X(t)$ are, on $[0, t]$, either

1. continuous; or
2. of bounded variation; or
3. bounded and Borel measurable.

Then, from the discussions in Section A.4 of Appendix A, the sample paths of $X^*(t)$ are right-continuous. Therefore, $X^*(t)$ is measurable.

A process $X(t)$ is

1. *Integrable* if $\sup_{t \in \mathsf{A}} E|X(t)| < \infty$;
2. *Square integrable* if $\sup_{t \in \mathsf{A}} E[X(t)]^2 < \infty$;
3. *Bounded* if there exists a finite constant $B > 0$ such that

$$P\big(\sup_{t \in \mathsf{A}} E|X(t)| < B\big) = 1.$$

Let $\{\mathscr{F}_t \subset \mathscr{F} : t \in \mathsf{A}\}$ be a family of sub-σ-algebras.

1. $\{\mathscr{F}_t\}$ is *increasing* if $\mathscr{F}_s \subset \mathscr{F}_t$ when $s \le t$. An increasing $\{\mathscr{F}_t\}$ is called a *filtration.*
2. $\{\mathscr{F}_t\}$ is *right-continuous* if $\mathscr{F}_t = \mathscr{F}_{t+}$ where the σ-algebra $\mathscr{F}_{t+} = \bigcap_{h>0} \mathscr{F}_{t+h}$.

A companion to $\mathscr{F}_{t+}$ is $\mathscr{F}_{t-}$ which is the smallest σ-algebra containing all sets in $\bigcup_{h>0} \mathscr{F}_{t-h}$. If $\{\mathscr{F}_t\}$ is a filtration, then

$$\mathscr{F}_{t-} = \sigma\Big\{\bigcup_n \mathscr{F}_{t_n}\Big\}, \tag{B.8}$$

where t_n is any sequence in A such that $t_n < t$ and , $t_n \uparrow t$. A *stochastic basis* is a probability space $(\Omega, \mathscr{F}, P)$ equipped with a right-continuous filtration $\{\mathscr{F}_t : t \in \mathsf{A}\}$. A stochastic basis is *complete* if $\mathscr{F}$ is complete and $\mathscr{F}_0$ contains all P-null sets of $\mathscr{F}$.

A stochastic process $X(t)$ is *adapted* to a filtration $\mathscr{F}_t$ if $X(t)$ is $\mathscr{F}_t$ measurable for each t.

If $X(t)$ and $Y(t)$ are both adapted to a right-continuous filtration $\mathscr{F}_t$, the paths of $X(t)$ are either right- or left- continuous, and the paths of $Y(t)$ are right-continuous and of bounded variation on finite intervals, then $\int_0^t X(s)dY(s)$ as a process indexed by t is adapted to $\mathscr{F}_t$.

A *counting process* $\{N(t) : t \ge 0\}$ is a stochastic process adapted to a filtration $\{\mathscr{F}_t : t \ge 0\}$ with $N(0) = 0$, $P(N(t) < \infty) = 1$ for each t, and with paths being, with probability one, right-continuous step functions with jump size 1.

For a probability space $(\Omega, \mathscr{F}, P)$ with a filtration $\{\mathscr{F}_t : t \in \mathsf{A}\}$, the σ-algebra on $\mathsf{A} \times \Omega$ generated by sets

$$[0] \times A, \quad A \in \mathscr{F}_0,$$

and

$$(a, b] \times A, \quad \text{for } a < b,\ a, b \in \mathsf{A},\ A \in \mathscr{F}_a,$$

is called the *predictable σ-algebra* generated by the filtration $\mathscr{F}_t$.

A process $\mathscr{X}$ is *predictable* with respect to a filtration $\mathscr{F}_t$ if the mapping $X(t, \omega) : \mathsf{A} \times \Omega \mapsto \mathsf{R}$ is measurable with respect to the predictable σ-algebra generated by that filtration. For brevity $\mathscr{X}$ is called an $\mathscr{F}_t$-predictable process.

If a process is adapted to a filtration $\mathscr{F}_t$ and left continuous, then it is $\mathscr{F}_t$-predictable. A deterministic measurable function is predictable with respect to any filtration.

If a process $X(t)$ is $\mathscr{F}_t$-predictable, then $X(t)$ is $\mathscr{F}_{t-}$-measurable for any $t > 0$.

B.4 Martingales

Let $\mathscr{X} = \{X(t) : t \in \mathrm{A}\}$ be a cadlag stochastic process adapted to a filtration $\{\mathscr{F}_t : t \in \mathrm{A}\}$. $\mathscr{X}$ is called a *martingale* with respect to $\mathscr{F}_t$ or, for brevity, $\mathscr{X}$ is an $\mathscr{F}_t$-martingale, if

1. $E|X(t)| < \infty$ for any $t \in \mathrm{A}$;

2. $$E[X(t+s)|\mathscr{F}_t] = X(t) \quad a.s. \quad \text{for all} \quad s,t \geq 0. \tag{B.9}$$

$\mathscr{X}$ is a *submartingale* if (B.9) is replaced by

$$E[X(t+s)|\mathscr{F}_t] \geq X(t) \quad a.s. \quad \text{for all} \quad s,t \geq 0,$$

and a *supermartingale* if (B.9) is replaced by

$$E[X(t+s)|\mathscr{F}_t] \leq X(t) \quad a.s. \quad \text{for all} \quad s,t \geq 0.$$

In probability books, the martingale definition does not always have the cadlag requirement. But it is often needed in other parts of statistical analysis and the processes being studied nearly always have this property. Thus it is included to simplify the presentation.

For a martingale $X(t)$, by the law of iterated expectations, $EX(t) = EX(s)$ for any $0 \leq s \leq t$. Thus martingale has constant expectation over time. Often that constant is 0.

For $t > 0$ and integers $n \geq 1$,

$$E[X(t)|\mathscr{F}_{t-t/2^n}] = X(t - t/2^n), \quad a.s.$$

Thus, by (B.9), (B.2) and the cadlag property of a martingale,

$$\begin{aligned} E[X(t)|\mathscr{F}_{t-}] &= \lim_n E[X(t)|\mathscr{F}_{t-t/2^n}] \\ &= \lim_n X(t - t/2^n) \\ &= X_-(t), \quad a.s. \end{aligned} \tag{B.10}$$

Suppose T, C are time to event and time to censoring, respectively. Define

$$X = T \wedge C, \delta = I(T \leq C)$$

and

$$\begin{aligned} N(t) &= I(X \leq t, \delta = 1), \\ N_C(t) &= I(X \leq t, \delta = 0), \\ \mathscr{F}_t &= \sigma\{N(s), N_C(s) : 0 \leq s \leq t\}. \end{aligned}$$

Let

$$M(t) = N(t) - \int_0^t I(X \geq s) d\Lambda(s), \tag{B.11}$$

where Λ is the cumulative hazard function of T. As shown in Section 11.2, $M(t)$ is an $\mathscr{F}_t$-martingale if and only if

$$\frac{-dP(T > t, T \leq C)}{P(T \geq t, C \geq t)} = d\Lambda(t), \tag{B.12}$$

for t such that $P(\min(T, C) \geq t) > 0$. Note that there is no assumption on the relationship between T and C. When T and C are independent, then (B.12) is satisfied.

The right-continuous process

$$A(t) = \int_0^t I(X \geq s) d\Lambda(s)$$

is $\mathscr{F}_t$-predictable. Intuitively, this is because $A(t)$ is obtained as a limit of left continuous processes. Loosely speaking, in survival analysis context, predictability means that the value of the process at t is determined given information up to but not including t.

From (B.11), subtraction of the predictable process $A(t)$ from the counting process $N(t)$ yields a martingale under (B.12). It turns out that martingales can be obtained more generally. A collection $\{X_t : t \in \Gamma\}$ of random variables is said to be *uniformly integrable* if

$$\lim_{n \to \infty} \sup_{t \in \Gamma} E\left[|X_t| I(|X_t| > n)\right] = 0.$$

It can be shown that $\{X_t : t \in \Gamma\}$ is uniformly integrable if and only if

1. $\sup_{t \in \Gamma} E|X_t| < \infty$;
2. For any $\varepsilon > 0$, there exists a $\delta > 0$ such that for any B with $P(B) < \delta$,

$$\sup_{t \in \Gamma} \int_B |X_t| dP < \varepsilon.$$

A nonnegative random variable ξ a *stopping time* with respect to a filtration $\{\mathscr{F}_t : t \in \mathsf{A}\}$. if

$$\{\xi \leq t\} \in \mathscr{F}_t \quad \text{for all} \quad t \in \mathsf{A}.$$

Let $\mathscr{X} = \{X(t) : t \in \mathsf{A}\}$ be a nonnegative submartingale adapted to a stochastic basis $\{\mathscr{F}_t : t \in \mathsf{A}\}$. Then there exists a unique increasing right-continuous predictable process $A(t)$ with $A(0) = 0$ and $EA(t) < \infty$ such that

$$M(t) = X(t) - A(t) \tag{B.13}$$

is a martingale. A is called the *compensator* for the submartingale X. Uniqueness of $A(t)$ is in the sense that if there is another decomposition, then the compensator and martingale from that decomposition are modifications of $A(t)$, $M(t)$ in (B.13), respectively. Moreover, if X is bounded, then M is uniformly integrable and A is integrable.

The decomposition result above is called the Doob-Meyer decomposition [65, 205, 206]. The version stated here is from Theorem 1.4.1 of Fleming and Harrington [82], for nonnegative submartingales. More general results are also available [188].

For any nonnegative increasing process $Q(t)$ adapted to a filtration $\{\mathscr{F}_t : t \geq 0\}$ with $EQ(t) < \infty$, since $Q(t+s) - Q(t) \geq 0$ for $s, t \geq 0$, it follows that $E[Q(t+s) - Q(t)|\mathscr{F}_t] \geq 0$, therefore $Q(t)$ is a submartingale. In particular, if $N(t)$ is a counting process adapted to a stochastic basis $\{\mathscr{F}_t : t \geq 0\}$ with $EN(t) < \infty$ for any t, then there exists a unique cadlag increasing $\mathscr{F}_t$-predictable process A such that $A(0) = 0$, $EA(t) < \infty$ and $M(t) = N(t) - A(t)$ is a $\mathscr{F}_t$-martingale.

Often, statistics can be written in the form $\sum_{i=1}^n \int_0^t H_i dM_i$, where for $1 \leq i \leq n$, $M_i = N_i - A_i$ is a martingales with respect to a right-continuous filtration $\mathscr{F}_t$, N_i is a counting process, and H_i is $\mathscr{F}_t$-predictable. In Section B.11 later, the counting process and martingale theory will be used for asymptotic analysis of various estimators or statistics.

B.5 Variation and Covariation Processes of Martingales

Since a martingale $M(t)$ has constant expectation over time, $EM(t) = 0$ for any t if $M(0) = 0$. It follows that in the Doob-Meyer decomposition of an $\mathscr{F}_t$- submartingale $N(t)$ with $N(0) = 0$, $EN(t) = EA(t)$. If M is a martingale with $EM^2(t) < \infty$, $t \geq 0$, then by Jensen's inequality, M^2 is a submartingale. Thus by the Doob-Meyer decomposition, M^2 has a compensator, denoted by $\langle M, M\rangle$, such that $\langle M, M\rangle(0) = 0$, $E\langle M, M\rangle(t) < \infty$, and $M^2(t) - \langle M, M\rangle(t)$ is a martingale. The compensator is called the *predictable quadratic variation process* of M or *predictable variation process* of M.

Similarly, if M_1 and M_2 are two martingales with respect to a right-continuous filtration $\{\mathscr{F}_t : t \geq 0\}$ with $EM_i^2(t) < \infty$, $t \geq 0, i = 1,2$, then by considering the martingale $M_1 + M_2$ and its predictable variation process, it can be shown that there exists a unique right-continuous predictable process $\langle M_1, M_2\rangle$ with $\langle M_1, M_2\rangle(0) = 0$ and $E\langle M_1, M_2\rangle(t) < \infty$, such that

1. $\langle M_1, M_2\rangle$ is the difference of two cadlag increasing predictable processes, and

2. $M_1M_2 - \langle M_1, M_2\rangle$ is a martingale.

$\langle M_1, M_2\rangle$ is called the *predictable covariation process* of M_1 and M_2.

From the above, M_1M_2 is a martingale if and only if $\langle M_1, M_2\rangle \equiv 0$, in which case M_1 and M_2 are said to be *orthogonal.* One practical importance of orthogonal martingales is that they are uncorrelated if $M_1(0)$ and $M_2(0)$ are.

B.6 Local Martingales

The theory related to martingales can be extended to processes that satisfy similar, but weaker conditions than those required for martingales. In particular, note that for the martingale generated from a counting process and the related square integrable martingale, two of the conditions required are $EN(t) < \infty$ and $EM^2(t) < \infty$, for any $t \geq 0$. These two conditions will be dropped in this section.

An increasing sequence of random variables $\xi_n, n = 1, \ldots,$ is a *localizing sequence* with respect to a filtration $\mathscr{F}_t$ if each ξ_n is an $\mathscr{F}_t$-stopping time and $\lim_n \xi_n = \infty$, *a.s.* A property for a process $X(t)$ is said to hold *locally* if there is a localizing sequence ξ_n such that for each n, the property holds for the process $\{X(t \wedge \xi_n) : t \in \mathsf{A}\}$. For example, an $\mathscr{F}_t$-process $X(t)$ is *locally bounded* if, for each n, the process $X(t \wedge \xi_n)$ is a bounded process in t. A cadlag $\mathscr{F}_t$-process $X(t)$ is locally bounded.

A cadlag process $M(t)$ is an $\mathscr{F}_t$-*local martingale* if there exists a localizing sequence ξ_n such that for each n, $M_n = \{M(t \wedge \xi_n) : t \in \mathsf{A}\}$ is an $\mathscr{F}_t$-martingale. If M_n is a martingale and also square integrable for each n, then M_n is a *square integrable martingale* and M a *local square integrable martingale.* Local submartingales and local supermartingales are defined analogously.

A martingale is a local martingale. Conversely, an $\mathscr{F}_t$-local martingale is a martingale if, for the localizing sequence ξ_n and any fixed t, $\{M(t \wedge \xi_n) : n \geq 1\}$ is uniformly integrable.

Let $\{X(t) : t \in \mathsf{A}\}$ be a nonnegative right-continuous $\mathscr{F}_t$-local submartingale with localizing sequence $\{\xi_n\}$, where $\mathscr{F}_t$ is a right-continuous filtration. Then there exists a unique increasing right-continuous predictable process $A(t)$ with $A(0) = 0$,

$P(A(t) < \infty) = 1$ for all $t \in \mathsf{A}$, such that

$$X(t) = M(t) + A(t), \tag{B.14}$$

where $M(t)$ is a right-continuous local martingale. $A(t)$ is called the compensator of $X(t)$. Also, $A(t) = \lim_n A_n(t)$, $a.s.$ for each t, with $A_n(t)$ the compensator for the stopped submartingale $\{X(t \wedge \tau_n) : t \in \mathsf{A}\}$. This is the extended Doob-Meyer decomposition [82, Theorem 2.2.3.]. Various versions of the Doob-Meyer decomposition are given in Liptser and Shiryayev [188].

Let N be a counting process. It can be shown that N is a local submartingale. Thus the extended Doob-Meyer decomposition applies. Moreover, the compensator A is a locally bounded process, $\Delta A(t) \leq 1, a.s.$ for each t, and $M = N - A$ is a local square integrable martingale. In addition, $EN(t) = EA(t)$ for each t. If $EA(t) < \infty$ for all t, then $M = N - A$ is a martingale.

If M is a right-continuous $\{\mathscr{F}_t : t \in \mathsf{A}\}$-local square integrable martingale with localizing sequence $\{\xi_n\}$, where $\{\mathscr{F}_t : t \in \mathsf{A}\}$ is a right-continuous filtration, then there exists a unique right-continuous increasing predictable process $\langle M, M\rangle$ with $\langle M, M\rangle(0) = 0$ and $\langle M, M\rangle(t) < \infty, a.s.$ for each t, such that

1. $\{M^2(t) - \langle M, M\rangle(t) : t \in \mathsf{A}\}$ is a local martingale;
2. $\langle M, M\rangle(t) = \lim_n \langle M(\cdot \wedge \xi_n), M(\cdot \wedge \tau_n)\rangle(t)$;
3. $EM^2(t) \leq E\langle M, M\rangle(t)$;
4. $EM^2(t) = E\langle M, M\rangle(t)$ if M is a martingale.

Similarly, if $M_1$and M_2 are two $\mathscr{F}_t$-local square integrable martingales with a right-continuous filtration $\mathscr{F}_t$. then there exists a unique cadlag predictable process $\langle M_1, M_2\rangle$ with $\langle M_1, M_2\rangle(0) = 0$, $\langle M_1, M_2\rangle(t) < \infty$ $a.s.$ for each t, such that $M_1 M_2 - \langle M_1, M_2\rangle$ is an $\mathscr{F}_t$-local martingale. $\langle M_1, M_2\rangle$ is given by

$$\langle M_1, M_2\rangle = \left[\langle M_1 + M_2, M_1 + M_2\rangle - \langle M_1, M_1\rangle - \langle M_2, M_2\rangle\right]/2.$$

B.7 Martingale Integrals

For a counting process N and a stochastic basis $\{\mathscr{F}_t\}$, let $M = N - A$ be the $\mathscr{F}_t$-local square integrable martingale from the extended Doob-Meyer decomposition. Let H be a locally bounded $\mathscr{F}_t$- predictable process. Then $\int_0^t H(s)dM(s)$ is a local square integrable martingale.

Suppose there are counting processes N_i, $\mathscr{F}_t$-local square integrable martingales M_i and locally bounded $\mathscr{F}_t$- predictable processes $H_{i,j}$ as described above,

$1 \le i \le n, \ell = 1,2$. Let

$$X_\ell(t) = \sum_{i=1}^{n} \int_0^t H_{i,\ell}(s) dM_i(s), \ 1 \le i \le n, \ \ell = 1,2.$$

Then

1. X_1, X_2 are local square integrable martingales and

$$\langle X_\ell, X_m \rangle(t) = \sum_{i=1}^{n} \sum_{j=1}^{n} \int_0^t H_{i\ell} H_{jm} d\langle M_i, M_j \rangle, \ \ell, m = 1,2.$$

2. If, in addition,

$$E \int_0^t H_{i,\ell}^2 d\langle M_i, M_i \rangle < \infty$$

for each t and $1 \le i \le n$, $\ell = 1,2$, then

   (a) X_ℓ is a martingale over $[0, t]$, and $EX_\ell(t) = 0$, $\ell = 1,2$.

   (b) $EX_\ell(t)X_m(u) = E\sum_{i=1}^{n}\sum_{j=1}^{n}\int_0^t H_{i\ell}H_{jm} d\langle M_i, M_j \rangle$, for any $0 \le t \le u < \infty$.

Note that the variance formula is obtained by setting $t = u$ and $\ell = m$ in property (2b) above.

These results show that for sums of martingale integrals, calculation of the variance and covariance boils down to integrals with respect to the processes $\langle M_i, M_j \rangle(t)$, $i, j = 1, \ldots, n$. The next section focuses on determination of those processes.

B.8 Continuous and Discontinuous Compensators

A p-variate process $\{N_1, \ldots, N_p\}$ is called a *multivariate counting process* if each N_j is a counting process, $1 \le j \le p$ and no two component processes jump at the same time. For such a process, if the compensator A_j for N_j is continuous, $1 \le j \le p$, then

1. $\langle M_j, M_j \rangle = A_j$. That is, A_j is the unique cadlag increasing predictable process with $A_j(0) = 0$, $A_j(t) < \infty$, *a.s.* for each t, and $M_j^2 - A_j$ is a local martingale, $1 \le j \le p$.

2. $\langle M_i, M_j \rangle = 0$ if $i \neq j$. That is, $M_i M_j$ is a local martingale.

3. $EM^2(t) \le EA(t)$ for each t.

4. If in addition, $EA(t) < \infty$, or equivalently $EN(t) < \infty$ for each t, then $M^2 - A$ is a martingale, thus $EM^2(t) = EA(t)$.

Let $\mathscr{F}_t$ be a right-continuous filtration and N_i's be $\mathscr{F}_t$-adapted counting processes with $\mathscr{F}_t$-predictable compensator A_i's, and $M_i = N_i - A_i, 1 \le i \le n$. Then

1. $\int_0^t \Delta M_i dM_i - \int_0^t (1 - \Delta A_i) dA_i$ is an $\mathscr{F}_t$-local martingale.
2. $\langle M_i, M_i \rangle(t) = \int_0^t (1 - \Delta A_i) dA_i$. That is, $M_i^2 - \int_0^t (1 - \Delta A_i) dA_i$ is a local martingale.
3. If $\{N_1, \ldots, N_n\}$ is a multivariate counting process, then

$$\langle M_i, M_j \rangle(t) = -\int_0^t \Delta A_i dA_j, \quad i \ne j.$$

4. Suppose $EN_i(t) < \infty$, $t \ge 0, 1 \le i \le n$. Then the local martingales in (1), (2) and (3) above are martingales.

When $\{N_1, \ldots, N_n\}$ is not a multivariate counting process, a technical assumption as stated below is needed for obtaining $\langle M_i, M_j \rangle$.

The conditional independence condition: For each $t \ge 0$, given $\mathscr{F}_{t-}$,

$$\Delta N_i(t),\ \Delta N_j(t) \text{ are uncorrelated}, \qquad i \ne j, 1 \le i,\ j \le n. \tag{B.15}$$

Since $\Delta N_i(t)$, $\Delta N_j(t)$ are binary, (B.15) is equivalent to them being independent. Also, the condition only gives pair-wise independence among the $\Delta N_i(t)$'s. Under this condition, some algebra gives

$$E[N_i(t) N_j(t) | \mathscr{F}_{t-}] = E[N_i(t) | \mathscr{F}_{t-}] E[N_j(t) | \mathscr{F}_{t-}].$$

This and predictability of A_i gives

$$E[M_i(t) M_j(t) | \mathscr{F}_{t-}] = M_{i-}(t) M_{j-}(t).$$

From these results it can be shown that, under the conditional independence assumption,

$$\langle M_i, M_j \rangle = 0, \ \ a.s. \text{ for } i \ne j.$$

B.9 Convergence of Random Variables and Vectors

Before describing convergence results of martingale integrals, we first summarize results regarding various convergence concepts for random variables or vectors. Suppose a random variable X and a sequence of random variables X_n, $n = 1, 2, \ldots$

are defined on a probability space, $(\Omega, \mathscr{F}, P)$. X_n converges to X *in probability* if

$$\lim_n P\big(|X_n - X| > \varepsilon\big) = 0$$

for any $\varepsilon > 0$, or equivalently, if

$$\limsup_n P\big(|X_n - X| > \varepsilon\big) < \xi$$

for any ε, $\xi > 0$. Convergence in probability can be naturally extended to a sequence of k-component vectors X_n, by simply replacing $|X_n - X|$ with the norm $\|X_n - X\|_0^\tau$ in the above conditions, where $\|a\|_0^\tau = \sqrt{\sum_{i=1}^k a_i^2}$ for $a \in \mathrm{R}^k$.

Convergence in probability, for either random variables or vectors, is denoted by

$$X_n \xrightarrow{P} X.$$

Often, a sequence X_n converging in probability to a zero vector is written as

$$X_n = o_p(1).$$

A related notation is

$$X_n = O_p(1),$$

for a sequence X_n bounded in probability. That is, for any $\varepsilon > 0$, there exist $B > 0$ and N such that

$$P\big(\|X_n\|_0^\tau > B\big) < \varepsilon \quad \text{for all } n > N.$$

A sequence of random vectors X_n *converges in distribution* to a random vector X if, for their corresponding CDFs F_n and F,

$$F_n(x) \to F(x) \quad \text{at each continuity point of } F.$$

In such a case the sequence F_n is said to *converge weakly* to F. Convergence in distribution is denoted by

$$X_n \xrightarrow{d} X,$$

or

$$X_n \xrightarrow{d} L,$$

where L is the law or distribution of X.

If the limit X assigns probability 1 to a constant $c \in \mathrm{R}^k$, then almost sure convergence, convergence in probability and convergence in distribution are denoted by $X_n \to c, a.s.$, $X_n \xrightarrow{P} c$, and $X_n \xrightarrow{d} c$, respectively. Note that for convergence in distribution of X_n to X, it is not required that $X_1, X_2, \ldots$ and X are defined on a common probability space. Convergence in distribution refers to the behavior of the CDFs associated with the random variables/vectors, not values of the random variables/vectors. However, for asymptotic analysis and to facilitate understanding of concepts, often it is possible to construct variables on a common probability space as described in property #8 below, in a list of some frequently used properties.

1. If $X_n \to X$, *a.s.*, then $X_n \xrightarrow{P} X$.

2. $X_n \xrightarrow{P} X$ if and only if each subsequence of X_n contains a further subsequence that converges to X almost surely.

3. If $X_n \xrightarrow{P} X$, then $X_n \xrightarrow{d} X$.

4. If $X_n \xrightarrow{d} c$, then $X_n \xrightarrow{P} c$.

5. If $X_n \xrightarrow{d} X$, $Y_n - X_n \xrightarrow{P} 0$, then $Y_n \xrightarrow{d} X$.

6. (*Slutsky's theorem*) Suppose $X_n \xrightarrow{d} X$ and $Y_n \xrightarrow{d} c$, where c is a constant vector. Then

   (a) $X_n + Y_n \xrightarrow{d} X + c$;

   (b) $Y_n \cdot X_n \xrightarrow{d} c \cdot X$, where "$\cdot$" denotes the dot product of vectors:

   $$a \cdot b = a_1 b_1 + \cdots + a_k b_k,$$

   if $a = (a_1, \ldots, a_k)^{\mathrm{T}}$ and $b = (b_1, \ldots, b_k)^{\mathrm{T}}$.

7. $X_n \xrightarrow{d} X$ if and only if $Ef(X_n) \to Ef(X)$ for any bounded continuous $f : \mathsf{R}^k \mapsto \mathsf{R}$.

8. If $X_n \xrightarrow{d} X$ and g is a continuous function from R^k to R^q, then $g(X_n) \xrightarrow{d} g(X)$.

9. If $X_n \xrightarrow{d} X$, then there exists random vectors $\widetilde{X}_n$, $n \geq 1$ and $\widetilde{X}$ defined on a common probability space $(\Omega, \mathscr{F}, P)$, such that $\widetilde{X}_n$ and X_n have the same distribution, $n \geq 1$, $\widetilde{X}$ and X have the same distribution, and $\widetilde{X}_n \to \widetilde{X}$, *a.s.*

B.10 Martingale Central Limit Theorem

The martingale and related concepts can be extended to vector-valued random variables. Suppose $X_j(t)$, $j = 1, \ldots, k$ are local square integrable martingales with predictable covariation processes $\langle X_j, X_\ell \rangle$, $1 \leq j, \ell \leq k$. Then $X(t) = \left(X_1(t), \ldots, X_k(t)\right)^{\mathrm{T}}$ is a vector-valued local square integrable martingale with predictable variation process $\langle X \rangle(t)$ that is a $k \times k$ matrix function with (j, ℓ) element $\langle X_j, X_\ell \rangle(t)$, $t \geq 0$.

For a given sample size n, let $M_i^{(n)}(t),\ t \in [0,\tau], 1 \le i \le n$, be local square integrable martingales obtained from counting processes with associated filtration $\mathscr{F}_t^{(n)}$ that may depend on n. Let $H_{ji}^{(n)}(t),\ 1 \le j \le k,\ 1 \le i \le n$ be locally bounded $\mathscr{F}_t^{(n)}$-predictable processes and $X^{(n)}(t) = \left(X_1^{(n)}(t),\ldots,X_k^{(n)}(t)\right)^{\mathrm{T}}$ where

$$X_j^{(n)}(t) = \sum_{i=1}^{n} \int_0^t H_{ji}^{(n)}(s)dM_i^{(n)}(s), j = 1,\ldots,k,\ t \in [0,\tau].$$

For a given $\varepsilon > 0$, define $X_\varepsilon^{(n)}(t) = \left(X_{1\varepsilon}^{(n)}(t),\ldots,X_{k\varepsilon}^{(n)}(t)\right)^{\mathrm{T}}$ where

$$X_{j\varepsilon}^{(n)}(t) = \sum_{i=1}^{n} \int_0^t H_{ji}^{(n)}(s)I\left(|H_{ji}^{(n)}(s)| > \epsilon\right)dM_i^{(n)}(s), j = 1,\ldots,k,\ t \in [0,\tau].$$

Note that $X_\varepsilon^{(n)}(t)$ is a vector-valued local square integrable martingale, with predictable variation process $\langle X_\varepsilon^{(n)}\rangle(t)$.

Suppose $V(t)$ is a $k \times k$ matrix of deterministic and continuous functions on $[0,\tau]$, such that $V(0) = 0$ and $V(t) - V(s)$ is positive semi-definite for $0 \le s \le t \le \tau$. The following martingale central limit result is based on Rebolledo [258]. A related version is given by Theorem II.5.1 of Andersen et al. [7]. Convergence of a sequence of random matrices is defined as convergence of random vectors obtained by arranging each matrix as a vector.

Theorem B.1. For $X^{(n)}(t)$ and $V(t)$ defined above, suppose that for a subset $A \subset [0,\tau]$, as $n \to \infty$,

1. $\langle X^{(n)}\rangle(t) \xrightarrow{P} V(t)$ for any $t \in \mathsf{A}$;

2. $\langle X_\varepsilon^{(n)}\rangle(t) \xrightarrow{P} 0$ for any $t \in \mathsf{A}$ and any $\varepsilon > 0$.

Then for any $t \in \mathsf{A}$,

$$X^{(n)}(t) \xrightarrow{d} N\left(0, V(t)\right).$$

More generally, for any $\left\{t_1,\ldots,t_k\right\} \subset A$ where $0 < t_1 < \cdots < t_r \le \tau$,

$$\left(X^{(n)}(t_1)^{\mathrm{T}},\ldots,X^{(n)}(t_r)^{\mathrm{T}}\right)^{\mathrm{T}} \xrightarrow{d} N\left(0,\Sigma\right),$$

where Σ is a $(kr) \times (kr)$ matrix consisting of $k \times k$ blocks:

$$\Sigma = \begin{bmatrix} V(t_1) & V(t_1) & \ldots & V(t_1) \\ V(t_1) & V(t_2) & \ldots & V(t_2) \\ \ldots & \ldots & \ldots & \ldots \\ V(t_1) & V(t_2) & \ldots & V(t_r) \end{bmatrix}.$$

Note that when Theorem B.1 is applied to the random censorship model, continuity of $V(t)$ requires the underlying survival function to be continuous. Convergence for discontinuous distributions is possible using other approaches, such as those in Gill [95] or Shorack and Wellner [279]. Results on convergence of stochastic processes, which will be presented in Appendix C, also allow the distributions to be discontinuous.

To verify the conditions needed for this central limit theorem, a result due to Lenglart [166] is often useful. The *Lenglart's inequality*, when specialized to a nonnegative $\mathscr{F}_t$-local submartingale $X(t)$ with compensator $A(t)$ over an interval $[0,\tau]$, states that for any $\varepsilon > 0$ and any $\delta > 0$,

$$P(\sup_{t\in[0,\tau]} X(t) > \varepsilon) \leq \frac{\delta}{\varepsilon} + P(A(\tau) > \delta). \tag{B.16}$$

In Proposition B.1 below, a convergence result is established for integrals of a sequence of processes. It can be used to verify the conditions needed for Theorem B.1.

Proposition B.1. *Let A be either a finite closed interval* $[0,a]$ *or* $[0,\infty)$, $X_n(t)$ *a sequence of measurable stochastic processes on A, and* μ *a finite measure on A, Suppose that conditions (a) and (b) below hold:*

(a)

$$\sup_n \sup_{t\in A} \left|X_n(t)\right| \leq C$$

for some $C < \infty$.

(b) There is a subset $B \subset A$, *such that* $\mu(B^c \cap A) = 0$ *and for any* $t \in B$, *as* $n \to \infty$,

$$X_n(t) \xrightarrow{P} g(t),$$

for a deterministic and Borel measurable function $g(t)$.

Then,

$$\int_A X_n d\mu \xrightarrow{P} \int_A g d\mu.$$

Note that the integration is with respect to the time variable t. For each fixed t, $X_n(t)$ is a random variable, i.e., a mapping from the probability space Ω to the real line. The dependence of

$$\int_A X_n d\mu$$

on $\omega \in \Omega$ is suppressed, which may cause confusion. The measure μ may be the Borel measure with A being a bounded interval $[0, \tau]$. That is,

$$\int_A X_n d\mu = \int_0^\tau X_n(t)dt.$$

Another possibility is

$$\int_A X_n d\mu = \int_0^\infty X_n(t)h(t)dt,$$

for a nonnegative function h with

$$\int_0^\infty h(x)dx < \infty.$$

One more example is

$$\int_A X_n d\mu = \int_0^\tau X_n(t)d\Lambda(t)$$

where Λ is a cumulative hazard function with $\Lambda(\tau) < \infty$, for some $\tau < \infty$.

If a stronger condition holds:

$$\sup_{t \in B} \left| X_n(t) - g(t) \right| \xrightarrow{P} 0,$$

then the conclusion of the proposition follows more easily, since

$$\begin{aligned}
&\left| \int_A X_n d\mu - \int_A g d\mu \right| \\
\leq\ & \sup_{t \in B} \left| X_n(t) - g(t) \right| \mu(B) + \int_{B^c \cap A} \left| X_n - g \right| d\mu \\
\leq\ & \sup_{t \in B} \left| X_n(t) - g(t) \right| \mu(B) + 2C\mu(B^c \cap A) \\
\xrightarrow{P}\ & 0.
\end{aligned}$$

However, in applications such as the study of weighted log-rank tests, the uniform convergence condition may not hold.

Proposition B.1 is for a more general measure μ and the proof is adapted from Gill [96] who considered $\int_0^\tau X_n(t)dt$. While condition (a) in Proposition B.1 is often satisfied, there are works in the literature that require weaker conditions and yield stronger results, such as Helland [112] and Gill [96] (see also [7, p.85]). These works involve more technical proofs, and interested readers are referred to them for further details.

Proof of Proposition B.1. Fix a $t \in B$. For any $\varepsilon > 0$,

$$\begin{aligned} E\big|X_n(t) - g(t)\big| &= E\big|X_n(t) - g(t)\big| I\big(\big|X_n(t) - g(t)\big| > \varepsilon\big) \\ &\quad + E\big|X_n(t) - g(t)\big| I\big(\big|X_n(t) - g(t)\big| \le \varepsilon\big) \\ &\le 2CP\big(\big|X_n(t) - g(t)\big| > \varepsilon\big) + \varepsilon. \end{aligned}$$

Thus

$$\limsup_n E\big|X_n(t) - g(t)\big| \le \varepsilon.$$

Since ε is arbitrary, $E\big|X_n(t)-g(t)\big| \to 0$. Note that we also have $E\big|X_n(t)-g(t)\big| \le 2C$. Thus by the dominated convergence theorem,

$$\int_A E\big|X_n(t) - g(t)\big| d\mu \to 0.$$

Interchanging the order of expectation and integration, we obtain

$$E\int_A \big|X_n(t) - g(t)\big| d\mu \to 0.$$

Now

$$\begin{aligned} P\Big(\Big|\int_A \{X_n(t) - g(t)\} d\mu\Big| > \varepsilon\Big) &\le \frac{1}{\varepsilon} E\Big|\int_A \{X_n(t) - g(t)\} d\mu\Big| \\ &\le \frac{1}{\varepsilon} E\int_A \big|X_n(t) - g(t)\big| d\mu. \end{aligned}$$

It follows that

$$\int_A X_n d\mu \xrightarrow{P} \int_A g d\mu.$$

□

Often, in addition to the asymptotic normality that can be established using Theorem B.1, a consistent estimator of the asymptotic covariance is required. The next proposition establishes the convergence of a class of integrals which is useful for this purpose.

Proposition B.2. *Let $A_n(t)$ and $B_n(t)$ be two sequences of processes on $[0,\tau]$ for some $\tau < \infty$. Assume that $B_n(t)$ is cadlag and of bounded variation, $V_0^\tau(B_n) = O_p(1)$, and*

$$\sup_{0 \le t \le \tau} \big|B_n(t) - B(t)\big| \xrightarrow{P} 0,$$

for a deterministic function $B(t)$ of bounded variation on $[0,\tau]$. Furthermore,

$$\sup_{0\le t\le\tau} |A_n(t) - A(t)| \xrightarrow{P} 0$$

for a deterministic function $A(t)$. Consider the following conditions (a) and (b):

(a) $A(t)$ is cadlag and of bounded variation on $[0,\tau]$.

(b) $A_n(t)$ is obtained from finitely many operations of addition and multiplication from processes A_{nj}, $j = 1,\ldots,J$, where for each j, the sequence A_{nj} is either cadlag or caglad, and

$$\sup_{0\le t\le\tau} |A_{nj}(t) - A_{0j}(t)| \xrightarrow{P} 0,$$

for a deterministic function $A_{0j}(t)$ on $[0,\tau]$.

Then, under the additional condition of either (a) or (b),

$$\sup_{0<s\le\tau} \left| \int_0^s A_n dB_n - \int_0^s A dB \right| \xrightarrow{P} 0.$$

Proof. To simplify notations, for any function $X(t)$ on $[0,\tau]$, define

$$\|X\|_0^\tau = \|X(\cdot)\|_0^\tau = \sup_{s\in[0,\tau]} |X(s)|.$$

We start by considering the more elaborate case under condition (b). Note that A must be obtained from $A_{01},\ldots,A_{0J}$ through the same operation as the one through which A_n is obtained from $A_{n1},\ldots,A_{nJ}$.

Suppose that A_{nj} is cadlag with limit A_{0j}. By property #2 in Section B.9 on convergence in probability, there is a subsequence along which the uniform convergence of A_{nj} occurs almost surely. Thus A_{0j} is also cadlag almost surely. Since a set of probability zero does not affect the conclusion of Proposition B.2, for simplicity, we can treat A_{0j} as being cadlag without loss of generality. We have

$$\int_0^s A_{nj} dB_n - \int_0^s A_{0j} dB = \phi_n(s) + \psi_n(s),$$

where

$$\phi_n(s) = \int_0^s (A_{nj} - A_{0j}) dB_n, \quad \psi_n(s) = \int_0^s A_{0j} d(B_n - B).$$

The ϕ_n part is simple:

$$\|\phi_n\|_0^\tau \le \|A_{nj} - A_{0j}\|_0^\tau \cdot \bigvee_0^\tau (B_n) = o_p(1),$$

For ψ_n, we need to show that for any $\varepsilon, \xi > 0$,

$$\limsup_n P(\|\psi_n\|_0^\tau > \varepsilon) < \xi. \tag{B.17}$$

Conditions on B_n and B imply that there exists a $C_0 > 0$ such that

$$\limsup_n P\Big\{\bigvee_0^\tau (B_n) + \bigvee_0^\tau (B) > C_0\Big\} < \xi. \tag{B.18}$$

For the fixed ε and C_0 in (B.17) and (B.18), there exists a cadlag step function f_ε with finitely many jump points $0 < a_1 < \cdots < a_L \le \tau$ such that

$$\|A_{0j} - f_\varepsilon\|_0^\tau < \varepsilon/(2C_0) \tag{B.19}$$

[24, p.122]. By the convergence of B_n,

$$\limsup_n P\Big\{\sum_{\ell=1}^L |\Delta(f_\varepsilon)(a_\ell)| \cdot |B_n(a_\ell) - B(a_\ell)| > \varepsilon/2\Big\} = 0. \tag{B.20}$$

Note that

$$\int_0^s f_\varepsilon d(B_n - B) = \sum_{\ell=1}^L I(a_\ell \le s)\Delta f_\varepsilon(a_\ell)\big[B_n(a_\ell) - B(a_\ell)\big].$$

Thus

$$\begin{aligned}
&\limsup_n P\Big(\Big\|\int_0^\cdot f_\varepsilon d(B_n - B)\Big\|_0^\tau > \varepsilon/2\Big) \\
\le\ &\limsup_n P\Big(\sum_{\ell=1}^L |\Delta(f_\varepsilon)(a_\ell)| \cdot |B_n(a_\ell) - B(a_\ell)| > \varepsilon/2\Big) \\
=\ &0.
\end{aligned}$$

From these results, we obtain

$$
\begin{aligned}
& \limsup_n P(\|\psi_n\|_0^\tau > \varepsilon) \\
\leq\ & \limsup_n P\Big(\Big\| \int_0^{\cdot} (\boldsymbol{A}_{0j} - f_\varepsilon) d(\boldsymbol{B}_n - B) \Big\|_0^\tau > \varepsilon/2\Big) \\
& + \limsup_n P\Big(\Big\| \int_0^{\cdot} f_\varepsilon d(B_n - B) \Big\|_0^\tau > \varepsilon/2\Big) \\
\leq\ & \limsup_n P\Big(\|\boldsymbol{A}_{0j} - f_\varepsilon\|_0^\tau \Big[\bigvee_0^\tau (B_n) + \bigvee_0^\tau (B)\Big] > \varepsilon/2\Big) + 0 \\
\leq\ & \limsup_n P\Big(\frac{\varepsilon}{2C_0}\Big[\bigvee_0^\tau (B_n) + \bigvee_0^\tau (B)\Big] > \varepsilon/2\Big) \\
=\ & \limsup_n P\Big(\bigvee_0^\tau (B_n) + \bigvee_0^\tau (B) > C_0\Big) \\
<\ & \xi.
\end{aligned}
$$

Thus

$$\Big\| \int_0^{\cdot} A_{nj} dB_n - \int_0^{\cdot} A_{0j} dB \Big\|_0^\tau = o_p(1).$$

Similarly, the case for a caglad A_{nj} can be handled, where the step function used in the approximation is left continuous.

To deal with a product $A_{nj}A_{nk}$ where A_{nj} and A_{nk} are cadlag and caglad, respectively, define $\widetilde{B}_n(t) = \int_0^t A_{nj} dB_n$. Then

$$\int_0^s A_{nj} A_{nk} dB_n = \int_0^s A_{nk} d\widetilde{B}_n,$$

Note that the limit A_{0j} is cadlag, hence bounded. It follows that

$$\|A_{nj}\|_0^\tau \leq \|A_{0j}\|_0^\tau + \|A_{nj} - A_{0j}\|_0^\tau = O_p(1),$$

and

$$\bigvee_0^\tau (\widetilde{B}_n) \leq \|A_{nj}\|_0^\tau \cdot \bigvee_0^\tau (B_n) = O_p(1).$$

Thus the previous results can be applied to A_{nk} and $\widetilde{B}_n$ to obtain convergence of $\int_0^s A_{nj} A_{nk} dB_n$. Because a product of cadlag/caglad functions is still cadlag/caglad, and A_n is obtained from a finite sum of products, the convergence of $\int_0^s A_n dB_n$ follows.

Next, consider the case under condition (a). We have

$$\begin{aligned}
&\int_0^s A_n dB_n - \int_0^s A dB \\
&= \int_0^s (A_n - A) dB_n + \int_0^s A d(B_n - B) \\
&= \int_0^s (A_n - A) dB_n + [A(B_n - B)]|_0^s - \int_0^s (B_{n-} - B_-) dA.
\end{aligned}$$

Note that from the convergence of B_n,

$$\sup_{0<t\le\tau} |B_{n-}(t) - B_-(t)| \le \sup_{0\le t\le\tau} |B_n(t) - B(t)| \xrightarrow{P} 0.$$

Thus the convergence result follows. □

B.11 Applications to Survival Analysis

B.11.1 Kaplan-Meier and Nelson-Aalen Estimators

Let $T_i, 1 \le i \le n$ be i.i.d. time-to-event variables with CDF $F(t)$, survival function $S(t)$ and cumulative hazard function $\Lambda(t)$. Due to censoring, the observed data are $(X_i, \delta_i), 1 \le i \le n$, where $X_i = T_i \wedge C_i$, $\delta_i = I(T_i \le C_i)$, and C_i is time to censoring, $1 \le i \le n$. Note that there is no assumption of independence between T_i and C_i at this point.

Let

$$\begin{aligned}
N_i(t) &= I(X_i \le t, \delta_i = 1) = I(T_i \le t \wedge C_i),\ 1 \le i \le n, \\
N_i^C(t) &= I(X_i \le t, \delta_i = 0),\ 1 \le i \le n, \\
Y_i(t) &= I(X_i \ge t),\ 1 \le i \le n,
\end{aligned}$$

and set

$$\mathscr{F}_t = \sigma\{N_i(s), N_i^C(s) : 0 \le s \le t, i = 1, \ldots, n\}.$$

It can be shown that $\mathscr{F}_t$, or any σ-algebra generated by counting processes, is a right-continuous filtration. Note that $N_i(t) + N_i^C(t) = I(X_i \le t) = 1 - Y_{i+}(t)$. Thus $\mathscr{F}_t$ can also be written

$$\mathscr{F}_t = \sigma\{N_i(s), Y_{i+}(s) : 0 \le s \le t, i = 1, \ldots, n\}. \tag{B.21}$$

Let

$$M_i = N_i - A_i, \text{ with } A_i(t) = \int_0^t Y_i(s)d\Lambda(s), 1 \le i \le n. \tag{B.22}$$

By results in Section 11.2, under the independent censoring condition (2.38), $M_i(t)$ is an $\mathscr{F}_t$-martingale, $1 \le i \le n$. From $\Delta A_i = Y_i d\Lambda$ and $Y_i^2 = Y_i$, it also follows that, for $1 \le i \le n$,

$$\langle M_i, M_i\rangle(t) = \int_0^t (1 - \Delta A_i)dA_i = \int_0^t Y_i(1 - Y_i\Delta\Lambda)d\Lambda = \int_0^t Y_i(1 - \Delta\Lambda)d\Lambda.$$

When Λ, or equivalently F, is continuous, then A_i's are continuous and $\{N_1, \ldots, N_n\}$ is a multivariate counting process, because with probability one there are no ties and therefore no two N_i's jump at the same time. From the previous section, $\langle M_i, M_j\rangle = 0$ if $i \ne j, 1 \le i, j \le n$. When Λ has discontinuities, as in the discrete or mixed case, under the conditional independence condition (B.15), we also have $\langle M_i, M_j\rangle = 0$ if $i \ne j, 1 \le i, j \le n$.

Let

$$X_\ell(t) = \sum_{i=1}^n \int_0^t H_{i\ell}(s)dM_i(s), \ \ell = 1, 2,$$

where $\mathscr{F}_t$, $M_i t)$ are in (B.21) and (B.22), respectively, and $H_{i\ell}$ is locally bounded and $\mathscr{F}_t$-predictable on $[0, \infty)$. Proposition B. 3 below summarizes some important results from the previous sections applied to X_1, X_2 under the independent censoring model.

Proposition B.3. *Suppose that the independent censoring condition (2.38) holds. In addition, assume that either Λ is continuous or the conditional independence condition (B.15) holds for $\mathscr{F}_t$ in (B.21). Then,*

(a) $X_1(t)$, $X_2(t)$ are local square integrable martingales and

$$\langle X_\ell, X_m\rangle(t) = \sum_{i=1}^n \int_0^t H_{i\ell}(s)H_{im}(s)Y_i(s)[1 - \Delta\Lambda(s)]d\Lambda(s).$$

(b) If, in addition, $E\int_0^t H_{i,\ell}^2(s)Y_i(s)[1 - \Delta\Lambda(s)]d\Lambda(s) < \infty$ for any $t > 0$ and $1 \le i \le n$, $\ell = 1, 2$. then $X_1(t)$, $X_2(t)$ are martingales over $[0, t]$ for any $t > 0$, $EX_\ell(t) = 0$, and

$$E[X_\ell(t)X_m(y)] = \sum_{i=1}^n \int_0^t EH_{i\ell}(s)H_{im}(s)Y_i(s)[1 - \Delta\Lambda(s)]d\Lambda(s)$$

for $0 \le t \le y$, $\ell, m = 1, 2$.

For the Nelson-Aalen estimator $\widehat{\Lambda}$ in (2.44) and the Kaplan-Meier estimator $\widehat{F}$

in (2.45), let

$$A_n(t) = \sqrt{n}\big[\widehat{\Lambda}(t) - \Lambda(t)\big],$$

$$B_n(t) = \sqrt{n}\big[\widehat{F}(t) - F(t)\big].$$

A sequence of random variables X_n is said to converge in probability to ∞, denoted by $X_n \xrightarrow{P} \infty$, if for any $C > 0$,

$$\limsup_n P(|X_n| < C) = 0.$$

Theorem B.2 below establishes consistency and asymptotic normality of $\widehat{\Lambda}$ and $\widehat{F}$. under the independent censoring model. Note that the consistency does not require F to be continuous but the weak convergence does. Various versions of such results and their proofs are available in the literature [95, 82, 279, 7]. To be more accessible, the results stated here use more streamlined notations and conditions, and the proof is more elementary, with additional details included for clarity.

Theorem B.2. *Suppose that the independent censoring condition (2.38) holds, and that τ is a fixed point such that*

$$\tau < \tau_F, \ \ \textit{and} \ \ K(\tau) \xrightarrow{P} \infty \tag{B.23}$$

for τ_F in (A.13) and the at-risk process $K(t)$ defined in (2.43).

(a) If, in addition, either F is continuous or the conditional independence condition (B.15) holds for $\mathscr{F}_t$ in (B.21), then

$$\sup_{t\in[0,\tau]} \big|\widehat{\Lambda}(t) - \Lambda(t)\big| \xrightarrow{P} 0, \ \ \textit{and} \ \ \sup_{t\in[0,\tau]} \big|\widehat{F}(t) - F(t)\big| \xrightarrow{P} 0. \tag{B.24}$$

(b) If F is continuous and (B.23) is strengthened to

$$\tau < \tau_F, \ \ \textit{and} \ \ \sup_{t\in[0,\tau]} \big|K(t)/n - \xi(t)\big| \xrightarrow{P} 0, \tag{B.25}$$

for a function $\xi(t)$ with $\xi(\tau) > 0$. then for any $0 < t_1 < \cdots < t_r \le \tau$,

$$\big(A_n(t_1), \ldots, A_n(t_r)\big)^T \xrightarrow{d} N\big(0, \Sigma_\Lambda\big), \tag{B.26}$$

and

$$\big(B_n(t_1), \ldots, B_n(t_r)\big)^T \xrightarrow{d} N\big(0, \Sigma_F\big), \tag{B.27}$$

where the (j,k)*-element of* Σ_Λ *is*

$$\sigma_\Lambda(t_j,t_k)=\int_0^{t_j}\frac{1}{\xi(x)}\left[1-\Delta\Lambda(x)\right]d\Lambda(x),\quad 1\le j\le k\le r, \tag{B.28}$$

and the (j,k)*-element of* Σ_F *is*

$$\sigma_F(t_j,t_k) = [1-F(t_j)][1-F(t_k)]\int_0^{t_j}\frac{1}{\xi}\frac{1-F_-}{1-F}[1-\Delta\Lambda]d\Lambda,\quad 1\le j\le k\le r. \tag{B.29}$$

Moreover,

$$\sup_{t\in[0,\tau]}\left|\widehat{\sigma}_\Lambda(t,t)-\sigma_\Lambda(t,t)\right|\xrightarrow{P}0,\qquad \sup_{t\in[0,\tau]}\left|\widehat{\sigma}_F(t,t)-\sigma_F(t,t)\right|\xrightarrow{P}0,$$

where

$$\widehat{\sigma}_\Lambda(t,t)=n\int_0^t\frac{1}{K(s)^2}\left[1-\frac{\Delta H(u)}{K(s)}\right]dH(s), \tag{B.30}$$

and

$$\widehat{\sigma}_F(t,t)=n[1-\widehat{F}(t)]^2\int_0^t\frac{1}{K(s)[K(s)-\Delta H(s)]}dH(s). \tag{B.31}$$

Proof. Let

$$M(t)=\sum_{i=1}^n M_i(t)=H(t)-\int_0^t K(x)d\Lambda(x),$$

where $H(t)$ is defined in (2.43). Let J be as defined in (A.13) and

$$\Phi(t)=\int_0^t\frac{J}{K}dM.$$

Note that J/K is a locally bounded $\mathscr{F}_t$- predictable process. Thus $\Phi(t)$ is a local square integrable martingale and

$$\langle\Phi,\Phi\rangle(t)=\int_0^t\left(\frac{J}{K}\right)^2d\langle M,M\rangle(x)=\int_0^t\frac{J}{K}[1-\Delta\Lambda]d\Lambda. \tag{B.32}$$

On $\{\tau\le L\}$ with L defined in (A.13), for any $t\in[0,\tau]$, we have $t<\tau_F$ and $t\le L$. Thus

$$\widehat{\Lambda}(t)-\Lambda(t)=\int_0^t\frac{dH}{K}-\Lambda(t)=\int_0^t\frac{dM}{K}=\Phi(t), \tag{B.33}$$

where the second last equality follows from the definition of $M(t)$ and the last one from the fact that $J(t) = 1$ for $t \le L$. Note that

$$P(\tau > L) \le P(K(\tau) = 0) \to 0. \tag{B.34}$$

Thus, to prove the first part of (B.24), it suffices to prove that

$$\sup_{t \in [0,\tau]} [\Phi(t)] \xrightarrow{P} 0. \tag{B.35}$$

These types of statements can be justified rigorously, as demonstrated in the proofs of Proposition C.1 and Theorem C.2 in Appendix C.

By the Lenglart's inequality applied to $\Phi^2(t)$, for any ε, $\delta > 0$,

$$P(\sup_{t \in [0,\tau]} \Phi^2(t) > \varepsilon) \le \frac{\delta}{\varepsilon} + P\Big(\int_0^\tau \frac{J}{K}[1 - \Delta\Lambda] d\Lambda > \delta\Big). \tag{B.36}$$

On $\{\tau \le L\}$, for any $t \in [0, \tau]$, by the monotonicity of $K(t)$,

$$\frac{J(t)}{K(t)} = \frac{1}{K(t)} \le \frac{1}{K(\tau)} = \frac{J(\tau)}{K(\tau)}. \tag{B.37}$$

Thus

$$\int_0^\tau \frac{J}{K}[1 - \Delta\Lambda] d\Lambda \le \frac{J(\tau)}{K(\tau)} \Lambda(\tau).$$

It follows that the second term on the right hand side of (B.36) converges to 0 for any $\delta > 0$. Since ε, δ are arbitrary, (B.35) follows from (B.36).

Now for $\widehat{F}(t)$, let

$$\Psi(t) = \int_0^t \frac{1 - \widehat{F}_-}{1 - F} \frac{J}{K} dM$$

for $t < \tau_F$. Then $\Psi(t)$ is a local square integrable martingale with

$$\langle \Psi, \Psi \rangle(t) = \int_0^t \Big(\frac{1 - \widehat{F}_-}{1 - F}\Big)^2 \frac{J}{K}(1 - \Delta\Lambda) d\Lambda. \tag{B.38}$$

From (A.14), on $\{\tau \le L\}$, for any $t \in [0, \tau]$,

$$\widehat{F}(t) - F(t) = [1 - F(t)]\Psi(t).$$

Thus similarly to the argument for $\widehat{\Lambda} - \Lambda$, to prove the second part of (B.24), it suffices to prove that

$$\sup_{t \in [0,\tau]} [\Psi(t)] \xrightarrow{P} 0.$$

This can be done similarly to the case for $\Phi(t)$, using the fact that

$$\Big[\frac{1 - \widehat{F}_-(t)}{1 - F(t)}\Big]^2 \le \frac{1}{[1 - F(\tau)]^2}$$

for $t \in [0,\tau]$. Thus the second part of (B.24) is established.

(b) Let

$$A^*(t) = \sqrt{n}\Phi(t) = \int_0^t \frac{\sqrt{n}J}{K}dM, \quad A^*_\varepsilon(t) = \int_0^t \frac{\sqrt{n}J}{K} I\Big(\Big|\frac{\sqrt{n}J}{K}\Big| > \varepsilon\Big)dM.$$

From (B.32), for any $t \in [0,\tau]$,

$$\langle A^*, A^*\rangle(t) = \int_0^t \frac{J}{K/n}[1-\Delta\Lambda]d\Lambda.$$

Condition (B.25) implies that $J[K(t)/n]^{-1}$ converges in probability to $1/\xi(t)$, uniformly for $t \in [0,\tau]$. This statement can be rigorously justified, similar to the proof of Proposition C.1 in Appendix C later.

Furthermore, the limit $1/\xi(t)$ is bounded for $t \in [0,\tau]$. Thus

$$\langle A^*, A^*\rangle(t) \xrightarrow{P} \int_0^t \frac{1}{\xi}[1-\Delta\Lambda]d\Lambda.$$

For $A^*_\varepsilon(t)$, note that

$$\langle A^*_\varepsilon, A^*_\varepsilon\rangle(t) = \int_0^t \frac{J}{K/n} I\Big(\Big|\frac{\sqrt{n}J}{K}\Big| > \varepsilon\Big)[1-\Delta\Lambda]d\Lambda.$$

On $\{\tau \le L\}$, by (B.37) and monotonicity of K, for $t \in [0,\tau]$,

$$0 \le \frac{J(t)}{K(t)/n} I\Big(\Big|\frac{\sqrt{n}J(t)}{K(t)}\Big| > \varepsilon\Big) \le \frac{J(\tau)}{K(\tau)/n} I\Big(K(\tau)/n < \frac{1}{\varepsilon\sqrt{n}}\Big).$$

It follows that

$$\langle A^*_\varepsilon, A^*_\varepsilon\rangle(t) \xrightarrow{P} 0.$$

From the martingale central limit theorem, for any $0 < t_1 < \cdots < t_r \le \tau$,

$$\big(A^*(t_1), \ldots, A^*(t_r)\big)^{\mathrm{T}} \xrightarrow{d} N\big(0, \Sigma_\Lambda\big), \tag{B.39}$$

where the expression for Σ_Λ in (B.28) is due to the martingale property. Now (B.26) follows from (B.39), (B.33) and (B.34). The assertion (B.27) can be proved similarly and the proof is omitted.

Note that

$$\widehat{\sigma}_\Lambda(t,t) = n\int_0^t \frac{1}{K(s)}\big[1-\Delta\widehat{\Lambda}(s)\big]d\widehat{\Lambda}(s),$$

which is obtained from $\sigma_\Lambda(t,t)$ by replacing $\xi(t)$ and $\Lambda(t)$ by $K(t)/n$ and $\widehat{\Lambda}(t)$, respectively. Similarly, $\widehat{\sigma}_F(t,t)$ is obtained from $\sigma_F(t,t)$ by replacing $\xi(t)$, $\Lambda(t)$ and $F(t)$ by $K(t)/n$, $\widehat{\Lambda}(t)$ and $\widehat{F}(t)$, respectively, using the fact that, from the definition of $\widehat{F}(t)$,

$$1-\widehat{F}(t)=[1-\widehat{F}_-(t)]\Big[1-\Delta\widehat{\Lambda}(t)\Big]=[1-\widehat{F}_-(t)]\Big[1-\frac{\Delta H(t)}{K(t)}\Big].$$

Furthermore, $\Delta\widehat{\Lambda}(t)=\widehat{\Lambda}(t)-\widehat{\Lambda}_-(t)$. Observe that the integrals are on $(0,t]$. To simplify notations, uniform convergence on $[0,\tau]$ of $\widehat{\Lambda}_-$ and $\widehat{F}_-$ can be obtained from that of $\widehat{\Lambda}$ and $\widehat{F}$ by defining

$$\Lambda_-(0)=\widehat{\Lambda}_-(0)=F_-(0)=\widehat{F}_-(0)=0.$$

Now consistency of $\widehat{\sigma}_\Lambda(t,t)$ and $\widehat{\sigma}_F(t,t)$ follows from Proposition B.2. □

From the proof, the factors $1-\Delta\Lambda$ and $[1-F_-]/[1-F]$ inside the integrals in (B.28), and (B.29), respectively, are inherited from the martingale compensator formula and (A.14), respectively, which are valid for possibly discontinuous F. However, one of the conditions for the weak convergence in Theorem B.3 is continuity of F, in which case the factors $1-\Delta\Lambda$ and $[1-F_-]/[1-F]$ are identically 1. Thus we have

$$\sigma_\Lambda(t_j,t_k)=\int_0^{t_j}\frac{1}{\xi(x)}d\Lambda(x),\quad 1\le j\le k\le r,$$

and

$$\sigma_F(t_j,t_k)=\big[1-F(t_j)\big]\big[1-F(t_k)\big]\int_0^{t_j}\frac{1}{\xi(x)}d\Lambda(x),\quad 1\le j\le k\le r.$$

Therefore, $\sigma_\Lambda(t,t)$ and $\sigma_F(t,t)$ can also be consistently estimated by $\widetilde{\sigma}_\Lambda(t,t)$ and $\widetilde{\sigma}_F(t,t)$, respectively, where

$$\widetilde{\sigma}_\Lambda(t,t)=n\int_0^t\frac{1}{K(s)^2}dH(s),\tag{B.40}$$

and

$$\widetilde{\sigma}_F(t,t)=n[1-\widehat{F}(t)]^2\int_0^t\frac{1}{K(s)^2}dH(s).\tag{B.41}$$

From Section 11.2, the random censorship model is an independent censoring model. It can also be shown that the model satisfies the conditional independence assumption (B.15) for $\mathscr{F}_t$ in (B.21). Thus Theorem B.2 applies and the following results can be obtained. Let G_i be the CDF of C_i, $i=1,\ldots,n$, and $G_{na}=\sum_{i=1}^n G_i/n$.

Corollary B.1. *Suppose that data are from the random censorship model defined in Section 2.4, and that τ is a fixed point such that*

$$\tau<\tau_F,\ \textit{and}\ \sup_{t\in[0,\tau]}|G_{na}(t)-G(t)|\to 0\tag{B.42}$$

for a function G with $G_-(\tau) < 1$. Then,

(a)

$$\sup_{t\in[0,\tau]} \left|\widehat{\Lambda}(t) - \Lambda(t)\right| \xrightarrow{P} 0, \quad and \quad \sup_{t\in[0,\tau]} \left|\widehat{F}(t) - F(t)\right| \xrightarrow{P} 0. \tag{B.43}$$

(b) If F is continuous, then for any $0 < t_1 < \cdots < t_r \le \tau$,

$$\left(A_n(t_1),\ldots,A_n(t_r)\right)^T \xrightarrow{d} N\left(0,\Sigma_\Lambda^*\right), \tag{B.44}$$

and

$$\left(B_n(t_1),\ldots,B_n(t_r)\right)^T \xrightarrow{d} N\left(0,\Sigma_F^*\right), \tag{B.45}$$

where the (j,k)-element of Σ_Λ^* is

$$\int_0^{t_j} \frac{[1-\Delta\Lambda(x)]d\Lambda(x)}{[1-F_-(x)][1-G_-(x)]}, \quad 1 \le j \le k \le r, \tag{B.46}$$

and the (j,k)-element of Σ_F^* is

$$\left[1-F(t_j)\right]\left[1-F(t_k)\right]\int_0^{t_j} \frac{[1-\Delta\Lambda(x)]d\Lambda(x)}{[1-F(x)][1-G_-(x)]}, \quad 1 \le j \le k \le r, \tag{B.47}$$

The estimators in (B.30), (B.31), (B.40) and (B.41) remain uniformly consistent for the limiting variance processes in (B.46) and (B.47), respectively.

Proof. Since $K(t) = \sum_{i=1}^n I(X_i \ge t)$ and all the indicator functions are bounded by 1, from the uniform strong law of large numbers [243, Theorem 8.3] and the assumption on G_{na},

$$\sup_{t\in[0,\tau]} \left|K(t)/n - (1-F_-(t))(1-G_-(t))\right| \to 0 \text{ almost surely,} \tag{B.48}$$

where the limit is decreasing and bounded below by $(1-F_-(\tau))(1-G_-(\tau)) > 0$. Thus condition (B.25) is satisfied and the results follow from Theorem B.2. □

Theorem B.2 can also be applies to data under type II censoring. For example, if the censoring variable is an order statistic $T_{(r)}$ corresponding to the sample pth percentile for a $p \in (0,1)$. Then

$$K(t) = \sum_{i=1}^n I(X_i \ge t) = I(T_{(r)} \ge t) \sum_{i=1}^n I(T_i \ge t).$$

If $\tau < F^{-1}(p)$, the pth percentile of F, then condition (B.25) is satisfied under proper conditions on F, and the results of Theorem B.3 apply. Interested readers are encouraged to fill in the details of the argument.

B.11.2 Weighted Log-Rank Tests

Note that in the subsection above, all the convergence results are established over a range $[0,\tau]$ such that $K(\tau) \xrightarrow{P} \infty$. Such range restriction is necessary for making inference on $\widehat{\Lambda}(t)$ and $\widehat{F}(t)$, as the estimators can be unstable near the upper end of the data range. This means that some of the data will not be used. On the other hand, for weighted log-rank test statistics, with properly chosen weights, typically the statistics behave much more stably, and all data can be used. Therefore, it is useful to establish convergence over the maximal possible range, the trial's duration.

Consider the weighted log-rank test statistics under the null hypothesis of equal distributions in the two groups. To establish their asymptotic normality with data over the entire trial duration range, we will restrict our attention to the random censorship model with i.i.d. censoring variables within each group. This setting is still quite general for applications in clinical trials. To illustrate why some restriction is necessary, we will point out some gaps in relevant works from the literature after the proof of the results.

Suppose there are two independent samples from the control and treatment groups, respectively. Let $T_1,\ldots,T_n$ be the time-to-event variables from the pooled sample, with the $n_1 < n$ control group variables arranged before the treatment group variables. Let $C_1,\ldots,C_n$ be the corresponding time-to-censoring variables. The observed data are independent pairs $(X_i,\ \delta_i), i = 1,\ldots,n$, with $X_i = T_i \wedge C_i$, $\delta_i = I(X_i = T_i)$. It is assumed that (T_i,C_i), $1 \le i \le n_1$, are i.i.d., and (T_i,C_i), $n_1+1 \le i \le n$, are i.i.d.

Let F_C and G_C be the CDFs of T_1 and C_1, respectively, and F_T and G_T be the CDFs of T_n and C_n, respectively. Denote by Λ_C and Λ_T the cumulative hazard functions corresponding to F_C and F_T, respectively. Recall from Section 2.8.2 the constants:

$$z_i = I(i > n_1), \qquad 1 \le i \le n.$$

The cumulative hazard function of T_i is $\Lambda_i = z_i\Lambda_T + (1-z_i)\Lambda_C$, $1 \le i \le n$.

Let

$$M_i = N_i - \int_0^t Y_i(s)d\Lambda_i(s), 1 \le i \le n, \tag{B.49}$$

where N_i, Y_i are the counting process and at-risk process of the ith individual, respectively. Then similarly to the one-sample case discussed in the previous subsection, $M_i(t)$ is a martingale, $1 \le i \le n$, and

$$\langle M_i, M_i\rangle(t) = \int_0^t Y_i(1-\Delta\Lambda_i)d\Lambda_i.$$

In addition, when F_C, F_T are continuous, $\langle M_i, M_j\rangle = 0$ if $i \ne j, 1 \le i, j \le n$.

Consider the null hypothesis

$$H_0 : F_T = F_C. \tag{B.50}$$

Let F be the common CDF of the two groups under H_0. Assume that $n_1/n \to p_C \in (0,1)$ and let $p_T = 1 - p_C$. From this and the strong law of large numbers, under H_0, for any $t \geq 0$, almost surely,

$$
\begin{aligned}
K_C(t)/n &\to k_C(t), \\
K_T(t)/n &\to k_T(t), \\
K(t)/n &\to k(t),
\end{aligned}
\tag{B.51}
$$

where

$$
\begin{aligned}
k_C(t) &= p_C[1-F_-(t)][1-G_{C-}(t)], \\
k_T(t) &= p_T[1-F_-(t)][1-G_{T-}(t)], \\
k(t) &= [1-F_-(t)][1-G_-(t)],
\end{aligned}
$$

with G_{C-}, G_{T-} being the left continuous versions of G_C, G_T, respectively, and

$$G = p_C G_C + p_T G_T.$$

Let

$$U_\Phi(t) = \sum_{i=1}^{n} \int_0^t \Phi(x)\left[z_i - \frac{K_T(x)}{K(x)}\right] dN_i(x),$$

for $t \geq 0$, where the at-risk processes K, K_T are as defined in (2.43) and (2.48), respectively. Theorem B.3 below establishes the asymptotic normality of the weighted log-rank test statistics under H_0.

Theorem B.3. *Suppose that two-sample survival data are obtained from the setting described above. Assume that conditions (a)—(d) below hold:*

(a) The null hypothesis (B.50) is true, with a continuous function Λ being the common cumulative hazard function of the two groups.

(b) τ^* is a fixed constant such that

$$C_i \leq \tau^*,\ i = 1, \ldots, n, \ \text{and}\ \ \tau^* < \tau_0, \tag{B.52}$$

where $\tau_0 = \sup\{t : \Lambda(t) < \infty\}$.

(c) Φ is predictable and nonnegative, and

$$\sup_n \sup_{t\in[0,\tau^*]} \Phi(t) \leq A, \ \text{and}\ \ \sup_{t\in[0,\tau^*]} |\Phi(t) - \phi(t)| \xrightarrow{P} 0,$$

for a constant $A < \infty$ and a function ϕ on $[0, \tau^*]$.

(d)

$$n_1/n \to p_C \in (0,1).$$

Then, for any $0 < t_1 < \cdots < t_r \le \tau^*$,

$$n^{-1/2}\big(U_\Phi(t_1),\ldots,U_\Phi(t_r)\big)^T \xrightarrow{d} N\big(0,\Sigma_\Phi\big), \tag{B.53}$$

where the (j,k)*-element of* Σ_Φ *is*

$$\sigma_\Phi(t_j,t_k) = \int_0^{t_j} \eta(x)d\Lambda(x), \quad 1 \le j \le k \le r, \tag{B.54}$$

with

$$\eta(t) = I\big(k(t)>0\big)\phi^2(t)\frac{k_C(t)k_T(t)}{k(t)}\big[1-\Delta\Lambda(t)\big],$$

for k_C, k_T, k *in (B.51).*

Moreover, $\sigma_\Phi(t,t)$ *can be consistently estimated by* $\widehat{\sigma}_\Phi(t,t)$, *where*

$$\widehat{\sigma}_\Phi(t,t) = \frac{1}{n}\int_0^t \Phi^2(x)\frac{K_C(x)K_T(x)}{K^2(x)}dH(x). \tag{B.55}$$

Proof. With some algebra, it can be shown that, under H_0,

$$\begin{aligned} U_\Phi(t) &= \sum_{i=1}^n \int_0^t \Phi(x)\Big[z_i - \frac{K_T(x)}{K(x)}\Big]dM_i(x) \\ &= \sum_{i=1}^n \int_0^t J^*(x)\Phi(x)\Big[z_i - \frac{K_T(x)}{K(x)}\Big]dM_i(x), \end{aligned} \tag{B.56}$$

where

$$J^*(x) = I\big(K(x)>0\big).$$

Note that the integrand in (B.56) is bounded and predictable. Thus $U_\Phi(t)$ is a local square integrable martingale. It is in fact a square integrable martingale, but this property is not needed yet.

Let

$$\begin{aligned} B_i(x) &= n^{-1/2}J^*(x)\Phi(x)\Big[z_i - \frac{K_T(x)}{K(x)}\Big], \\ D^*(t) &= \sum_{i=1}^n \int_0^t B_i(x)dM_i(x), \\ D_\varepsilon^*(t) &= \sum_{i=1}^n \int_0^t B_i(x)I\big(|B_i(x)|>\varepsilon\big)dM_i(x), \end{aligned}$$

where $\varepsilon > 0$. Then $D^*(t) = n^{-1/2}U_\Phi(t)$. Under H_0,

$$\langle D^*, D^*\rangle(t) = \sum_{i=1}^{n}\int_0^t B_i^2 Y_i[1-\Delta\Lambda]d\Lambda,$$

$$\langle D_\varepsilon^*, D_\varepsilon^*\rangle(t) = \sum_{i=1}^{n}\int_0^t B_i^2 I\big(|B_i| > \varepsilon\big)Y_i[1-\Delta\Lambda]d\Lambda.$$

Since $K = K_T + K_C$ for K_C in (2.48), some algebraic simplification leads to

$$\begin{aligned}\langle D^*, D^*\rangle(t) &= n^{-1}\int_0^t J^*\Phi^2\Big(\frac{K_T}{K}\Big)^2 K_C[1-\Delta\Lambda]d\Lambda \\ &\quad + n^{-1}\int_0^t J^*\Phi^2\Big(\frac{K_C}{K}\Big)^2 K_T[1-\Delta\Lambda(x)]d\Lambda \\ &= \int_0^t \eta_n(x)d\Lambda(x). \qquad (B.57)\end{aligned}$$

where

$$\eta_n(x) = J^*(x)\Phi^2(x)\frac{K_C(x)}{n}\frac{K_T(x)}{K(x)}[1-\Delta\Lambda(x)],\ x \le \tau^*.$$

By condition (b), $G(\tau^*) = 1$. Let

$$\tau = \inf\{t : G(t) = 1\}.$$

Then $\tau \le \tau^*$, and $G(\tau) = 1$. The latter also implies that $G_C(\tau) = G_T(\tau) = 1$. Thus with probability 1,

$$\max_i X_i \le \max_i C_i \le \tau. \qquad (B.58)$$

If $\tau < \tau^*$, fix an $x \in (\tau, \tau^*]$. By (B.58), with probability 1, $K(x) = 0$. Thus $k(x) = 0$ as well. For any $\varepsilon > 0$,

$$P\Big(I\big(K(x) > 0\big) > \varepsilon\Big) = P\big(K(x) > 0\big) = 0,$$

Thus

$$J^*(x) \xrightarrow{P} 0. \qquad (B.59)$$

Note that since $K_C/n \le 1$, $K_T/K \le 1$, we have $\eta_n(x) \le A^2 J^*(x)$. It follows that $\eta_n(x) \xrightarrow{P} 0 = \eta(x)$.

Now for any $x < \tau$, we have $k(x) > 0$. Note that $J^*(x) = I\big(K(x)/n > 0\big)$. Thus $J^*(x) \xrightarrow{P} 1$. From conditions (b) and (c), we have

$$\eta_n(x) \xrightarrow{P} \eta(x).$$

Putting the above results together, we have proved that

$$\eta_n(x) \xrightarrow{P} \eta(x) \text{ for } x \in [0,\tau^*],\ x \neq \tau. \tag{B.60}$$

Note that $\eta_n \leq A^2$, $\int_0^{\tau^*} d\Lambda(x) < \infty$ and $\int_0^{\tau^*} I(x=\tau)d\Lambda(x) = 0$. By Proposition B.1,

$$\langle D^*, D^*\rangle(t) \xrightarrow{P} \int_0^t \eta(x)d\Lambda(x), \tag{B.61}$$

for all $t \in [0,\tau^*]$.

Now for $\langle D_\varepsilon^*, D_\varepsilon^*\rangle(t)$, some algebra yields

$$\langle D_\varepsilon^*, D_\varepsilon^*\rangle(t) = \int_0^t \eta_{n1\varepsilon}(x)d\Lambda(x) + \int_0^t \eta_{n2\varepsilon}(x)d\Lambda(x), \tag{B.62}$$

where

$$\begin{aligned}
\eta_{n1\varepsilon} &= J^*\Phi^2\Big(\frac{K_T}{K}\Big)^2\frac{K_C}{n}I\Big(\frac{J^*\Phi}{\sqrt{n}}\frac{K_T^2}{K^2} > \varepsilon\Big)[1-\Delta\Lambda], \\
\eta_{n2\varepsilon} &= J^*\Phi^2\Big(\frac{K_C}{K}\Big)^2\frac{K_T}{n}I\Big(\frac{J^*\Phi}{\sqrt{n}}\frac{K_C^2}{K^2} > \varepsilon\Big)[1-\Delta\Lambda].
\end{aligned}$$

At a fixed $x < \tau$, the indicators involving ε in $\eta_{n1\varepsilon}(x)$ and $\eta_{n2\varepsilon}(x)$ converge in probability to 0. Thus

$$\eta_{nj\varepsilon}(x) \xrightarrow{P} 0,\ j = 1,2.$$

For $x > \tau$, as shown earlier, $J^*(x) \xrightarrow{P} 0$. Therefore we also have the convergence to zero in probability of $\eta_{nj\varepsilon}(x)$, $j = 1,2$. It follows that

$$\eta_{nj\varepsilon} \xrightarrow{P} 0 \text{ for } x \in [0,\tau^*],\ x \neq \tau,\ j = 1,2.$$

By Proposition B.1 again,

$$\langle D_\varepsilon^*, D_\varepsilon^*\rangle(t) \xrightarrow{P} 0. \tag{B.63}$$

From (B.61), (B.63) and the martingale central limit theorem, for any $0 < t_1 < \cdots < t_r \leq \tau$,

$$n^{-1/2}\big(U_\Phi^*(t_1),\ldots,U_\Phi^*(t_r)\big)^{\mathrm{T}} \xrightarrow{d} N(0,\Sigma_\Phi), \tag{B.64}$$

with the (j,k) element $\sigma_\Phi(t_j,t_k)$ of Σ_Φ given by (B.54).

For consistency of $\widehat{\sigma}_\Phi(t,t)$, consider the martingale

$$Q(t) = \sum_{i=1}^n \int_0^t J^*(x)\Phi^2(x)\frac{K_C(x)K_T(x)}{K^2(x)}dM_i(x).$$

Similarly to the proof of weak convergence of $n^{-1/2}U_\Phi(t)$ above, it can be shown that for any $0 < t \le \tau^*$,

$$n^{-1/2} Q(t) \xrightarrow{d} N(0, \sigma_Q(t)),$$

where the limiting variance $\sigma_Q(t)$ is finite. It follows that $Q(t)/n \xrightarrow{P} 0$. That is,

$$\frac{1}{n}\int_0^t J^* \Phi^2 \frac{K_C K_T}{K^2} dH - \frac{1}{n}\int_0^t J^* \Phi^2 \frac{K_C K_T}{K}[1-\Delta\Lambda] d\Lambda \xrightarrow{P} 0.$$

Since H has no jumps on the interval where $K = 0$, the above result can be re-written as

$$\widehat{\sigma}_\Phi(t,t) - \frac{1}{n}\int_0^t J^* \Phi^2 \frac{K_C K_T}{K}[1-\Delta\Lambda] d\Lambda \xrightarrow{P} 0.$$

From this and (B.61), consistency of $\widehat{\sigma}_\Phi(t,t)$ follows. □

Since $\eta_n \le A^2$, by (B.57), $E\langle D^*, D^*\rangle(t) < \infty$ for any $t \le \tau^*$. Thus by Theorem B.2,

$$E\left[D^*(t)\right]^2 = E\langle D^*, D^*\rangle(t).$$

Thus

$$Var\left(n^{-1/2} U_\Phi\right) = E\left[D^*(t)\right]^2 = E\widehat{\sigma}_\Phi(t,t), \tag{B.65}$$

where the last equality follows from the fact that $EQ(t) = EQ(0) = 0$.

Thus $\widehat{\sigma}_\Phi(t,t)$ is also an unbiased estimator of the variance of $n^{-1/2} U_\Phi(t)$. For U_Φ and V_Φ in (2.51) and (2.53) of Section 2.8.2, respectively, since the N_i's have no mass beyond $[0, \tau^*]$, we have

$$V_\Phi = n\widehat{\sigma}_\Phi(\tau^*, \tau^*), \qquad U_\Phi = U_\Phi(\tau^*, \tau^*).$$

Therefore, the result (B.65) with $t = \tau^*$ shows that V_Φ is an unbiased estimator of the variance of U_Φ in (2.51).

Regarding the estimator (2.52) of Section 2.8.2, by Proposition 3.2.2 of Gill [95],

$$\int_0^t (\Delta H - 1) dH - \int_0^t K(K-1)\Delta\Lambda d\Lambda$$

is a martingale. From this and (B.49), for a bounded predictable f,

$$\begin{aligned} M_1^*(t) &= \int_0^t \frac{I(K>1)f}{K-1}(\Delta H - 1) dH - \int_0^t I(K>1) f K \Delta\Lambda d\Lambda, \\ M_2^*(t) &= \int_0^t I(K>1) f dH - \int_0^t I(K>1) f K d\Lambda \end{aligned}$$

are both zero mean martingales, since $I(K > 1)f/(K-1)$ and $I(K > 1)f$ both are bounded and predictable. From

$$M_2^*(t) - M_1^*(t) = \int_0^t I(K>1) f\Big(1 - \frac{\Delta H - 1}{K-1}\Big) dH - \int_0^t I(K>1) f K(1-\Delta\Lambda) d\Lambda,$$

it follows that

$$E\int_0^t I(K>1) f\Big(1 - \frac{\Delta H - 1}{K-1}\Big) dH = E\int_0^t I(K>1) f K(1-\Delta\Lambda) d\Lambda. \tag{B.66}$$

In particular, for $f = \Phi^2(x) K_C(x) K_T(x) [K^2(x)]^{-1}$, we have

$$\begin{aligned} & E\int_0^t I(K>1)\Phi^2(x)\frac{K_C(x)K_T(x)}{K^2(x)}\Big(1 - \frac{\Delta H - 1}{K-1}\Big) dH \\ = \;& E\int_0^t I(K>1)\Phi^2(x)\frac{K_C(x)K_T(x)}{K^2(x)} K(1-\Delta\Lambda) d\Lambda. \end{aligned} \tag{B.67}$$

Note that when $K \le 1$, K is either 0 or 1. When $K(x) = 1$, there is a single observation among the X_i's that is the largest observation. Thus $K_C(x)$ or $K_T(x)$ must be zero and $\Phi^2(x)K_C(x)K_T(x)/K^2(x) = 0$ by the convention $0/0 = 0$. Similarly, $\Phi^2(x)K_C(x)K_T(x)/K^2(x) = 0$ when $K = 0$. Thus the factor $I(K>1)$ can be omitted from both sides of the equation in (B.67). With $t = \tau^*$, this shows that the estimator in (2.52) of Section 2.8.2 is an unbiased estimator of the variance of $n^{-1/2}U_\Phi$.

Theorem B.3 establishes convergence over the entire trial follow-up interval $[0, \tau^*]$ without relying on a common assumption in the literature that censoring distributions have positive mass at τ^*. In the typical staggered entry scenarios, that assumption requires a positive probability of entering the trial at time 0. The assumptions in Theorem B.3 are more flexible.

The proof of Theorem B.3 addresses certain gaps in an argument in Andersen et al. [7, p.367] with the use of Proposition B.1 and the assumed conditions on censoring. Specifically, the convergence

$$K(t)/n \to k(t)$$

in general does not necessarily imply

$$I(K(t)/n > 0)[K(t)/n]^{-1} \xrightarrow{P} I(k(t) > 0)[k(t)]^{-1}$$

over the interval where $k(t) = 0$. As a simple example to illustrate the issue, let $f_n(t)$ and $f(t)$ be functions on $[0,1]$ that are defined to be constants $1/n$ and 0, respectively, for $n = 1, \cdots$. Then $f_n(t)$ converges uniformly over $[0,1]$ to $f(t)$, yet

$$I(f_n(t) > 0) = 1 \neq 0 = I(f(t) > 0), \qquad t \in [0,1].$$

For weighted log-rank tests, some common choices of the weight Φ include the Gehan weight

$$\Phi(t) = \frac{1}{n} K(t),$$

and the $G^{\rho,\gamma}$ family of weights

$$\Phi(t) = S_{-}^{\rho}(t)\left[1 - S_{-}^{\gamma}(t)\right],$$

where S_{-} is the left limit version of the Kaplan-Meier estimator S based on the pooled sample. By (B.43) and Corollary B.1, these weights satisfy condition (c) of Theorem B.4. Therefore, the corresponding weighted log-rank statistics are asymptotically normal under H_0 as established by Theorem B.4. Note that the Gehan weight here is properly scaled with a factor $1/n$ compared with the form mentioned in Section 2.6.3.

B.12 Martingales and Covariation Processes in Trials with Staggered Entry

A significant technical challenge in survival data analysis is the presence of censoring. In the previous sections, it has been shown how applications of the martingale theory lead to simple mean, variance and covariance formulas for martingale integrals with predictable integrands.

In clinical trials, participants often enter the study in a staggered fashion. If statistical analysis is performed at a single time point, censoring due to loss to follow-up and administrative censoring can be combined, and results from previous sections apply. However, interim analysis requires joint distributions of test statistics at different calendar times. The staggered entry phenomenon gives rise to an additional level of complexity.

In this section, we consider martingales relevant to interim monitoring. To simplify the presentation, We will only consider the two-sample problem described in Section 10.8, with the additional assumption that the survival functions S_C, S_T are continuous.

Let

$$\begin{aligned}
\widetilde{N}_i(t) &= I(T_i \le \widetilde{C}_i \wedge t), \quad 1 \le i \le n, \\
\widetilde{Y}_i(t) &= I(T_i \wedge \widetilde{C}_i \ge t), \quad 1 \le i \le n, \\
\widetilde{M}_i(t) &= \widetilde{N}_i(t) - \int_0^t \widetilde{Y}_i(s)\, d\Lambda(s; Z_i), \quad 1 \le i \le n, \qquad \text{(B.68)}
\end{aligned}$$

for $\Lambda(s;Z_i)$ in (10.53): $\Lambda(s;Z_i) = \left[Z_i\Lambda_T(s) + (1-Z_i)\Lambda_C(s)\right]$. Define

$$\widetilde{\mathscr{F}}_t = \sigma\left\{Z_i, \widetilde{N}_i(s), \widetilde{Y}_{i+}(s) : 0 \le s \le t, i = 1, \ldots, n\right\}. \tag{B.69}$$

From results in Sections B.8 and B.11, and Section 11.4, $\widetilde{M}_i(t)$ is a martingale with respect to $\{\widetilde{\mathscr{F}}_t : t \ge 0\}$, with covariation processes

$$\langle \widetilde{M}_i, \widetilde{M}_k\rangle(t) = I(i=k)\int_0^t \widetilde{Y}_i(s)d\Lambda(s;Z_i), \;\; i,k = 1,\ldots,n. \tag{B.70}$$

Now enlarge the σ-algebra $\widetilde{\mathscr{F}}_t$ by adding information on the trial starting times $\xi_1,\ldots,\xi_n$. This yields the σ-algebra

$$\mathscr{F}_t^* = \sigma\left\{\xi_i, Z_i, \widetilde{N}_i(s), \widetilde{Y}_{i+}(s) : 0 \le s \le t, i = 1, \ldots, n\right\}. \tag{B.71}$$

By the independence of ξ_i's from other variables, $\widetilde{M}_i(t)$ is also a martingale with respect to $\{\mathscr{F}_t^* : t \ge 0\}$, with the same covariation processes as in (B.70).

Let $H_j(t) = I\left((x_j - \xi_i)^+ \ge t\right)$. Then, for the processes $N_{i,j}(t)$ and $M_{i,j}(t)$ defined in (10.57) and (10.59), respectively, we have

$$\begin{aligned}
M_{i,j}(t) &= I\left(T_i \wedge \widetilde{C}_i \wedge (x_j - \xi_i)^+ \wedge t\right) \\
&\quad - \int_0^t I\left(T_i \wedge \widetilde{C}_i \wedge (x_j - \xi_i)^+ \ge s\right) d\Lambda(s;Z_i) \\
&= \widetilde{N}_i\left(t \wedge (x_j - \xi_i)^+\right) \\
&\quad - \int_0^t I\left((x_j - \xi_i)^+ \ge s\right)\widetilde{Y}_i(s) d\Lambda(s;Z_i) \\
&= \int_0^t H_j(s) d\widetilde{M}_i(s).
\end{aligned} \tag{B.72}$$

Since the left continuous $H_j(t)$ is predictable with respect to $\{\mathscr{F}_t^* : t \ge 0\}$, from results in Section B.7, $M_{i,j}(t)$ is a $\mathscr{F}_t^*$- martingale, with the covariation processes

$$\langle M_{i,j}, M_{i,\ell}\rangle(t) = \int_0^t H_j(s)H_\ell(s) d\langle \widetilde{M}_i, \widetilde{M}_k\rangle(s), j, \ell = 1, \ldots, J. \tag{B.73}$$

Note that $H_j(s)H_\ell(s) = H_j(s)$ for $j \le \ell$, and $K_j(t)$ and $K_{T,j}(t)$ in (10.55) are predictable with respect to $\{\mathscr{F}_t^* : t \ge 0\}$. Thus the process $\mathscr{M}_j(t)$ in (10.61) is an $\mathscr{F}_t^*$-

martingale with covariation processes

$$\begin{aligned}
\langle \mathcal{M}_j, \mathcal{M}_\ell \rangle(t) &= \sum_{i=1}^{n} \int_0^t \left[Z_i - \frac{K_{T,j}(s)}{K_j(s)} \right] \left[Z_i - \frac{K_{T,\ell}(s)}{K_\ell(s)} \right] d\langle M_{i,j}, M_{i,\ell} \rangle(s) \\
&= \sum_{i=1}^{n} \int_0^t \left[Z_i - \frac{K_{T,j}(s)}{K_j(s)} \right] \left[Z_i - \frac{K_{T,\ell}(s)}{K_\ell(s)} \right] \\
&\quad \cdot H_j(s) H_\ell(s) d\langle \widetilde{M}_i, \widetilde{M}_i \rangle(s) \\
&= \sum_{i=1}^{n} \int_0^t \left[Z_i - \frac{K_{T,j}(s)}{K_j(s)} \right] \left[Z_i - \frac{K_{T,\ell}(s)}{K_\ell(s)} \right] \\
&\quad \cdot I(X_{i,j} \geq s) d\Lambda(s; Z_i), \qquad \text{(B.74)}
\end{aligned}$$

for $j \leq \ell \leq J$, where $X_{i,j}$ is defined in (10.54). From this, with some algebra, we obtain

$$\begin{aligned}
\langle \mathcal{M}_j, \mathcal{M}_\ell \rangle(t) &= \int_0^t \frac{K_{C,j} K_{C,\ell}}{K_j K_\ell} K_{T,j} d\Lambda_T \\
&\quad + \int_0^t \frac{K_{T,j} K_{T,\ell}}{K_j K_\ell} K_{C,j} d\Lambda_C. \qquad \text{(B.75)}
\end{aligned}$$

C

Convergence of Random Functions

C.1 Introduction

Asymptotic analysis provides a rigorous framework for justifying large-sample properties of parameter estimators and test statistics. These properties serve as the basis for widely used approximations for statistical procedures, including confidence intervals and hypothesis testing. Often, asymptotic analysis involves random variables and vectors in R^k, as briefly reviewed in Section B.10. However, to address more challenging problems, it is necessary and often advantageous to analyze random functions in spaces more abstract and larger than R^k. Here a brief summary is provided for various concepts of convergence for these random functions and their applications in asymptotic analysis.

Classic books on these topics include Billingsley [24], Shorack and Wellner [279], and Pollard [242, 243]. More recent references include Van der Vaart and Wellner [310] and Kosorok [139], where the former provides a rigorous and comprehensive treatment of the topics and the latter gives a graduate textbook level presentation with applications to semiparametric inference. Also, the book by Van der Vaart [309] illustrates applications of empirical process methods to various statistical problems.

Convergence of stochastic processes and random functions is often studied using advanced results from probability theory and functional analysis, therefore grasping the definitions and understanding the results can be challenging. Moreover, there are different versions of the theory that emerged over decades of research progress.

This appendix aims to present a reader-friendly and up-to-date overview of the basic concepts and some commonly used results, with a focus on their applications to survival analysis. Therefore, older definitions, more technical terminologies, and less often used properties are omitted. The focus is primarily on the setup of i.i.d. observations, although results are available in the literature for independent but not identically distributed or even dependent observations.

For more properties and technical details, readers can refer to the more recent references [243, 310, 139].

DOI: 10.1201/9780429324437-C

After the overview of the empirical process theory in Sections C.1 through C.6, Section C.7 presents some general convergence results that are particularly useful in various applications to survival analysis.

C.2 Empirical Processes

To help understand the concepts and ideas, it is helpful to review the convergence definitions and related results in Section B.10 of Appendix B for random variables or vectors in $\mathbb{R}^k$, $k \geq 1$. It is also useful to look at a specific example. Let ξ_n be a sequence of i.i.d. uniform random variables on $[0,1]$ with common CDF $F(x) = x, 0 \leq x \leq 1$. Consider the empirical CDF

$$\tilde{F}_n(x) = \frac{1}{n}\sum_{i=1}^{n} I(\xi_i \leq x), \quad -\infty < x < \infty.$$

Let $G_n(x) = \sqrt{n}\left[\tilde{F}_n(x) - x\right]$. By the central limit theorem,

$$G_n(x) \xrightarrow{d} N\big(0, x(1-x)\big) \quad \text{for any } x \in [0,1], \tag{C.1}$$

where $N\big(0, x(1-x)\big)$ is the normal distribution with mean zero and variance $x(1-x)$.

When $\tilde{F}_n(x)$ is needed for multiple values of x, the multivariate central limit theorem strengthens (C.1) to

$$\big(G_n(x_1), \ldots, G_n(x_k)\big) \xrightarrow{d} N(0, V), \quad \text{for any } x_1, \ldots, x_k \in [0,1],\ k \geq 1, \tag{C.2}$$

where $N(0,V)$ denotes the k-variate normal distribution with mean vector zero and covariance matrix V whose (i,j)-element is $x_i \wedge x_j - x_i x_j$, $i, j = 1, \ldots, k$.

For goodness-of-fit test of the uniform distribution, we may need uniform convergence result for $\sup_x |G_n(x)|$, which involves behavior of $G_n(x)$ for x in the entire range $[0,1]$. To study such quantities, we need extensions of random vectors and associated convergence properties to a more abstract setting.

Recall that a random variable is a map from $(\Omega, \mathscr{F}, P)$ to $\mathbb{R}$ with the Borel σ-algebra $\mathscr{B}(\mathbb{R})$. More generally, a map η from $(\Omega, \mathscr{F}, P)$ to a measure space A can be considered. Suppose $\eta_1, \ldots, \eta_n$ are i.i.d. copies of η from $(\Omega, \mathscr{F}, P)$ to A, then the *empirical measure* $\mathbb{P}_n$ is defined by

$$\mathbb{P}_n(B) = \frac{1}{n}\sum_{i=1}^{n} I(\eta_i \in B) = \frac{\#\{i \leq n : \eta_i \in B\}}{n}, \tag{C.3}$$

For any measurable set B in A. For a measurable function $f : \mathsf{A} \mapsto \mathsf{R}$,

$$\int f d\mathbb{P}_n = \frac{1}{n}\sum_{i=1}^{n} f(\eta_i),$$

which is a random variable. For a simpler notation, $\int f d\mathbb{P}_n$ will be written $\mathbb{P}_n f$.

If F is a collection of functions from A to R, then a collection of random variables $\{\mathbb{P}_n f : f \in \mathsf{F}\}$ is obtained. Such a collection of random variables on a common probability space and indexed by a class of functions is called a stochastic process. This extends the definition of a stochastic process in Appendix B to a collection indexed by a class of functions. An *empirical process* is a stochastic process based on a sample, such as $\{\mathbb{P}_n f : f \in \mathsf{F}\}$.

Let $\mathbb{P} = P \circ \eta^{-1}$, the probability measure on A induced by η:

$$\mathbb{P}(B) = P(\eta \in B),$$

for a measurable set B. $\int f d\mathbb{P}$ will be abbreviated to $\mathbb{P}f$.

Assume that $\mathbb{P}f$ exists for any $f \in \mathsf{F}$. The centered and scaled empirical process $\mathbb{G}_n$, defined by

$$\mathbb{G}_n = \sqrt{n}(\mathbb{P}_n - \mathbb{P}), \tag{C.4}$$

is the focus of the empirical process theory. For each $f \in \mathsf{F}$,

$$\mathbb{G}_n f = \sqrt{n}(\mathbb{P}_n - \mathbb{P})f = \sqrt{n}\left[\frac{1}{n}\sum_{i=1}^{n} f(\eta_i) - \mathbb{P}f\right]. \tag{C.5}$$

When it is necessary to specify the index set, the collection of random variables $\{\mathbb{G}_n(f) : f \in \mathsf{F}\}$ is referred to as the empirical process indexed by F.

For a fixed $f \in \mathsf{F}$, by the law of large numbers and central limit theorem,

$$\begin{aligned} \mathbb{P}_n f &\to \mathbb{P}f \ a.s., \text{ if } \mathbb{P}f \text{ exists}, \\ \mathbb{G}_n f &\xrightarrow{d} N(0, \mathbb{P}(f - \mathbb{P}f)^2), \text{ if } \mathbb{P}f^2 < \infty, \end{aligned}$$

respectively. For various statistical analyses, it is necessary to establish uniform convergence results over $f \in \mathsf{F}$ in a certain sense. The precise statements and conditions required are the main objectives in this overview.

It is helpful to see how these definitions connect with the empirical CDF example. For $\mathsf{A} = [0,1]$ and $\eta_i = \xi_i, 1 \le i \le n$, the empirical measure is the probability measure corresponding to the empirical CDF $\tilde{F}_n(x)$. Furthermore, if $\mathsf{F} = \{f_t : t \in [0,1]\}$ where $f_t(x) = I(x \le t)$, then

$$\{\mathbb{G}_n(f) : f \in \mathsf{F}\} = \{G_n(x) : x \in [0,1]\}.$$

C.3 Weak Convergence in Metric Spaces

A *metric space* is a pair (D, d) where D is a set and d is a metric or distance function $\mathsf{D} \times \mathsf{D} \mapsto [0, \infty)$ satisfying

1. $d(x, y) = d(y, x)$ for any $x, y \in \mathsf{D}$;
2. $d(x, z) \leq d(x, y) + d(y, z)$ for any $x, y, z \in \mathsf{D}$;
3. $d(x, y) = 0$ if and only if $x = y$.

The metric space will be referred to as D when the metric d is clear from the context or is not emphasized. A semimetric on D satisfies all requirements of a metric except (3).

Examples of D include $D[0, 1]$, the collection of cadlag functions on $[0, 1]$, and $\ell^{\infty}(\mathsf{F})$, where F is the index set and $\ell^{\infty}(\mathsf{F})$ denotes the collection of all bounded functions $\mathsf{F} \mapsto \mathsf{R}$. For both $D[0, 1]$ and $\ell^{\infty}(\mathsf{F})$, the metric is the uniform metric:

$$d(x, y) = \sup_{t \in [0,1]} |x(t) - y(t)|$$

and

$$d(x, y) = \sup_{t \in \mathsf{F}} |x(t) - y(t)|,$$

respectively. Often the index set F itself is a metric or semimetric space. The two metric spaces $D[0, 1]$ and $\ell^{\infty}(\mathsf{F})$ may arguably be the two most frequently encountered in statistical applications.

For sets D_1, D_2, the product set is $\mathsf{D}_1 \times \mathsf{D}_2 = \{(x, y) : x \in \mathsf{D}_1, y \in \mathsf{D}_2\}$. For two metric spaces (D_1, d_1), (D_2, d_2), the product metric space is $\mathsf{D}_1 \times \mathsf{D}_2$ equipped with

$$d\big((x_1, y_1), x_2, y_2)\big) = \sqrt{d_1(x_1, x_2)^2 + d_2(y_1, y_2)^2}, \quad (x_i, y_i) \in \mathsf{D}_1 \times \mathsf{D}_2, i = 1, 2.$$

The definition can be extended to a product of more than two component metric spaces in an obvious way.

Some basic concepts related to a metric space are listed below.

1. The open ball about $a \in \mathsf{D}$ of radius r is the set $B_r(a) = \{x \in \mathsf{D} : d(a, x) < r\}$.
2. A subset $S \subset \mathsf{D}$ is an open set if, for any $a \in S$ there is a ball $B_r(a) \subset S$.
3. S is *totally bounded* if, for every $\epsilon > 0$, there exists a finite collection $\{x_1, \ldots, x_k\} \subset S$ such that $S \subset \bigcup_j B_\varepsilon(x_j)$.
4. A sequence in S is *Cauchy* if $d(x_n, x_m) \to 0$ as $n, m \to \infty$.
5. S is *complete* if every Cauchy sequence in S has a limit in S.

6. S is *compact* if it is complete and totally bounded.

7. A metric space is *separable* if it has a countable dense subset: there is a countable $A \subset \mathsf{D}$ such that any open subset of D contains at least one element of A.

8. A function f from D to R is continuous at a fixed $x \in \mathsf{D}$ if, for any $\epsilon > 0$ there exists a $\delta > 0$ such that $|f(x) - f(y)| < \epsilon$ when $d(x, y) < \delta$. Note that δ here depends on ϵ and the fixed x.

9. f is *continuous* if it is continuous at all $x \in \mathsf{D}$.

10. f is *uniformly continuous* if, for any $\epsilon > 0$ there exists a $\delta > 0$ such that $|f(x) - f(y)| < \epsilon$ whenever $d(x, y) < \delta$, $x, y \in \mathsf{D}$.

A subset $C \subset \mathsf{D}$ is *separable* if (C, d) is a separable metric space. Compactness and total boundedness of a subset $S \subset \mathsf{D}$ can be defined analogously. These and the continuity definitions can also be extended to a semimetric space.

The Borel σ-algebra $\mathscr{B}(\mathsf{D})$ on (D, d) is the σ-algebra generated by all open sets in (D, d). A map from Ω to a metric space (D, d) is called a *random element* if it is Borel measurable. A random element X or its induced probability measure $\mathsf{P} = PX^{-1}$ on D is *separable* if $P(X \in C) = 1$ for a separable $C \subset \mathsf{D}$.

Let

$$C_b(\mathsf{D}) = \{f \mid f : \mathsf{D} \mapsto \mathsf{R},\ f \text{ is bounded and continuous}\}.$$

Then weak convergence of random elements can be defined using property #6 in Section B.10: A sequence of random elements X_n *converges weakly* to the random element X if

$$Ef(X_n) \to Ef(X) \text{ for any } f \in C_b(\mathsf{D}).$$

In measure theory, although measurability of a function or set is usually required, it may not draw much attention since non-measurable sets or functions only occur in very pathological examples. However, as illustrated by Billingsley [24, pp. 152–153], some simple maps such as the empirical CDF may not be Borel measurable in the metric space $D[0,1]$. If X is not Borel measurable, then $f(X)$ may not be measurable and $Ef(X)$ may not be defined.

To extend weak convergence definition to arbitrary maps, the first step is to define outer expectation. Let $H : \Omega \mapsto [-\infty, \infty]$, which is not necessarily Borel measurable. The outer expectation is

$$E^* H = \inf\{EU \mid U : \Omega \mapsto \mathsf{R} \text{ measurable},\ U \geq H,\ EU \text{ exists}\},$$

where EU can be $-\infty$ or ∞. Similarly, the outer probability $P^*(A)$ for a possibly non-measurable set A is

$$P^*(A) = \inf\{P(B) : A \subset B \subset \Omega, B \text{ measurable}\}.$$

The companion inner probability $P_*(A)$ is

$$P_*(A) = 1 - P^*(A^c),$$

where A^c is the complement of A. It can be shown that

$$P^*\left(\bigcup_{k=1}^{K} A_k\right) \le \sum_{k=1}^{K} P^*(A_k)$$

for a finite K.

Note that E^* and P^* reduce to the usual expectation and probability when the map or the set is measurable.

Now a sequence of random maps $X_n : \Omega_n \mapsto \mathsf{D}$ is said to *converge weakly* to a random element X in D if

$$E^* f(X_n) \to Ef(X) \text{ for any } f \in C_b(\mathsf{D}). \tag{C.6}$$

Such convergence is denoted by $X_n \rightsquigarrow X$. If P_n and P are the probability measure induced by X_n and X, respectively, the weak convergence is equivalently denoted by $\mathsf{P}_n \rightsquigarrow \mathsf{P}$ or $X_n \rightsquigarrow \mathsf{P}$. Weak convergence is also called convergence in distribution or convergence in law.

Note that the limit X must be a random element although X_n may not be. Also note that Ω_n depends on n, but dependence on n of E^* is suppressed. The notation of Ω_n implies that X_n and X may be defined on different probability spaces, but they all have the same range space D.

Let D, E be two metric spaces. Some important properties of weak convergence are given below.

1. If $\mathsf{D}_0 \subset \mathsf{D}$ and the two spaces have the same metric, and X_n, X as maps to D take values in D_0, then $X_n \rightsquigarrow X$ as maps in D_0 if and only if $X_n \rightsquigarrow X$ as maps in D.

2. (*Continuous mapping theorem*) Suppose $g : \mathsf{D} \mapsto \mathsf{E}$ is continuous at all points in $\mathsf{D}_0 \subset \mathsf{D}$ and X is a random element taking values in D_0. Then $X_n \rightsquigarrow X$ implies $g(X_n) \rightsquigarrow g(X)$.

3. (*Slutsky's theorem*) Suppose $X_n \rightsquigarrow X$ and X is separable, and $Y_n \rightsquigarrow c$. Then $(X_n, Y_n) \rightsquigarrow (X, c)$. From this and the continuous mapping theorem, it follows that

   (a) $X_n + Y_n \rightsquigarrow X + c$;

   (b) $Y_n \cdot X_n \rightsquigarrow c \cdot X$ if X_n and Y_n are R^k random vectors, where "$\cdot$" denotes the dot product of vectors.

   (c) $Y_n X_n \rightsquigarrow cX$ if c is a scalar.

A random element X in D is *tight* if, for any $\epsilon > 0$, there exists a compact set $K \subset$ D such that $P(X \in K) > 1 - \epsilon$. If X is tight, then it is separable. The two properties are the same if the metric space is complete.

A stochastic process Q indexed by F is *Gaussian* if the finite dimensional marginal distribution of $\big(Q(f_1), \ldots, Q(f_k)\big)$ is multivariate normal for any $\{f_1, \ldots, f_k\} \subset \mathsf{F}$, $k \geq 1$.

For a random element X in D and a class F of functions from D to R, suppose $\mathbb{P} = P \circ X^{-1}$ and $\mathbb{P}|f| = E|f(X)| < \infty$ for any $f \in \mathsf{F}$. Thus gives rise to a stochastic process $\{\mathbb{P}f : f \in \mathsf{F}\}$. X is Gaussian if this induced process is Gaussian.

Assume that $\mathbb{P}f^2 = Ef^2(X) < \infty$ for $f \in \mathsf{F}$. For $f,\ g \in \mathsf{F}$, define a semimetric on F by

$$\rho_{\mathbb{P}}(f, g) = \sqrt{Var\big[f(X) - g(X)\big]} = \sqrt{\mathbb{P}(f-g)^2 - \big[\mathbb{P}(f-g)\big]^2}. \tag{C.7}$$

For a random element X in $\ell^\infty(\mathsf{F})$, the following statements (a) and (b) are equivalent:

(a) X is tight.

(b) There exists a semimetric ρ such that (F, ρ) is totally bounded and almost all sample paths of X are in $UC(\mathsf{F}, \rho)$, the space of uniformly continuous functions from F to R under the semimetric ρ.

Furthermore, if X is a Gaussian random element in $\ell^\infty(\mathsf{F})$, then tightness of X is equivalent to F being totally bounded with the semimetric $\rho_{\mathbb{P}}$ and X having almost all sample paths in $UC(\mathsf{F}, \rho_{\mathbb{P}})$.

The following theorem is a fundamental result and various versions have been given including those in Pollard [243], Van der Vaart and Wellner [310] and Kosorok [139].

Theorem C.1. *A sequence of random maps $X_n : \Omega_n \mapsto \ell^\infty(\mathsf{F})$ converges weakly to a tight random element X in $\ell^\infty(\mathsf{F})$ if and only if*

1. $\big(X_n(f_1), \ldots, X_n(f_k)\big) \xrightarrow{d} \big(X(f_1), \ldots, X(f_k)\big)$ *for any integer k, and any* $\{f_1, \ldots, f_k\} \subset \mathsf{F}$*; and*

2. *There exists a semimetric ρ for which* F *is totally bounded and*

$$\lim_{\delta \downarrow} \limsup_n P^* \Big\{ \sup_{s,t \in \mathsf{F},\ \rho(s,t) < \delta} |X_n(s) - X_n(t)| > \varepsilon \Big\} = 0, \tag{C.8}$$

For any $\varepsilon > 0$.

Furthermore, if X_n converges weakly to a random element X in $\ell^\infty(\mathsf{F})$, and ρ is a semimetric making F *totally bounded, then (C.8) is equivalent to X having almost all sample paths in $UC(\mathsf{F}, \rho)$.*

C.4 Other Types of Convergence

Other convergence modes can also be defined. X_n converges *in probability* to X if

$$P^*\left[d(X_n, X) > \varepsilon\right] \to 0, \quad \text{for any } \varepsilon > 0,$$

Or equivalently, if

$$\limsup_n P^*\left[d(X_n, X) > \varepsilon\right] < \xi, \quad \text{for any } \varepsilon,\ \xi > 0.$$

This is denoted by $X_n \xrightarrow{P} X$. When X_n and Y_n are close to each other in the sense that $d(X_n, Y_n) \xrightarrow{P} 0$, for convenience X_n and Y_n are said to be *asymptotically equivalent* to each other. A sequence of random quantities A_n from Ω to R is said to be bounded in probability if, for any $\varepsilon > 0$, there exists a constant B such that

$$\limsup_n P^*\left[|A_n| > B\right] < \varepsilon.$$

Such a sequence of quantities will be denoted by $A_n = O_P(1)$.

X_n converges *outer almost surely* to X if there exists a sequence of random variables Δ_n such that

$$d(X_n, X) \le \Delta_n \text{ for all } n \text{ and } P\left(\limsup_n \Delta_n = 0\right) = 1.$$

This is denoted by $X_n \xrightarrow{as*} X$. Note that even if X_n, X are random elements, $d(X_n, X)$ may not be a random variable.

Assume that X is a random element and that c is a fixed element or "constant" in D. In the results below, c is also viewed as the probability measure assigning probability 1 to that fixed element. Relationships among the convergence concepts are very similar to those for random variables/vectors in Section B.10:

1. $X_n \xrightarrow{as*} X$ implies $X_n \xrightarrow{P} X$;
2. $X_n \xrightarrow{P} X$ implies $X_n \rightsquigarrow X$;
3. $X_n \xrightarrow{P} c$ if and only if $X_n \rightsquigarrow c$;
4. $X_n \xrightarrow{P} X$ if and only if each subsequence of X_n contains a further subsequence that converges to X outer almost surely.
5. if $X_n \rightsquigarrow X$ and $d(X_n, Y_n) \xrightarrow{P} 0$, then $Y_n \rightsquigarrow X$.
6. (*Almost sure representation*) Let $X_n : \Omega_n \mapsto$ D be a sequence of maps and X a Borel measurable and separable random element on D. If $X_n \rightsquigarrow X$, then there exists a probability space $(\widetilde{\Omega}, \widetilde{\mathcal{F}}, \widetilde{P})$, maps $\widetilde{X}_n : \widetilde{\Omega} \mapsto$ D and $\widetilde{X} : \widetilde{\Omega} \mapsto$ D such that

(a) $\widetilde{X}_n \xrightarrow{as*} \widetilde{X}$;

(b) $E^* f(\widetilde{X}_n) = E^* f(X_n)$, $n \geq 1$, and $E^* f(\widetilde{X}) = E^* f(X)$ for every bounded $f : \mathsf{D} \mapsto \mathsf{R}$.

7. (*Continuous mapping theorem*) Suppose $g : \mathsf{D} \mapsto \mathsf{E}$ is continuous on a Borel subset $\mathsf{D}_0 \subset \mathsf{D}$, X_n and X are maps taking values in D, and X is a random element with $P(X \in \mathsf{D}_0) = 1$. Then

   (a) $X_n \xrightarrow{as*} X$ implies $g(X_n) \xrightarrow{as*} g(X)$;

   (b) $X_n \xrightarrow{P} X$ implies $g(X_n) \xrightarrow{P} g(X)$;

C.5 Donsker and Glivenko-Cantelli Classes

Recall the empirical process $\mathbb{G}_n$ indexed by F in (C.5). Since the random variables $\eta_1, \ldots \eta_n$ in the definition of $\mathbb{G}_n$ are functions of $\omega \in \Omega$, $\mathbb{G}_n f$ is a function of (ω, f). Assume that for any $x \in \mathsf{A}$,

$$\sup_{f \in \mathsf{F}} |f(x) - \mathbb{P} f| < \infty, \tag{C.9}$$

Then for each ω, as f varies over F, $\mathbb{G}_n$ is a bounded function from F to R. That is, the sample paths of $\mathbb{G}_n$ are in the space $\ell^\infty(\mathsf{F})$. A class F of measurable functions $f : \mathsf{A} \mapsto \mathsf{R}$ is *Donsker* if

$$\mathbb{G}_n \rightsquigarrow \mathbb{G} \ \text{ in } \ell^\infty(\mathsf{F}) \text{ for a tight random element } \mathbb{G}.$$

The Donsker property depends on the measure $\mathbb{P}$, thus it is can also be called "$\mathbb{P}$-Donsker" more precisely. By Theorem C.1, weak convergence implies finite-dimensional convergence in distribution. Since the limit of the finite-dimensional convergence of $\mathbb{G}_n$ is normal by the multivariate central limit theorem, the limit process is necessarily tight Gaussian for a Donsker class. From the previous results on tightness, F is totally bounded with the semimetric $\rho_{\mathbb{P}}$, and $\mathbb{G}$ has almost all sample paths in $UC(\mathsf{F}, \rho_{\mathbb{P}})$.

A class of functions F is $\mathbb{P}$-*Glivenko-Cantelli*, or Glivenko-Cantelli for short, if

$$\sup_{f \in \mathsf{F}} |\mathbb{P}_n f - \mathbb{P} f| \to 0,$$

in probability or outer almost surely. A Donsker class is a Glivenko-Cantelli class in probability by the Slutsky's theorem. Furthermore, A Donsker class is also a Glivenko-Cantelli class outer almost surely. Thus we will mainly present results for Donsker class here.

Theorem C.1 can be used to show that a particular class F is Donsker. This would in general involve heavy-duty tools from advanced stochastic process theory. Fortunately, there are some basic Donsker classes and also various properties that help build up new Donsker classes from existing or simpler ones.

A vector space is a set on which scalar multiplication and addition are defined with the usual arithmetic properties. A finite-dimensional vector space V is

$$V = \{a_1 v_1 + \cdots + a_k v_k : (a_1, \ldots, a_k) \in \mathsf{R}^k\}$$

for some fixed $v_1, \ldots, v_k$ and $k \geq 1$. Some commonly encountered Donsker classes are listed below:

1. a class of finitely many functions;
2. A subset of a Donsker class;
3. a bounded subset of a finite-dimensional vector space;
4. the class
$$BBV_K(A) = \left\{f : A \mapsto \mathsf{R} \mid \sup_{a \in A} |f(a)| + \bigvee(f) \leq K\right\}, \tag{C.10}$$
where $A \subset \mathsf{R}$ is an interval, $\bigvee(f)$ is the total variation of f on A, and $K > 0$ is a constant;
5. a monotone random process $X(t)$ on $[a, b]$ (as a class of functions when t varies over $[a, b]$), with $\mathbb{P}[X^2(a) + X^2(b)] < \infty$;
6. indicator functions for half-space
$$\{I(x \in \mathsf{R}^k : a_1 x_1 + \cdots + a_k x_k \leq c) \mid (a_1, \ldots, a_k)^{\mathrm{T}} \in \mathsf{R}^k, c \in \mathsf{R}\};$$
7. $\{f_\theta : \mathsf{X} \mapsto \mathsf{R} \mid \theta \in \boldsymbol{T}\}$, where $\boldsymbol{T} \subset \mathsf{R}^k$ is bounded and
$$|f_{\theta_1}(x) - f_{\theta_2}(x)| \leq m(x) \|\theta_1 - \theta_2\|_0^\tau$$
with $\mathbb{P}m^2 < \infty$ for some m;
8. $\phi \circ \mathsf{F}$ for $\mathsf{F} = \mathsf{F}_1 \times \cdots \times \mathsf{F}_k$, defined as the class $\{\phi(f) : f = (f_1, \ldots, f_k) \in \mathsf{F}_1 \times \cdots \times \mathsf{F}_k\}$, where $\sup_j \sup_{f \in \mathsf{F}_j} |\mathbb{P}f| < \infty$, and ϕ satisfies
$$|\phi(f(x)) - \phi(g(x))| \leq K \sum_{i=1}^{k} |f_i(x) - g_i(x)|,$$
for all $f, g \in \mathsf{F}_1 \times \cdots \times \mathsf{F}_k$ and $x \in \mathsf{A}$ for some $K < \infty$, and $\mathbb{P}(\phi \circ f)^2 < \infty$ for at least one $f \in \mathsf{F}_1 \times \cdots \times \mathsf{F}_k$.

From this, it follows that if F, G are two Donsker classes with $\sup_{h \in \mathsf{F} \cup \mathsf{G}} |\mathbb{P}h| < \infty$, then the following classes are Donsker:

(a) $\mathsf{F} \vee \mathsf{G} = \{f \vee g : f \in \mathsf{F}, g \in \mathsf{G}\}$ where $\vee$ denotes maximum;

(b) $\mathsf{F} \wedge \mathsf{G} = \{f \wedge g : f \in \mathsf{F}, g \in \mathsf{G}\}$ where $\wedge$ denotes minimum;

(c) $\mathsf{F} + \mathsf{G} = \{f + g : f \in \mathsf{F}, g \in \mathsf{G}\}$;

(d) $\mathsf{FG} = \{fg : f \in \mathsf{F}, g \in \mathsf{G}\}$ if F, G are bounded.

An often used convergence result for Donsker class is that if F is $\mathbb{P}$-Donsker and a sequence f_n, $n = 1, \ldots,$ of random functions taking values in F is such that

$$\rho_{\mathbb{P}}(f_n, f_0) \xrightarrow{P} 0$$

with $\rho_{\mathbb{P}}$ in (C.7) and $\mathbb{P}f^2 < \infty$, then

$$\mathbb{G}_n(f_n - f_0) \xrightarrow{P} 0 \text{ and } \mathbb{G}_n f_n \rightsquigarrow \mathbb{G} f_0. \tag{C.11}$$

This follows from the uniform continuity of sample paths under $\rho_{\mathbb{P}}$.

C.6 Functional Delta Method

To describe the functional delta method, some basic concepts are needed. A normed space D is a vector space on which a norm is defined. A norm is a function $\|\cdot\| : \mathsf{D} \mapsto [0, \infty)$ satisfying

1. $\|x\| \geq 0$ for any $x \in \mathsf{D}$, and $\|x\| = 0$ implies $x = 0$;
2. $\|ax\| = |a|\|x\|$ for any $x \in \mathsf{D}$ and any real a;
3. $\|x + y\| \leq \|x\| + \|y\|$ for any $x, y \in \mathsf{D}$.

A normed space is also a metric space with $d(x, y) = \|x - y\|$.

A linear operator $T : \mathsf{D} \mapsto \mathbb{E}$ between two normed spaces is a map satisfying $T(ax + by) = aT(x) + bT(y)$. For brevity $T(x)$ will be denoted by Tx. When $\mathbb{E} = \mathsf{R}$, T is called a linear functional. T is a bounded linear operator if

$$\sup_{x \in \mathsf{D}, \|x\| \leq 1} \|Tx\| < \infty.$$

The supremum on the left above is denoted by $\|T\|$ and called the norm of T. Since a normed space is also a metric space with the norm induced metric, continuity of an operator is defined.

The following are equivalent:

1. T is a bounded linear operator;

2. T is continuous at one point $x_0 \in \mathsf{D}$;

3. T is continuous at all points of D.

A function $\phi : \mathsf{D}_\phi \subset \mathsf{D} \mapsto \mathsf{E}$ is *Hadamard differentiable* at $a \in \mathsf{D}_\phi$, tangentially to $\mathsf{D}_0 \subset \mathsf{D}$ if there is a continuous linear operator $\phi'_a : \mathsf{D}_0 \mapsto \mathsf{E}$ such that

$$\lim_n \frac{\phi(a + t_n h_n) - \phi(a)}{t_n} = \phi'_a(h),$$

for any scalar sequence $t_n \to 0$ and any $h_n \to h \in \mathsf{D}_0$, where $h_n \in \mathsf{D}$ and $a + t_n h_n \in \mathsf{D}_\phi$, $n \geq 1$. There is a functional delta method that extends the ordinary delta method to more abstract spaces.

Functional Delta Method. Suppose that

1. D, E are two normed spaces;

2. $\phi : \mathsf{D}_\phi \subset \mathsf{D} \mapsto \mathsf{E}$ is Hadamard differentiable at $a \in \mathsf{D}_\phi$, tangentially to $\mathsf{D}_0 \subset \mathsf{D}$;

3. $\sqrt{n}(X_n - a) \rightsquigarrow X$ where X_n takes values in D_ϕ and X is a tight process taking values in D_0.

Then

$$\sqrt{n}\left[\phi(X_n) - \phi(a)\right] \rightsquigarrow \phi'_a(X).$$

In addition, if $\mathsf{D}_0 = \mathsf{D}$, then

$$\sqrt{n}\left[\phi(X_n) - \phi(a)\right] - \phi'_a\left(\sqrt{n}(X_n - a)\right) \xrightarrow{P} 0.$$

The scaling factor $\sqrt{n}$ in the theorem can be replaced by a more general $r_n \to \infty$, but $\sqrt{n}$ is the appropriate one in almost all applications due to its connection with the usual central limit theorem.

C.7 Applications to Survival Analysis

In survival analysis, martingale integrals are frequently encountered. The martingale central limit theorem is the most widely used tool for traditional asymptotic analysis of these integrals. This approach requires that the integrands are predictable and the time-to-event variables have continuous distributions. When either condition fails, asymptotic results can be obtained using empirical process theory.

In asymptotic analysis, sequences of processes on an interval are often encountered. A nicely behaved sequence is typically one that exhibits uniform convergence in some sense. Often, additional conditions on total variations are also necessary. For clarity and easy reference, we will define below some classes of functions and sequence of processes.

For any function f on $[0,\tau]$, where $\tau > 0$ is a fixed point, recall the notation

$$\|f\|_0^\tau = \sup_{t\in[0,\tau]} |f(t)|$$

and the class $BBV_K([0,\tau])$ from (C.10). Note that

$$\begin{aligned} & \bigcup_{K=1}^{\infty} BBV_K([0,\tau]) \\ = & \left\{f : [0,\tau] \mapsto \mathrm{R} \mid \|f\|_0^\tau + \bigvee_0^\tau (f) < \infty\right\} \\ = & \left\{f : [0,\tau] \mapsto \mathrm{R} \mid \bigvee_0^\tau (f) < \infty\right\}, \end{aligned}$$

which will be denoted by $BV([0,\tau])$.

For a sequence of random functions A_n on $[0,\tau]$, let us call it *regularly convergent* if

$$\bigvee_0^\tau (A_n) = O_p(1) \text{ and } \|A_n - A_0\|_0^\tau \xrightarrow{P} 0, \tag{C.12}$$

with $A_0 \in BV([0,\tau])$. Note that there are no continuity or cadlag/caglad assumptions on A_n and A_0. Proposition C.1 below provide some useful properties for regularly convergent sequences.

Proposition C. 1. *Let $A_n(t)$ and $B_n(t)$ be two regularly convergent sequences of processes on $[0,\tau]$ for some $\tau < \infty$. Then new regularly convergent sequences can be obtained:*

(a) $A_n(t)B_n(t)$ and $A_n(t)+B_n(t)$;

(b) $J_n(t)/A_n(t)$, if $|A_0(t)| \geq c_0$ on $[0,\tau]$ for some $c_0 > 0$, where $J_n(t) = I(A_n(t) \neq 0)$.

(c) $\int_0^t A_n dB_n$, if B_n is cadlag, A_n either is cadlag or satisfies condition (b) in Proposition B.2.

Proof. (a) For $A_n(t)B_n(t)$, since $\|A_n\|_0^\tau$ and $\|B_n\|_0^\tau$ are both bounded in probability due to their convergence, we have

$$\begin{aligned} & \|A_nB_n - A_0B_0\|_0^\tau \\ = \; & \|(A_n - A_0)B_n + A_0(B_n - B_0)\|_0^\tau \\ \le \; & \|B_n\|_0^\tau \cdot \|A_n - A_0)\|_0^\tau + \|A_0\|_0^\tau \cdot \|B_n - B_0)\|_0^\tau \xrightarrow{P} 0. \end{aligned}$$

In addition, $A_0B_0 \in BV([0,\tau])$ and

$$\bigvee_0^\tau (A_nB_n) \le \|A_n\|_0^\tau \cdot \bigvee_0^\tau (B_n) + \|B_n\|_0^\tau \cdot \bigvee_0^\tau (A_n) = O_p(1).$$

Thus A_nB_n is regularly convergent. The case for $A_n + B_n$ is similar and simpler.

(b) By the convergence of A_n,

$$\limsup_n P^*\left(\|A_n - A_0\|_0^\tau \ge c_0/2\right) = 0. \tag{C.13}$$

By the triangle inequality,

$$\begin{aligned} |A_n(t)| \; & \ge \; |A_0(t)| - |A_n(t) - A_0(t)| \\ & \ge \; |A_0(t)| - \|A_n - A_0\|_0^\tau \end{aligned}$$

Thus

$$v_n \ge c_0 - \|A_n - A_0\|_0^\tau, \tag{C.14}$$

where $v_n = \inf_{t \in [0,\tau]} |(A_n(t)|$.

On $v_n > c$ for a constant $c > 0$,

$$\left|\frac{J_n(y)}{A_n(y)} - \frac{J_n(x)}{A_n(x)}\right| = \frac{|A_n(y) - A_n(x)|}{|A_n(y)A_n(x)|} \le \frac{|A_n(y) - A_n(x)|}{c^2}, \qquad x, y \in [0,\tau].$$

Thus on $v_n > c$,

$$\bigvee_0^\tau \left(\frac{J_n}{A_n}\right) \le c^{-2} \bigvee_0^\tau (A_n).$$

For any $\varepsilon > 0$, there exists a $\Gamma_0 >$ such that

$$\limsup_n P^*\left((c_0/2)^{-2} \bigvee_0^\tau (A_n) > \Gamma_0\right) < \varepsilon. \tag{C.15}$$

For the total variation of J_n/A_n, we have

$$\begin{aligned}
& P^*\Big(\bigvee_0^\tau\Big(\frac{J_n}{A_n}\Big) > \Gamma_0\Big) \\
\le\ & P^*\Big(\bigvee_0^\tau\Big(\frac{J_n}{A_n}\Big) > \Gamma_0, \nu_n > c\Big) + P^*\Big(\bigvee_0^\tau\Big(\frac{J_n}{A_n}\Big) > \Gamma_0, \nu_n \le c\Big) \\
\le\ & P^*\Big(c^{-2}\bigvee_0^\tau(A_n) > \Gamma_0, \nu_n > c\Big) + P^*\Big(\nu_n \le c\Big) \\
\le\ & P^*\Big(c^{-2}\bigvee_0^\tau(A_n) > \Gamma_0\Big) + P^*\Big(c_0 - \|A_n - A_0\|_0^\tau \le c\Big) \\
=\ & P^*\Big(c^{-2}\bigvee_0^\tau(A_n) > \Gamma_0\Big) + P^*\Big(\|A_n - A_0\|_0^\tau \ge c_0 - c\Big),
\end{aligned}$$

where (C.14) has been used to obtain the last inequality. Thus, with $c = c_0/2$, by (C.13) and (C.15),

$$\begin{aligned}
& \limsup_n P^*\Big(\bigvee_0^\tau\Big(\frac{J_n}{A_n}\Big) > \Gamma_0\Big) \\
\le\ & \limsup_n P^*\Big((c_0/2)^{-2}\bigvee_0^\tau(A_n) > \Gamma_0\Big) + \limsup_n P^*\Big(\|A_n - A_0\|_0^\tau \ge c_0/2\Big) \\
<\ & \varepsilon + 0.
\end{aligned}$$

Therefore,

$$\bigvee_0^\tau\Big(\frac{J_n}{A_n}\Big) = O_p(1).$$

A similar argument shows that

$$\Big\|\frac{J_n}{A_n} - \frac{1}{A_0}\Big\|_0^\tau \xrightarrow{P} 0$$

and that $1/A_0 \in BV([0,\tau])$. Thus the assertion is proved.

(c) This result follows from Proposition B.2 and an argument analogous to case (a) above. Note that the limit of a uniformly convergent sequence of cadlag functions is also cadlag. □

Throughout this book, particularly in Chapters Two, Five through Seven, and Eleven, integrals with respect to martingales are frequently encountered and studied, such as in the analysis of Nelson-Aalen estimators, Kaplan-Meier estimators, weighted log-rank tests, the Cox multiplicative models, and the model of short-term and long-term hazard ratios. To rigorously justify the asymptotic results, demonstrate the empirical process approach for asymptotic analysis, and present a general convergence result useful for various applications, we establish a weak convergence result for martingale integrals. For simplicity, we focus on the one-sample case, though the results and proofs can be adapted to two-sample and regression settings.

Assume that the pairs $(T_1, C_1), \ldots, (T_n, C_n)$, are i.i.d. copies of (T, C), where T, C are independent random variables representing time to event and time to censoring, respectively. The observed data are i.i.d. copies $\eta_i = (X_i,\ \delta_i), i = 1, \ldots, n$, of $\eta = (X,\ \delta)$, where

$$X_i = T_i \wedge C_i,\ \delta_i = I(X_i = T_i),\ 1 \le i \le n, \quad \text{and} \quad X = T \wedge C,\ \delta = I(X = T).$$

Note this is simply the random censorship model with i.i.d. censoring variables. Let F and G be The CDFs of T and C, respectively, and Λ the cumulative hazard function corresponding to F. The martingale M_i associated with the ith individual is

$$M_i(t) = \delta_i I(X_i \le t) - \int_0^t I(X_i \ge x) d\Lambda(x), \qquad i = 1, \ldots, n. \tag{C.16}$$

Theorem C.2 below provides general conditions for weak convergence of integrals with respect to the martingales in (C.16) and consistency of an estimator for the limit covariance function.

Theorem C.2. *Assume that:*

1. *The data are from the i.i.d. random censorship model described above;*
2. $\tau > 0$ *is a fixed point such that* $F_-(\tau) < 1,\ G_-(\tau) < 1$;
3. Y_n *is a sequence of maps from a probability space to* $\ell^\infty[0, \tau]$, *defined by*

$$Y_n(t) = n^{-1/2} \sum_{i=1}^n \int_0^t A_n(x) dM_i(x),$$

for a regularly convergent sequence A_n *with limit* A_0.

Then,

(a) Y_n *converges weakly to a Gaussian random element* Y *on* $\ell^\infty[0, \tau]$ *with mean zero and covariance*

$$\sigma(s, t) = \int_0^s A_0^2(x)[1 - G_-(x)][1 - \Delta\Lambda(x)] dF(x),\ 0 \le s \le t \le \tau. \tag{C.17}$$

(b) Suppose A_n *is obtained from finitely many operations of addition and multiplication from functions* $A_{nj},\ j = 1, \ldots, J$, *where for each* j, *the sequence* A_{nj}

is a regularly convergent sequence and either cadlag or caglad. Then

$$\sup_{s,t\in[0,\tau]} |\widehat{\sigma}(s,t)-\sigma(s,t)| \xrightarrow{P} 0, \tag{C.18}$$

where

$$\widehat{\sigma}(s,t) = \frac{1}{n}\int_0^s A_n^2(x)K(x)[1-\Delta\widehat{\Lambda}(x)]d\widehat{\Lambda}(x),\ 0\le s\le t\le\tau,$$

for the at-risk process $K(x)$ in (2.43) and the Nelson-Aalen estimator $\widehat{\Lambda}$ in (2.44).

For integrals of the type considered in Theorem C.2, several different approaches are possible using the empirical process theory. One option is to express the integrals as Hadamard differentiable functionals of basic empirical processes, as demonstrated for the special case of the Nelson-Aalen estimator by both Van der Vaart and Wellner [310] and Kosorok [139]. Another approach involves using the almost sure representation when the limiting process has continuous sample paths, as shown in Lin et al. [177] and Yang and Prentice [344].

A further option is to apply weak convergence of related processes along with an extended version of (C.11), as illustrated by Pollard [243], who considered the case of the Nelson-Aalen estimator with non-random constant censoring variables. The proof here follows a similar approach to that used by Pollard.

Proof of Theorem C.2. (a) For $A\in BV([0,\tau])$, define an associated function A^* by

$$A^*(t) = \int_0^t A(x)d\Lambda(x),\ t\in[0,\tau].$$

Define a class of functions $\mathsf{F} = \{f=(t,A): t\in[0,\tau], A\in BV([0,\tau])\}$, where

$$\begin{aligned} f(\eta_i) &= \int_0^t A(x)dM_i(x) \\ &= \delta_i I(X_i\le t)A(X_i) - A^*(X_i\wedge t). \end{aligned}$$

It can be verified that $\mathbb{P}f = Ef(\eta)=0$, thus the corresponding centered and scaled empirical process $\{\mathbb{G}_n(f): f\in\mathsf{F}\}$ is given by

$$\mathbb{G}_n(f) = n^{-1/2}\sum_{i=1}^n\int_0^t A(x)dM_i(x).$$

Note that each $\mathbb{G}_n(f)$ is well defined, but sample paths of the process may not be in $\ell^\infty(\mathsf{F})$.

Now for any B, consider a subset F_B of F defined by

$$\mathsf{F}_B = \{f = (t, A) : t \in [0, \tau], \|A\|_0^\tau + \bigvee_0^\tau (A) \le B\}.$$

Then, for $f \in \mathsf{F}_B$,

$$|f(\eta_i)| \le \|A\|_0^\tau \cdot [1 + \Lambda(\tau)] \le B[1 + \Lambda(\tau)].$$

Thus $\{\mathbb{G}_n(f) : f \in \mathsf{F}_B\}$ is a sequence of random maps in $\ell^\infty(\mathsf{F}_B)$. Note that for these maps,

$$f(\eta_i) = \delta_i I(X_i \le t) A(X_i) - I(X_i \le t) A^*(X_i) - I(X_i > t) A^*(t),$$

and

$$\|A^*\|_0^\tau + \bigvee_0^\tau (A^*) \le 2\Lambda(\tau)\|A\|_0^\tau \le 2B\Lambda(\tau).$$

Therefore, by properties #1 and #4 in Section C.5, $f(\eta_i)$ is obtained from bounded Donsker classes through additions and multiplications (note that $\{A^*(t)\}$ is a bounded class of constants and thus a degenerate Donsker class). From properties #8(c) and #8(d) in Section C.5, F_B is Donsker for $\{\mathbb{G}_n(f) : f \in \mathsf{F}_B\}$. The semimetric $\rho_{\mathbb{P}}$ in (C.7) is given by $\rho_{\mathbb{P}}^2(f_1, f_2) = \mathbb{P}(f_1 - f_2)^2$ for $f_j = (t_j, \kappa_j) \in \mathsf{F}_B, j = 1, 2$. In particular, for any $t \in [0, \tau]$,

$$\begin{aligned} &\rho_{\mathbb{P}}^2\big((t, \kappa_1), (t, \kappa_2)\big) \\ = \quad & Var\Big(\int_0^t [\kappa_1(x) - \kappa_2(x)] dM_i(x)\Big) \\ = \quad & \int_0^t [\kappa_1(x) - \kappa_2(x)]^2 [1 - F_-(x)][1 - G_-(x)][1 - \Delta\Lambda(x)] d\Lambda(x) \\ \le \quad & \Big(\|\kappa_1 - \kappa_2\|_0^\tau\Big)^2, \end{aligned} \tag{C.19}$$

where the last equality follows from the fact that $\int_0^t [\kappa_1(x) - \kappa_2(x)] dM_i(x)$ is a martingale in t since $\kappa_1 - \kappa_2$ is deterministic and therefore predictable.

Next define a $\ell^\infty[0, \tau]$ process Y_n^0 by

$$Y_n^0(t) = n^{-1/2} \sum_{i=1}^n \int_0^t A_0(x) dM_i(x).$$

Intuitively, Y_n should be close to Y_n^0 due to the uniform convergence of A_n to A_0. We will make this precise by proving that

$$Y_n - Y_n^0 \xrightarrow{P} 0 \quad \text{in } \ell^\infty[0, \tau]. \tag{C.20}$$

That is, for any ε, $\xi > 0$,

$$\limsup_n P^*\left(\| Y_n - Y_n^0 \|_0^\tau > \varepsilon\right) < \xi.$$

By condition (C.12) for A_n, there exists a $B_0 > 0$ such that

$$\limsup_n P^*(\mathbb{A}^c) < \xi/2, \tag{C.21}$$

where $\mathbb{A}$ is a subset of the probability space Ω defined by

$$\mathbb{A} = \left\{ \| A_n \|_0^\tau + \bigvee_0^\tau (A_n) \le B_0 \right\}.$$

Let K_0 be a constant such that the limit A_0 of A_n satisfies

$$\| A_0 \|_0^\tau + \bigvee_0^\tau (A_0) \le K_0.$$

Then, on $\mathbb{A}$, (t, A_0) and any realization of (t, A_n) are all in $\mathsf{F}_{B_0+K_0}$. Since $\mathsf{F}_{B_0+K_0}$ is Donsker for $\{\mathbb{G}_n(f) : f \in \mathsf{F}_{B_0+K_0}\}$, by Theorem C.1 there exists a $v_0 > 0$ such that for any $v \le v_0$,

$$\limsup_n P^*\left\{ \sup_{a,b \in \mathsf{F}_{B_0+K_0},\ \rho_{\mathbb{P}}(a,b) < v} |\mathbb{G}_n(a) - \mathbb{G}_n(b)| > \varepsilon \right\} < \xi/2. \tag{C.22}$$

Now define a subset $\mathbb{B}$ of Ω by

$$\mathbb{B} = \left\{ \| A_n - A_0 \|_0^\tau < v_0 \right\}.$$

By condition (C.12) on A_n,

$$\limsup_n P^*(\mathbb{B}^c) = 0. \tag{C.23}$$

Note that

$$Y_n(t) - Y_n^0(t) = \mathbb{G}_n\big((t, A_n)\big) - \mathbb{G}_n\big((t, A_0)\big).$$

Furthermore, on $\mathbb{A} \cap \mathbb{B}$, sample paths of A_n are in $BBV_{B_0+K_0}([0,\tau])$, and

$\rho_{\mathbb{P}}\big((t,A_n),(t,A_0)\big) < \nu_0$ by (C.19). Thus from (C.21) through (C.23),

$$\begin{aligned}
&\limsup_n P^*\Big(\sup_{t\in[0,\tau]}|Y_n(t)-Y_n^0(t)|>\varepsilon\Big)\\
\le\ &\limsup_n P^*\Big(\sup_{t\in[0,\tau]}|Y_n(t)-Y_n^0(t)|>\epsilon,\mathbb{A}\cap\mathbb{B}\Big)\\
&+\limsup_n P^*\left(\mathbb{A}^c\right)+\limsup_n P^*\left(\mathbb{B}^c\right)\\
<\ &\limsup_n P^*\Big(\sup_{a,b\in \mathsf{F}_{B_0+K_0},\ \rho_{\mathbb{P}}(a,b)<\nu_0}|\mathbb{G}_n(a)-\mathbb{G}_n(b)|>\varepsilon,\mathbb{A}\cap\mathbb{B}\Big)+\xi/2+0\\
<\ &\xi. \qquad\qquad (C.24)
\end{aligned}$$

This proves (C.20).

Similar to the case for $\{\mathbb{G}_n f : f\in \mathsf{F}_B\}$, the class $\{t : t\in[0,\tau]\}$ can be shown to be Donsker for $\{Y_n^0(t) : t\in[0,\tau]\}$. Also, from Appendix B, $\{Y_n^0(t) : t\in[0,\tau]\}$ is a martingale with predictable variation process

$$\frac{1}{n}\sum_{i=1}^{n}\int_0^t A^2(x)I(X_i\ge x)[1-\Delta\Lambda(x)]d\Lambda(x).$$

Thus the limit process Y of Y_n^0 is Gaussian with mean zero and covariance given by (C.17). This, combined with (C.20) and property #5 in Section C.4, implies the assertion in Theorem C.2 (a).

(b) By the uniform strong law of large numbers [243, Theorem 8.3],

$$\sup_{t\in[0,\tau]}\left|K(t)/n-(1-F_-(t))(1-G_-(t))\right|\to 0\ a.s. \qquad (C.25)$$

From this result, Proposition C.1, and the condition on τ, we can conclude that for J defined in (A.1), nJK^{-1} is regularly convergent on $[0,\tau]$.

Similarly to (C.25), for the function $H(t)$ in (2.43),

$$\sup_{t\in[0,\tau]}\left|H(t)/n-\int_0^t[1-G_-(x)]dF(x)\right|\to 0\quad a.s.$$

Thus the cadlag H/n is regularly convergent. Note that

$$\widehat{\Lambda}(t)=\int_0^t\frac{J(x)}{K(x)/n}d[H(x)/n],$$

and $\widehat{\Lambda}$ is increasing from $\widehat{\Lambda}(0)=0$. From Proposition C. 1, the cadlag $\widehat{\Lambda}$ is regularly convergent. Now the consistency follows from Proposition B.2, similar to the consistency proof for Theorem B.2. □

The proof uses martingale properties to derive (C.19) and the form (C.17) for the asymptotic covariance matrix. Without reference to martingales, it is simple to obtain an inequality similar to (C.19), using

$$
\begin{aligned}
& Var\Big(\int_0^t a(x)dM_i(x)\Big) \\
= \quad & Var\Big(\delta_i a(X_i)I(X_i \le t) - \int_0^t I(X_i \ge x)a(x)d\Lambda(x)\Big) \\
\le \quad & 2(\|a\|_0^\tau)^2[1+\Lambda^2(\tau)],
\end{aligned}
$$

for $t \in [0,\tau]$. Using this result instead of (C.19), the weak convergence can be established similarly. However, covariance calculation without utilizing the martingale property can be tedious.

To illustrate applications of Theorem C.2, consider the Nelson-Aalen estimator $\widehat{\Lambda}$ and the Kaplan-Meier estimator $\widehat{F}$ in (2.44) and (2.45), respectively. Corollary C.1 below establishes consistency and asymptotic normality of $\widehat{\Lambda}$ and $\widehat{F}$. Note that one of the conditions for $\widehat{\Lambda}$ is $F_-(\tau) < 1$, while the counterpart for $\widehat{F}$ is $F(\tau) < 1$, due to the factor $1 - F$ in the denominator.

Corollary C.1. *Assume that the observed data follow the i.i.d. random censorship model.*

(a) Suppose that τ is a fixed point such that $F_-(\tau) < 1$, $G_-(\tau) < 1$. Then, $\sqrt{n}(\widehat{\Lambda} - \Lambda)$ as a process on $[0,\tau]$ converges weakly to a Gaussian process with mean zero and covariance

$$\sigma_\Lambda(s,t) = \int_0^s \frac{[1-\Delta\Lambda(x)]d\Lambda(x)}{[1-F_-(x)][1-G_-(x)]} \quad 0 \le s \le t \le \tau. \tag{C.26}$$

Furthermore,

$$\sup_{s,t\in[0,\tau]} |\widehat{\sigma}_\Lambda(s,t) - \sigma_\Lambda(s,t)| \xrightarrow{P} 0,$$

where

$$\widehat{\sigma}_\Lambda(s,t) = \int_0^s \frac{n[1-\Delta\widehat{\Lambda}_n(x)]d\widehat{\Lambda}_n(x)}{K(x)}, \quad 0 \le s \le t \le \tau.$$

(b) Suppose that τ is a fixed point such that $F(\tau) < 1$, $G_-(\tau) < 1$. Then, $\sqrt{n}(\widehat{F} - F)$ as a process on $[0,\tau]$ converges weakly to a Gaussian process with mean zero and covariance

$$\sigma_F(s,t) = [1-F(s)][1-F(t)]\int_0^s \frac{[1-\Delta\Lambda(x)]d\Lambda(x)}{[1-F(x)][1-G_-(x)]} \quad 0 \le s \le t \le \tau. \tag{C.27}$$

Furthermore,

$$\sup_{s,t\in[0,\tau]} |\widehat{\sigma}_F(s,t) - \sigma_F(s,t)| \xrightarrow{P} 0,$$

where

$$\widehat{\sigma}_\Lambda(s,t) = [1-\widehat{F}(s)][1-\widehat{F}(t)]\int_0^s \frac{nd\widehat{\Lambda}_n(x)}{K(x)[1-\Delta\widehat{\Lambda}_n(x)]}, \qquad 0 \le s \le t \le \tau.$$

Proof. (a) From (B.33), on $\{\tau \le \max_i X_i\}$, for any $t \in [0,\tau]$,

$$\sqrt{n}[\widehat{\Lambda}(t) - \Lambda(t)] = \sqrt{n}\int_0^t \frac{JdM}{K} = n^{-1/2}\sum_{i=1}^n \int_0^t \frac{nJ}{K}dM_i \tag{C.28}$$

for J defined in (A.13). From the proof for part (b) of Theorem C.2, nJK^{-1} is regularly convergent on $[0,\tau]$. Therefore, by Theorem C.2, the last quantity in (C.28) converges weakly to a Gaussian process with mean zero and covariance in (C.26).

For any $\varepsilon > 0$,

$$\begin{aligned} &P\Big(\sup_{t\in[0,\tau]}\Big|\sqrt{n}[\widehat{\Lambda}(t) - \Lambda(t)] - n^{-1/2}\sum_{i=1}^n\int_0^t \frac{nJ}{K}dM_i\Big| > \varepsilon\Big) \\ \le\ & P\big(\tau > \max_i X_i\big) \\ &\to 0, \end{aligned}$$

by (B.34). That is,

$$\sqrt{n}[\widehat{\Lambda}(t) - \Lambda(t)] - n^{-1/2}\sum_{i=1}^n\int_0^t \frac{nJ}{K}dM_i \xrightarrow{P} 0 \quad \text{in } \ell^\infty[0,\tau].$$

Thus, the weak convergence result and the consistency of the variance estimator follow from Theorem C. 2.

(b) The uniform convergence of $\widehat{F}$ to F on $[0,\tau]$ is needed in the proof for weak convergence, and it has been is established in part (a) of Theorem B.2 using the Lenglart's inequality. Note that the conditional independence condition (B.15) is satisfied for the i.i.d. random censorship model. Here, we provide a proof of consistency without relying on the counting process and martingale setup.

From (A.14), for any $t \in [0,\tau]$,

$$\widehat{F}(t) - F(t) = S(t)\int_0^t \frac{1-\widehat{F}_-}{1-F}d(\widehat{\Lambda} - \Lambda) = S(t)A(t), \tag{C.29}$$

where

$$A(t) = \int_0^t (1 - \widehat{F}_-) dB$$

with

$$B(t) = \int_0^t \frac{1}{S} d(\widehat{\Lambda} - \Lambda).$$

Integrating by parts yields

$$A(t) = \left[1 - \widehat{F}(t)\right] B(t) + \int_0^t B d\widehat{F}.$$

Thus

$$\|A\|_0^\tau \leq 2\|B\|_0^\tau. \tag{C.30}$$

Since

$$\begin{aligned} B(t) &= \frac{\widehat{\Lambda}(t) - \Lambda(t)}{S(t)} - \int_0^t [\widehat{\Lambda}_- - \Lambda_-] d\frac{1}{S} \\ &= \frac{\widehat{\Lambda}(t) - \Lambda(t)}{S(t)} + \int_0^t [\widehat{\Lambda}_- - \Lambda_-] \frac{1}{SS_-} dS, \end{aligned}$$

we have

$$\|B\|_0^\tau \leq \frac{\|\widehat{\Lambda} - \Lambda\|_0^\tau}{S(\tau)} + \frac{\|\widehat{\Lambda} - \Lambda\|_0^\tau}{S(\tau)S_-(\tau)}.$$

Thus from the uniform consistency of $\widehat{\Lambda}$ on $[0,\tau]$ established in part (a) before,

$$\|B\|_0^\tau \xrightarrow{P} 0. \tag{C.31}$$

The uniform consistency of $\widehat{F}$ on $[0,\tau]$ follows from (C.29)–(C.31), thus $\widehat{F}_-$ is regularly convergent (define $\widehat{F}_-(0) = 0$).

On $\{\tau \leq \max_i X_i\}$,

$$\sqrt{n}\left[\widehat{F}(t) - F(t)\right] = [1 - F(t)]\sqrt{n} \int_0^t \frac{1 - \widehat{F}_-}{1 - F} \frac{J}{K} dM = n^{-1/2} \sum_{i=1}^n \int_0^t \frac{1 - \widehat{F}_-}{1 - F} \frac{nJ}{K} dM_i.$$

The weak convergence of the last quantity follows from Theorem C.2.

Since $P\left(\tau > \max_i X_i\right) \to 0$, $\sqrt{n}\left[\widehat{F}(t) - F(t)\right]$ converges weakly to the same limit. Consistency of the variance estimator can be established similarly to the proofs of part (a) and Theorem B.2. □

The uniform consistency of $\widehat{\Lambda}$ on $[0,\tau]$ and the weak convergence of $\sqrt{n}\left[\widehat{\Lambda}(t) - \Lambda(t)\right]$ in $\ell^\infty[0,\tau]$ are established in the proof for part (b) of Theorem C.2 and in Corollary C.1, respectively, using the strong law of large numbers. These results can also be obtained with an alternative proof that does not rely on the strong law.

Let

$$\Phi_n(t) = K(t)/n - (1 - F_-(t))(1 - G_-(t)).$$

Note that $\{\sqrt{n}\Phi_n(t) : t \in [0,\tau]\}$ is a centered and scaled empirical process based on the sample $X_1, \cdots, X_n$, with the index set $\mathsf{F} = \{f_t : t \in [0,\tau]\}$, where $f_t(x) = I(x \geq t)$. By properties #4 and #2 in Section C.5, $\sqrt{n}\Phi_n(t)$ converges weakly in $\ell^\infty[0,\tau]$. Thus

$$\|\Phi_n\|_0^\tau \xrightarrow{P} 0.$$

Since $K(t)/n$ is monotone and takes values in $[0,1]$, it is regularly convergent. From the assumption (2) of Theorem C.2 and Proposition C.1, $nJ(t)/K(t)$ is also regularly convergent. Similarly, it can be shown that $H(t)/n$ is regularly convergent. It follows from Proposition C.1 that

$$\|\widehat{\Lambda}(t) - \Lambda(t)\|_0^\tau \xrightarrow{P} 0.$$

From the proof of Corollary C.1, the regular convergence of $nJ(t)/K(t)$ also yields the weak convergence of $\sqrt{n}[\widehat{\Lambda}(t) - \Lambda(t)]$ in $\ell^\infty[0,\tau]$.

Although this argument establishes uniform consistency and weak convergence without using the strong law of large numbers, an approach based on the latter can yield the strong uniform consistency of $\widehat{\Lambda}(t)$:

$$\|\widehat{\Lambda}(t) - \Lambda(t)\|_0^\tau \to 0, \ a.s.$$

Bibliography

[1] O. O. Aalen. Statistical inference for a family of counting processes. Ph. D. Thesis, University of California, Berkeley, 1975.

[2] O. O. Aalen. Nonparametric inference for a family of counting processes. *Annals of Statistics*, 6(4):701–726, 1978.

[3] O. O. Aalen. Discussion on the paper by Zeng and Lin. *Journal of the Royal Statistical Society: Series B*, 69:537–539, 2007.

[4] H. Akaike. A new look at the statistical model identification. *IEEE Transactions on Automatic Control*, 19:716–723, 1974.

[5] J. E. Andersen, T. A. Louis, N. V. Holm, and B. Harvald. Time-dependent association measures for bivariate survival distributions. *Journal of the American Statistical Association*, 87:641–650, 1992.

[6] P. K. Andersen. Comparing survival distributions via hazard ratio estimates. *Scand. J. Statist.*, 10:77–85, 1983.

[7] P. K. Andersen, O. Borgan, R. D. Gill, and N. Keiding. *Statistical Models Based on Counting Processes.* Springer-Verlag, 1993.

[8] P. K. Andersen and R. D. Gill. Cox's regression model for counting processes: a large sample study. *Annals of Statistics*, 10(4):1100–1120, 1982.

[9] R. B. Ash. *Real Analysis.* Academic Press, 1972.

[10] P. C. Austin and J. P. Fine. Practical recommendations for reporting Fine-Gray model analyses for competing risk data. *Statistics in Medicine*, 36:4391–4400, 2017.

[11] S. Axler. *Measure, Integration & Real Analysis.* Springer Nature, 2020.

[12] N. Balakrishnan and M. Kateri. On the maximum likelihood estimation of parameters of Weibull distribution based on complete and censored data. *Statistics and Probability Letters*, 78:2971–2975, 2008.

[13] T. A. Balan and H. Putter. A tutorial on frailty models. *Statistical Methods in Medical Research*, 29:3424–3454, 2020.

[14] H. Bang and A. A. Tsiatis. Median regression with censored cost data. *Biometrics*, 58:643–649, 2003.

[15] W. E. Barlow and R. L. Prentice. Residuals for relative risk regression. *Biometrika*, 75:65–74, 1988.

[16] A. Bathke, M. Kim, and M. Zhou. Combined multiple testing by censored empirical likelihood. *Journal of Statistical Planning and Inference*, 139:814–827, 2009.

[17] I. Bebu and J. M. Lachin. Large sample inference for a win ratio analysis of a composite outcome based on prioritized components. *Biostatistics*, 17:178–187, 2016.

[18] J. M. Begun and N. Reid. Estimating the relative risk with censored data. *Journal of the American Statistical Association*, 78:337–341, 1983.

[19] S. Bennett. Analysis of survival data by the proportional odds model. *Statistics in Medicine*, 2(2):273–277, 1983.

[20] R. Beran. Minimum Hellinger distance estimates for parametric models. *Annals of Statistics*, 5:445–463, 1977.

[21] P. J. Bickel, C. A. Klaassen, Y. Ritov, and J. A. Wellner. *Efficient and Adaptive Estimation for Semiparametric Models*. Baltimore: Johns Hopkins University Press, 1993.

[22] Y. Bilias, M. Gu, and Z. Ying. Towards a general asymptotic theory for Cox model with staggered entry. *Annals of Statistics*, 25:662–682, 1997.

[23] P. Billingsley. *Probability and Measure*. Wiley, 3rd edition, 1995.

[24] P. Billingsley. *Convergence of Probability Measures*. Wiley, 2nd edition, 1999.

[25] M. Bobbio, B. Demichelis, and G. Giustetto. Completeness of reporting trial results: effect on physicians' willingness to prescribe. *The Lancet*, 343:1209–1211, 1994.

[26] G. P. Box and D. R. Cox. An analysis of transformations (with discussion). *Journal of the Royal Statistical Society: Series B*, 26:211–252, 1964.

[27] N. E. Breslow and N. E. Day. *Statistical Methods in Cancer Research 2. The Design and Analysis of Cohort Studies*. LARC, Lyon, 1972.

[28] N. E. Breslow, L. Elder, and L. Berger. A two sample censored-data rank test for acceleration. *Biometrics*, 40:1042–1069, 1984.

[29] J. Buckley and I. James. Linear regression with censored data. *Biometrika*, 66(3):429–436, 1979.

[30] M. Buyse. Generalized pairwise comparisons of prioritized outcomes in the two-sample problem. *Statistics in Medicine*, 29:3245–3257, 2010.

[31] S. Buyske, R. Fagerstrom, and Z. Ying. A class of weighted log-rank tests for survival data when the event is rare. *Journal of the American Statistical Association*, 95(449):249–258, 2000.

[32] J. Cai and R. L. Prentice. Estimating equations for hazard ratio parameters based on correlated failure time data. *Biometrika*, 82:151–184, 1995.

[33] J. Cai and R. L. Prentice. Regression estimation using multivariate failure time data and a common baseline hazard function model. *Lifetime Data Analysis*, 3:197–213, 1997.

[34] J. Cai and D. E. Schaubel. Marginal means/rates models for multiple type recurrent event data. *Lifetime Data Analysis*, 10:121–138, 2004.

[35] T. Cai, L. J. Wei, and M. Wilcox. Semiparametric regression analysis for clustered failure time data. *Biometrika*, 87:867–878, 2000.

[36] A. Chan, A. Hrobjartsson, M. T. Haahr, P. C. Gotzsche, and D. G. Altman. Empirical evidence for selective reporting of outcomes in randomized trials: comparison of protocols to published articles. *Journal of the American Medical Association*, 291:2457–2465, 2004.

[37] A. Charles-Nelson, S. Katsahian, and C. Schramm. How to analyze and interpret recurrent events data in the presence of a terminal event: An application on readmission after colorectal cancer surgery. *Statistics in Medicine*, 38:3476–3502, 2019.

[38] K. Chen, Z. Jin, and Z. Ying. Semiparametric analysis of transformation models with censored data. *Biometrika*, 89:659–668, 2002.

[39] Y. Chen, K. Chen, and Z. Ying. Analysis of multivariate failure time data using marginal proportional hazards model. *Statistica Sinica*, 20:1025–1041, 2010.

[40] Y. Q. Chen and N. P. Jewell. On a class of semiparametric hazards regression models. *Biometrika*, 88:687–702, 2001.

[41] Y. Q. Chen and M. C. Wang. Analysis of accelerated hazards model. *Journal of the American Statistical Association*, 95:608–618, 2000.

[42] S. C. Cheng, L. J. Wei, and Z. Ying. Analysis of transformation models with censored data. *Biometrika*, 82:835–845, 1995.

[43] S. C. Choi, P. J. Smith, and D. P. Becker. Early decision in clinical trials when treatment differences are small. *Controlled Clinical Trials*, 6:280–288, 1985.

[44] D. Clayton. A model for association in bivariate life tables and its applications in epidemilogical studies of familial tendency in chronic disease incidence. *Biometrika*, 65:141–151, 1978.

[45] D. Clayton and J. Cuzick. The semi-parametric pareto model for regression analysis of survival times. *Proceedings of the 45th Session of the International Statistical Institute*, 23:1–18, 1985.

[46] L. X. Clegg, J. Cai, and P. K. Sen. A marginal mixed baseline hazards model for multivariate failure time data. *Biometrics*, 55:805–812, 1999.

[47] A. C. Cohen. Maximum likelihood estimation in the Weibull distribution based on complete and on censored samples. *Technometrics*, 7:579–588, 1965.

[48] R. J. Cook and J. F. Lawless. Marginal analysis of recurrent events and a terminating event. *Statistics in Medicine*, 16:911–924, 1997.

[49] R. J. Cook and J. F. Lawless. *Multistate Models for the Analysis of Life History Data*. Chapman & Hall/CRC, New York, 2018.

[50] S. R. Cosslett. Nonparametric maximum likelihood methods. *Handbook of Statistics*, 15:385–404, 1997.

[51] D. R. Cox. Regression models and life-tables. *Journal of the Royal Statistical Society. Ser B*, 34(2):187–220, 1972.

[52] D. R. Cox. Partial likelihood. *Biometrika*, 62:269–276, 1975.

[53] D. R. Cox and D. V. Hinkley. *Theoretical Statistics*. Chapman & Hall, 1974.

[54] D. R. Cox and D. Oakes. *Analysis of Survival Data*. Chapman & Hall, London, 1984.

[55] H. Cramér. *Mathematical Methods of Statistics*. Princeton Univ. Press, 1946.

[56] M. Crowder. *Classical Competing Risks*. Chapman & Hall, Boca Raton, 2001.

[57] J. Cuzick. Rank regression. *Annals of Statistics*, 16:1369–1389, 1988.

[58] D. M. Dabrowska and K. A. Doksum. Estimation and testing in the two-sample generalized odds-rate model. *Journal of the American Statistical Association*, 83:1–23, 1988.

[59] D. L. DeMets. Futility approaches to interim monitoring by data monitoring committees. *Clinical Trials*, 3:522–529, 2006.

[60] D. L. DeMets and K. K. G. Lan. Interim analysis: The alpha spending function approach. *Statistics in Medicine*, 13:1341–1352, 1994.

[61] G. Diao, A. N. Vidyashankar, S. Zohar, and S. Katsahian. Competing risks model with short-term and long-term covariate effects for cancer studies. *Statistics in Biosciences*, 13:142–159, 2021.

[62] G. Diao, D. Zeng, and S. Yang. Efficient semiparametric estimation of short-term and long-term hazard ratios with right-censored data. *Biometrics*, 69(4):840–849, 2013.

[63] A. Dmitrienko and M. D. Wang. Bayesian predictive approach to interim monitoring in clinical trials. *Statistics in Medicine*, 25:2178–2195, 2006.

[64] J. L. Doob. The limiting distributions of certain statistics. *Annals of Mathematical Statistics*, 6:160–169, 1935.

[65] J. L. Doob. *Stochastic Processes*. Wiley, 1953.

[66] L. Duchateau and P. Janssen. *The Frailty Model*. Springer, 2008.

[67] J. W. Eaton, D. Bateman, S. Hauberg, and R. Wehbring. GNU Octave: a high-level interactive language for numerical computations. https://docs.octave.org/octave.pdf Last accessed December 2024.

[68] B. Efron. The two sample problem with censored data. In *Proceedings of the Fifth Berkeley Symposium On Mathematical Statistics and Probability*, pages 831–853. Prentice-Hall, 1967.

[69] B. Efron. Prediction, estimation, and attribution. *Journal of the American Statistical Association*, 115(530):636–655, 2020.

[70] B. Efron and R. Tibshirani. *An Introduction to the Bootstrap*. Chapman & Hall/CRC, 1993.

[71] S. S. Ellenberg, T. R. Fleming, and D. L. DeMets. *Data Monitoring Committees in Clinical Trials: A Practical Perspective*. Willey, 2002.

[72] S. S. Emerson and T. R. Fleming. Symmetric group sequential test designs. *Biometrics*, 45:905–932, 1989.

[73] European Medicines Agency. Guideline on adjustment for baseline covariates in clinical trials. https://www.ema.europa.eu/en/documents/scientific-guideline/guideline-adjustment-baseline-covariates-clinical-trials_en.pdf. Last accessed May 2022.

[74] J. Fan, R. L. Prentice, and L. Hsu. A class of weighted dependence measures for bivariate failure time data. *Journal of the Royal Statistical Society Series B*, 62:181–190, 2000.

[75] W. Feller. On boundaries and lateral conditions for the Kolmogorov differential equations. *Annals of Mathematics*, 65:527–570, 1957.

[76] J. P. Fine and R. J. Gray. A proportional hazards model for the subdistribution of a competing risk. *Journal of the American Statistical Association*, 94:496–509, 1999.

[77] J. P. Fine, H. Jiang, and R. Chappell. On semi-competing risks data. *Biometrika*, 88:907–919, 2001.

[78] J. P. Fine, Z. Ying, and L. J. Wei. On the linear transformation model for censored data. *Biometrika*, 85:980–986, 1998.

[79] D. M. Finkelstein and D. A. Schoenfeld. Combining mortality and longitudinal measures in clinical trials. *Statistics in Medicine*, 18:1341–1354, 1999.

[80] L. D. Fisher and D. Y. Lin. Time-dependent covariates in the cox proportional-hazards regression model. *Annual Review of Public Health*, 20:145–157, 1999.

[81] T. Fleming and D. L. DeMets. Monitoring of clinical trials: Issues and recommendations. *Controlled Clinical Trials*, 14:183–197, 1993.

[82] T. R. Fleming and D. P. Harrington. *Counting Processes and Survival Analysis*. Wiley, 2nd edition, 2005.

[83] T. R. Fleming, D. P. Harrington, and M. O'Sullivan. Supremum versions of the log-rank and generalized Wilcoxon statistics. *Journal of the American Statistical Association*, 82:312–320, 1987.

[84] L. M. Friedman, C. D. Furberg, and D. L. DeMets. *Fundamentals Of Clinical Trials*. Springer, 4th edition, 2010.

[85] M. Fygenson and Y. Ritov. Monotone estimating equations for censored data. *Annals of Statistics*, 22:732–746, 1994.

[86] J. N. Gastwirth. The use of maximum efficiency robust tests in combining contingency tables and survival analysis. *Journal of the American Statistical Association*, 80:380–384, 1985.

[87] E. A. Gehan. A generalized Wilcoxon test for comparing arbitrarily singly-censored samples. *Biometrika*, 52:203–223, 1965.

[88] S. Geisser. On the curtailment of sampling. *Canadian Journal of Statistics*, 20:297–309, 1992.

[89] C. Genest, K. Ghoudi, and L. Rivest. A semiparametric estimation procedure of dependence parameters in multivariate families of distributions. *Biometrika*, 82:543–552, 1995.

[90] C. Genest and J. MacKay. The joy of Copulas: bivariate distributions with uniform marginals. *The American Statistician*, 40:280–283, 1986.

[91] C. Genest and L. Rivest. Statistical inference procedures for bivariate Archimedean Copulas. *Journal of the American Statistical Association*, 88:1034–1043, 1993.

[92] D. Ghosh and D. Y. Lin. Nonparametric analysis of recurrent events and death. *Biometrics*, 56:554–562, 2000.

[93] D. Ghosh and D. Y. Lin. Marginal regression models for recurrent and terminal events. *Statistica Sinica*, 12:663–688, 2002.

[94] D. Ghosh and D. Y. Lin. Semiparametric analysis of recurrent events data in the presence of dependent censoring. *Biometrics*, 59:877–885, 2003.

[95] R. D. Gill. *Counting Processes and Survival Analysis.* Mathematical Centre Tracts 124, Mathematisch Centrum, Amsterdam, 1980.

[96] R. D. Gill. Discussion of the papers by Helland and Kurtz. *Bulletin of the International Statistical Institute*, 50:239–243, 1983.

[97] R. D. Gill. Large sample behaviour of the product-limit estimator on the whole line. *Annals of Statistics*, 11:49–58, 1983.

[98] R. D. Gill. *Lectures on survival analysis.* Lectures on Probability Theory, Springer, 1994.

[99] R. D. Gill and S. Johansen. A survey of product-integration with a view toward application in survival analysis. *Annals of Statistics*, 18(4):1501–1555, 1990.

[100] R. D. Gill and M. Schumacher. A simple test of the proportional hazards assumption. *Biometrika*, 74(2):289–300, 1987.

[101] D. Glidden. A two-stage estimator for the dependence parameter for the Clayton- Oakes model. *Lifetime Data Analysis*, 6:141–156, 2000.

[102] B. Gompertz. On the nature of the function expressive of the law of human mortality. *Philosophical Transactions of the Royal Society (London)*, 115:513–583, 1825.

[103] G. Gong and F. J. Samaniego. Pseudo maximum likelihood estimation: theory and applications. *Annals of Statistics*, 9:861–869, 1981.

[104] R. J. Gray. A Class of K-sample tests for comparing the cumulative incidence of a competing risk. *Annals of Statistics*, 16:1141–1154, 1988.

[105] M. Greenwood. The natural duration of cancer. *Reports of Public Health and Related Subjects*, 33:1–26, 1926.

[106] Gastrointestinal Tumor Study Group. A comparison of combination chemotherapy and combined modality therapy for locally advanced gastric carcinoma. *Cancer*, 49:1771–1777, 1982.

[107] M. Gu and T. Lai. Weak convergence of time-sequential censored rank statistics with applications to sequential testing in clinical trials. *Annals of Statistics*, 19:1403–1433, 1991.

[108] J. A. Hanley and B. J. McNeil. The meaning and use of the area under a receiver operating characteristic (ROC) curve. *Radiology*, 143:29–36, 1982.

[109] D. P. Harrington and T. R. Fleming. A class of rank test procedures for censored survival data. *Biometrika*, 69:133–143, 1982.

[110] J. L. Haybittle. Repeated assessment of results in clinical trials of cancer treatment. *British Journal of Radiology*, 44:793–797, 1971.

[111] J. J. Heckman and B. E. Honore. The identifiability of the competing risks model. *Biometrika*, 76:325–330, 1989.

[112] I. S. Helland. Applications of central limit theorems for martingales with continuous time. *Bulletin of the International Statistical Institute*, 50:239–243, 1983.

[113] J. L. Hodges and E. L. Lehmann. Estimates of location based on rank tests. *Annals of Mathematical Statistics*, 34:598–611, 1963.

[114] R. V. Hogg, J. W. McKean, and A.T. Craig. *Introduction to Mathematical Statistics*. Pearson, 2019.

[115] P. Hougaard. A class of multivariate failure time distributions. *Biometrika*, 73:671–678, 1986 (Correction in 75: 395, 1988).

[116] P. Hougaard. Frailty models for survival data. *Lifetime Data Analysis*, 1:255–273, 1995.

[117] P. Hougaard. *Analysis of Multivariate Survival Data*. Springer-Verlag, New York, 2000.

[118] L. Hsu and R. L. Prentice. On assessing the strength of dependency between failure time variates. *Biometrika*, 83:491–506, 1996.

[119] C. Y. Huang and M. C. Wang. Joint modeling and estimation for recurrent event processes and failure time data. *Journal of the American Statistical Association*, 99:1153–1165, 2004.

[120] International Council for Harmonisation of Technical Requirements for Pharmaceuticals for Human Use. ICH Guidelines. https://www.ich.org/page/ich-guidelines. Last accessed May 2022.

[121] J. O. Irwin. The standard error of an estimate of expectational life. *Journal of Hygiene*, 47:188–189, 1949.

[122] M. Jacobsen. *Statistical Analysis of Counting Processes*. Lecture Notes in Statistics 12, Springer-Verlag, 1982.

[123] C. Jennison and B. W. Turnbull. *Group Sequential Methods with Applications to Clinical Trials*. Chapman & Hall/CRC, 1999.

[124] J. Jennison and B. W. Turnbull. Statistical approaches to interim monitoring of medical trials: a review and commentary. *Statistical Science*, 5:299–317, 1990.

[125] Z. Jin. M-estimation in regression models for censored data. *Journal of Statistical Planning and Inference*, 137:3894–3903, 2007.

[126] Z. Jin. Semiparametric accelerated failure time model for the analysis of right censored data. *Communications for Statistical Applications and Methods*, 23:467–478, 2016.

[127] Z. Jin, D. Y. Lin, L. J. Wei, and Z. Ying. Rank-based inference for the accelerated failure time model. *Biometrika*, 90:341–353, 2003.

[128] Z. Jin, D. Y. Lin, and Z. Ying. On least-squares regression with censored data. *Biometrika*, 93:147–161, 2006.

[129] N. L. Johnson and S. Kotz. *Distributions in Statistics: Continuous Univariate Distributions, Vol. 1*. Houghton Mifflin, Boston, 1970.

[130] J. D. Kalbfleisch and R. L. Prentice. Estimation of average hazard ratio. *Biometrika*, 68:105–112, 1981.

[131] J. D. Kalbfleisch and R. L. Prentice. *The Statistical Analysis of Failure Time Data*. Wiley, 2nd edition, 2002.

[132] E. L. Kaplan and P. Meier. Nonparametric estimation from incomplete observations. *Journal of the American Statistical Association*, 53(282):457–481, 1958.

[133] T. G. Karrison. Versatile tests for comparing survival curves based on weighted log-rank statistics. *The Stata Journal*, 16(3):678–690, 2016.

[134] Kay, R. A Markov model for analysing cancer markers and disease states in survival studies. *Biometrics*, 42:855–865, 1986.

[135] T. L. Kelley. *Crossroads in the Mind of Man: A Study of Differentiable Mental Abilities.* Stanford University Press, 1928.

[136] K. Kim and D. L. DeMets. Design and analysis of group sequential tests based on the type I error spending rate function. *Biometrika*, 74:149–154, 1987.

[137] M. T. Koller, H. Raatz, E. W. Steyerberg, and M. Wolbers. Competing risks and the clinical community: irrelevance or ignorance? *Statistics in Medicine*, 31:1089–1097, 2012.

[138] A. N. Kolmogrov and S. V. Fomin. *Introductory Real Analysis.* Dover Publications, Inc., 1970.

[139] M. R. Kosorok. *Introduction to Empirical Processes and Semiparametric Inference.* Springer Publishing Company, 2008.

[140] M. R. Kosorok, B. L. Lee, and J. P. Fine. Robust inference for univariate proportional hazards frailty regression models. *Annals of Statistics*, 32:1448–1491, 2004.

[141] M. R. Kosorok and C. Y. Lin. The versatility of function-indexed weighted log-rank statistics. *Journal of the American Statistical Association*, 94:320–332, 1999.

[142] H. Koul and T. DeWet. Minimum distance estimation in a linear regression model. *Annals of Statistics*, 11:921–932, 1983.

[143] H. Koul, V. Susarla, and J. Van Ryzin. Regression analysis with randomly right censored data. *Annals of Statistics*, 9(6):1276–1288, 1981.

[144] H. Koul and S. Yang. Minimum sample scale problem: Uncensored and censored data. In *Recent Developments in Statistics and Their Applications, Proceedings of the Ohio State-Korea University Conference, 1987*, pages 117–134. Seoul: Freedom Academy Publishing Company, 1989.

[145] J. M. Lachin. A review of methods for futility stopping based on conditional power. *Statistics in Medicine*, 24:2747–2764, 2005.

[146] J. M. Lachin and M. A. Foulkes. Evaluation of sample size and power for analyses of survival with allowance for nonuniform patient entry, losses to follow-up, noncompliance, and stratification. *Biometrics*, 42:507–519, 1986.

[147] Z. L. Lai and Z. Ying. Large sample theory of a modified Buckley-James estimator for regression analysis with censored data. *Annals of Statistics*, 19:1370–1402, 1991.

[148] Z. L. Lai and Z. Ying. Rank regression methods for left-truncated and right-censored data. *Annals of Statistics*, 19:531–556, 1991.

[149] E. Lakatos. Sample sizes based on the log-rank statistic in complex clinical trials. *Biometrics*, 44:229–241, 1988.

[150] K. K. G. Lan and D. L. DeMets. Discrete sequential boundaries for clinical trials. *Biometrika*, 70(3):659–663, 1983.

[151] K. K. G. Lan and D. L. DeMets. Changing frequency of interim analysis in sequential monitoring. *Biometrics*, 45:1017–1020, 1989.

[152] K. K. G. Lan and D. L. DeMets. Group sequential procedures: Calendar versus information time. *Statistics in Medicine*, 8:1191–1198, 1989.

[153] K. K. G. Lan, R. Simon, and M. Halperin. Stochastically curtailed tests in long-term clinical trials. *Communications in Statistics, Series C*, 1:207–219, 1982.

[154] B. Lau, S. R. Cole, and S. J. Gange. Competing risk regression models for epidemiologic data. *American Journal of Epidemiology*, 170:244–256, 2009.

[155] J. F. Lawless and C. Nadeau. Some simple robust methods for the analysis of recurrent events. *Technometrics*, 37:158–168, 1995.

[156] J. F. Lawless, C. Nadeau, and R. J. Cook. Analysis of mean and rate functions for recurrent events. In *Proc. 1st Seattle Symp. Biostatistics: Survival Analysis*, pages 37–49. Springer, New York, 1997.

[157] L. Le Cam. Locally asymptotically normal families of distributions. *University of California Publications in Statistics*, 3:37–98, 1960.

[158] L. Le Cam and G. L. Yang. *Asymptotics in Statistics: Some Basic Concepts.* Springer, 2000.

[159] E. W. Lee, L. J. Wei, and D. A. Amato. Cox-type regression analysis for large numbers of small groups of correlated failure time observations. *Survival Analysis: State of the Art*, Kluwer Academic Publishers, 237–247, 1992.

[160] E. W. Lee, L. J. Wei, and Z. Ying. Linear regression analysis for highly stratified failure time data. *Journal of the American Statistical Association*, 88:557–565, 1993.

[161] J. W. Lee. Some versatile tests based on the simultaneous use of weighted log-rank statistics. *Biometrics*, 52:721–725, 1996.

[162] J. W. Lee. On the versatility of the combination of weighted log-rank statistics. *Computational Statistics and Data Analysis*, 51:6557–6564, 2007.

[163] S.H. Lee and S. Yang. Checking the censored two-sample accelerated life model using integrated cumulative hazard difference. *Lifetime Data Analysis*, 13(3):371–380, 2007.

[164] E. L. Lehmann. The power of rank tests. *Annals of Mathematical Statistics*, 24:23–43, 1953.

[165] E. L. Lehmann. Robust estimation in analysis of variance. *Annals of Mathematical Statistics*, 34:957–966, 1963.

[166] E. Lenglart. Relation de domination entre deux processus. *Ann. Inst. Henri Poincaré*, 13:171–179, 1977.

[167] F. Leroy, J. Dauxois, and P. Tubert-Bitter. On the parametric maximum likelihood estimator for independent but non-identically distributed observations with application to truncated data. *Journal of Statistical Theory and Applications*, 15:96–107, 2016.

[168] Y. Li, R. L. Prentice, and X. Lin. Semiparametric maximum likelihood estimation in normal transformation models for bivariate survival data. *Biometrika*, 95:947–960, 2008.

[169] D. Y. Lin. Goodness-of-fit analysis for the Cox regression model based on a class of parameter estimators. *Journal of the American Statistical Association*, 86(415):725–728, 1991.

[170] D. Y. Lin. Cox regression analysis of multivariate failure time data: the marginal approach. *Statistics in Medicine*, 13:2233–2247, 1994.

[171] D. Y. Lin. Nonparametric inference for cumulative incidence functions in competing risks studies. *Statistics in Medicine*, 16:901–910, 1997.

[172] D. Y. Lin. Regression analysis of incomplete medical cost data. *Statistics in Medicine*, 22:1181–1200, 2003.

[173] D. Y. Lin. On the Breslow estimator. *Lifetime Data Analysis*, 13:471–480, 2007.

[174] D. Y. Lin, T. R. Fleming, and L. J. Wei. Confidence bands for the survival curves under the proportional hazards model. *Biometrika*, 81(1):73–81, 1994.

[175] D. Y. Lin, W. Sun, and Z. Ying. Nonparametric estimation of the gap time distributions for serial events with censored data. *Biometrika*, 86:59–70, 1999.

[176] D. Y. Lin and L. J. Wei. The robust inference for the Cox proportional hazards model. *Journal of the American Statistical Association*, 84:1074–1078, 1989.

[177] D. Y. Lin, L. J. Wei, I. Yang, and Z. Ying. Semiparametric regression for the mean and rate functions of recurrent events. *Journal of the Royal Statistical Society, Ser. B.*, 62:711–730, 2000.

[178] D. Y. Lin, L. J. Wei, and Z. Ying. Checking the cox model with cumulative sums of martingale-based residuals. *Biometrika*, 80(3):557–572, 1993.

[179] D. Y. Lin, L. J. Wei, and Z. Ying. Accelerated failure time model for counting processes. *Biometrika*, 85:605–618, 1998.

[180] D. Y. Lin, L. J. Wei, and Z. Ying. Semiparametric transformation models for point processes. *Journal of the American Statistical Association*, 96:620–628, 2001.

[181] D. Y. Lin, Q. Yao, and Z. Ying. A general theory on stochastic curtailment for censored survival data. *Journal of the American Statistical Association*, 94:510–521, 1999.

[182] D. Y. Lin and Z. Ying. A simple nonparametric estimator of the bivariate survival function under univariate censoring. *Biometrika*, 80:573–582, 1993.

[183] D. Y. Lin and Z. Ying. Semiparametric analysis of the additive risk model. *Biometrika*, 81:61–71, 1994.

[184] D. Y. Lin and Z. Ying. Semiparametric analysis of general additive-multiplicative intensity models for counting processes. *Annals of Statistics*, 23:1712–1734, 1995.

[185] D. Y. Lin and Z. Ying. Semiparametric inference for the accelerated life model with time-dependent covariates. *Journal of Statistical Planning and Inference*, 44:47–63, 1995.

[186] R. S. Lin, J. Lin, S. Roychoudhury, and et al. Alternative analysis methods for time to event endpoints under nonproportional hazards: a comparative analysis. *The Stata Journal*, 12:187–198, 2020.

[187] W. Lin. Agnostic notes on regression adjustments to experimental data: Reexamining Freedman's critique. *Annals of Applied Statistics*, 7:295–318, 2013.

[188] R. S. Liptser and A. N. Shiryayev. *Statistics of Random Processes I, General Theory.* Springer-Verlag, 1977.

[189] L. Liu, R. A. Wolfe, and X. Huang. Shared frailty models for recurrent events and a terminal event. *Biometrics*, 60:747–756, 2004.

[190] T. A. Louis. Non-parametric analysis of an accelerated failure time model. *Biometrika*, 68:381–390, 1981.

[191] X. Luo, J. Qiu, S. Bai, and H. Tian. Weighted win loss approach for analyzing prioritized outcomes. *Statistics in Medicine*, 36:2452–2465, 2017.

[192] X. Luo, M. C. Wang, and C. Huang. A comparison of various rate functions of a recurrent event process in the presence of a terminal event. *Statistical Methods in Medical Research*, 19:167–182, 2010.

[193] R. C. MacCallum, S. Zhang, K. J. Preacher, and D. D. Rucker. On the practice of dichotomization of quantitative variables. *Psychological Methods*, 7:19–40, 2002.

[194] W. M. Makeham. On the law of mortality and the construction of annuity tables. *Journal of the Institute of Actuaries (London)*, 8(6):301–310, 1860.

[195] N. Mantel. Evaluation of survival data and two new rank order statistics arising in its consideration. *Cancer Chemotherapy Reports*, 50(3):163–170, 1966.

[196] L. Mao. On the alternative hypotheses for the win ratio. *Biometrics*, 75:347–351, 2019.

[197] L. Mao. Nonparametric inference of general while-alive estimands for recurrent events. *Biometrics*, 79:1749–1760, 2023.

[198] L. Mao. On restricted mean time in favor of treatment. *Biometrics*, 79:61–72, 2023.

[199] L. Mao and D. Y. Lin. Semiparametric regression for the weighted composite endpoint of recurrent and terminal events. *Biostatistics*, 17:390–403, 2016.

[200] A. W. Marshall and I. Olkin. Families of multivariate distribution. *Journal of the American Statistical Association*, 83(445):834–841, 1988.

[201] A. J. McNeil and J. Nešlehová. Multivariate Archimedean copulas, d-monotone functions and l_1-norm symmetric distributions. *Annals of Statistics*, 37:3059–3097, 2009.

[202] K. McPherson. Sequential stopping rules in clinical trials. *Statistics in Medicine*, 9:595–600, 1990.

[203] P. Meier. Estimation of a distribution function from incomplete observations. *Perspectives in Statistics (J. Gani, ed.)*, pages 67–87. Academic, London, 1975.

[204] Meira-Machado, L. and de Uña-Álvarez, J. and Cadarso-Suárez, C. and Andersen, P. K. Multi-state models for the analysis of time-to-event data. *Statistical Methods in Medical Research*, 18:195–222, 2009.

[205] P. A. Meyer. A decomposition theorem for supermartingales. *Illinois Journal of Mathematics*, 6:193–205, 1962.

[206] P. A. Meyer. Decomposition of supermartingales: the uniqueness theorem. *Illinois Journal of Mathematics*, 7:1–17, 1963.

[207] R. Miller and J. Halpern. Regression with censored data. *Biometrika*, 69:521–531, 1982.

[208] M. Miloslavsky, S. Keles, M. J. Van Der Laan, and S. Butler. Recurrent events analysis in the presence of time-dependent covariates and dependent censoring. *Journal of the Royal Statistical Society, Ser. B*, 66:239–257, 2004.

[209] S. A. Murphy, A. J. Rossini, and A. W. van der Vaart. Maximal likelihood estimation in the proportional odds model. *Journal of the American Statistical Association*, 92:968–976, 1997.

[210] S. A. Murphy and A. W. van der Vaart. On profile likelihood. *Journal of the American Statistical Association*, 95:449–485, 2000.

[211] R. B. Nelsen. An introduction to copulas. In *Lecture Notes in Statistics*, volume 139. Springer-Verlag, 1999.

[212] W. Nelson. Theory and applications of hazard plotting for censored failure data. *Technometrics*, 14(4):945–966, 1972.

[213] D. Oakes. Bivariate survival models induced by frailties. *Journal of the American Statistical Association*, 84:487–493, 1989.

[214] D. Oakes. On the win-ratio statistic in clinical trials with multiple types of event. *Biometrika*, 103:742–745, 2016.

[215] P. C. O'Brien and T. R. Fleming. A multiple testing procedure for clinical trials. *Biometrics*, 35:549–556, 1979.

[216] W. J. Padgett and L. J. Wei. Estimation of the ratio of scale parameters in the two sample problem with arbitrary right censorship. *Biometrika*, 69:252–256, 1982.

[217] D. Pak and S. Yang. ClinicalTrialSummary: summary measures for clinical trials with survival outcomes. Version 1.1.1. https://cran.r-project.org/web/packages/ClinicalTrialSummary/index.html. Last accessed December 2024.

[218] D. Pak and S. Yang. EventWinRatios: event-specific win ratios for terminal and non-terminal events. Version 1.0.0. https://cran.r-project.org/web/packages/EventWinRatios/index.html. Last accessed December 2024.

[219] D. Pak and S. Yang. YPInterimTesting: interim monitoring using adaptively weighted log-rank test in clinical trials. Version 1.0.3. https://cran.r-project.org/web/packages/YPInterimTesting/index.html. Last accessed December 2024.

[220] D. Pak and S. Yang. YPmodelPhreg: the short-term and long-term hazard ratio model with proportional adjustment. Version 1.0.0. https://cran.r-project.org/web/packages/YPmodelPhreg/index.html. Last accessed December 2024.

[221] W. C. Parr and W. R. Schucany. Minimum distance and robust estimation. *Journal of the American Statistical Association*, 75:616–624, 1980.

[222] M. Paukner and R. Chappell. Window mean survival time. *Statistics in Medicine*, 40:5521–5533, 2021.

[223] L. Peng and J. P. Fine. Regression modeling of semicompeting risks data. *Biometrics*, 63:96–108, 2007.

[224] M. S. Pepe and J. Cai. Some graphical displays and marginal regression analyses for recurrent failure times and time dependent covariates. *Journal of the American Statistical Association*, 88:811–820, 1993.

[225] M. S. Pepe and T. R. Fleming. Weighted Kaplan-Meier statistics: A class of distance tests for censored survival data. *Biometrics*, 45:497–507, 1989.

[226] M. S. Pepe and M. Mori. Kaplan-Meier, marginal or conditional probability curves in summarizing competing risks failure time data? *Statistics in Medicine*, 12:737–751, 1993.

[227] J. Peron, P. Roy, B. Ozenne, and et al. The net chance of a longer survival as a patient-oriented measure of treatment benefit in randomized clinical trials. *JAMA Oncology*, 2(7):901–905, 2016.

[228] R. Peto and J. Peto. Asymptotically efficient rank invariant test procedures (with discussion). *Journal of the Royal Statistical Society. Ser A*, 135:185–206, 1972.

[229] R. Peto, M. C. Pike, P. Armitage, and et al. Design and analysis of randomized clinical trials requiring prolonged observation of each patient. I. Introduction and design. *British Journal of Cancer*, 34:586–612, 1976.

[230] A. N. Pettitt. Proportional odds models for survival data and estimates using ranks. *Journal of the Royal Statistical Society. Ser C*, 33:169–175, 1984.

[231] A. Philippou and G. Roussas. Asymptotic normality of the maximum likelihood estimate in the independent not identically distributed case. *Annals of the Institute of Statistical Mathematics*, 27:45–55, 1975.

[232] S. Piantadosi and C. L. Meinert, editors. *Principles and Practice of Clinical Trials*. Springer, Switzerland, 2022.

[233] M. Pintilie. *Competing Risks: A Practical Perspective*. Wiley, Chichester, 2006.

[234] B. Pitt, M. Pfeffer, S. Assmann, and et al. Spironolactone for heart failure with preserved ejection fraction. *The New England Journal of Medicine*, 370:1383–1392, 2014.

[235] S. J. Pocock. Group sequential methods in the design and analysis of clinical trials. *Biometrika*, 64:191–199, 1977.

[236] S. J. Pocock. *Clinical trials: a practical approach*. Wiley, Chichester, 1983.

[237] S. J. Pocock. Statistical and ethical issues in monitoring clinical trials. *Statistics in Medicine*, 12:1459–1469, 1993.

[238] S. J. Pocock, C. A. Ariti, T. J. Collier, and D. Wang. The win ratio: a new approach to the analysis of composite endpoints in clinical trials based on clinical priorities. *European Heart Journal*, 33(2):176–182, 2012.

[239] S. J. Pocock, T. C. Clayton, and G. W. Stone. Challenging issues in clinical trial design: part 4 of a 4-part series on statistics for clinical trials. *Journal of the American College of Cardiology*, 66:2886–2898, 2015.

[240] S. J. Pocock and Lubsen J. More on subgroup analyses in clinical trials. *The New England Journal of Medicine*, 358:2076, author reply 2076–2077, 2008.

[241] S. J. Pocock, McMurray J. J. V., and T. J. Collier. Statistical controversies in reporting of clinical trials. *Journal of the American College of Cardiology*, 66:2648–2662, 2015.

[242] D. Pollard. *Convergence of Stochastic Processes*. Springer-Verlag, 1984.

[243] D. Pollard. *Empirical Processes: Theory and Applications*. NSFCBMS Regional Conference Series in Probability and Statistics, Institute of Mathematical Statistics and American Statistical Association, 1990.

[244] J. L. Powell. Least absolute deviations estimation for the censored regression model. *Journal of Econometrics*, 25:303–325, 1984.

[245] R. L. Prentice. Linear rank tests with right censored data. *Biometrika*, 65:167–179, 1978.

[246] R. L. Prentice and J. Cai. Covariance and survivor function estimation using censored multivariate failure time data. *Biometrika*, 79:495–512, 1992.

[247] R. L. Prentice and L. Hsu. Regression on hazard ratios and cross ratios in multivariate failure time analysis. *Biometrika*, 84:349–363, 1997.

[248] R. L. Prentice, J. D. Kalbfleisch, A. V. Peterson Jr, N. Flournoy, V. T. Farewell, and N. E. Breslow. The analysis of failure times in the presence of competing risks. *Biometrics*, 34:541–554, 1978.

[249] R. L. Prentice, R. Langer, M.L. Stefanick, B. V. Howad, M. Pettinger, G. Anderson, D. Barad, D. Curb, J. Kotchen, L. Kuller, M. Limacher, J. Wacawski-Wende, and Women's Health Initiative Investigators. Combined postmenopausal hormone therapy and cardiovascular disease: toward resolving the discrepancy between observational studies and the women's health initiative clinical trial. *American Journal of Epidemiology*, 162(5):404–414, 2005.

[250] R. L. Prentice, M. Pettinger, and G. Anderson. Statistical issues arising in the Women's Health Initiative. *Biometrics*, 61:899–941, 2005.

[251] R. L. Prentice and S. G. Self. Asymptotic distribution theory for Cox-type regression models with general relative risk form. *Annals of Statistics*, 11:804–813, 1983.

[252] R. L. Prentice, B. J. Williams, and A. V. Peterson. On the regression analysis of multivariate failure time data. *Biometrika*, 68:373–379, 1981.

[253] M. A. Proschan, K. K. G. Lan, and J. Wittes. *Statistical Monitoring of Clinical Trials: A Unified Approach.* Springer, 2006.

[254] M.A. Proschan, D.A. Follmann, and M.A. Waclawiw. Effects of assumption violations on type I error rate in group sequential monitoring. *1131–1143*, 48, 1992.

[255] H. Putter, M. Fiocco, and R. B. Geskus. Tutorial in biostatistics: Competing risks and multi-state models. *Statistics in Medicine*, 26:2389–2430, 2007.

[256] H. Putter, J. van der Hage, G. H. de Bock, R. Elgalta, and C. J. H. van de Velde. Estimation and prediction in a multi-state model for breast cancer. *Biometrical Journal*, 48:366–380, 2006.

[257] C. R. Rao. Information and the accuracy attainable in the estimation of statistical parameters. *Bulletin of the Calcutta Mathematical Society*, 37:81–89, 1945.

[258] R. Rebolledo. Central limit theorem for local martingales. *Z Wahrsch Verw Gebiete*, 51:269–286, 1980.

[259] N. Reid. A conversation with Sir David Cox. *Statistical Science*, 9:439–455, 1994.

[260] J. J. Ren and M. Zhou. Full likelihood inferences in the Cox model: an empirical likelihood approach. *Annals of the Institute of Statistical Mathematics*, 63:1005–1018, 2011.

[261] Y. Ritov. Estimation in a linear regression model with censored data. *Annals of Statistics*, 18:303–328, 1990.

[262] D. Rizopoulos. *Joint Models for Longitudinal and Time-to-Event Data*. Chapman & Hall/CRC, 2012.

[263] J. M. Robins, A. Rotnitzky, and L. P. Zhao. Estimation of regression coefficients when some regressors are not always observed. *Journal of the American Statistical Association*, 89:846–866, 1994.

[264] J. M. Robins and A. A. Tsiatis. Semiparametric estimation of an accelerated failure time model with time-dependent covariates. *Biometrika*, 79:311–319, 1992.

[265] H. L. Royden and P. M. Fitzpatrick. *Real Analysis*. Prentice Hall, 4th edition, 2010.

[266] P. Royston, D. G. Altman, and W. Sauerbrei. Dichotomizing continuous predictors in multiple regression: a bad idea. *Statistics in Medicine*, 25:127–141, 2006.

[267] P. Royston and M. K. Parmar. The use of restricted mean survival time to estimate the treatment effect in randomized clinical trials when the proportional hazards assumption is in doubt. *Statistics in Medicine*, 30(19):2409–2421, 2011.

[268] W. Rudin. *Principles of Mathematical Analysis*. McGraw-Hill, 3rd edition, 1976.

[269] D. O. Scharfstein, A. A. Tsiatis, and P. B. Gilbert. Semiparametric efficient estimation in the generalized odds-rate class of regression models for right-censored time-to-event data. *Lifetime Data Analysis*, 4:355–391, 1998.

[270] D. E. Schaubel and J. Cai. Analysis of clustered recurrent event data with application to hospitalization rates among renal failure patients. *Biostatistics*, 6:404–419, 2005.

[271] D. E. Schaubel, D. Zeng, and J. Cai. A semiparametric additive rates model for recurrent event data. *Lifetime Data Analysis*, 12:389–406, 2006.

[272] I. J. Schoenberg. Contributions to the problem of approximation of equidistant data by analytic functions. *Quarterly of Applied Mathematics*, 4:45–99, 1946.

[273] D. A. Schoenfeld. The asymptotic properties of nonparametric tests for comparing survival distributions. *Biometrika*, 68:316–319, 1981.

[274] D. A. Schoenfeld. Sample-size formula for the proportional-hazards regression model. *Biometrics*, 39(2):499–503, 1983.

[275] G. E. Schwarz. Estimating the dimension of a model. *Annals of Statistics*, 6:461–464, 1978.

[276] T. Sellke and D. Siegmund. Sequential analysis of the proportional hazards model. *Biometrika*, 70:315–326, 1983.

[277] P. A. Shaw. Use of composite outcomes to assess risk–benefit in clinical trials. *Clinical Trials*, 15:352–358, 2018.

[278] J. H. Shih and T. A. Louis. Inferences on the association parameter in copula models for bivariate survival data. *Biometrics*, 51:1384–1399, 1995.

[279] G. R. Shorack and J. A. Wellner. *Empirical Processes with Applications to Statistics.* Wiley, New York, 1986.

[280] A. Sklar. Fonctions de répartition à n dimensions et leurs marges. *Publ. Inst. Stataist. Univ. Paris*, 9:229–231, 1959.

[281] E. V. Slud. Sequential linear rank tests for two-sample survival data. *Annals of Statistics*, 12:551–571, 1984.

[282] E. V. Slud and L. J. Wei. Two-sample repeated significance tests based on the modified Wilcoxon statistic. *Journal of the American Statistical Association*, 77:862–868, 1982.

[283] S. Snapinn, M. G. Chen, Q. Jiang, and T. Koutsoukos. Assessment of futility in clinical trials. *Pharmaceutical Statistics*, 5:273–281, 2006.

[284] Soutinho, G. and Meira-Machado, L. Methods for checking the Markov condition in multi-state survival data. *Computational Statistics*, 37:751–780, 2022.

[285] D. J. Spiegelhalter, L. S. Freedman, and P. R. Blackburn. Monitoring clinical trials: Conditional or predictive power? *Controlled Clinical Trials*, 7:8–17, 1986.

[286] C. F. Spiekerman and D. Y. Lin. Marginal regression models for multivariate failure time data. *Journal of the American Statistical Association*, 93:1164–1175, 1998.

[287] R. Sposto, D. Stablein, and S. Carter-Campbell. A partially grouped logrank test. *Statistics in Medicine*, 16:695–704, 1997.

[288] G. R. Stablein and Koutrouvelis I. A. A two-sample test sensitive to crossing hazards in uncensored and singly censored data. *Biometrics*, 41(3):643–652, 1985.

[289] S. M. Stigler. The epic story of maximum likelihood. *Statistical Science*, 22(4):598–620, 2007.

[290] C. A. Struthers and J. D. Kalbfleisch. Misspecified proportional hazard models. *Biometrika*, 73:93–108, 1986.

[291] J. Sun and S. Yang. YPmodel: the short-term and long-term hazard ratio model for survival data. Version 1.4. https://cran.r-project.org/web/packages/YPmodel/index.html. Last accessed January 2023.

[292] K. P. Suresh. An overview of randomization techniques: An unbiased assessment of outcome in clinical research. *Journal of Human Reproductive Sciences*, 4:8–11, 2011.

[293] R. E. Tarone. On the distribution of the maximum of the logrank statistic and the modified Wilcoxon statistic. *Biometrics*, 37:79–85, 1981.

[294] L. Thabane, L. Mbuagbaw, S. Zhang, and et al. A tutorial on sensitivity analyses in clinical trials: the what, why, when and how. *BMC Medical Research Methodology*, https://doi.org/10.1186/1471-2288-13-92, 2013.

[295] The SPRINT Research Group. A randomized trial of intensive versus standard blood-pressure control. *The New England Journal of Medicine*, 373:2103–2116, 2015.

[296] The Women's Health Initiative Study Group. Design of the women's health initiative clinical trial and observational study. *Controlled Clinical Trials*, 19:61–109, 1998.

[297] T. M. Therneau, P. M. Grambsch, and T. R. Fleming. Martingale-based residuals for survival models. *Biometrika*, 77:147–160, 1990.

[298] L. Tian, L. Zhao, and L. J. Wei. Predicting the restricted mean event time with the subject's baseline covariates in survival analysis. *Biostatistics*, 15(2):222–233, 2014.

[299] A. C. Titman and H. Putter. General tests of the Markov property in multistate models. *Biostatistics*, 23:380–396, 2022.

[300] A. Tsiatis. A nonidentifiability aspect of the problem of competing risks. *Proceedings of the National Academy of Sciences*, 72:20–22, 1975.

[301] A. Tsiatis. Repeated significance testing for a general class of statistics used in censored survival analysis. *Journal of the American Statistical Association*, 77:855–861, 1982.

[302] A. A. Tsiatis. Estimating regression parameters using linear rank tests for censored data. *Annals of Statistics*, 18:354–372, 1990.

[303] A. A. Tsiatis and M. Davidian. Joint modeling of longitudinal and time-to-event data: an overview. *Statistica Sinica*, 14:809–834, 2004.

[304] A. A. Tsiatis, G. L. Rosner, and C. R. Mehta. Exact confidence intervals following a group sequential test. *Biometrics*, 40:797–803, 1984.

[305] A. D. Tsodikov, J. G. Ibrahim, and A. Y. Yakovlev. Estimating cure rates from survival data. *Journal of the American Statistical Association*, 98:1063–1078, 2003.

[306] H. Uno and M. Horiguchi. Ratio and difference of average hazard with survival weight: New measures to quantify survival benefit of new therapy. *Statistics in Medicine*, 42:936–952, 2023.

[307] U.S. Food and Drug Administration. Adjusting for covariates in randomized clinical trials for drugs and biological products. https://www.fda.gov/media/148910/download. Last accessed December 2024.

[308] U.S. Food and Drug Administration. Multiple Endpoints in Clinical Trials; Guidance for Industry; Availability. https://www.federalregister.gov/documents/2022/10/21/2022-22882/multiple-endpoints-in-clinical-trials-guidance-for-industry-availability.

[309] A. W. van der Vaart. *Asymptotic Statistics*. Cambridge University Press, Cambridge, 1998.

[310] A. W. van der Vaart and J. A. Wellner. *Weak Convergence and Empirical Processes: With Applications in Statistics*. Springer-Verlag, 1996.

[311] J. W. Vaupel, K. G. Manton, and E. Stallard. The impact of heterogeneity in individual frailty on the dynamics of mortality. *Demography*, 16:439–454, 1979.

[312] V. Volterra and B. Hostinsky. *Operations Infinitesimales Lineaires*. Gauthier-Villars, Paris, 1938.

[313] J. Wagner, J. Thompson, S. Carter, and et al. Effect of graft-versus-host disease prophylaxis on 3-year disease-free survival in recipients of unrelated donor bone marrow (T-cell Depletion Trial): a multi-centre, randomised phase II–III trial. *Lancet*, 366:733–741, 2005.

[314] M. C. Wang, J. Qin, and C. T. Chiang. Analyzing recurrent event data with informative censoring. *Journal of the American Statistical Association*, 96:1057–1965, 2001.

[315] E. J. Wegman and I. W. Wright. Spline in statistics. *Journal of the American Statistical Association*, 78:351–365, 1983.

[316] J. Wei, T. Mütze, A. Jahn-Eimermacher, and J. Roger. Properties of two while-alive estimands for recurrent events and their potential estimators. *Statistics in Biopharmaceutical Research*, 15:257–267, 2023.

[317] L. J. Wei. The accelerated failure time model: a useful alternative to the Cox regression model in survival analysis. *Statistics in Medicine*, 11:1871–1879, 1992.

[318] L. J. Wei and M. H. Gail. Nonparametric estimation for a scale-change with censored observations. *Journal of the American Statistical Association*, 78:382–388, 1983.

[319] L. J. Wei and J. M. Lachin. Two-sample asymptotically distribution-free tests for incomplete multivariate observations. *Journal of the American Statistical Association*, 79:653–661, 1984.

[320] L. J. Wei, D. Y. Lin, and L. Weissfeld. Regression analysis of multivariate incomplete failure time data by modeling marginal distributions. *Journal of the American Statistical Association*, 84:1065–1073, 1989.

[321] L. J. Wei, Z. Ying, and D. Y. Lin. Linear regression analysis of censored survival data based on rank tests. *Biometrika*, 77:845–851, 1990.

[322] R. L. Wheeden and A. Zygmund. *Measure and Integral: An Introduction to Real Analysis.* CRC Press, 2nd edition, 2015.

[323] A. Wienke. *Frailty Models in Survival Analysis.* Chapman & Hall/CRC, 2010.

[324] Writing group for the Women's Health Initiative investigators. Risks and benefits of estrogen plus progestin in healthy postmenopausal women: principal results from the women's health initiative randomized controlled trial. *Journal of the American Medical Association*, 288(3):321–333, 2002.

[325] C. O. Wu. Estimating the real parameter in a two-sample proportional odds model. *Annals of Statistics*, 23:376–395, 1995.

[326] J. Xu, J. D. Kalbfleisch, and B. Tai. Statistical analysis of illness–death processes and semi-competing risks data. *Biometrics*, 66:716–725, 2010.

[327] S. Yang. Semiparametric analysis of treatment effect via the failure probability ratio and the ratio of cumulative hazards. *Contemporary Developments in Statistical Theory*, Springer Proceedings in Mathematics & Statistics, 329–351, 2014.

[328] S. Yang. Minimum Hellinger distance estimation of parameter in the random censorship model. *Annals of Statistics*, 19(2):579–602, 1991.

[329] S. Yang. Some inequalities about the Kaplan-Meier estimator. *Annals of Statistics*, 20(1):535–544, 1992.

[330] S. Yang. A central limit theorem of the integrated square error of the kernel density estimators with randomly censored data. *Journal of Statistical Planning and Inference*, 37(2):127–143, 1993.

[331] S. Yang. A central limit theorem for functionals of the Kaplan-Meier estimator. *Statistics and Probability Letters*, 21:337–345, 1994.

[332] S. Yang. Weighted empiricals and the product-limit estimator in the multiplicative hazard and time transfer regression model. *Statistics and Probability Letters*, 30:17–24, 1996.

[333] S. Yang. Extended weighted log-rank estimating functions in censored regression. *Journal of the American Statistical Association*, 92(439):977–984, 1997.

[334] S. Yang. A generalization of the product-limit estimator with an application to censored regression. *Annals of Statistics*, 25(3):1088–1108, 1997.

[335] S. Yang. Some scale estimators and lack-of-fit tests for the censored two-sample accelerated life model. *Biometrics*, 54(3):1040–1052, 1998 (Correction in 56: 324, 2000).

[336] S. Yang. Censored median regression using weighted empirical survival and hazard functions. *Journal of the American Statistical Association*, 94(445):137–145, 1999.

[337] S. Yang. Semiparametric inference on the absolute risk reduction and the restricted mean survival difference in clinical trial. *Lifetime Data Analysis*, 19(2):219–241, 2013.

[338] S. Yang. Improving testing and description of treatment effect in clinical trials with survival outcomes. *Statistics in Medicine*, 38(4):530–544, 2019.

[339] S. Yang. Interim monitoring using the adaptively weighted log-rank test in clinical trials for survival outcomes. *Statistics in Medicine*, 38(4):601–612, 2019.

[340] S. Yang. Testing and estimation of treatment effects in clinical trials for terminal and non-terminal events subject to competing risks. *Statistics in Medicine*, 44(18–19):e70205, 2025. https://doi.org/10.1002/sim.70205.

[341] S. Yang, W. T. Ambrosius, L. J. Fine, A. P. Bress, W. C. Cushman, D. S. Raj, S. Rehman, and L. Tamariz. A new modeling and inference approach for the sprint trial outcomes. *Clinical Trials*, 15(3):305–312, 2018.

[342] S. Yang, L. Hsu, and L. Zhao. Combining asymptotically normal tests: case studies in comparison of two groups. *Journal of Statistical Planning and Inference*, 133(1):139–158, 2005.

[343] S. Yang and R. L. Prentice. Semiparametric inference in the proportional odds regression model. *Journal of the American Statistical Association*, 94(445):125–136, 1999.

[344] S. Yang and R. L. Prentice. Semiparametric analysis of short-term and long-term hazard ratios with two-sample survival data. *Biometrika*, 92(1):1–17, 2005.

[345] S. Yang and R. L. Prentice. Improved logrank-type tests for survival data using adaptive weights. *Biometrics*, 66(1):30–38, 2010.

[346] S. Yang and R. L. Prentice. Estimation of the 2-sample hazard ratio function using a semiparametric model. *Biostatistics*, 12(2):354–368, 2011.

[347] S. Yang and R. L. Prentice. Assessing potentially time-dependent treatment effect from clinical trials and observational studies for survival data, with applications to the women's health initiative combined hormone therapy trial. *Statistics in Medicine*, 34(11):1801–1817, 2015.

[348] S. Yang and J. Troendle. Event-specific win ratios and testing with non-terminal and terminal events. *Clinical Trials*, 18(3):180–187, 2021.

[349] S. Yang, J. Troendle, D. Pak, and E. Leifer. Event-specific win ratios for inference with terminal and non-terminal events. *Statistics in Medicine*, 41(7):1225–1241, 2022.

[350] S. Yang and Y. Zhao. Testing treatment effect by combining weighted log-rank tests and using empirical likelihood. *Statistics and Probability Letters*, 77:1385–1393, 2007.

[351] S. Yang and Y. Zhao. Checking the short-term and long-term hazard ratio model for survival data. *Scandinavian Journal of Statistics*, 39(3):554–567, 2012.

[352] J. Ye. On measuring and correcting the effects of data mining and model selection. *Journal of the American Statistical Association*, 93(441):120–131, 1998.

[353] Y. Ye, J. D. Kalbfleisch, and Schaubel. D. E. Semiparametric analysis of correlated recurrent and terminal events. *Biometrics*, 63:78–87, 2007.

[354] Z. Ying. Minimum Hellinger-type distance estimation for censored data. *Annals of Statistics*, 20:1361–1390, 1992.

[355] Z. Ying. A large sample study of rank estimation for censored regression data. *Annals of Statistics*, 21:76–99, 1993.

[356] Z. Ying, S. H. Jung, and L. J. Wei. Survival analysis with median regression models. *Journal of the American Statistical Association*, 90(429):178–184, 1995.

[357] Z. Ying, L. J. Wei, and J. S. Lin. Prediction of survival probability based on a linear regression model. *Biometrika*, 79:205–209, 1992.

[358] G. Yung and Y. Liu. Sample size and power for the weighted log-rank test and Kaplan-Meier based tests with allowance for nonproportional hazards. *Biometrics*, 76:939–950, 2020.

[359] D. Zeng and D. Y. Lin. Efficient estimation of semiparametric transformation models for counting processes. *Biometrika*, 93:627–640, 2006.

[360] D. Zeng and D. Y. Lin. Efficient estimation for the accelerated failure time model. *Journal of the American Statistical Association*, 102:1387–1396, 2007.

[361] D. Zeng and D. Y. Lin. Maximum likelihood estimation in semiparametric regression models with censored data. *Journal of the Royal Statistical Society, Series B*, 69:507–564, 2007.

[362] D. Zeng and D. Y. Lin. Semiparametric transformation models with random effects for joint analysis of recurrent and terminal events. *Biometrics*, 65:746–752, 2009.

[363] L. Zhao, B. Claggett, L. Tian, H. Uno, M. A. Pfeffer, S. D. Solomon, L. Trippa, and L. J. Wei. On the restricted mean survival time curve in survival analysis. *Biometrics*, 72(1):215–221, 2016.

[364] L. Zhao, L. Tian, B. Claggett, M. A. Pfeffer, D. H. Kim, S. D. Solomon, and L. J. Wei. Estimating treatment effect with clinical interpretation from a comparative clinical trial with an end point subject to competing risks. *J. Amer. Med. Assoc. Cardiology*, 3:357–358, 2018.

[365] L. Zhou. A simple censored median regression estimator. *Statistica Sinica*, 16:1043–1058, 2006.

[366] M. Zhou. M-estimation in censored linear models. *Biometrika*, 79:837–841, 1992.

[367] M. Zhou. Empirical likelihood analysis of the rank estimator for the censored accelerated failure time model. *Biometrika*, 92:492–498, 2005.

[368] M. Zhou and G. Li. Empirical likelihood analysis of the Buckley-James estimator. *Journal of Multivariate Analysis*, 99:649–664, 2008.

[369] D. A. Zipkin, C. A. Umscheid, N. L. Keating, and et al. Evidence-based risk communication: a systematic review. *Annals of Internal Medicine*, 161:270–280, 2014.

[370] D. M. Zucker. Restricted mean life with covariates: modification and extension of a useful survival analysis method. *Journal of the American Statistical Association*, 93(442):702–709, 1998.

[371] D. M. Zucker and E. Lakatos. Weighted log rank type statistics for comparing survival curves when there is a time lagnin the effectiveness of treatments. *Biometrika*, 77:853–864, 1990.

[372] D. M. Zucker and S. Yang. Inference for a family of survival models encompassing the proportional hazards and proportional odds models. *Statistics in Medicine*, 25(6):995–1014, 2006.

Index

For Product Safety Concerns and Information please contact our EU representative GPSR@taylorandfrancis.com Taylor & Francis Verlag GmbH, Kaufingerstraße 24, 80331 München, Germany